Department of Family Medicine (R700)
University of Miami School of Medicine
P. O. Box 016700
Miami, Florida 33101

James M. Gall, M.D., C.C.F.P.
Department of Family Medicine
University of Miami School of Medicine
P. O. Box 016700
Miami, Florida 33101

FAMILY PRACTICE
Foundation of Changing
Health Care

James M. Gall, M.D., C.C.F.P.
Department of Family Medicine
University of Miami School of Medicine
P. O. Box 016700
Miami, Florida 33101

FAMILY PRACTICE
Foundation of Changing Health Care

John P. Geyman, M.D.

Professor and Chairman
Department of Family Medicine
School of Medicine
University of Washington
Seattle, Washington

APPLETON-CENTURY-CROFTS/NEW YORK

80 81 82 83 84 / 10 9 8 7 6 5 4 3 2 1

Prentice-Hall International, Inc., London
Prentice-Hall of Australia, Pty. Ltd., Sydney
Prentice-Hall of India Private Limited, New Delhi
Prentice-Hall of Japan, Inc., Tokyo
Prentice-Hall of Southeast Asia (Pte.) Ltd., Singapore
Whitehall Books Ltd., Wellington, New Zealand

Library of Congress Cataloging in Publication Data

Geyman, John P   1931–
    Family practice.

    Portions of this book are based on the author's The modern
family doctor and changing medical practice, published
in 1971.
    Bibliography: p.
    Includes index.
    1. Family medicine.   2. Family medicine—United
States.   I. Title.
R729.5.G4G46   616   79–18290
ISBN 0–8385–2537–7

Text design: Meryl Sussman Levavi

Cover design: Meryl Sussman Levavi

PRINTED IN THE UNITED STATES OF AMERICA

To
My wife Gene
and
our sons Matt, Cal and Sabin,
whose encouragement and support have
made this book possible

CONTENTS

Department of Family Medicine (R700)
University of Miami School of Medicine
P. O. Box 016700
Miami, Florida 33101

James M. Gall, M.D., C.C.F.P.
Department of Family Medicine
University of Miami School of Medicine
P. O. Box 016700
Miami, Florida 33101

	Preface	xi
	Acknowledgments	xiii
1	The History of General Practice	1
2	Family Practice as a Specialty	13
3	Supply and Distribution of Physicians	27
4	Barriers to Health Care	51
5	Perspectives in Primary Care	69
6	The Changing Health Care System	89
7	Changing Trends in Medical Education	115
8	Undergraduate Education for Family Practice	141
9	Graduate Education for Family Practice	159
10	Continuing Education in Family Practice	185
11	Clinical Content of Family Practice	203
12	The Family in Family Practice	225
13	Practice Patterns of Family Physicians	249
14	Family Practice as a Career Option	277
15	Research in Family Practice	297

16   Progress in the 1970s   321
     Epilogue   341

Appendices
 1   National Health Planning Guidelines   345
 2   Essentials for Family Practice Residencies   361
 3   Family Practice Teaching Programs   369
 4   ACOG-AAFP Agreement for Curriculum and Hospital
     Privileges in Obstetrics-Gynecology   441
 5   The Virginia Study
     David W. Marsland, M.D., Maurice Wood, M.B.,
     Fitzhugh Mayo, M.D.
     Part I: Rank Order of Diagnosis by Frequency   446
     Part II: Diagnosis by Disease Category
     and Age/Sex Distribution   462
 6   Conversion Code from RCGP to ICHPPC
     Classification System   481
     Ronald Schneeweiss, M.B., H. Winston Stuart, Jr.,
     Jack Froom, M.D., Maurice Wood, M.B.,
     Herbert L. Tindall, M.D., Jenny D. Williamson
 7   Preventive Medicine Approaches:
     A Lifetime Health-Monitoring Program—
     Goals and Professional Services   491
     Flow Sheet for Health Screening of Adults   496
 8   Community Resources:
     Available Community Resources   499
     Selected List of Voluntary Health Agencies   502
 9   Glossary for Primary Care: Report of the
     North American Primary Research Group
     (NAPCRG) Committee on Standard Terminology   507
10   Research Workbook: A Guide for Initial Planning
     of Clinical, Social, and
     Behavioral Research Objectives   517
     Michael J. Gordon, Ph.D.

     Index   531

PREFACE

Ten years have now passed since the recognition in 1969 of family practice as the twentieth specialty in American medicine. The 1970s were a period of intense activity as the organizational, educational, and clinical elements of this new specialty were defined and established. Many of the initial questions facing the specialty in its beginning years were largely resolved, and new issues are being raised as the specialty enters its next stage of maturation and further development in the 1980s.

It is important at this point in the development of family practice to describe and reassess its progress, current status, and future directions. The purpose of this book is therefore threefold: (1) to provide an overview of the specialty as presently defined, including its historical context and future projections; (2) to describe progress in the field during the 1970s in terms of clinical, educational, research, and organizational perspectives; and (3) to show how the specialty relates to medicine as a whole and to the community after 10 years.

The 1970s witnessed increased sharpness and clarity in the definition of family medicine as an academic discipline and family practice as its applied clinical specialty. In 1966 McWhinney* proposed four essential criteria for the definition of any academic discipline: (1) a distinguishable body of knowledge; (2) a unique field of action; (3) an active area of research; and (4) a training

* McWhinney IR: General practice as an academic discipline. *Lancet* 1:419–23, 1966.

which is intellectually rigorous. The field will be viewed and profiled in terms of these criteria.

I write this book from the vantage point of one who was trained in a one-year rotating internship and a two-year general practice residency in preparation for six years of rural family practice in Mount Shasta, California. Since leaving practice in 1969, my experience in academic family medicine has been based in both community hospital and medical school settings in California, Utah and, since late 1976, at the University of Washington.

The book is being written primarily for medical students, family practice residents, family physicians, and medical educators, but hopefully it will be of interest and value to others, both inside and outside of medicine, interested in the emerging role of family practice in modern health care and in changing trends in medical education and medical practice. An updated view of family practice should be of particular interest to medical students considering their own roles in medicine from 1980 into the twenty-first century.

An earlier book,* forms the basis for a small portion of this book. Several chapters are drawn from that book and updated here. However, since family practice had no formal place in medical education in the United States before 1969, and since such remarkable progress has been made in the field during the last ten years, the contents are almost entirely new, and draw principally from the experience and literature in the field during the 1970s.

Initial attention will be directed to the history of general practice and the nature of family practice as a new kind of specialty. The general background of medical practice and medical education in the United States will then be considered in terms of physician manpower, problems of health care delivery, the changing health care system, and changing trends in medical education. The content, objectives and methods of education for family practice will next be described for a continuum of education at undergraduate, graduate, and postgraduate levels. Subsequent chapters will deal with various aspects of family practice, including clinical content, patterns of practice, research, and requisites and personal satisfactions of the family physician. Finally, an overview of progress will be presented for the field during the 1970s and some of the specialty's current needs outlined as it enters its next stage of further evolution in the 1980s.

Attention has deliberately been focused on changing patterns of health care delivery and the structure of medical practice, for family practice has developed in direct response to major problems within the health care system. Fundamental changes are under way in American medicine, and any specific field of medicine must be examined in the context of these changes. The development of family practice and the national emphasis on expansion and improvement of primary care are important dimensions of present trends.

JOHN P. GEYMAN, M.D.
Seattle, Washington

* Geyman JP: *The Modern Family Doctor and Changing Medical Practice.* New York, Appleton, 1971.

ACKNOWLEDGMENTS

This book has been made possible by the support and help of many. I am especially indebted to my family, who allowed me to devote many nights and weekends to this task without complaint, and whose encouragement helped me past any temporary arrests of progress.

Thanks are also due to the colleagues and fellow faculty members who have reviewed manuscripts and offered helpful suggestions. The following reviewers of selected chapters contributed to their value:

Dr. Robert Van Citters, Dean, School of Medicine, University of Washington, Seattle

Dr. Thomas Grayston, Vice President for Health Sciences, University of Washington, Seattle

Dr. Ted Phillips, Dr. C. Kent Smith, Dr. Gabriel Smilkstein, and Dr. Robert Rosenblatt, Department of Family Medicine, University of Washington, Seattle

Dr. Stephen Shortell and Dr. Ira Moscovice, School of Public Health and Community Medicine, University of Washington, Seattle

Dr. Edward Neal, practicing family physician, Healdsburg, California

I would also like to gratefully acknowledge the efforts of Jenny Freece for her patience and care in typing the manuscript through several revisions, and Lurie Pracht for her review of the entire manuscript.

Finally, I would like to thank the staff of Appleton-Century-Crofts, particularly Richard Lampert and Margaret Willard, for their diligence and skill in publishing this book. I am especially indebted to David Stires, president of Appleton-Century-Crofts and publisher of *The Journal of Family Practice*, for his advice and persistent encouragement, and for his early awareness of the importance of the specialty of family practice to the health care of the American people.

JOHN P. GEYMAN, M.D.

FAMILY PRACTICE
Foundation of Changing Health Care

CHAPTER ONE

The History of General Practice

There is something wrong with our value system in medicine and in society if the consultant who solves a complex problem in 90 minutes is regarded higher than the family physician who may have seen six of his patients for less complicated complaints in the same period. There should be no greater reward for any service in medicine than for care of the sick, direct or indirect, immediate or delayed, of a general or highly specialized nature. The status of scientist has its glories; but medicine's ultimate responsibility is to people.

Hiram B. Curry[1]

Since the specialty of family practice has taken root from the field of general practice, a brief review of the history of general practice provides a necessary background upon which profiles of family practice can be described and understood. There is a natural tendency today, as in previous times, to consider our problems as unique and special to our own time and place. This is usually not the case, and such a perception obscures our larger understanding of problems at hand and limits our capacity to solve these problems.

The interaction and balance between the generalist and specialist in medical practice have been the subject of continued interest and recurrent debate in many cultures for hundreds of years. The generalist/specialist interface has been a dynamic one featured by shifting trends in one or the other direction. At no time, however, has the need for the generalist disappeared from the process of medical care.

This chapter starts with a historical perspective of the generalist in medicine and then focuses on the evolution of general practice in the United States from 1900 to 1969, when family practice was recognized as the twentieth specialty in American medicine. The growth of specialization and the decline of general practice will be summarized, together with the resultant vacuum in primary care which led to major changes in medical care and medical education in the 1970s.

HISTORICAL PERSPECTIVE

Herodotus, describing medical practice in the Nile valley of Egypt before 2000 B.C., made the following observation: "The art of medicine is thus divided: each physician applies himself to one disease only and not more. All places abound in physicians; some are for the eyes, others for the head, others for the teeth, others for the intestines, and others for internal disorders." [2]

A similar concern was reflected in this country almost 4000 years later at the start of the twentieth century. In 1900, when at least 80 percent of physicians were in general practice, the following editorial comment appeared in *The Journal of the American Medical Association*[3]: "In these days of specialization the field of the general practitioner is becoming greatly restricted. In fact, there is some danger that in many instances the so-called general practitioner ultimately may come to perform the functions of a mere business agent of the specialists, and to act as the local distributor for the patients in his community. At the same time, as the value and the need of genuine specialists in medicine are fully recognized and established, there cannot be too strong a warning uttered against a tendency noticeable in some quarters to carry specialization to a degree of refinement beyond all reason."

At the start of this century in the United States, medical education commonly lacked both quality and content. There was a deficit of formal education and a stress on experiential training through preceptorships, and the sale of fake medical licenses and diplomas was by no means rare.[4]

The Flexner Report of 1910 was instrumental in the reform of medical education in the United States. Widespread improvements were brought about in medical schools, and many inferior schools were closed. At the same time, premedical education was introduced and postgraduate training in the form of an internship was required.[5] The Flexner Report also led to increased emphasis in the medical schools on the biomedical sciences as a foundation for medical practice. The inevitable result of these changes was the subsequent development of biomedical research, specialty boards, and formal residency training programs in the various specialties.

The growth of specialization has been the dominant feature of American medicine in the last 50 years, and this trend was especially accelerated after

World War II. This has involved a remarkable growth of scientific medical knowledge and the fractionation of the medical profession into many specialties and subspecialties with increasingly narrow concerns.

In predictable response to the problems and effects of specialization, the late 1960s saw the pendulum begin to swing back toward rebuilding the role of the generalist in medicine. As pointed out by Phillips[6] in 1971, "It would appear that we are now seeing history repeat itself—we are returning to emphasis on application of accumulated knowledge to the recipient of medical care. It is in this context that we are seeing renewed interest in the role of the family physician, and in education for family practice."

GROWTH OF SPECIALIZATION

The concern with specialization in American medicine was not a new phenomenon. In 1869, a resolution was passed by the House of Delegates of the American Medical Association as follows[7]:

> Resolved, that this Association recognizes specialties as proper and legitimate fields of practice.
> Resolved, that specialists shall be governed by the same rules of professional etiquette as have been laid down for general practitioners.
> Resolved, that it shall not be proper for specialists publicly to advertise themselves as such or to assume any title not specially granted by a regularly scheduled college.

There was no attempt at that time, and for almost 50 years afterward, to define specialties.

The first specialty to be defined and to be made official by a Board was ophthalmology in 1917. Curiously, only two years later, at the 1919 meeting of the American Medical Association, a resolution was introduced recommending the encouragement of ". . . the designation of the practice of general medicine or 'family physicians' as a distinct specialty." But the proposal was defeated.[8] The reluctance of the medical profession to recognize so broad a field as a definitive specialty continued for 50 more years. It is noteworthy that in 1941, some 22 years after the initial attempt, a resolution was again introduced before the House of Delegates of the American Medical Association calling for a Board of General Practice. Once again the resolution was rejected, but in 1946, the AMA Section on General Practice was formed.[5]

A look at the beginnings of the specialty boards is interesting in terms of the sequence of their appearance (Table 1-1). It can be noted that some of the specialty boards were defined by anatomy (e.g., ophthalmology and dermatology), one by sex (obstetrics–gynecology), two by age (pediatrics and internal medicine), and many by basic approach to management (e.g., most surgical specialties). It can also be seen that the two most general of the specialties (pediatrics and internal medicine) were both established in the mid-1930s.

TABLE 1-1.   YEAR OF ORGANIZATION OF
SPECIALTY BOARDS

BOARD	YEAR
1. Ophthalmology	1917
2. Obstetrics–gynecology	1930
3. Dermatology	1932
4. Pediatrics	1933
5. Psychiatry–neurology	1934
6. Otolaryngology	1934
7. Radiology	1934
8. Orthopedic surgery	1934
9. Colon–rectal surgery	1934
10. Urology	1935
11. Pathology	1936
12. Internal medicine	1936
13. Plastic surgery	1937
14. Surgery	1937
15. Anesthesiology	1937
16. Neurologic surgery	1940
17. Physical medicine and rehabilitation	1947
18. Preventive medicine	1948
19. Thoracic surgery	1948
20. Family practice	1969
21. Allergy and immunology	1971
22. Nuclear medicine	1971

The dramatic change in the ratio between general practitioners and specialists between 1931 and 1967 can be seen in Table 1-2.[9] The total number of physicians increased by 95 percent from 1931 to 1967. During this same period, the number of specialists in private practice increased by 469 percent.

The university medical centers and large teaching hospitals were at the hub of increasing specialization, particularly after the 1940s. Advances in medical technology were implanted and applied in tertiary care centers, which grew more distant from the everyday practice of medicine in the community. Simultaneously, the curricula in medical schools placed major emphasis on the study of disease and technical competence, while humanistic aspects of medical care were relatively neglected.[10] The educational experiences of medical students were focused more on the clinical problems of patients referred to tertiary care centers than on the study and care of patients in primary care settings in the community.

Although specialization within the medical profession has clearly brought great benefits to the public through the possibility of increased quality of medical care, the net effects of this process are both positive and negative. In a thoughtful paper examining the division of labor within medicine, Menke summarizes the dilemma of specialization in these words[11]:

Specialization is both a product of and a contributor to the scientific information explosion in medicine. It subdivides both doctor and patient, increases the difficulty of attaining a clear sense of medical identity for students and young physicians, and places additional strain on the traditional doctor–patient relationship. Specialization emphasizes the science of medicine and its rational processes in the treatment of disease and contributes to depersonalization, aggravates patient anxieties, and implicitly encourages quackery. It is probably the major factor disturbing traditional ethical and economic patterns in medicine, and it dominates medical education and research and medical practice, promotes jurisdictional disputes within the profession, and weakens organizational strength and professional power.

DECLINE OF GENERAL PRACTICE

Although any discussion of general practice in recent years tends to center on its decline in numbers and influence, this discussion should not overlook the large role played by general practice in the improvement of health care in the post-Flexner era in the United States. Many well-trained physicians entered general practice and translated their knowledge and skills into nationwide quality patient care. These general practitioners brought modern surgery, obstetrics, anesthesia, medicine, and pediatrics directly to people everywhere, often employing great skill as they practiced their healing arts. Most deliveries were done by general practitioners, and the maternal and infant mortality rates dropped sharply as modern techniques were broadly applied.

General practitioners functioned as family doctors, giving continuing care to the entire family, and establishing a public image that has been unequaled by later developments in American medicine. This type of personal care became

TABLE 1–2. DISTRIBUTION OF PHYSICIANS IN THE UNITED STATES, 1931–1967

YEAR	TOTAL NUMBER OF PHYSICIANS	TOTAL IN PRIVATE PRACTICE	GENERAL PRACTITIONERS IN PRIVATE PRACTICE	SPECIALISTS IN PRIVATE PRACTICE
1931	150,425 (100%)	134,274 (89.2%)	112,116 (74.5%)	22,158 (14.7%)
1940	165,290 (100%)	142,939 (86.5%)	109,272 (66.1%)	33,667 (20.4%)
1949	191,577 (100%)	150,417 (78.5%)	95,526 (49.9%)	54,891 (28.7%)
1959	225,772 (100%)	160,592 (71.1%)	81,957 (36.3%)	78,635 (34.8%)
1967	294,072 (100%)	190,079 (64.6%)	62,757 (21.3%)	127,222 (43.3%)

Source: *GP* 40:193, 1969.

symbolic of what people expect of the physician and what they often fail to find in modern medicine as it grows progressively more depersonalized.

General practice probably reached its zenith in the 1930s and early 1940s. During that era, graduates of medical schools and rotating internships were able to practice a high quality of medicine. The progressive technical advances in medicine during and after World War II, however, brought with them the rise of specialist practice and the consequent decline of general practice.

In 1900, there was one general practitioner for every 600 people.[12] By the late 1960s, there was only one for every 3000 people. The ratio of general practitioners to specialists had been completely reversed over a period of 40 years, from about 80 percent general practitioners to 20 percent specialists in 1930 to about 20 percent:80 percent in 1970. The shortage of generalists was even more serious, since almost half of the physicians in general practice in 1969 were over 55 years old,[13] and no more than 10 percent of graduates from medical schools planned careers in general practice.

Many explanations have been advanced for the decline of general practice. The Millis Commission isolated three major reasons for the decline of general practice[14]:

1. General practice, once the mainstay of medicine, has gradually lost prestige as the specialties have risen in honor and accomplishments. In deciding upon his own career, the young physician may never see excellent examples of comprehensive, continuing care of highly qualified and prestigious primary physicians. He is certain, however, to see a variety of specialists and to observe that they usually enjoy higher prestige, greater hospital privileges, and more favorable working conditions than do general practitioners.
2. Educational opportunities that would serve to interest students in family practice and provide interns and residents with appropriate training are few in number and often poorer in quality than the programs leading to the specialties.
3. The conditions of practice for a general practitioner or a physician interested in family practice are thought to be less attractive than the conditions and privileges enjoyed by a specialist.

The Millis Commission called "... for a revolution, not a few patchwork adaptations ..." to overcome these disadvantages.[14]

Haggerty, in 1963, listed the following as reasons for the decline in general practice[15]:

1. Medical school admissions committees, made up of specialists, favor scientifically oriented students.
2. Lack of departments of family medicine in medical schools.
3. Shortage of university-affiliated residencies in family medicine.
4. Increasing proportion of straight internships.

5. Specialists receive special consideration in such matters as military service and insurance coverage.
6. The general practitioner's lack of status in the hospital, long hours, night calls, desire to live in a city.

James Bryan, as Executive Secretary of the American Federation of Clinical Research, in 1967 called attention to the paucity of ongoing meaningful research in patient care, particularly in the functions of the family physician. In his words, "Everything about medicine is the subject of highly sophisticated research effort, amply supported by public funds—everything, that is, except the art and science of caring for people." [16]

Although there were many reasons for the decline of general practice in past years, the four most important reasons in my judgment, were the following:

1. Lack of definition as a specialty whereby the academic, educational and research elements of the field could be developed for the clinical discipline.
2. Deemphasis of general practice and primary care in the medical schools, where medical students were traditionally exposed almost entirely to the model of the specialist. Most students made the decision to enter a specialty during their medical school years, although many entering freshman medical students were greatly interested at first in general practice.[15,16]
3. Value system predominating within medicine and society favoring the development and application of complex technical procedures and in-depth medical knowledge in narrow areas. Students in medical schools learned to perceive these as more interesting and of greater value than the care of common clinical problems or the uniqueness of the patient as a person.
4. Predominance of solo practice among general practitioners, who, after several years, often developed uncontrolled practices. Among those general practitioners who left general practice for a specialty residency, overwork was usually the major reason given, and many were reluctant to give up the variety, interest, and personal satisfactions of general practice.

The above discussion points out the increasing separation of the medical student from the practicing family physician over a 40-year period to the end of the 1960s. At the graduate level, the record is likewise unimpressive. A small number of two-year general practice residencies were started in community hospitals during the 1950s and 1960s. This effort, however, was a relatively minor one compared to the need and represented a patchwork approach without the kinds of coordinated, fundamental changes that were required to reverse the trend away from general practice. Some exceptional programs filled their residency staffs over the years, but the average number of general practice residents was only about 400 to 500 each year, compared with totals of 20,000 specialty residents in 1960 and over 35,000 in 1968.[17,18] Table 1-3 lists the number of residencies by specialty in the United States for 1968.[18] It can be seen that only 45 percent of general practice residencies were filled.

TABLE 1-3.   NUMBER OF RESIDENCIES BY SPECIALTY IN 1968

SPECIALTY	NUMBER OF APPROVED PROGRAMS	TOTAL POSITIONS OFFERED SEPT. 1, 1968	TOTAL POSITIONS FILLED SEPT. 1, 1968	POSITIONS VACANT SEPT. 1, 1968	POSITIONS FILLED SEPT. 1, 1968 (%)
Anesthesiology	193	1,919	1,502	417	78
Colon–rectal surgery	14	34	29	5	85
Dermatology	79	541	512	29	95
General practice	154	902	402	500	45
Internal medicine	419	7,169	6,163	1,006	86
Neurologic surgery	86	547	504	43	92
Neurology	94	837	684	153	82
Obstetrics–gynecology	358	2,872	2,503	369	87
Ophthalmology	159	1,291	1,238	53	96
Orthopedic surgery	234	1,871	1,573	113	94
Otolaryngology	106	923	873	50	95
Pathology	639	3,573	2,230	1,343	62
Pediatrics	260	2,539	2,185	354	86
Pediatric allergy	41	87	65	22	75
Pediatric cardiology	53	156	125	31	80
Physical medicine	65	477	277	200	58
Plastic surgery	73	218	201	17	92
Psychiatry	260	4,844	3,620	1,224	75
Psychiatry, child	117	664	473	191	71
Radiology	272	2,637	2,240	397	85
Surgery	570	6,739	6,064	675	90
Thoracic surgery	93	308	279	24	91
Urology	179	958	867	91	91
Total	4,518	42,106	34,794	7,312	83
Other than hospitals					
Aerospace medicine	4	116	78	37	68
General preventive medicine	21	206	104	102	50
Occupational medicine					
academic	7	48	18	40	45
In-plant	21	28	2	26	7
Public health	24	100	40	60	40
Forensic pathology	19	29	11	20	35
Total	96	527	253	285	48
Grand total	4,614	42,633	35,047	7,597	82

Source: *JAMA* 210:1498, 1969. Reprinted with permission from the American Medical Association.

IMPACT ON PRIMARY CARE

The continued decline in the numbers of general practitioners was increasingly evident to the public and to the medical profession during the 1950s and 1960s. It was becoming progressively more difficult to obtain the services provided by the family physician: first-contact care, point of entry to other health-care services, and continuity of care over time with an understanding of the patient's family and social context. As a result, the public perceived health-care services as increasingly fragmented, episodic, impersonal, disease-oriented, inaccessible, costly, and complex.[19]

The public's demand for the services of the family physician remained strong. Medical societies throughout the country were constantly receiving calls for a physician willing to render primary care. In 1966, among callers to the Chicago Medical Society's Referral Service specifically requesting a field of practice, calls for general practitioners were about four times more frequent than for internists or gynecologists, and other fields were requested to an even lesser extent.[20] The American Medical Association Placement Service's experience for 1968 showed that approximately one-third of all opportunities registered were for general practice, but only 8 percent of physician registrants were in general practice. Table 1-4 shows the supply and demand in different fields for 1968.[21]

James Bryan,[16] a speaker at the conference of the Family Health Foundation of America in 1967, succinctly summed up the situation in these words: "What confronts us today is a societal monstrosity; a profession that is standing on its head. Its management function—its generalist coordinator—lies at the bottom of the heap—we must somehow right this pyramid and stand it on its base."

By the late 1960s, only one physician in five was in general practice. Although both internal medicine and pediatrics were growing rapidly, there was a severe shortage of primary care physicians. In 1969, there was one internist for every 14,000 people in the United States; many of these were in subspecialty practice, while most of them practiced in the more affluent cities and over one-quarter were located in New York or California.[22] Although the number of pediatricians rose from 1600 in 1931 to 10,500 in 1962, the child population increased at an even greater rate. In 1963, a pediatric manpower study showed a decline from 96 practitioners per 100,000 children (under 15) in 1940 to 50 per 100,000 in 1961, considering the combined effect of an increased number of pediatricians and a decreased number of general practitioners.[23]

The field of surgery was also growing rapidly during the 1960s, despite the feeling by many that this was already an overcrowded field. In 1966, there were 6010 residents in surgical residencies, as compared to 494 residents in general practice residencies. At the same time, 3 percent of all opportunities reported to the American Medical Association Placement Service were for general surgeons, while 38 percent of all such opportunities were for general practitioners.[24]

As of January 1, 1970, the number of residents in specialty fields showed a continuing shift away from primary care. Compared to 717 residents in general practice residencies, there were approximately eleven times as many in psy-

TABLE 1–4.   ANNUAL STATISTICAL REPORT, PHYSICIAN'S PLACEMENT SERVICE, 1968

SPECIALTY	PHYSICIANS SEEKING OPPORTUNITIES		OPPORTUNITIES OFFERED	
	No.	%	No.	%
General practice	208	8	1060	29
Allergy	16	1	25	1
Anesthesiology	63	2	85	2
Dermatology	58	2	44	1
ENT–EENT	77	3	138	4
Internal medicine	528	20	635	18
Miscellaneous*	211	8	389	11
Neurologic surgery	21	1	23	1
Obstetrics–gynecology	224	8	158	4
Ophthalmology	117	4	111	3
Orthopedics	121	5	128	4
Pathology	106	4	37	1
Pediatrics	128	5	306	8
Psychiatry–neurology	104	4	108	3
Radiology	82	3	75	2
Surgery	448	17	170	5
Urology	123	5	108	3
Total	2635	100	3600	100

*These files break down into four principal categories: occupational medicine, pharmaceutical medicine, public health, and school health.

Source: *JAMA* 210:1058, 1969. Reprinted with permission from the American Medical Association.

chiatry, four times as many in obstetrics–gynecology and pediatrics, and two to three times as many in anesthesiology, ophthalmology, orthopedic surgery, pathology, and radiology.[25]

An additional drain on physicians available for primary care was reflected by the following increases in other areas between 1949 and 1967[26]: physicians in federal service—up 120 percent; physicians in hospital-based practice—up 138 percent; physicians in administration, research, and medical education—up 362 percent. During this same period, the total number of physicians in private practice increased by only 26 percent, and the number of general practitioners decreased by 34 percent.

THE AMERICAN ACADEMY OF GENERAL PRACTICE

Alarmed by the developing shortage of physicians for primary care, a group of approximately 150 family doctors met in June 1947 in Atlantic City, New Jersey, and organized the American Academy of General Practice. By 1970, this group had grown to become a strong force in American medicine, with a membership of about 31,000 members, second only to the American Medical Association in size. The founders of the Academy formulated the following objectives[27]:

1. To promote and maintain the highest standards of general practice.
2. To encourage medical students to become qualified family doctors.
3. To preserve the general practitioner's right to practice medicine to the full extent of his ability.
4. To provide postgraduate training opportunities for the family doctor.
5. To advance the science of medicine and the nation's health and welfare, and to preserve the right of free choice of physician by the patient.

Early emphasis was placed on continuing medical education, and the Academy was the first medical organization to require postgraduate education of its membership. Each member was required to complete 150 hours of accredited study every three years. There were active county chapters all over the country, each with a monthly scientific program.

The Academy continued to stress the importance and necessity of the family doctor and recognized in the early 1960s that the nature of general practice was evolving toward the newer concept of family practice. It was increasingly apparent that medical practice varied widely in different parts of the country. One feature of this variability was the surgical content of general practice, which was actually eliminated in certain parts of the country. From 1950 to the mid-1960s, the proportion of the Academy's membership performing major surgery decreased from 68 percent to less than 33 percent.[28]

Following the monumental Millis, Willard, and Folsom reports in 1966 (which will be described more fully in the next chapter), the Academy worked closely with the AMA Council on Medical Education and the AMA Section on General Practice. "Essentials of Residency Training in Family Practice" were drawn up.[29] As new family practice programs began to appear across the country, the continued work of the Academy was instrumental in establishing the American Board of Family Practice, and the field came into being as a specialty in breadth in 1969.

REFERENCES

1. Curry HB: Phoenix in flight: All systems go! JAMA 222:823, 1972
2. Margotta R: The Story of Medicine. New York, Golden Press, 1968, p 25
3. Editorial, JAMA 232:1420, 1900
4. Canfield PR: Family medicine: An historical perspective. J Med Educ 51:904, 1976
5. Shaw WJ: Evolution of a specialty. JAMA 186:575, 1963
6. Phillips TJ: Education and training for family practice: Historical perspective. Northwest Med 70:31, 1971

7. Greenwood G, Frederickson RF: Specialization in the Medical and Legal Professions. Chicago, Callaghan, 1964, p 12

8. Greenwood G, Frederickson RF: Specialization in the Medical and Legal Professions. Chicago, Callaghan, 1964, p 45

9. Editorial: 1931–1967 distribution of physicians in the U.S. by major professional activity and specialty. GP 40:193, 1969

10. Engel G: Care and feeding of the medical student. JAMA 215:1135, 1971

11. Menke WG: Divided labor: The doctor as specialist. Ann Int Med 72:943, 1970

12. Silver GA: Family practice: Resuscitation or reform? JAMA 185:188, 1963

13. What's ahead? Med Economics, Sept. 2, 1969, p 16

14. Millis Commission: The Graduate Education of Physicians: The Report of the Citizens Commission on Graduate Medical Education. Chicago, AMA, 1966, p 179

15. Haggerty RJ: Etiology of decline of general practice. JAMA 185:180, 1963, p 179

16. Bryan JE: A summary report on the regional conferences on comprehensive medical care for the American family. GP (suppl): 17, 1967

17. Angrist A: Plea for two-year mixed internship for family physician and specialist. JAMA 173:1642, 1960

18. Editorial: Annual report on graduate medical education in the United States. JAMA 210:1498, 1969

19. Lewis CE: Family practice: The primary care specialty. In Lewis CE, Fein R, Mechanic D (eds): A Right to Health: The Problem of Access to Primary Medical Care. New York, Wiley, 1976, p 77

20. Marchmont-Robinson H: Today's challenge. JAMA 204:247, 1968

21. Editorial: Annual report on graduate medical education in the United States. JAMA 210:1508, 1969

22. Rutstein DD: The Coming Revolution in Medicine. Cambridge, Massachusetts, MIT, 1967, p 66

23. Knowles JH: The quantity and quality of medical manpower: A review of medicine's current efforts. J Med Educ 44:102, 1969

24. Editorial. More and better GP's, fewer and better surgeons. Calif GP 18:15, 1967

25. AMA Mailing Service, December 1969, personal communication

26. Editorial: 1931–1967 distribution of physicians in the U.S. by major professional activity and specialty. GP 40:193, 1969

27. Truman SR: The History of the Founding of the American Academy of General Practice. St. Louis, Green, 1969, p 43

28. Annual Report of the American Academy of General Practice. Kansas City, Missouri, American Academy of General Practice, 1968, p 10

29. Education for Family Practice. Kansas City, Missouri, Commission on Education, American Academy of General Practice, 1969, Appendix

CHAPTER TWO

Family Practice as a Specialty

While specialization is an unquestioned benefit in every phase of clinical medicine, it greatly sharpens the need for a parallel development of the synthesizing and integrative functions required to understand and treat humans and their diseases. Concentration on an organ system or technique too often produces an insensitivity to distress signals elsewhere in the body or in the person.

Edmund D. Pellegrino[1]

The adequacy of care available from the family physician, and his sense of responsibility, will in large measure determine the effectiveness with which the whole structure of medical care serves the patient.

Robert R. Huntly[2]

In the 1950s, the idea of family practice as a recognized, definable specialty was a visionary one in the minds of a few. The specialty was formally recognized by the end of the 1960s with the formation of the American Board of Family Practice in 1969. Today, after its first decade of vigorous development in medical education, clinical practice, and beginning efforts in research, the specialty is well established as a major element of the country's expanding primary care base within medicine.

Viewed in a larger context, the development of family practice at this particular stage in the evolution of American society is both logical and inevitable. We traced in the last chapter the inexorable growth of specialization and subspecialization, which was accelerated after the 1940s. The increasing emphasis on the technology of medicine led to problems of access and cost of care, fragmentation of the doctor–patient relationship, and growing confusion and even resentment by an increasing part of the population as to the role of the physician and the medical profession. The 1960s and 1970s in the United States witnessed widespread changes throughout many parts of society, with a fundamental theme reflecting concern for what Lewis Mumford has termed "the primacy of the person." In his words: "Our machines have become gigantic, powerful, self-operating, inimical to truly human standards and purposes: our men, devitalized by this very process, are now dwarfed, paralyzed, impotent. Only by restoring primacy to the person—and to the experience and disciplines that go into the making of persons—can the fatal imbalance be overcome." [3]

The natural climate favoring the genesis of family practice is well stated by McWhinney as follows[4]:

It is no accident that family medicine is emerging at a time when the inter-relatedness of all things is being rediscovered, when the importance of ecology is being forced on one's awareness, when the limitations of the closed-system way of thinking are being more and more appreciated, and when scientists, especially those in the life sciences, are beginning to react to the scientific bias against integration, synthesis and teleology. Nor is it coincidence that this movement of ideas is taking place at a time when the virtues of economic growth are being questioned, when bigness for its own sake is ceasing to be considered good, when human values are being asserted over technology, and when the importance of enduring and stable human relations is being discovered anew.

The shift toward family practice, with the attendant reappraisal of medical education, represents a positive step by the medical profession to respond directly to the changing needs of society. This shift can be viewed as one away from primary concern for diseases and organ systems toward the whole patient as a person, his/her family, and the community.

EVOLUTION OF FAMILY PRACTICE AS A SPECIALTY

The complete history of the formation of the twentieth specialty could be a book in itself, and only a brief summary will be presented here. It must be said that the final event was the culmination of the work of many people after many meetings and conferences over the years. In an excellent review article, Walsh described in some detail the history and organizational process of family practice as a specialty.[5]

As early as 1947, some of the leaders in the American Academy of General Practice and the AMA Section on General Practice favored board certification. One of the leading proponents in the 1950s was Dr. Ward Darley, who was especially farsighted in seeing the need for board certification and the redefinition of the modern family physician, as well as the development of more appropriate training programs.[6]

However, it was in the 1960s that support for the new specialty became widespread, and the American Academy of General Practice is to be credited with exerting strong leadership in this direction. National and regional conferences were held, and the course to certification was charted.

In a span of one hundred days during 1966, four reports were released that gave the greatest thrust toward the new specialty of family practice. The most impressive thing about these reports is that they all came to very similar conclusions yet had been prepared over a long period of time by completely independent groups. These reports called for basic changes throughout the structure of medical education.

The National Commission on Community Health Services, also known as the Folsom Commission, stressed the need for every individual to have a *personal* physician for easy access to health care on a coordinated, comprehensive, and continuing basis. This physician would be skilled in preventive medicine and the use of community resources.[7]

The report of the Citizens Commission on Graduate Medical Education (Millis Commission) called for a similar physician, but by the name of *primary* physician. This group underscored the crucial importance of comprehensive health care and decried the lack of appreciation of this vital area in the medical schools. The following excerpts are taken from this report[8]:

> In the academic world, it is customary to put a greater premium on depth of knowledge in a specialized area than on more comprehensive wisdom covering a larger field. . . . Perhaps these attitudes are proper among scientists or in the university, where the men most honored are the ones who are extending the frontiers of knowledge. But medicine, although intimately based upon science, is not science. It is an application of science.

Specific recommendations made by the Millis Commission include the following[9]:

1. Simple rotation among several services, in the manner of the classical rotating internship, though extending over a longer period of time, will not be sufficient. Knowledge and skill in several areas are essential, but the teaching should stress continuing and comprehensive patient responsibility rather than the episodic handling of acute conditions in the several areas.
2. Experience in the management of emergency cases and knowledge of specialized care required before and following surgery should be included.

3. A new body of knowledge should be taught in addition to the medical specialties that constitute the bulk of the program.
4. There should be ample opportunities for individual variation in the graduate program.
5. The level of training should be on a par with that of other specialties. A two-year graduate program is not sufficient.
6. Each teaching hospital should organize its staff, through an educational council, a committee on graduate education, or some similar means, so as to make its programs of graduate medical education a corporate responsibility rather than the individual responsibilities of particular medical or surgical services or heads of services.
7. The internship, as a separate and distinct portion of medical education, should be abandoned, and the internship and residency years should be combined into a single period of graduate medical education called a residency and planned as a unified whole.
8. State licensure acts and statements of certification requirements should be amended to eliminate the requirement of a separate internship and an appropriately described period of graduate medical education should be substituted therefor.
9. Graduation from medical school should be recognized as the end of general medical education, and specialized training should begin with the start of graduate medical education.

The Millis Commission viewed national health priorities in this way[10]:

> What is wanted is comprehensive and continuing health care, including not only the diagnosis and treatment of illness, but also its prevention and the supportive and rehabilitative care that helps a person to maintain, or to return to, as high a level of physical and mental health and well being as he can attain.

The report of the Ad Hoc Committee on Education for Family Practice of the Council on Medical Education (Willard Report) labeled the new specialist in comprehensive health care the *family* physician. The committee recognized the need for ". . . significant reorientation of medical education and change in the attitudes of the medical profession." Seeing the preparation of a large number of family physicians as the first order of business for American medicine at this time, the committee felt that ". . . a major national need exists, that such an approach is justified, and that it should be initiated promptly." [11]

The Ad Hoc Committee felt that family practice is truly a specialty, because both the composite body of knowledge used by the family practitioner and his function are significantly different from other specialists. The Willard Report made the following further recommendations[12]:

1. Keynotes in family practice programs should be excellence comparable to programs in other specialties and flexibility to permit the design of training programs that will meet the needs and interests of individual physicians.

2. Medical schools and teaching hospitals should explore the possibility of developing models of family practice in cooperation with the practicing profession.
3. Recognition and status equivalent to other specialties should be accorded to family practice.
4. Study should be made of the effect of premedical programs and the admission procedures, curricula, and student evaluation policies of medical schools upon the production of family physicians.
5. An adequate graduate training program in family practice can be provided in three years if it is properly designed and incorporates experience in a suitable model of practice under the supervision of family practice physicians.

The report of the Committee on Requirements for Certification of the American Academy of General Practice was the fourth major report of 1966 that was of monumental importance to the new specialty of family practice.[13] This committee formulated the core content of family medicine, which served as the take-off point for emerging residency programs in family practice.

As a logical subsequent step in the evolution of family practice, the American Academy of General Practice became the American Academy of Family Physicians in 1971. The Academy has continued to play a vital role in the development of the new specialty, particularly in the facilitation of education programs at all levels and through liaison with other specialties and various levels of government.

THE AMERICAN BOARD OF FAMILY PRACTICE

The American Board of Family Practice since 1969 has been responsible for development and implementation of certification and recertification procedures. The board thereby has an important responsibility for setting and maintaining high standards of performance in the field.

The American Board of Family Practice is noteworthy from several standpoints. Most important, perhaps, is that it has provided recognition for the specialized knowledge and skills of the generalist as a family physician. Second, this was the first board to require recertification by examination, which was established at six-year intervals. Third, this board was the first to include specialists from other clinical fields in its membership. * Finally, no grandfather clause was permitted. To be eligible for examination, a candidate must have completed an approved family practice residency program or have been in

---

* The membership of the American Board of Family Practice is constituted as follows: five members representing the American Academy of Family Physicians; five members representing the AMA Section on General/Family Practice; five members representing other specialty boards (one representative each from internal medicine, pediatrics, psychiatry and neurology, obstetrics–gynecology, and surgery).

active family practice for a minimum of six years and completed at least 300 hours of continuing study acceptable to the board. This kind of practice eligibility was permitted only until 1978; thereafter, all candidates were required to have satisfactorily completed a three-year family practice residency program.

The first examinations were given on a pilot basis to 2087 candidates at a number of places throughout the country in February, 1970. A profile of these first candidates for board certification is shown in Table 2-1.[14] Examina-

---

TABLE 2-1.   PROFILE OF FIRST CANDIDATES FOR BOARD CERTIFICATION IN FAMILY PRACTICE

99% were members of The American Academy of General Practice.
99% had never taken any other board examination.
93% were in private practice.
81% passed the examination.
50% had residency training ranging from less than one year to more than four years.
35% reported doing part-time teaching.
 4% reported teaching or research as major activities.
 1% were graduates of approved three-year family practice residencies.

---

tions have been given annually since 1970, and by 1978 there were over 19,000 diplomates of the American Board of Family Practice.

The certification examination is a full two-day examination that covers the breadth of family practice and tests both clinical knowledge and problem-solving skills. Three basic kinds of questions are included: multiple choice, pictorial, and patient management problems. The recertification examination includes a one-day cognitive examination and self audit of twenty of the physician's actual patients. This audit is subject to review by the board and involves the in-depth audit of four patients from any five of the following twenty categories:

1. Abnormal vaginal bleeding
2. Acute cystitis
3. Acute duodenal ulcer
4. Appendicitis
5. Chronic bronchial asthma
6. Chronic obstructive pulmonary disease
7. Colitis
8. Congestive heart failure
9. Coronary artery disease
10. Depression
11. Diabetes mellitus
12. Hypertension
13. Lumbar disk disease
14. Normal pregnancy through delivery
15. Obesity
16. Otitis media
17. Pediatric patient
18. Postoperative carcinoma of breast
19. Rheumatoid arthritis
20. Vaginitis

SOME BASIC DEFINITIONS

Family Physician

The American Academy of Family Physicians (AAFP) and the American Board of Family Practice (ABFP) defined the family physician as one who

> . . . provides health care in the discipline of family practice. His training and experience qualify him to practice in the several fields of medicine and surgery.
>
> The family physician is educated and trained to develop and bring to bear in practice unique attitudes and skills which qualify him or her to provide continuing, comprehensive health maintenance and medical care to the entire family regardless of sex, age or type of problems, be it biological, behavioral or social. This physician serves as the patient's or family's advocate in all health-related matters, including the appropriate use of consultants and community resources.

A closely related definition has been developed by the American Medical Association, which views the family physician as one who

> . . . serves the public as a physician of first contact and means of entry into the health care system; evaluates his patients' total health care needs; assumes responsibility for his patients' comprehensive and continuing health care and acts as coordinator of his patients' health services; and accepts responsibility for his patients' total health care, including the use of consultants, within the context of their environment, including the community and the family or comparable social unit.

Family Practice

The common definition jointly held by the AAFP and ABFP for family practice is:

> Family practice is comprehensive medical care with particular emphasis on the family unit, in which the physician's continuing responsibility for health care is not limited by the patient's age or sex nor by a particular organ system or disease entity.
>
> Family Practice is the specialty in breadth which builds upon a core of knowledge derived from other disciplines—drawing most heavily on internal medicine, pediatrics, obstetrics and gynecology, surgery and psychiatry—and which establishes a cohesive unit, combining the behavioral sciences with the traditional biological and clinical sciences. The core of knowledge encompassed by the discipline of family practice prepares the family physician for a unique role in patient management, problem solving, counseling and as a personal physician who coordinates total health care delivery.

Family Medicine

There was early agreement that *family medicine* constitutes the academic discipline that is applied in *family practice*. In the first several years of family practice development, however, there was considerable controversy on the more specific definition of the academic discipline. Some felt that family medicine should be defined only in terms of its *unique content,* as different from all other clinical disciplines. This approach tended to focus principally on the behavioral and ecologic interactions of the family as a unit, and it was even argued by some that family medicine is more a behavioral than a clinical discipline.[15,16]

Recent years have seen a consensus that a *functional* definition of family medicine is required. In functional terms, *family medicine* can be satisfactorily defined as that body of knowledge and skills applied by the family physician as he/she provides primary, continuing, and comprehensive health care to patients and their families regardless of their age, sex, or presenting complaint. It is a horizontal discipline, sharing portions of all other clinical and related disciplines from which it is derived but applying these derivative portions in a unique way to families. In addition, family medicine includes new, incompletely developed elements, such as family dynamics in health and disease and its own areas of developing research.[17]

FUNCTIONAL ELEMENTS OF FAMILY PRACTICE

Family practice is thus the broadest of clinical specialties in medicine by inclusion of portions of the other clinical disciplines and other areas related to the ongoing care of the whole patient and his/her family. All other specialties have defined their areas by exclusion, on the basis of anatomy, organ system, age, sex, or basic kind of management (i.e., most surgical fields). As Bryan[18] has stated, "... the family physician's aim is to broaden his concern, to widen his skill, to accept responsibility, not merely to pass it along .... his is the task of synthesizing where his fellows particularize."

Family practice cuts across the territorial boundaries of all of the traditional specialties, and varies somewhat in its application by each family physician based upon his/her own training, interests, and skills, as well as the community of practice and the proximity to other medical resources.[19] Spitzer has proposed the conceptual schema shown in Figure 2-1 to illustrate these points.[20]

Millis has called this a horizontal kind of specialization, and has seen the need for all physicians not only to specialize, but also to remain open to future changes in their specialized areas. In his words, "It is inevitable that as time runs, we must deal with greater amounts of knowledge and that choices will have to be made as to that portion of knowledge that we will make our own."[21]

The comparative differences in breadth and depth of clinical knowledge and skills between family practice and the more limited clinical specialties are well illustrated in Figure 2-2. It can be seen that a consulting discipline requires great depth in several limited areas related to the physician's chosen field and necessarily yields comprehensiveness to that end.[22]

Family practice can be further described as: (1) including an area of clinical competency to deal definitively with those common clinical problems that constitute approximately 95 percent of all patient visits to primary-care physi-

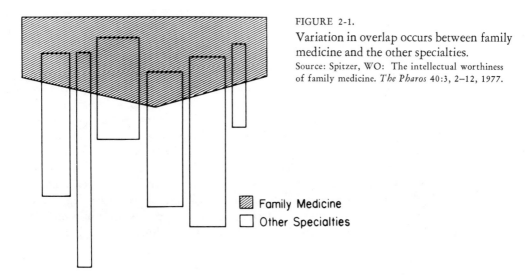

FIGURE 2-1.

Variation in overlap occurs between family medicine and the other specialties.

Source: Spitzer, WO: The intellectual worthiness of family medicine. *The Pharos* 40:3, 2–12, 1977.

cians[23–25]; (2) including responsibility for continuity of patient care both in and out of the hospital, with the emphasis on more effective ambulatory care; (3) involving the responsibility to arrange and coordinate consultation or referral to other specialists and community resources as indicated; and (4) requiring team-work with other members of the health care team. Although

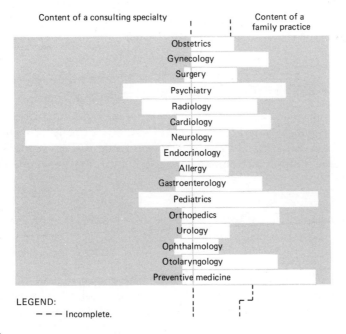

FIGURE 2-2.

Comparison of content between family practice and a consulting specialty, neurology.

Source: Rakel RE: *Principles of Family Medicine.* Philadelphia, WB Saunders, Company, 1977, p. 12.

there may be some differences between the actual practices of individual family physicians in different parts of the country and different community settings, the *sine qua non* of family practice, as Stephens [26] suggests, is "the knowledge and skill which allow the family physician to confront relatively large numbers of unselected patients with unselected conditions and to carry on therapeutic relationships with patients over time."

As is true of other primary care physicians (i.e., general pediatrics and general internal medicine), the family physician's practice is featured by five key elements: (1) accessibility, (2) continuity of care, (3) comprehensiveness of services, (4) coordination of total health care, and (5) accountability, or ongoing responsibility for the patient's welfare. One of these elements, comprehensive health care, has been the subject of some attention as to the appropriate range of the physician's concerns. Dr. George James, as Commissioner of Health in New York City, in 1963 suggested the following four basic categories of health care which help to clarify this issue[27]:

Stage I. Foundations of disease. This stage includes many factors that individually or in combination may later be responsible for disease and that are subject to preventive care of the individual or his family. Examples of such factors include genetic heritage of the individual, dietary patterns, activity habits, smoking, and housing conditions.

Stage II. Preclinical disease. This stage is defined as "the stage when a health problem is developing but is not yet far enough advanced to make the victim aware." [27] In this stage, detection is possible but often neglected. Examples include prediabetes, premalignant lesions, and asymptomatic glaucoma.

Stage III. Treatment of symptomatic disease. Third-stage medicine constitutes the bulk of traditional clinical medicine and forms the basis for existing patterns of medical practice.

Stage IV. Rehabilitation and management of medical conditions for which biologic cure is not possible. James calls this stage the "control of disability" [27] and stresses rehabilitation during this stage. Examples are individuals with chronic disease, stable posttraumatic sequelae, and other handicapping problems.

On the basis of such a framework as the James stages, comprehensive health care can then be viewed as including:

• Health education
• Assessment of foundations of disease and the degree of risk for individual patients and their families, with planning of appropriate followup care
• Periodic physical examinations and laboratory screening; multiphasic screening as indicated
• Emergency care
• Care of acute symptomatic disease

- Care of chronic conditions, including rehabilitation
- Counseling, on an individual or family basis, for such conditions as (a) marital or family problems, (b) individual emotional problems, (c) genetic problems, and (d) nutritional problems

It is obvious that there are environmental factors important in stage I that need attention by society in general and by the community in particular (e.g., air pollution, housing, poverty) but that are usually beyond the capability of the physician himself. It is also clear that the individual family physician's practice will vary in the mix of emphasis by James stage and by clinical content based upon many variables, such as the demography of the practice and community, the health beliefs and behavior of the community, third-party reimbursement policies, and many other related factors. An example of the breakdown of services by James stages in family practice is shown in Table 2-2,

TABLE 2-2. SERVICES PROVIDED BY FAMILY PHYSICIANS IN THE ROCHESTER REGION

James Stage		Percent of Services*
I.	Health maintenance	9.0
II.	Preclinical disease	21.0
III.	Symptomatic disease	66.5
IV.	Rehabilitation	25.0

* Adds up to more than 100 percent because some patients receive multiple services.
Source: Proceedings of a seminar held at Columbus, Ohio. Ohio Academy of Family Physicians, 1968, p. 43.

which is based on a study of 370 family physicians in an eleven-county area around Rochester, New York.[28]

The foregoing discussion of the functional elements of family practice is not complete without reemphasis of the centrality of the individual patient as person and the family itself as patient. As McWhinney points out, the personal commitment of the family physician to his/her patient "involves 'staying with' the patient whatever his problem may be." To the family physician, "problems become interesting and important not only for their own sake but because they are Mr. Smith's or Mrs. Jones' problem. Very often in such relations there is not even a very clear distinction between a medical problem and a nonmedical one. The patient defines the problem." [29]

The centrality of the family as the object of care is important for many reasons. Perhaps the major reason is that the physician needs to apply health care to the smallest unit that at the same time allows optimal results of health care. Many individual illnesses are illnesses of the family as well, ranging from communicable disease to behavioral problems. The management of the individual patient with a disease must involve the understanding and assistance of other members of the family. Though the family as a unit has undergone evolutionary changes in recent decades, it remains the primary social group out of which all other social groupings are formed. Dennis[30] has brought this perspective to the subject:

> It is within the family milieu, and very early in life, that we find the genesis of social or antisocial human behavior, mental health, or illness, many communicable diseases, and the nutritional and other factors that ultimately lead to many of the chronic degenerative and disabling disorders of later life. It is not possible to separate poor mental and physical health, ignorance, and poverty from the pathology of the family.

COMMENT

Having traced the progressive decline of general practice over the last 40 years in the preceding chapter, it is logical to ask why we can expect family practice to grow and develop as a foundation of future primary health care in the United States. Some of the reasons that allow us to project a bright future for family practice are:

1. Increased realization that the quality and quantity of health care actually delivered in this country fall far short of the public's needs and medicine's potential.
2. Disenchantment with increasing specialism among many medical students.
3. Commitment of today's medical student to improved delivery of health care.
4. Development of departments of family practice in a majority of the nation's medical schools.
5. Development of numerous new residencies in family practice.
6. Progress toward development of an active research base in the field.
7. Board certification in family practice.
8. Growing emphasis on group practice, which can afford family physicians an opportunity for a full family and personal life outside of medicine.

As new graduates from the expanding number of family practice residencies have joined the ranks of board-certified family physicians drawn from general practice, the pendulum is swinging back to a more desirable balance with the other specialties. The 1960s were a decade of formative change, the 1970s were a decade for implementation, and the 1980s will be a decade of vigorous growth and further development of a specialty responding to the needs of the times.

We are surrounded daily with ample evidence that modern health care in this country is excessively fragmented, uncoordinated, wasteful, impersonal, and confusing to the public. There is an urgent need for synthesis amidst this disarray. As Magraw[31] has said in his pleas for synthesis in medicine: "Integration and synthesis do not occur in an institution—they only occur within a man and not between men." And to James, the family physician is "the man responsible for the navigation of human beings through the problems and difficulties involved in the maintenance of their health through each of the four stages of the natural history of disease. He is the key generalist of the future of medicine, and is the most indispensable of all." [11,32]

REFERENCES

1. Pellegrino ED: The generalist function in medicine. JAMA 198:541, 1966
2. Huntly RR: Epidemiology of family practice. JAMA 185:175, 1963
3. Mumford L: The Transformation of Man. New York, Harper and Row, 1956
4. McWhinney IR: Family medicine in perspective. N Engl J Med 293:4, 1975
5. Walsh JG: New specialty—family practice. JAMA 212:1191, 1970
6. Darley W: An educator's approach to training for comprehensive medical care. GP Aug. (suppl): 22, 1967
7. Health is a Community Affair. The Report of the National Commission on Community Health Services. Cambridge, Massachusetts, Harvard University Press, 1966
8. The Graduate Education of Physicians. The Report of the Citizens Commission of Graduate Medical Education. Chicago, AMA, 1966, p 40
9. The Graduate Education of Physicians. The Report of the Citizens Commission of Graduate Medical Education. Chicago, AMA, 1966, p 48
10. The Graduate Education of Physicians. The Report of the Citizens Commission of Graduate Medical Education. Chicago, AMA, 1966, p 36
11. Meeting the Challenge of Family Practice. The Report of the Ad Hoc Committee on Education for Family Practice of the Council on Medical Education. Chicago, AMA, 1966, p 1
12. Meeting the Challenge of Family Practice. The Report of the Ad Hoc Committee on Education for Family Practice of the Council on Medical Education. Chicago, AMA, 1966, p 49
13. Editorial: The core content of family medicine, report of the committee on requirements for certification. GP 34:225, 1966
14. Editorial: GP and the hospital. Hosp Pract 112, 1970
15. Carmichael LP: Psychiatry and family medicine. New Physician 19:525, 1970
16. Ransom DC, Vandervoort HE: The development of family medicine: problematic trends. JAMA 225:1098, 1973
17. Geyman JP: Family medicine as an academic discipline. J Med Educ 46:815, 1971
18. Bryan JE: A summary report on the regional conferences on comprehensive medical care for the American family. GP Aug. (suppl): 20, 1967
19. Geyman JP: Family practice in evolution: Progress, problems and projections. N Engl J Med 298:593, 1978
20. Spitzer WO: The intellectual worthiness of family medicine. Pharos p 2, July 1977
21. Millis JS: A re-examination of assumptions in medical education. GP (suppl), p 46, August 1967
22. Rakel RE: Principles of family medicine. Philadelphia, Saunders, 1977, p 12
23. Schmidt DD: Referral patterns in an individual family practice. J Fam Pract 5:401, 1977

24. Geyman JP, Brown TC, Rivers K: Referrals in family practice: A comparative study by geographic region and practice setting. J Fam Pract 3:163, 1976
25. Metcalfe DH, Sishy D: Patterns of referral from family practice. J Fam Pract 1:34, 1974
26. Stephens GG: The intellectual basis of family practice. J Fam Pract 2:423, 1975
27. James G: The general practitioner of the future. N Engl J Med 27:1287, 1963
28. Haggerty RJ: The role of the university in education for family practice. Proceedings of a seminar held at Columbus, Ohio. Columbus, Ohio. Ohio Academy of Family Physicians, 1968, p 43
29. McWhinney IR: Family medicine in perspective. N Engl J Med 293:176, 1975
30. Dennis JL: Medical education, physician manpower, the state and community. J Med Educ 4:21, 1969
31. Magraw RM: The increasing ferment in medicine in comprehensive medical care. GP (suppl.), p 33, 1967
32. James G: The general practitioner of the future. N Engl J Med 27:1291, 1963

CHAPTER THREE

Supply and Distribution of Physicians

In my judgment, all of us concerned with health manpower problems—and I include the Congress, the Executive Branch, the medical schools, and everyone else who is in a position to influence national policy—have to recognize that simply increasing the aggregate supply of doctors has not and will not solve the problems we face in making health services available to the people of this country.

Charles C. Edwards[1]

The adequacy of the number of doctors in the United States cannot be reasonably determined apart from issues such as their geographic distribution, the allocation of tasks among medical specialties, the rise of other health workers, and the general scope of medical care. The number of physicians relative to the population is generally an uninformative statistic by itself.

David Mechanic[2]

Since the development of family practice represents a direct response to systemic problems in the health care system in the United States, it is useful to examine the general context of these problems to better understand the future role of family practice in this country. This is the first of three chapters that will deal with general background issues. We will focus first on trends and problems related to the supply and distribution of physicians.

The supply of physicians has been an important and controversial subject especially during the last 30 years in the United States. Although there was general agreement throughout the 1950s and 1960s that a physician shortage existed as a serious problem, there was considerable debate as to how to relieve this shortage and the number of physicians needed. The 1970s saw increasing pessimism among health planners and policy makers that simply increasing the total number of physicians would effectively address the problems of delivery of health care, and there was some evidence that these problems were even aggravated by the growing supply of physicians. The end of the 1970s saw a growing consensus that the physician shortage of earlier years would become a physician surplus in the 1980s and that the real problems of physician supply involved geographic and specialty maldistribution.

The purpose of this chapter is threefold: (1) to discuss briefly the various factors affecting the adequacy of physician supply; (2) to outline the trends in total numbers of physicians, together with their geographic and specialty distribution; and (3) to review past and current approaches to the problems of physician supply and distribution.

VARIABLES AFFECTING PHYSICIAN SUPPLY

It is now apparent that the total number of physicians available to provide health care is only one of many factors important in any analysis of the relation between supply and demand of health care services. In a comprehensive review of medicine's efforts concerning the quantity and quality of medical manpower in this country, Knowles [3] in 1969 listed the following factors in connection with any appraisal of the physician supply:

1. Specification of the type of physician involved (by field), the actual use of his/her time (practice, research, administration), and in his/her location (rural–urban, hospital, medical school).
2. Effectiveness of recruitment of workers into the field.
3. The training capacity of hospitals and medical schools.
4. The restraining or facilitating functions of state and specialty board licensure.
5. Analysis of training expense.
6. Degree of retention of doctors once in school, hospital, or practice.
7. The productivity of the physician.
8. The accessibility and availability of physicians.
9. The ability to substitute other health workers in roles previously assumed by the physician.

More recently, Howard Stambler, as Chief of the Manpower Analysis Branch of the Bureau of Health Manpower, in 1975 suggested four additional important factors influencing the adequacy of physician supply[4]:

1. Changes in the organization and delivery of health care (e.g., introduction and expansion of prepaid group practice plans).
2. Changes in the financial structure of the health care delivery system (e.g., Medicare, Medicaid, a possible future national health insurance).
3. Effects of technological breakthroughs of virtually unknown dimensions.
4. Major legislation or policy changes, such as those related to licensing and credentialling of health manpower, changes affecting immigration of foreign medical graduates, or unforeseen state and federal laws.

Certainly many other factors can have important affects on the adequacy (or lack thereof) of the physician supply, but the range of the factors listed above points to the complexity of any analysis of physician manpower needs and projections. The demand for health care services is likewise subject to many factors, such as[3]:

1. Age, sex, race, geographic location, education, and income of the population being considered.
2. The extent of health information.
3. Availability of physician and other health workers, equipment, and facilities.
4. Social legislation and financing mechanisms.

Knowles has pointed out the important observation that demand is by no means synonymous with need for health care services.[3] It is clear that many needs for health care are not being demanded by certain segments of our population. On the other side of the coin, it can likewise be argued that the demand, as represented by health services delivered, may also exceed genuine needs. Mechanic[5] has observed that: "Medical care is a highly discretionary activity; and physicians can generate considerable work that they would not be inclined to do if there were more demand for their services." McNerney[6] has documented that the more hospital beds or surgeons in a community, the higher the rates of hospital admissions and of surgical procedures.

Pursuing the definition of *medical needs* further, Mechanic[8] suggests that they include the following three components:

1. Those needs recognized by medical personnel and also by the recipients as requiring care.
2. Those needs recognized by medical personnel as needing care but not so recognized by the recipients (e.g., outreach work and health education).
3. Those needs defined by the consumer but not evident in medical screening or community assessments.

The examination of our physician supply is therefore a complex task. In a 1967 report by the American Medical Association's Department of Survey Research, the statement was made that[7]:

> Appraising the adequacy of the present distribution necessitates the evaluation of health care requirements in each community. No commonly accepted standard exists that can be applied nationally for such an evaluation. Some have utilized physician–population ratios toward this end. The use of ratios alone, however, does not constitute an adequate measure of the quantity or quality of health care received by the American public.

AGGREGATE NUMBER OF PHYSICIANS

At this writing, there are over 410,000 M.D.s in the United States. This number represents an 86 percent increase since 1950, a 58 percent increase since 1960, and a 22 percent increase since 1970. Such an increase in the aggregate number of physicians is the inevitable result of the concerted efforts of government, medical schools, and other groups that focused primarily on the *number* of physicians as the principal factor to consider. Table 3-1 provides an interesting historical perspective of some of the major assessments of the physician supply between 1953 and 1970.[9]

A significant part of the increase in numbers of physicians is due to rapid expansion of enrollments in United States medical and osteopathic schools;

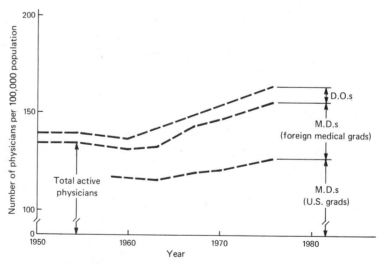

FIGURE 3-1.

Rapid increase in the supply of physicians. Most of the increase was due to the immigration of foreign medical graduates.

Source: *Physicians for the Future. Report of the Macy Commission.* New York, Josiah Macy, Jr. Foundation, 1976, p. 80.

current first-year enrollments are more than double 1966 levels. A second major part of the growth in the aggregate number of physicians is the influx of foreign medical graduates. By 1973, active foreign medical graduates numbered 68,000, or one-fifth of all practicing physicians, and the annual increase in licensed foreign medical graduates has nearly equalled the increase in United States trained licensed physicians.[10] Figure 3-1 illustrates these trends during the last 25 years.[11]

Projections of trends existing during the late 1970s concerning the growth in total numbers of physicians showed a 50 percent increase between 1974 and the year 2000 when the physician-to-population ratio would likely reach 255/100,000 (Figure 3-2).[12] In an excellent review of the implications of this kind of increase, Morrow and Edwards suggest reduction in the numbers of foreign medical graduates entering the United States for the following reasons: (1) mounting concern about the impact on the quality of health care related to heavy reliance on foreign medical graduates, many of whom are considered less well trained than their United States counterparts; (2) the need to reduce future projected physician-to-population ratios while preserv-

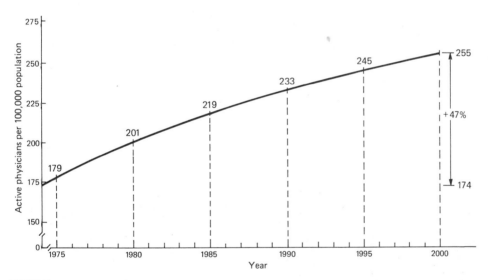

FIGURE 3-2.

Projected growth in the number of physicians (M.D.s and D.O.s) per 100,000 population in the United States, 1974 to 2000. Assumptions: (1) No further growth beyond 1975 in first-year enrollments of United States medical and osteopathic schools. (2) Foreign medical graduate physicians entering the United States equals 8000 annually. (3) One-quarter of foreign medical graduates entering the United States will leave upon completing their graduate education. (4) Annual rate of deaths and retirements of active physicians equals 2 percent of the total, reflecting relative youth of current and rapidly growing physician population. (5) Series E population projections.

Source: Morrow, J.H., and Edwards, A.B.: U.S. health manpower policy: Will the benefits justify the costs? *Journal of Medical Education* 51:792, 1976.

TABLE 3–1.   SUMMARY OF REPORTS ON THE PHYSICIAN SHORTAGE

DATE OF PUBLICATION	REPORTING BODY	ESTIMATED SHORTAGE OR FUTURE NEED FOR PHYSICIANS	STANDARD USED FOR ESTIMATED NEED
1953	President's Commission on the Health Needs of the Nation	For 1960, US needs: 7,000 more	To maintain the 1940 physician-population ratio of 133 per 100,000.
		11,000 more	To maintain the 1949 physician-population ratio of 135 per 100,000.
		24,000 more	To maintain the 1949 ratio and also meet projected military needs.
		43,000 more	To have one private physician per 1,000 civilian population and maintain 1949 levels in hospitals, schools and military.
		35,000 more	To bring all geographical areas with low physician-population ratios up to the national average.
		62,000 more	To bring all geographical areas up to a ratio of 166 physicians per 100,000 population.
			All estimates based on projected 1960 population of 171,176,000.
1959	Surgeon General's Consultant Group on Medical Education (The Bane Committee)	Need to graduate 3,600 more per annum	To maintain the 1959 physician-population ratio of 141 per 100,000 through 1975. Estimated 1975 population—235,246,000.
1965	President's Commission on Heart Disease, Cancer, and Stroke	Existing shortage of 20,000 physicians. Need to graduate 1,000 more per annum and increase to 1,300 more by 1975 to raise total by 57,000.	Based on standard of one private physician per 1,000 civilian population. To maintain the 1965 physician-population ratio of 149 per 100,000. Based on estimated 1975 population of 230,000,000.

Year	Organization	Finding	Standard
1967	Task Force on Health Manpower	Existing shortage of 35,900 physicians. Need for 54,800 more by 1975.	To bring every low state's physician-population ratio up to the national average. To maintain the 1965 physician-population ratio of 153 per 100,000. Based on estimated 1975 population of 232,221,000.
1967	US Public Health Service	Existing shortage of 53,000 physicians in 1966. Need for 103,000 more by 1975.	Based on standards of 100 physicians exclusive of hospital staff per 100,000 population, which is average ratio of prepaid group practice plans.
1967	National Advisory Commission on Health Manpower	Shortage exists because physician productivity is not keeping pace with demand for services. Future needs will depend on improvements in health-care system and physician productivity.	No numerical standard given for number of physicians in population.
1970	Carnegie Commission on Higher Education	Existing shortage of 50,000. Increase medical school entrants by 52% by 1978.	Quotes Dr. Roger Egeberg. To achieve physician-population ratios of 161.4 per 100,000 by 1977 and 216.4 per 100,000 by 2002.

Source: Senior, B. and Smith, B.A.: The number of physicians as a constraint on delivery of health care: How many physicians are enough? *JAMA* 222:179, 1972. Reprinted with permission from the American Medical Association.

ing opportunities for graduate medical education for qualified foreign medical graduates; and (3) prevention of the need to reverse previous inducements offered to United States schools to expand.[12] The result of reduction of the number of foreign medical graduates remaining in the United States to 1000 each year after 1980 is shown in Figure 3-3.[13]

By the late 1970s, there was growing consensus among medical educators, health planners, and policymakers that the expansion of United States medical

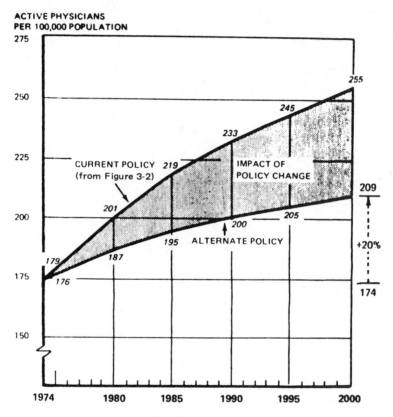

FIGURE 3-3.

Impact of reducing foreign medical graduate inflow on projected growth in the number of active physicians per 100,000 population, 1974 to 2000. Alternate policy assumptions: (1) No further growth beyond 1975 in first-year enrollments of U.S. medical and osteopathic schools. (2) Number of foreign medical graduates entering the United States declines from 8000 in 1974 to 1000 by 1980 and remains at that level. (3) One-quarter of foreign medical graduates entering the United States leave upon completing their graduate education. (4) Annual rate of deaths and retirements of active physicians equals 2 percent through 1979, 2.1 percent from 1980 to 1989, and 2.2 percent from 1990 to 2000. (5) Series E population projections.

Source: Morrow, JH, and Edwards, AB: U.S. health manpower policy: Will the benefits justify the costs? *Journal of Medical Education* 51: 801, 1976.

and osteopathic schools should be stopped and existing enrollments stabilized. In 1976, Stambler [14] observed that:

> In general, our projected supply estimates indicate very clearly that before long the Nation will be better supplied with health manpower than at any time in our history, placing the U.S. near the top of all the industrialized nations in terms of overall supply. For example, by 1990, the average physician/population ratio for the U.S. as a whole may be higher than the current ratio in even the most well-supplied State.

The lack of correlation between the number of physicians and the outcome of health care has been well documented by many observers. For example, the infant mortality rate, general mortality rate, or morbidity rate for chronic diseases are no lower in the Middle Atlantic states, a region of relatively high physician-to-population ratio, than in the Rocky Mountain states, a region with a lower ratio. Further, the general mortality rate in the United States in 1900, when the physician-to-population ratio was 157/100,000, was 17.2/1000, whereas the general mortality rate had fallen to 9.4/1000 in 1967, when the physician-to-population ratio had dropped to 153/100,000.[15] As Petersdorf [16] has noted, "the physician-to-population ratio is one of the more fallacious health-care indexes to which we have been subjected."

GEOGRAPHIC DISTRIBUTION

It has been generally recognized that geographic maldistribution among physicians has existed for years both in total numbers of physicians and in specialty distribution by region, state, or size of community. The data show extreme variations by geographic area. Over 45 million Americans live in areas where the delivery of health care services are inadequate or nonexistent, at least 120 rural counties are without a physician, and many people in the cities find that private physicians are unavailable.[17]

Table 3-2 shows the distribution of physicians by aggregate number and by specialty in the United States in 1973. It can be seen that the total number of physicians in the East South Central region was then little more than one-half the number of physicians in the Middle Atlantic region and that considerable variations existed for specialty distribution.[18]

With the exception of family practice residency programs, most of the nation's efforts in graduate medical education during the past 25 years have aggravated, and even partly caused, the chronic patterns of geographic maldistribution of physicians. There has been a strong tendency for residency graduates in most specialties to establish practice in populous, high-income areas of the country. For example, the state of New York, which accounted for over 20 percent of all residents in training in 1970, has the largest density of physicians-to-population, well in excess of 200 physicians per 100,000 people.[19]

Although the relative supply among physicians is strongly influenced by the influx of foreign medical graduates (Figure 3-4),[20] foreign graduates have not

TABLE 3-2. DISTRIBUTION OF SPECIALISTS (M.D.) BY GEOGRAPHIC DIVISION, 1973

GEOGRAPHIC DIVISION	PHYSICIANS PER 100,000 POPULATION	PERCENT IN EACH FIELD OF SPECIALIZATION						
		All	General practice	Medicine and pediatrics	Surgery	Anesthesiology, Pathology, Radiology	Psychiatry, Neurology	Other and Not Classified
United States	148	100	17	25	27	12	8	11
Middle Atlantic*	190	100	13	28	26	11	10	12
New England	189	100	11	29	26	12	11	10
Pacific	180	100	18	24	27	12	9	10
South Atlantic	138	100	15	26	29	11	8	11
Mountain	135	100	19	24	29	12	7	9
East North Central	129	100	18	24	27	12	7	11
West North Central	124	100	21	23	27	11	8	10
West South Central	114	100	21	22	30	12	6	9
East South Central	103	100	21	22	31	11	5	10

Source: Computed from Warner and Aherne. *Profile of Medical Practice, 1973;* In: *Physicians for the Future, Report of the Macy Commission.* New York, Josiah Macy, Jr. Foundation, 1976, p. 71.

* Includes New York and New Jersey.

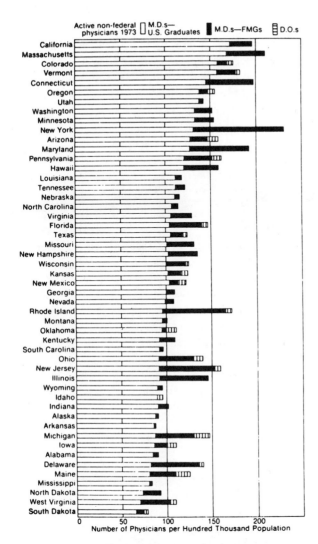

FIGURE 3-4.

Influence on the relative supply of physicians among the states by the location of foreign medical graduates. Source: *Physicians for the Future. Report of the Macy Commission.* New York, Josiah Macy, Jr. Foundation, 1976, p. 68.

helped, and have even aggravated, existing geographic maldistribution of physicians, since few practice in underserved areas of the country.[21] For example, in 1970, foreign medical graduates comprised the highest percentage of physicians in New York (35 percent) and Rhode Island (30 percent), both states having high physician-to-population ratios. A large proportion of foreign medical graduates have been employed by hospitals or other institutions. Only about one-third of all foreign medical graduates in 1970 were in office-based practice, compared with about two-thirds of active physician graduates of United States and Canadian schools.[22]

Although significant efforts are being made to address the problem of geographic maldistribution of physicians (e.g., National Health Service Corps, scholarship and loan repayment programs), there is little evidence to date that this problem will be effectively solved. Federal projections for the distribution of physicians in 1990 are shown in Table 3-3.[23] At a minimum, it is projected that 5 percent of physician graduates will practice in nonmetropolitan areas; even an optimistic estimate of 15 percent of physician graduates settling in nonmetropolitan areas leaves these areas relatively short of physicians.[23]

SPECIALTY DISTRIBUTION

There is ample evidence that maldistribution of physicians by specialty was an increasing problem during the last several decades that reached serious proportions by the end of the 1970s. The first chapter traced the decline of the generalist role in American medicine before the advent of family practice as a specialty and outlined the resultant vacuum in primary care. Although family practice is the fastest growing specialty in United States medicine, the deficits in primary care are so severe that continued major readjustments in the specialty distribution of physicians will be required over a long period of time to redress the balance.

At a symposium sponsored by the Bureau of Health Manpower in 1977 dealing with policy analysis for physician manpower planning, Wessen[24] summed up the problem in this way:

> Especially prominent has been the relative dearth of primary care physicians—a lack the general public regularly testifies to when they complain about difficulties in obtaining physician services. Until very recently, at least, the maldistribution of physicians by specialty has been scarcely affected by the quantitative leap in production of doctors of medicine—approximately a 200% increase in the last twenty years, and of about 70% during the last decade.

Examples of the magnitude of this problem are plentiful. Whereas there was an 8.4 percent reduction in the total number of physicians in general/family practice, internal medicine, and pediatrics between 1965 and 1972, there was an increase of 19.6 percent in the number of surgical specialists and an increase of 33.6 percent in the number of other specialists during the same period.[25] Although in 1970 the average neurosurgeon in this country is believed to have performed only five or six major operations per month,[26] the number of filled first-year residency positions in that specialty increased from 101 in 1960 to 143 in 1973.[27] An extensive study conducted by the American College of Surgeons and the American Surgical Association, *Surgery in the United States*, recommended in 1975 that the number of residency graduates in the surgical specialties be reduced from 2600 per year to between 1600 and 2000 per year.[28]

TABLE 3-3. METROPOLITAN/NONMETROPOLITAN SUPPLY OF PATIENT CARE M.D.s—1975–1990

	ACTUAL 1973	ASSUMED GEOGRAPHIC LOCATION OF NEW SUPPLY (%)	PROJECTED 1990
Total practicing nonfederal patient care M.D.s (includes interns and residents)	270,412 (129/100,000)		449,376 (179/100,000)
Metropolitan	235,375 (149/100,000)	95 85	410,036 (217/100,000) 384,444 (204/100,000)
Nonmetropolitan	35,037 (68/100,000)	5 15	38,312 (62/100,000) 65,252 (105/100,000)

Source: Kindig DA: Health manpower—The right places. In *Health Manpower Issues*. DHEW Publication No. (HRA) 76–40, 1976, p. 25.

As is the case for geographic maldistribution of physicians, graduate medical education to date has contributed to the increasing specialty maldistribution of physicians, rather than helping to alleviate the problem. To date, the number and type of residency positions in the various specialties has been determined solely by the respective specialties without a coordinated effort to "rationalize the mix" at any level. The "territorial imperative" often operates at the level of the individual residency program, whereby programs are unnecessarily expanded or continued at the same level past a time when a clear need exists for more graduates in the field. Many hospitals have relied on residents for their service function, which may be considered cheaper than hiring staff physicians. Residents have also been depended upon for teaching by clinical departments in medical schools and the larger teaching hospitals.

The influx of foreign medical graduates is again part of the specialty maldistribution problem. The number of foreign medical graduates in this country increased from 36,569 in 1963 to 77,660 in 1973, an increase of 112.3 percent, compared with a growth rate of 21 percent for United States medical graduates over the same period.[29] In recent years, the annual growth of licensed foreign medical graduates became almost as large as the increase in United States trained licensed physicians and by 1973 represented one-fifth of all practicing physicians.[10] Of the approximately 2000 foreign medical graduates entering the United States each year for surgical training, 1500 remain as surgeons and only about 400 become board certified.[30] Foreign medical graduates occupy over 50 percent of filled residency positions in anesthesiology, pathology, and physical medicine and rehabilitation,[31] and only a very small number enter the primary care specialties. In addition, the quality of care provided by many foreign medical graduates has been seriously questioned by a number of observers. Weiss and his colleagues, for example, observed that "a large number of FMG's are functioning in a medical underground delivering patient care in an unsupervised and unregulated fashion." [31] Some estimates have been made that the number of unlicensed foreign medical graduates may exceed 10,000.[32]

Dr. Robert Knouss,[33] as Director of the Division of Medicine of the Bureau of Health Manpower, in 1976 summarized the end result of these trends in these words:

> Specialization, which has been stimulated by shifts toward hospital care and uncontrolled because of a lack of adequate planning, has also been accompanied by an increased fragmentation of medical care. Furthermore, specialization as a general phenomenon appears to have been associated with observable inefficiencies in the delivery of services. Underutilization, overtraining, duplication and varying levels of compensation for the performance of similar tasks have all been cited as factors in rising health care costs, the forces of inflation aside.

And further, this should not be interpreted "as an argument for despecialization, it is, instead, a plea for achieving a balance between generalism and specialism, for improved efficiency in the delivery of services, and for a move away from fragmentation."

APPROACHES TO PHYSICIAN MANPOWER PROBLEMS

New Directions in the 1970s

The foregoing makes it clear that the main theme in most thinking and re- sponses to address physician manpower problems during recent years in this country focused primarily on efforts to increase the total numbers of physi- cians. By the mid-1970s, however, there was general consensus that these efforts had failed and that other kinds of intervention to address geographic and specialty maldistribution were needed. Some new initiatives have been taken at several levels since the mid-1970s that have especially involved organized medicine, academic medicine, and government in an increasingly collaborative manner. An overall perspective of these new initiatives can be developed by brief review of some of the policy statements of several of the major orga- nizations.

The Association of American Medical Colleges (AAMC) Task Force on Foreign Medical Graduates in 1974 proposed a series of actions that would reduce the influx of foreign medical graduates without adopting discriminatory policies. The following steps were recommended[34]:

1. Limit the number of first-year positions in approved residency programs of graduate medical education "so as to exceed only slightly the expected number of graduates from domestic medical schools and to provide suffi- cient opportunities to highly qualified FMG's."
2. Apply the same standards of admission to residency programs to foreign and United States graduates.
3. Close the loopholes in licensure of foreign medical graduates by state medi- cal boards.

The mid-1970s saw the formation of two new bodies with broad responsi- bilities for improving the coordination of medical education—the Coordinating Council on Medical Education (CCME) and the Liaison Committee on Gradu- ate Medical Education (LCGME).* These groups included wide representation within medicine in the hope that the overall needs of medical education could be better served, particularly through accreditation decisions. In 1975, the CCME rcommended[35]:

---

* The Liaison Committee for Graduate Medical Education includes representatives from the AMA, AAMC, the American Hospital Association (AHA), the Council of Medical Specialty Societies (CMSS), and the American Board of Medical Specialties (ABMS).

> As a national goal, schools of medicine should be encouraged to accept voluntarily the responsibility for providing an appropriate environment that will motivate students to select careers related to the teaching and practice of primary care. An initial national target of having 50% of graduating medical students choose careers as primary care specialists appears reasonable.

This goal had the support of the House of Delegates of the American Medical Association, many professional organizations, and the federal government.

At the federal level, the Health Professions Educational Assistance Act of 1976 (Public Law 94–484) also established new directions from previous legislation. This act extended federal support for the training of physicians, dentists, and other health personnel to 1980 with new provisions to more directly affect: (1) the kinds of health professionals being trained and (2) where they will practice. Among the various provisions of the law were the following[36]:

1. Capitation grants to medical schools provided that percentages of filled first-year residency positions in direct or affiliated residency programs in primary care (family medicine, general internal medicine, and general pediatrics) exceeded 35 percent in 1978, 40 percent in 1979, and 50 percent in 1980.
2. Project grants provided to help establish academic administrative units in family medicine in medical and osteopathic schools.
3. Matching construction grants for ambulatory primary care teaching facilities.
4. Revision of the Immigration and Nationality Act to restrict the entry of foreign medical graduates.
5. New student assistance programs of insured loans and scholarships for needy health professions students.
6. Increased authorizations for National Health Service Corps (NHSC) scholarships with obligated service conditions broadened to include private practice.
7. Categorical support for teaching programs in general dentistry, since a problem of excess specialization has taken place in dentistry as in medicine.

After intensive study, the Institute of Medicine of the National Academy of Sciences in 1978 released a comprehensive report, *An Integrated Manpower Policy for Primary Care*. Among its specific recommendations were the following[37]:

1. For the present, the number of entrants to medical school should remain at the current annual level.
2. For the present, the number of nurse practitioners and physician assistants trained should remain at the current annual level.

3. A substantial increase should be made in the national goal for percentage distribution of first-year residents in primary care fields (although a definite level was not recommended, there was a general feeling that 60 to 70 percent of first-year residency positions in primary care specialties may be indicated instead of the lower 50 percent figure).
4. Third-party reimbursement by federal and state programs and private insurers of all physicians should be at the same level of payment for the same primary care service, and consideration should be given to narrowing the differentials in payment levels between primary care and nonprimary care procedures.
5. Medical schools should provide all students with some clinical experience in a primary care setting.
6. The curriculum of undergraduate medical education should include epidemiology and the behavioral and social sciences.
7. In selecting among applicants for admission, medical schools should give weight to likely indicators of primary-care selections.

Another important contribution to physician manpower planning during the late 1970s was the excellent report of the Macy Commission, *Physicians for the Future*. This group made the following observations[38]:

> The responsibility for the nation's health programs is so fragmented that the programs are not being carried out with maximal effectiveness. It also became clear, after careful review of existing professional organizations, that no one agency is at this time "putting it all together"—coordinating and giving unified direction to the numerous current efforts aimed at the improvement of health.

The commission noted further that "Differences of opinion among the parent organizations and the lack of independent status and staff have thus far limited the CCME's effectiveness in dealing with current problems."

The Macy Commission therefore called for the formation of an independent, broadly representative National Commission of Medical Education, Manpower and Services, which would concern itself with[39]:

1. The nation's need for physicians.
2. The expansion of existing medical schools and the number and location of new schools.
3. The apportionment of graduates among the various specialties and their geographical distribution.
4. The flow of foreign medical graduates and United States foreign medical graduates.
5. The financing of medical education, so that federal support will meet reasonable needs.
6. The nation's need for nurse practitioners and physicians' assistants.

Redistribution of Graduate Medical Education

Although it is clear that redistribution of residency positions in graduate medical education cannot as an isolated measure solve complex physician manpower problems, it is generally agreed that this is a vital and indispensable part of any effective response to these problems. Mechanisms are being developed whereby analysis and redistribution can be accomplished to rationalize the mix of medical graduates by specialty.

It is both appropriate and likely that redistribution of graduate medical education will take place in the context of specific limits in the total number of residency positions as well as reduction in the number of foreign medical graduates entering the country for graduate training. Although there is room for some debate with respect to the precise proportions by individual specialties, all agree that the three primary-care specialties of family medicine, general internal medicine, and general pediatrics (particularly the first two) are in relatively short supply, while many of the other specialties are, or soon will be, in surplus.

In an excellent paper addressing the subject of United States health manpower policy, Morrow and Edwards [40] propose the approximate allocation of first-year graduate medical education positions by specialty as shown in Table 3-4. This proposal calls for 50 percent of graduate medical education positions in primary-care specialties, with 25 percent of all positions in family practice. This kind of reallocation appears to be a logical response to the specialty maldistribution problem based on presently available data.

In order to obtain the reapportionment of residency positions along the lines noted above, continued expansion is required for family practice residency programs. Conversion will be required for many existing internal medicine residency positions from subspecialty/fellowship positions to general medicine positions. The reduction of many other specialty residencies will involve either decreasing the size of existing programs or terminating some currently operational programs. Such an approach will prevent increasing surpluses in many of the limited specialties and subspecialties. These changes will require reorientation of teaching and service functions in both community hospitals and the larger teaching hospitals, with full-time staff physicians and/or faculty often replacing many of the functions previously carried by residents in the limited specialties.

COMMENT

Restructuring of graduate medical education in these directions can go a long way toward relieving both geographic and specialty maldistribution of physicians, but must be accompanied by related changes in medical education and clinical practice to be maximally effective. A variety of important issues must be addressed simultaneously, such as financing mechanisms for medical educa-

TABLE 3–4. APPROXIMATE ALLOCATION BY SPECIALTY OF 16,500 FIRST–YEAR RESIDENCY POSITIONS

SPECIALTY	1973–1974 LEVEL*	ACTIONS INDICATED†	APPROXIMATE ALLOCATION
Family/general practice	942	Substantially increase	4,000
Medical specialties			
Internal medicine	3,955‡	Essentially maintain (emphasize general internal medicine)	3,700
Pediatrics	1,699§	Reduce	1,300
Dermatology	234	Reduce	200
Surgical specialties			
First-year general surgery	2,698	Reduce	2,175
General surgery (including colon and rectal)	(1,074)¶	Reduce	(900)
Neurological surgery	(143)	Substantially reduce	(100)
Orthopedic surgery	(591)	Reduce	(450)
Otolaryngology	(266)	Reduce	(200)
Plastic surgery	(174)	Substantially reduce	(125)
Thoracic surgery	(130)	Reduce	(100)
Urology	(320)	Essentially maintain	(300)
Obstetrics–gynecology	1,003	Essentially maintain	900
Ophthalmology	495	Essentially maintain	450
Other specialties			
Anesthesiology	797	Reduce	650
Neurology	357	Reduce	300
Psychiatry	1,472**	Essentially maintain	1,350
Pathology	898††	Substantially reduce	600
Physical medicine and rehabilitation	135	Essentially maintain	125
Radiology (total)	1,076	Substantially reduce	750
Total	15,761	Essentially maintain	16,500

* Based on *Directory of Approved Internships and Residencies 1974-75,* AMA, Table 11, adjusted as noted below to minimize double counting.

† Essentially maintain = ±10 percent; reduce = −10 percent to −25 percent; substantially reduce = −25 percent or more.

‡ Half of first-year dermatology and physical medicine and rehabilitation residents subtracted on the assumption that their first-year of residency training was in internal medicine.

§ Does not include pediatric allergy and pediatric cardiology.

¶ To estimate the number of first-year residents who will remain in general surgery, first-year residents in neurological surgery, orthopedic surgery, otolaryngology, plastic surgery, thoracic surgery, and urology were subtracted from total of first-year residents in general surgery.

** Does not include child psychiatry.

†† Does not include forensic pathology and neuropathology.

Source: Morrow, J.H. and Edwards, A.B.: U.S. health manpower policy: Will the benefits justify the costs? *Journal of Medical Education* 51:803, 1976.

tion, reimbursement policies, and remodeling of the existing health care delivery system around a stronger primary-care base. As Petersdorf [41] suggests:

> We should aim to make the practice of primary care medicine—whether it be by family practitioners, general internists, or pediatricians—as attractive, prestigious, and rewarding as subspecialty practice. This should be the major goal of medical schools, professional organizations, accrediting bodies, and government. If it can be reached, many of our health manpower problems will be relieved.

Although some will say that we do not yet have the information or capability to "fine tune" the mix of physicians by specialty, this is not the issue at this point. The pendulum has swung so far in this country toward subspecialization that the problems are major and call for "rough tuning" or equally major actions to rebalance the health care delivery system. Stevens [42] has observed that two revolutionary periods have already occurred in American medicine during the twentieth century—the revolution in undergraduate medical education between 1905 and 1910 and that involving the development of specialist education and certification in the 1930s. She sees the inevitable need for a "third period of radical education and manpower reform in the 1970's and 1980's in response to organizational and economic pressures, whether through national health insurance or government financing of medical education."

Only time will tell whether the currently accepted target of 50 percent for the three primary care specialties will meet the needs of the public. In my view, this is short of the mark, and a target at or above 60 percent may be required. The critical question concerning the effectiveness of any such target, however, is the extent to which the long-standing trend toward subspecialization in internal medicine and pediatrics can be altered toward primary care roles. Academic departments and faculty in internal medicine and pediatrics are predominantly oriented to the subspecialties, and there is considerable evidence that the trends toward subspecialization remain strong. As Somers [43] observes:

> The primary care issue is not just a matter of numbers or how the doctor is listed in the medical directories. It involves the physician's basic value system, his philosophy of patient care, and his personal professional priorities. The effective primary care physician must be prepared—not only technically, but philosophically and temperamentally—to assume continuing responsibility for the patient's overall health needs, including health maintenance. Medical school and residency training, and attitudes inculcated in those settings, must be reasonably consistent with the end-product that Congress and the public are demanding, or avoidable conflict and frustrations will continue to plague the profession and its educational institutions.

Family practice represents the essential foundation of the strengthening primary-care base in American medicine. Today's family physician is well prepared clinically and attitudinally to carry the major responsibility for the primary care of families. Family practice has already demonstrated its capability of addressing the problem of geographic maldistribution of physicians—over

50 percent of graduates of family practice residencies have established practice in communities of less than 30,000 population, and the remainder are evenly distributed in larger communities.[44] Although the present goal for 25 percent of the nation's future physicians to enter family practice may be reasonable in the short run, a larger proportion of family physicians may ultimately be required.

Today's problems of physician maldistribution took over 40 years to develop in this country, and cannot be solved in 5 or 10 years. As Knouss[45] points out:

> Over the next few years, a quantum increase in information and understanding of the issues will be necessary before fine adjustments in the distribution of resources can be made. And efforts to achieve short-term improvements must be weighed against their impact on health manpower over the next several decades.

REFERENCES

1. Edwards CC: A candid look at health manpower problems. J Med Educ 49:21, 1974
2. Mechanic D: Relationships between medical need and responsiveness of care: A framework for developing policy options. In Lewis CE, Fein R, Mechanic D (eds): A Right to Health: The Problem of Access to Primary Medical Care. New York, Wiley, 1976, p 30
3. Knowles JH: The quantity and quality of medical manpower: A review of medicine's current efforts. J Med Educ 44:84, 1969
4. Stambler HV: Health manpower—the right number. In Health Manpower Issues, DHEW Publication No. (HRA) 76–40, 1976, p 12
5. Mechanic D: Relationships between medical need and responsiveness of care: A framework for developing policy options. In Lewis CE, Fein R, Mechanic D (eds): A Right to Health: The Problem of Access to Primary Medical Care. New York, Wiley, 1976, p 31
6. McNerney W: Why does medical care cost so much? N Engl J Med 282:1458, 1970
7. Distribution of Physicians, Hospitals and Hospital Beds in the U.S. Chicago, AMA, 1967, p 5
8. Mechanic D: Relationships between medical need and responsiveness of care: A framework for developing policy options. In Lewis CE, Fein R, Mechanic D (eds): A Right to Health: The Problem of Access to Primary Medical Care. New York, Wiley, 1976, p 31
9. Senior B, Smith BA: The number of physicians as a constraint on delivery of health care: How many physicians are enough? JAMA 222:179, 1972
10. Stambler HV: Health manpower—the right number. In Health Manpower Issues, DHEW Publication No. (HRA) 76–40, 1976, p 9
11. Physicians for the Future. Report of the Macy Commission. New York, Josiah Macy, Jr. Foundation, 1976, p 80
12. Morrow JH, Edwards AB: U.S. health manpower policy: Will the benefits justify the costs? J Med Educ 51:792, 1976

13. Morrow JH, Edwards AB: U.S. health manpower policy: Will the benefits justify the costs? J Med Educ 51:801, 1976

14. Stabler HV: Health manpower—the right number. In Health Manpower Issues, DHEW Publication No. (HRA) 76–40, 1976, p 11

15. Senior B, Smith BA: The number of physicians as a constraint on delivery of health care: How many physicians are enough? JAMA 222:180, 1972

16. Petersdorf RG: Health manpower: Numbers, distribution, quality. Ann Intern Med 82:695, 1975

17. Physicians for the Future. Report of the Macy Commission, New York, Josiah Macy, Jr. Foundation, 1976, p 6

18. Physicians for the Future. Report of the Macy Commission, New York, Josiah Macy, Jr. Foundation, 1976, p 71

19. Rousselot LM: Federal efforts to influence physician education, specialization distribution projections and options. Am J Med 55:124, 1973

20. Physicians for the Future. Report of the Macy Commission, New York, Josiah Macy, Jr. Foundation, 1976, p 68

21. Physicians for the Future. Report of the Macy Commission, New York, Josiah Macy, Jr. Foundation, 1976, p 19

22. Progress and Problems in Medical and Dental Education: Federal Support versus Federal Control. Report of the Carnegie Foundation for the Advancement of Teaching. San Francisco, Jossey-Bass, 1976, p 27

23. Kindig DA: Health manpower—the right place. In Health Manpower Issues. DHEW Publication No. (HRA) 76–40, 1976, p 25

24. Wessen AF: On the demand for graduate medical education positions by specialty. In Policy Analysis for Physician Manpower Planning. DHEW Publication No. (HRA) 78–2, 1978, p 63

25. Holden WD: Attitudes of the Coordinating Council on Medical Education toward physician manpower. Bull NY Acad Med 52:1078, 1976

26. Odom GL: Neurological surgery in our changing times: The 1972 AANS presidential address. J Neurosurg 37:255, 1972

27. Physicians for the Future. Report of the Macy Commission, New York, Josiah Macy, Jr. Foundation, 1976, p 79

28. Surgery in the United States. A Joint Study by the American College of Surgeons and the American Surgical Association (n.p.:n.p., 1975)

29. Distribution of Physicians in the United States, 1973. Chicago, AMA, Center for Health Services Research and Development, 1974, p 42

30. Petersdorf RG: Health Manpower: Numbers, distribution, quality. Ann Intern Med 82:696, 1975

31. Weiss RJ et al: Foreign medical graduates and the medical underground. N Engl J Med 290:1408, 1974

32. Holden WD: Developments in graduate medical education. In Purcell EF, ed: Recent Trends in Medical Education. New York, Josiah Macy, Jr. Foundation, 1976, p 257

33. Knouss RF: Health manpower—the right kind. In Health Manpower Issues. DHEW Publication No. (HRA) 76–40, 17–18, 1976

34. Graduates of foreign medical schools in the United States: A challenge to medical education. J Med Educ 49:809, 1974

35. Coordinating Council on Medical Education: Physician Manpower and Distribution: The Primary Care Physician. Chicago, Coordinating Council on Medical Education, 1975, p 6

36. Whiteside DF: Training the nation's health manpower—the next 4 years. Public Health Rep 92:2, 1977

37. An Integrated Manpower Policy for Primary Care. Washington, D.C., Institute of Medicine of the National Academy of Sciences, 1978

38. Physicians for the Future. Report of the Macy Commission, New York, Josiah Macy, Jr. Foundation, 1976, p 34

39. Physicians for the Future. Report of the Macy Commission, New York, Josiah Macy, Jr. Foundation, 1976, p 36

40. Morrow JH, Edwards AB: U.S. health manpower policy: Will the benefits justify the costs? J Med Educ 51:803, 1976

41. Petersdorf RG: Health manpower: Numbers, distribution, quality. Ann Intern Med 82:701, 1975

42. Stevens R: Trends in medical specialization in the United States. Inquiry 8:18, 1971

43. Somers AR, Somers HM: Health and Health Care: Policies in Perspective. Germantown, Maryland, Aspen Systems Corporation, 1977, p 441

44. Geyman JP: Family practice in evolution: Progress, problems and projections. N Engl J Med 298:593, 1978

45. Knouss RF: Health manpower—the right kind. In Health Manpower Issues, DHEW Publication No. (HRA) 76–40, 17–18, 1976, p 23

CHAPTER FOUR

Department of Family Medicine (R700)
University of Miami School of Medicine
P. O. Box 016700
Miami, Florida 33101

James M. Gall, M.D., C.C.F.P.
Department of Family Medicine
University of Miami School of Medicine
P. O. Box 016700
Miami, Florida 33101

Barriers to Health Care

The perceived crisis (in health care) stems not from our lack of technical capacity, but from our failure to ensure that all citizens have equal access to the promise that medical science has made possible and to humane and responsive care. The perceived crisis is a constellation of attitudes. To many with lower incomes, the barriers are economic and relate to the hardships of purchasing necessary care. For middle-class persons, a frequent concern is the possibility of a catastrophic illness and its consequences for the economic viability of the family. For the aged, increasing inflation and gaps in the Medicare program, requiring personal expenditures from their meager resources, are a source of worry. And people in general express concern about improved medical care and inadequate interest in the patient as a person.

David Mechanic [1]

One of the premises of this book is that the medical profession does not exist in a vacuum, but in a complex society of changing needs. Our central commitment as health professionals must be to understand these needs and to respond maximally to them. In medicine, we must learn what leaders in business and industry learned long ago—to expect change—and to plan ahead for anticipated future changes and perhaps even to innovate change.

In the preceding chapter, geographic and specialty maldistribution of physicians was found to represent a major problem. There is another critical problem being recognized in recent years—the vast extent of unmet health needs of a large number of people in this country. An understanding of current barriers to delivery of health care services is essential to any efforts to extend available knowledge and health resources to our entire population.

BACKGROUND

As White and his colleagues [2] pointed out in their classic paper on the ecology of medical care in 1961, approximately three-fourths of the population have an acute or chronic illness in any given month that leads to some action, such as the restriction of activity or the taking of medication. Among those people reporting an illness during the month, about one-third seek medical care. Many of these people are immediately confronted with a number of barriers that tend to limit access to adequate medical care.

Various estimates have been made that between 30 and 50 million Americans do not have access to medical care equal to that of the majority of citizens. This large segment of the population is a diverse group, including the poor, the "working poor," many older people, and people living in underserved areas. Mechanic sums up the problem of access to medical care in this way[3]:

> As medicine has demonstrated greater efficacy, all segments of the population have gained greater appreciation of the high standard of medical care possible in the United States. With heightened expectations the failure to find accessible and responsive services has become a bitter pill to swallow, especially among more deprived groups who see their difficulties as one more manifestation of their exclusion from the mainstream of American society. Innumerable studies support these perceptions by demonstrating that the poor have a greater prevalence of illness, disability, chronicity, and restriction of activity because of health problems than those of higher status and that they have less accessibility to many health services and receive lower quality care.

Among the many studies of the health problems of lower socioeconomic groups, for example, one study commissioned by Blue Cross revealed that the incidence of serious illness in the poverty group was two to three times higher than that for the population as a whole. Of the poor households, 70 percent had current medical problems, whereas only 44 percent of total households had reported such problems. Seventy percent of the poor considered medical facilities available to them as inadequate, and 54 percent did not even know where they would turn in a medical emergency.[4]

We have no accurate way of measuring the proportion of Americans who are receiving adequate comprehensive care for their families, but it surely must be a disappointingly low figure. Certainly the poor are not the only group of our population receiving less than adequate health care. Despite remarkable increases in medical resources in recent years, many people with the ability to pay and with close proximity to medical resources cannot find a personalized source of ongoing care for everyday problems. We saw in the last chapter that there is a serious deficit of primary care physicians in this country. It is now germane to look at some of the major barriers to adequate health care that presently exist.

BARRIERS TO HEALTH CARE

Examination of 12 important barriers between the patient and the health provider is useful to a clearer understanding of present deficiencies of medical practice. Obviously, many often exist concurrently and consideration of each alone is somewhat artificial.

Consumer-Related Barriers

SOCIOECONOMIC BARRIER

This barrier can be looked on as a twofold problem involving (1) the large part of our population that is poor or has difficulty in paying the costs of medical care and (2) the spiraling costs of health care services.

Although about 80 percent of Americans have some kind of health insurance for general hospital care, many do not have coverage for drugs, diagnostic studies, nursing home, and dental expenses. Figure 4-1 shows the percentages of people with private health insurance in 1974 by type of benefit.[5] For the family just above poverty levels by existing formulas, health care is difficult to purchase. Often such families have no insurance coverage, and can afford only the rudiments of acute care.

There is some evidence that access to health care services has improved for disadvantaged groups over the last 20 years, at least as measured by increased utilization of these services. Figure 4-2 shows significant gains in access to health care of medium- and low-income people in the United States since 1963.[6]

Elimination of the financial barrier to services, however, has been shown not to be effective in itself for improving the health of the concerned group. Thus, in Buffalo, New York, among children 5 to 9 years old, 73 percent of children in the upper class had obtained measles immunization as compared to only 19 percent in the lower economic stratum, despite the free availability of the vaccine through health department clinics.[7] Similar observations have been made after 15 years of experience in England with the National Health Service, where the higher-income groups have made better use of available health services both in and out of the hospital, including psychiatric care.[8, 9]

The poor have been noted to behave differently from people in higher socioeconomic strata. They often define illness in different terms and tend to seek health care on an episodic basis and relatively late after the onset of illness. They

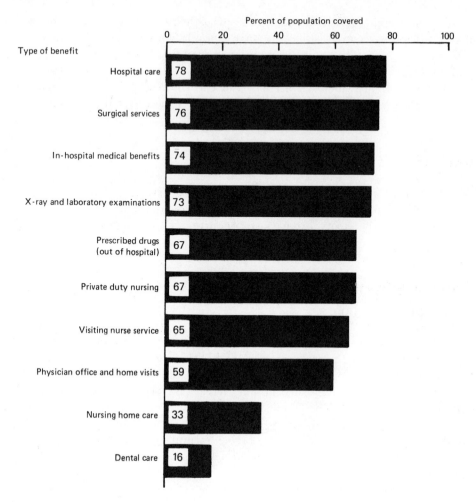

FIGURE 4-1.

Percent of persons with private health insurance, by type of benefit (United States, 1974), based on estimates of the net number of different persons insured for each benefit.

Source: Mueller, MS, and Piro, PA: Private health insurance in 1973: A review of coverage, enrollment, and financial experience. *Social Security Bulletin* 39:4, March 1976, Table 1.

are more likely to seek care from subprofessionals or marginal practitioners often available in their neighborhoods.[10]

Income and educational level have been shown to correlate adversely with such outcomes of care as infant mortality rate, as shown in Figure 4-3.[11] Likewise, the number of some types of visits to physicians are negatively related to income levels, particularly with respect to visits for preventive care (Figure 4-4).[12]

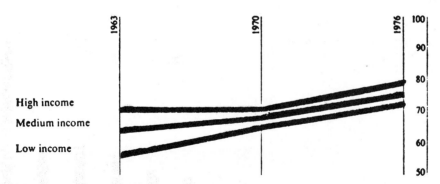

FIGURE 4-2.

Utilization of health care services by income level.

Source: *America's Health System: A Portrait. Special Report.* The Robert Wood Johnson Foundation, Princeton, New Jersey, No. 1, 1978, p. 8.

Although improved access to health care services by 1976 resulted in 4.6 physician visits per person per year for low-income people compared to 3.8 visits per person per year for high-income people, the poor were still relatively disadvantaged with respect to need for medical services. For example, when measured in terms of the ratio of visits per 100 disability days, the poor had a lower ratio in 1976 than those above the poverty line (10.3 and 16.4 visits per 100 disability days for these two groups, respectively).[13]

Social class and socioeconomic status can also be directly related to other dimensions of health-seeking behavior. Table 4-1 shows the percentage of respondents who recognized specific symptoms as requiring medical attention,[14]

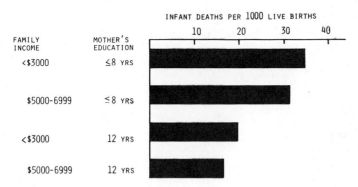

FIGURE 4-3.

Infant mortality rates, for white mothers by family income and mother's education (United States, 1964–1966).[10]

Source: U.S. National Center for Health Statistics: *Infant Mortality Rates: Socioeconomic Factors, United States.* Washington, D.C., Series 22, No. 14, Department of Health, Education and Welfare Publication No. (HSM) 72–1045, March 1972.

FIGURE 4-4.

Relative number of physician visits per person per year by income and type of visits (United States, 1971).

Source: U.S. National Center for Health Statistics: *Physician Visits—Volume and Interval Since Last Visit: U.S.—1971.* Rockville, Maryland, Public Health Service, Series 10, No. 97, March 1975, Table 17, p. 31.

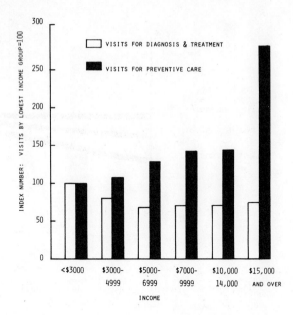

TABLE 4-1. PERCENT OF RESPONDENTS WHO RECOGNIZED SPECIFIED SYMPTOMS AS REQUIRING MEDICAL ATTENTION BY SOCIAL CLASS OR SOCIOECONOMIC STATUS OF RESPONDENTS (REGIONVILLE)

SYMPTOMS	*PERCENT RECOGNIZING SYMPTOM AS REQUIRING MEDICAL ATTENTION*	
	*Class I**	*Class II*
Loss of appetite	57	20
Persistent backache	53	19
Continued coughing	80	23
Persistent joint and muscle pains	80	19
Blood in stool	98	60
Blood in urine	100	69
Excessive vaginal bleeding	92	54
Swelling of ankles	77	23
Loss of weight	80	21
Bleeding of gums	79	20
Chronic fatigue	80	19
Shortness of breath	77	21
Persistent headaches	80	22
Fainting spells	80	33
Pain in chest	80	31
Lump in breast	94	44
Lump in abdomen	92	34

*The "higher" of the two social classes or socioeconomic groupings.

Source: Koos, E.L.: Data on the recognition of symptoms. *The Health of Regionville.* New York, Columbia University Press, 1954.

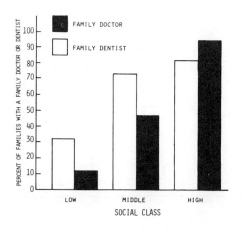

FIGURE 4-5.

Percent of families with a family doctor and with a family dentist by social class in "Regionville," a rural community in New York State (1954).
Source: Koos, EL, *The Health of Regionville*. New York: Columbia University Press, 1954, Fig. 9, p. 33; Fig. 15, p. 119.

while Figure 4-5 shows the comparative frequency of choice of a family doctor and family dentist by social class.[15]

Health care services have priced themselves out of the market for many people. Between 1960 and 1974, while the gross national product increased by 172 percent, expenditures for health care increased by 303 percent. National health expenditures rose from 5.2 percent of the GNP to almost 9 percent of the GNP in 1978.[16] While medical services as a whole increased 39 percent faster than all other services in the economy from 1965 to 1976, the daily room charges in hospitals increased 182 percent more sharply.[17] Figure 4-6 shows the percent increase in medical care and several other major components of the consumer price index from 1950 to 1970 in the United States.[18]

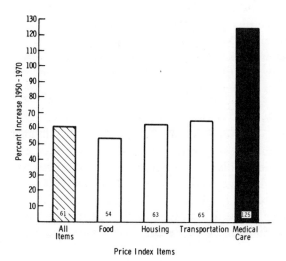

FIGURE 4-6.

Percent increase in medical care and other major components in the consumer price index (United States, 1950–1970).
Source: U.S. Department of Commerce, Bureau of the Census: *Statistical Abstract of the United States, 1971*. Washington, D.C., U.S. Government Printing Office, 1971, no. 534, p. 339.

EDUCATIONAL BARRIER

Increasing levels of education are correlated with utilization of a wider breadth of health services. People with more education use more preventive services, and show a higher average use of medical facilities than people with less education.[19] For example, a nationwide study of patterns of prenatal care has shown that the amount of prenatal care was even more closely related to educational level than to income. College graduates recorded almost twice as many prenatal visits, on the average, than mothers with an elementary education or less and sought care at an earlier time.[20] The value of prenatal care has been amply demonstrated in many studies. Nearly one-half of the babies born in our public hospitals have mothers who have received no prenatal care. Among these, 22 percent are born prematurely, 5 percent are mentally retarded at birth, and 9 percent will be mentally retarded by 12 years of age.[21] A child born into a poor family in this country is twice as likely to die in the first year of life as a child born to middle-class parents.[22] Figure 4-3 shows the higher infant mortality rate that is associated with lower levels of the mother's education.

INFORMATIONAL BARRIER

The informational barrier is, of course, often related to the educational barrier but may be influential in limiting utilization of available services even in well-educated groups. In a time of proliferating agencies and medical and community resources, an individual family often does not know where to seek appropriate help for a particular health problem. Language differences often constitute additional problems. Serious illnesses with innocuous-appearing initial symptoms may frequently be ignored. We are seeing increasing emphasis today on patient education in response to these problems.

PSYCHOLOGIC BARRIER

All practicing physicians can recount many examples of patients who either delayed or failed entirely to seek medical care for a multitude of psychologic reasons. We all have seen patients who have avoided seeing a physician because of fear of a disease such as cancer, anxiety about particular diagnostic or therapeutic procedures, apprehension at seeing the doctor, and a variety of other reasons. McWhinney has suggested that many patients do not seek medical attention until their limits to tolerate anxiety are reached.[23]

CULTURAL BARRIER

It is incumbent on health professionals to understand the cultural and religious beliefs of the people in their communities. Beyond the frequently coexistent language barrier, there are often widely disparate interpretations of disease or method of treatment on a cultural basis. In order to extend adequate care to such groups, physicians should be able to make their services acceptable to the people involved and understandable in terms of their own culture. In some ethnic groups, for instance, it may be considered "weak" for a man and head of a household to seek psychiatric counseling, or even any preventive medical care. Sickness may be interpreted as a threat to his male self image.

RACIAL BARRIER

Certain racial groups regularly have lower income and educational levels than whites, and have not always been accorded ready access to first-class medical care even if other barriers were not present. Unemployment tends to be higher and salaries lower in minority groups.

Although some improvements have been made in access to health care for minority groups in recent years (Figure 4-7),[24] life expectancy at birth is still significantly longer for whites than nonwhites. Maternal mortality rates for nonwhite mothers are three to four times those for white mothers.[25] Figure 4-8 shows comparative infant mortality rates for whites and blacks based on a study in New York City in 1968.[26]

GEOGRAPHIC BARRIER

Most studies show that the utilization of health services (especially preventive services) decreases with increasing distance from medical resources.[27] This is easy to comprehend in view of the sometimes great distances and poor roads that must be negotiated to get to a medical facility in many rural areas. But the geographic alienation from medical care can be just as great in the urban ghetto, where transportation is often not available though distances are short.

Provider-Related Barriers

LACK OF FACILITIES AND MANPOWER

The lack of uniform distribution of physician manpower has been seen in the last chapter. A similar situation exists for other health personnel and facilities. The number of general hospital beds in Appalachia is 15 percent below the national average, and extended care facilities are even more scarce.[28]

OPERATIONAL FEATURES OF SERVICE

The physical and operational features of many medical facilities, especially for the poor, often discourage their use. Such aspects as inconvenient clinic hours, disrespectful eligibility procedures, long waits, frequent changes of physicians and nurses, and impersonal care tend to work against comprehensive family health care and to meet only basic needs for the more acute illnesses.

FRAGMENTED CARE

Fragmentation of health care services, a severe problem for the poverty group, also permeates much of our population. Patients without a family doctor often see multiple physicians for a given illness and never receive comprehensive evaluation or care.

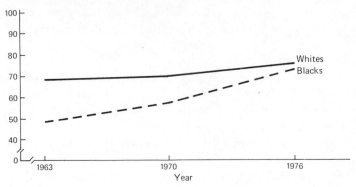

FIGURE 4-7.

Utilization of health care services by racial group.

Source: *America's Health System: A Portrait. Special Report.* The Robert Wood Johnson Foundation, Princeton, New Jersey, No. 1, 1978, p. 7.

County public health departments have developed many programs to meet specific needs within their locales, but few such services are comprehensive. Thus, we have the well-baby clinic, where immunizations are also provided, but no sick care; or the family planning clinic, where the postpartum mother is seen, but not her baby.

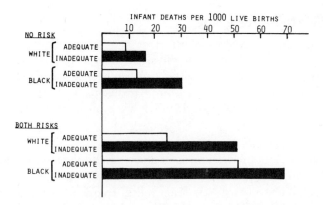

FIGURE 4-8.

Infant mortality rates by risk category (sociodemographic and medical-obstetric), health services index, and race (New York City, 1968). The health services index is a three-factor indicator of maternal health services (time of first prenatal visit; number of prenatal visits; and hospital service, whether ward or private) used to classify health services received by the woman as adequate, intermediate, or inadequate.

Source: Kessner, DM, et al.: *Infant Death: An Analysis by Maternal Risk and Health Care,* Washington, D.C., Institute of Medicine, National Academy of Sciences, 1973, Table 1–2, p. 23. Reproduced with permission of the National Academy of Sciences.

DOLLAR SHORTAGE

A report by the Committee on the Role of Medicine in Society of the California Medical Association in 1970 made the following observations, which summarize this barrier well and are equally true today[29]:

> It is unreasonable to expect that all the dollars needed can ever be assigned to health care, and their comparative lack will therefore always be a barrier to the quality as well as the quantity and availability of services. It will be necessary to combat this by improving methods of identifying what quality and quantity of services are needed, exposing and correcting waste and inefficiency in governmental and non-governmental programs and negotiating programs, and negotiating for sufficient funding from public and private sources.

ORGANIZATIONAL INERTIA

It is clear that important changes are taking place across all levels of our society. Planning for even the short-term future is difficult. Our governmental, professional, business, and educational organizations inevitably encounter considerable inertia in attempting to adapt to these changes. The result is another barrier to health care in a setting wherein we have never quite caught up with the demands for our services.[29]

SPECIAL PROBLEMS OF THE POOR

Dr. H. J. Geiger,[30] as Director of the Tufts-Delta Health Center in Mound Bayou, Mississippi, in 1969 made these comments in an excellent essay, "The Endlessly Revolving Door": "The health of the poor in this country is an ongoing national disaster. It's a grim fact of life in these United States that the poor are likelier to be sick, the sick are likelier to be poor, and, without intervention, the poor get sicker and the sick get poorer."

Many, if not all, of the 12 barriers to health care that have been described often are operating at the interface between the poor patient and the health provider. Extension of health care to this large part of our population represents a most difficult challenge to our health care system. Whatever progress is made in this direction should be helpful in reducing barriers to care for other neglected segments of our population.

The higher incidence of chronic illness and disability in the poor compared to the affluent has been documented by many studies. Figure 4-9 shows striking examples of these differences for various disease categories.[30]

Although the Medicaid program has improved the access to medical care for many poor people in recent years, many of the poor do not qualify for Medicaid or live in states where the benefits are minimal.[31] Dr. J. T. English[32] has described the health problems of the poor in these terms:

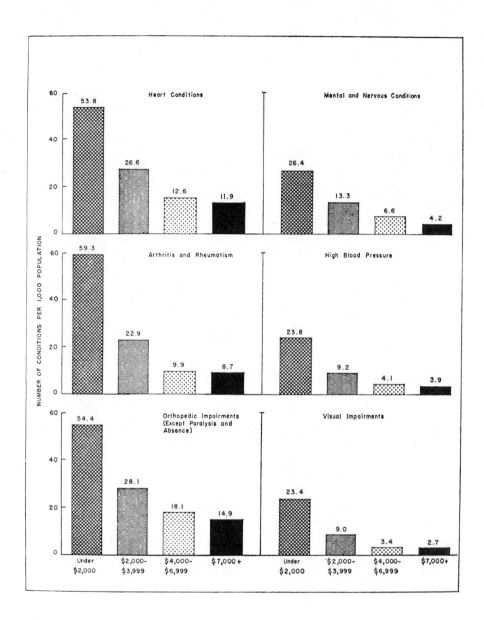

FIGURE 4-9.

Chronic conditions by family income.

Source: White: *Inquiry* 5:19, 1968. Copyright 1968 by the Blue Cross Association. All rights reserved. (Data from a survey conducted in fiscal 1963 by The National Center for Health Statistics, USPHS.)

Being poor means more than simply being without money—or without enough money. It means living, as most low income families do, under conditions that undermine both physical and mental health. Residents of poverty areas struggle with malnutrition, with inadequate housing, heating, and sanitary facilities, with substandard working conditions—sometimes, with rats. These unsatisfactory living conditions breed illness or make it worse. And the vicious cycle continues, since the poor who are also sick are handicapped in their efforts to take advantage of the educational and employment opportunities that might lift them above the poverty threshold.

SPECIAL PROBLEMS OF THE ELDERLY

People over 65 years of age represent a steadily increasing proportion of the population. Since 1900, this age group has increased from three million people to twenty-nine million people today. The age group over 75 years of age has grown particularly rapidly and now represents 38 percent of people over 65, compared to 31.4 percent of people over 65 in 1950.[33] Figure 4-10 illustrates the changing demography of the older population since 1900.

The elderly have special problems with respect to health care. People over 65 years of age now comprise 10 percent of the total population in the United States but represent 27 percent of the total expenditures for health care.[33] Figure 4-11 illustrates the increasing incidence of limitation of activity and of mobility with advancing age.[34]

The economic barrier to health care is a major one for many older people. Their postretirement incomes are sharply reduced at a time when their needs for health care tend to increase considerably. Medicare is of some help, but it by no means covers the costs. In 1975, for example, Medicare paid for 72 percent of hospital expenditures for the elderly, but only 54 percent of physicians' fees, 3 percent of the costs of skilled nursing care, and 4 percent of all other costs.[35] Medicare imposes higher cost-sharing and other limitations on ambulatory care than on hospital care.

SPECIAL PROBLEMS OF RURAL INHABITANTS

According to the 1970 census, 54 percent of the United States population lives in communities with populations of 25,000 or less. These communities represent about 95 percent of the 20,821 cities and towns in the United States.[36] Almost one-half of all rural Americans live in areas designated by the Department of Health, Education and Welfare as medically underserved. Over 15 million people in rural America have access to at most one physician per 4000 people, and 145 counties have no physicians.[37]

Inhabitants of rural areas encounter special problems with respect to health care. The following observations suggest the complexity of those interrelated problems and the extent to which they act as barriers to health care[38]:

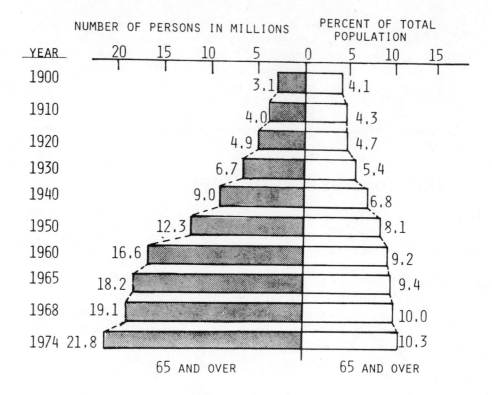

FIGURE 4-10.

Aged persons—number and percent of total population (United States, 1900–1974).
Sources: (1) For 1900–1960: U.S. Department of Commerce, Bureau of the Census. *1960 Census of Population, Vol. 1, Characteristics of Population, Part A. U.S. Summary,* Washington, D.C., 1961, Table 47, p. 1. (2) For 1965: U.S. Department of Commerce, Bureau of the Census. *Population Estimates,* Current Population Reports, Series P-25, No. 329. (3) For 1968: U.S. Department of Commerce, Bureau of the Census. *Population Estimates,* Current Population Reports, Series P-25, No. 400. (4) For 1974: U.S. Bureau of the Census. *Statistical Abstract of the United States, 1975.* 96th edition, Washington, D.C., U.S. Government Printing Office, 1975, Series P-25, No. 539, p. 32.

- Twenty-one percent of rural inhabitants have incomes below federally defined poverty levels (double the urban figure).
- There are nine dependents for every ten working-age adults in rural areas compared to seven dependents in urban settings.
- Rural areas experience special environmental, occupational, and social health hazards (e.g., 60 percent of all substandard housing in the United States is in rural areas).
- Rural areas have fewer health care resources despite their critical needs.
- Regulatory and reimbursement policies tend to disregard the special problems of rural hospitals.
- Rates of reimbursement for rural Medicare and Medicaid patients are substantially below those for urban providers (e.g., in 1973, the average Medi-

caid expenditure per poor child was $76 in metropolitan areas and only $5 in nonmetropolitan areas).

- Transportation costs are often barriers to health care in rural areas due to poor roads and inadequate public and private transportation.[39]
- The number of physician visits per person-year in 1976 for rural farm inhabitants was only 2.7, compared to 4.6 physician visits per person-year for central-city dwellers.

COMMENT

The measurement of access to health care is viewed by Mechanic [40] in the following way:

> Access is measured by the availability of services in the community, the obtainability of services by any and all subgroups of the population, and the comprehensiveness of services offered by the sources of first-contact care or facilities linked with it. . . . To the extent that the source of first-contact care is too narrow in orientation or poorly developed in skills and judgmental capacities, the probability is lower that the problem will be properly assessed and adequately managed.

Family practice has much to contribute to effectively dealing with the various barriers to health care that have been outlined. Well-trained family physicians have the broadest range of clinical knowledge and skills of anyone in

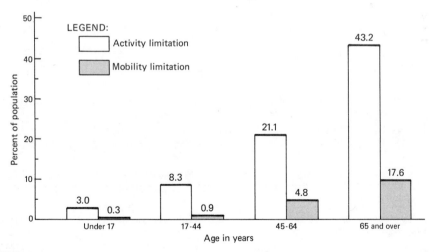

FIGURE 4-11.

Percentage of population with limitation of activity or mobility due to chronic disease.

Source: From the U.S. Department of Health, Education and Welfare, Public Health Service, Health Resources Administration, National Center for Health Statistics, National Health Survey Series 10, Number 96. Limitation of activity and mobility due to chronic conditions. United States, 1972.

medicine. Small groups of family physicians are the most flexible of physician groups and can locate anywhere from the rural community to the metropolitan area. Working in small groups, family physicians can be available 24 hours a day. In addition to serving as a ready source of entry into our health care system, they can provide "one-stop medical care" for about 95 percent of their patients' reasons for physicians' visits. Family physicians can provide this service at a reasonable cost and offer more personal, comprehensive, and better coordinated health care than other approaches. As many of the existing barriers to health care are reduced in coming years, the need and demand for the family physician can be expected to increase sharply.

REFERENCES

1. Mechanic D: The problem of access to medical care. In Lewis CE, Fein R, Mechanic D (eds): A Right to Health Care: The Problem of Access to Primary Medical Care. New York, Wiley, 1976, p 7
2. White K, Williams F, Greenberg B: The ecology of medical care. N Engl J Med 265:885, 1961
3. Mechanic D: The problem of access to medical care. In Lewis CE, Fein R, Mechanic D (eds): A Right to Health Care: The Problem of Access to Primary Health Care. New York, Wiley, 1976, p 7
4. McNerney WJ: Changing the health care system. Am J Nurs 69:2428, 1969
5. Mueller MS, Piro PA: Private health insurance in 1973: A review of coverage, enrollment and financial experience. Social Security Bull 39:4, 1976
6. America's Health System: A Portrait. Special Report. The Robert Wood Johnson Foundation, No. 1, 1978, p 8
7. Bergner L, Yerby AS: Low income and barriers to use of health services. N Engl J Med 278:541, 1968
8. Morris JN: Uses of Epidemiology. Edinburgh, Livingstone, 1957
9. Titmuss RM: Role of redistribution in social policy. Social Security Bull 28:14, June 1965
10. Bergner L, Yerby AS: Low income and barriers to the use of health services. N Engl J Med 278:543, 1968
11. U.S. National Center for Health Statistics. Infant Mortality Rates: Socioeconomic Factors, United States. Series 22, No. 14, DHEW Publication No. (HSM) 72–1045, 1972
12. U.S. National Center for Health Statistics. Physician Visits—Volume and Interval Since Last Visit: U.S.—1971. Series 10, No. 97. Rockville, Maryland, Public Health Service, 1975, p 31
13. Aday L: Economic and non-economic barriers to the use of needed medical services. Med Care p 13, June 1975
14. Koos EL: Data on the Recognition of Symptoms. In The Health of Regionville. New York, Columbia University Press, 1954
15. Koos EL: Data on the Recognition of Symptoms. In The Health of Regionville. New York, Columbia University Press, 1954, pp 33 and 119
16. Knouss RF: Health manpower—the right kind. In Health Manpower Issues. DHEW Publication No. (HRA) 76–40, 1976, p 17

17. Somers AR, Somers HM: Health and Health Care: Policies in Perspective. Germantown, Pennsylvania, Aspen Systems, 1976, p 236
18. Statistical Abstract of the United States. no. 534, p 339. Washington, D.C., U.S. Department of Commerce, Bureau of the Census, 1971
19. Mechanic D: Relationships between medical need and responsiveness of care. In Lewis CE, Fein R, Mechanic D (eds): A Right to Health: The Problem of Access to Primary Medical Care. New York, Wiley, 1976, p 17
20. Socio-Economic Report. San Francisco, Bureau of Research and Planning, Calif Med Assoc, Vol 8, No 12, November 1968
21. Notes from Airlie House Conferences held by Regional Medical Programs in Warrenton, Virginia, September 1969
22. English JT: The dimensions of poverty. Am J Nurs 69:2426, 1969
23. McWhinney IR: Beyond diagnosis—an approach to the integration of behavioral science and clinical medicine. N Engl J Med 287:384, 1972
24. America's Health System: A Portrait. Special Report. The Robert Wood Johnson Foundation, No. 1, 1978, p 7
25. English JT: The dimensions of poverty. Am J Nurs 69:2424, 1969
26. Kessner DM et al: Infant Death: An Analysis by Maternal Risk and Health Care. Washington, D.C., Institute of Medicine, National Academy of Sciences, 1973, p 23
27. Weiss JE, Greenlick MR, Jones JF: Determinants of medical care utilization: The impact of spatial factors. Inquiry 8:50–57, 1971
28. English JT: The dimensions of poverty. Am J Nurs 69:2428, 1969
29. California Medical Association Committee on the Role of Medicine in Society: Fifth progress report—The concept of mainstream medicine for all Californians. Calif Med 112:68, February 1970
30. Geiger HJ: The endlessly revolving door. Am J Nurs 69:2436, 1969
31. Davis K: Financing medical care: Implications for access to primary care. Paper presented at the Sun Valley Forum on National Health, Sun Valley, Idaho, June 28, 1973
32. English JT: The dimensions of poverty. Am J Nurs 69:2426, 1969
33. Brotman H: Facts and Figures on Older Americans. State Trends 1950–1971. Administration on Aging HE 1.209:6. Washington, D.C., Superintendent of Documents, 1971
34. National Center for Health Statistics. National Health Survey. Limitation of activity and mobility due to chronic conditions, United States—1972. DHEW Publication (HRA) Series 10, No. 96, 1972
35. Somers AR, Somers HM: Health and Health Care: Policies in Perspective. Germantown, Aspen Systems, 1977, p 434
36. Sparks RD: Our concern for rural health. In Proceedings of the 30th National Conference on Rural Health, Seattle, Washington, AMA, 1977, p 77
37. Schoen C: Financing rural health care. In Proceedings of the 30th National Conference on Rural Health, Seattle, Washington, AMA, 1977, p 29
38. Shortell SM: Factors associated with the utilization of health services. In Torres P, Williams S (eds): New York, Wiley, 1979
39. Schoen C: Financing rural health care. In Proceedings of the 30th National Conference on Rural Health, Seattle, Washington, AMA, 1977, p 28
40. Mechanic D: The problem of access to medical care. In Lewis CE, Fein R, Mechanic D (eds): A Right to Health Care: The Problem of Access to Primary Care. New York, Wiley, 1976, p 11

CHAPTER FIVE

Perspectives in Primary Care

It is ironic that widespread criticism of the medical profession and medical care institutions should develop precisely at the time when such care is technically better and more accessible than ever before. Indeed it is precisely the knowledge of the high quality and partial availability of superb medical care that causes the patient so often to feel let down, frustrated, dehumanized—in short, abandoned.

The patient's plea for personalized care is heard in many accents and with varying degrees of sophistication. His complaint is probably the most widely expressed criticism of medical care today, more urgent in the minds of many than even the rising costs of care. When the two are linked together in personal experience—high costs of ineffective impersonal care—the result is often a bitterness that bodes ill for patients and providers alike.

Anne R. Somers[1]

The last three chapters have traced various aspects of the reemphasis of primary care within American medicine in recent years. This has come at a time when the expectations and demand for health services have increased exponentially. With the emergence of Medicare, Medicaid, and increased levels of coverage by private health insurance programs, for example, the number of outpatient visits doubled between 1962 and 1970 in the United States, and increased by another 38 percent between 1970 and 1974. During this latter period, the utilization of hospitals' emergency rooms increased by 50 percent, partly as a symptom of the deficit of primary-care physicians.[2]

As the interest in primary care has grown at various levels both within and outside of medicine, so has confusion been generated on a number of basic issues related to its definition, content, and process. The purpose of this chapter is threefold: (1) to outline various definitions of primary care, (2) to describe briefly the basic elements of primary care, and (3) to discuss several current issues with respect to primary care in this country.

DEFINITIONS OF PRIMARY CARE

One of the most debated of terms in recent years is the term *primary care* itself. There has been a tendency by many disciplines and groups to claim major investments in primary care from their various perspectives, and the issues become cloudy in short order unless some basic definitions are established. We have seen a number of definitions proposed, and it is now possible to clarify the fundamental issues. The following definition suggested by Alpert draws from the contributions of many [3-7] and represents a general consensus within medicine.[8]

> Primary care can be defined as being within the personal rather than the public health system, and is therefore focused on the health needs of individuals and families—it is family-oriented. Primary care is "first-contact" care, and thus should be separated from secondary care and tertiary care, which are based on referral rather than initial contact.
>
> Primary care assumes longitudinal responsibility for the patient regardless of the presence or absence of disease. The primary care physician holds the contract for providing personal health services over a period of time. Specifically, primary care is neither limited to the course of a single episode of illness nor confined to the ambulatory setting. It serves as the "integrationist" for the patient. When other health resources are involved, the primary care physician retains the coordinating role. He or she cares for as many of the patient's problems as possible, and, where referral is indicated, fulfills his longitudinal responsibility as the integrationist.

Figures 5-1 and 5-2 illustrate conceptual views of primary care based upon the frequency, character of onset, duration, complexity, and diversity of conditions, and the requisite ties to the community.[9]

Although much of primary care takes place in ambulatory settings, primary care is not synonymous with ambulatory care. For example, many hospitalized patients will remain under the continuing primary care of the primary-care physician, while many ambulatory patients may be receiving secondary-care services (e.g., radiation therapy). Primary care is defined by the American

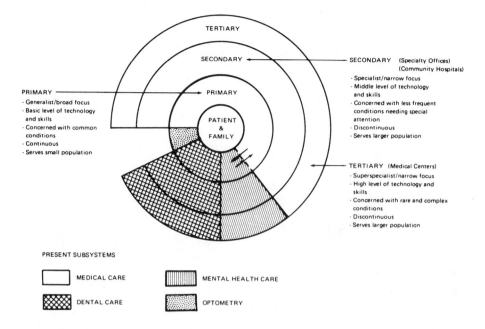

PRIMARY
- Generalist/broad focus
- Basic level of technology and skills
- Concerned with common conditions
- Continuous
- Serves small population

SECONDARY (Specialty Offices) (Community Hospitals)
- Specialist/narrow focus
- Middle level of technology and skills
- Concerned with less frequent conditions needing special attention
- Discontinuous
- Serves larger population

TERTIARY (Medical Centers)
- Superspecialist/narrow focus
- High level of technology and skills
- Concerned with rare and complex conditions
- Discontinuous
- Serves larger population

PRESENT SUBSYSTEMS

MEDICAL CARE
MENTAL HEALTH CARE
DENTAL CARE
OPTOMETRY

FIGURE 5-1.

Personal health care system levels of care.

Source: Parker AW: The dimensions of primary care: Blueprints for change. Andreopoulous S (ed.): *Primary Care: Where Medicine Fails*. New York, John Wiley and Sons, 1974, p. 19.

Academy of Family Physicians (AAFP) and the American Board of Family Practice (ABFP) as:

. . . a form of medical care delivery which emphasizes first contact care and assumes ongoing responsibility for the patient in both health maintenance and therapy of illness. It is personal care involving a unique interaction and communication between the patient and the physician. It is comprehensive in scope, and includes the overall coordination of the care of the patient's health problems, be they biological, behavioral or social. The appropriate use of consultants and community resources is an important part of effective primary care.

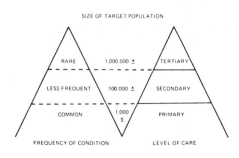

FIGURE 5-2.

Frequency of condition and size of target population as related to level of care.

Source: Parker AW: The dimensions of primary care: Blueprints for change. Andreopoulos S (ed.): In *Primary Care: Where Medicine Fails*, New York, John Wiley and Sons, 1974, p. 20.

A further description of the functions of primary care is added by the ABFP:

1. It is "first-contact" care serving as point-of-entry for the patient into the health-care system;
2. It includes continuity by virtue of caring for patients over a period of time in both sickness and in health;
3. It is comprehensive care, drawing from all the traditional major disciplines for its functional content;
4. It serves a coordinative function for all the health-care needs of the patient;
5. It assumes continuing responsibility for individual patient follow-up and community health problems; and
6. It is a highly personalized type of care.

ELEMENTS OF PRIMARY CARE

The above definitions are broad and leave room for various interpretations of the precise nature of primary care. In an attempt to introduce greater specificity to the definition of primary care, the Institute of Medicine has developed a checklist for primary care (Table 5-1), which categorizes desirable indicators of good primary care under its five major elements: (1) accessibility, (2) comprehensiveness, (3) coordination, (4) continuity, and (5) accountability.[10]

TABLE 5-1. CHECKLIST FOR PRIMARY CARE

A. Are services accessible?
   1. Are services available to patients?
     *a. Is access to primary care services provided 24 hours a day, seven days a week?
     *b. Is there an opportunity for a patient to schedule an appointment?
     c. Are scheduled office hours compatible with the work and way of life of most of the patients?
     d. Can most (90 percent) medically urgent cases be seen within one hour?
     e. Can most patients (90 percent) with acute but not urgent problems be seen within one day?
     f. Can most (90 percent) appropriate requests for routine appointments, such as preventive exams, be met within one week?
   2. Are services convenient to patients?
     a. Is the practice unit conveniently located, so that most patients can reach it by public or private transportation?
     b. Is the practice unit so designed that handicapped or elderly patients are not inconvenienced?
     c. Does the practice unit accept patients who have a means of payment, regardless of source (Medicare, Medicaid)?
   3. Are services acceptable to patients?
     *a. Is the waiting time for most (90 percent) of the scheduled appointments less than one-half hour?

---

* Essential to provision of primary care.

TABLE 5-1. CHECKLIST FOR PRIMARY CARE (cont.)

*b. If a substantial minority (25 percent) of patients has a special language or other communication barrier, does the office staff include people who can deal with this problem?

c. Are waiting accommodations comfortable and uncrowded?

d. Does the practice staff consistently demonstrate an interest in and appreciation of the culture, background, socioeconomic status, work environment, and living circumstances of patients?

e. Is simple, understandable information provided to patients about fees, billing procedures, scheduling of appointments, contacting the unit after hours, and grievance procedures?

f. Are patients encouraged to ask questions about their illness and their care, to discuss their health problems freely, and to review their records, if desired?

g. Does the practice unit accept patients without regard to race, religion, or ethnic origin?

B. Are services comprehensive?

*1. Within the patient population served, and realizing that this might be restricted to a certain age (pediatrics) or sex (obstetrics–gynecology), is the practice unit willing to handle, without referral, the great majority (over 90 percent) of the problems arising in this population (for example, general complaints such as fever or fatigue, minor trauma, sore throat, cough, and chest pain)?

*2. Are appropriate primary and secondary preventive measures used for those people at risk (for example, immunizations for tetanus, polio; early detection of hypertension; control of risk factors for coronary disease)?

*3. Are the practitioners in the unit willing, if appropriate, to admit and care for patients in hospitals?

*4. Are the practitioners in the unit willing to admit and care for patients in nursing homes or convalescent homes?

*5. Are the practitioners in the unit willing, if appropriate, to visit the patient at home?

*6. Are patients encouraged and assisted in providing for their own care and participating as allies in their own health care plan (for example, through instruction in nutrition, diet, exercise, accident prevention, family planning, and adolescent problems)?

7. Do the practitioners in the unit provide support to those agencies and organizations promoting community health (for example, health education programs for the public, disease detection programs, school health and sports medicine programs, emergency care training)?

C. Are services coordinated?

*1. Do the practitioners in the unit furnish pertinent information to other providers serving the patient, actively seek relevant feedback from consultants and other providers, and serve as the patient's ombudsmen in contacts with other providers?

*2. Is a summary or abstract of the patient's record provided to other physicians when needed?

*3. Do the practitioners in the unit develop a treatment plan with the patient that reflects consideration of the patient's understanding? Do the practitioners use a variety of tactics to ensure that the patient will cooperate in the treatment? Does the plan of treatment reflect the patient's physical, emotional, and financial ability to carry it out?

4. Is another source of care recommended when a patient moves to another geographic area?

D. Are services continuous?

*1. Can a patient who so desires make subsequent appointments with the same provider?

(cont.)

TABLE 5-1. CHECKLIST FOR PRIMARY CARE (cont.)

    *2. Are complete records maintained in a form easily retrievable and accessible?

    *3. Are relevant items or problems in the patient's record highlighted, regularly reviewed, and used in planning care?

    4. Is each patient reminded of his or her next appointment?

E. Is the unit accountable?

    *1. Do the practitioners in the unit assume responsibility for alerting proper authorities if a patient problem reveals a health hazard that may affect others in the community (for example, discovery of exposure to toxic chemicals in an industrial plant, discovery of a communicable disease)?

    2. Is there a patient–disease and age–sex registry maintained that can provide the basis of a practice audit?

    3. Is there a system for regular review of the quality of the *process* of medical care (for example, reviews for completeness of therapeutic programs and follow-up of acute illnesses)?

    4. Is there a system for regular assessment of the outcomes of the care offered (for example, review of outcome of treatment of specific illnesses, review of level of satisfaction of patients with the services provided, review of compliance with recommendations)?

    5. Is there evidence that the unit regularly assesses the capability of the staff and provides opportunity for continuing education?

    6. Are patients appropriately informed about the nature of their condition, the benefits and risks of available treatments, and the expected outcomes? Are they provided the opportunity to ask questions and discuss their medical record?

    7. If unexpected or undesired outcomes occur, are they made known and adequately explained to patients, and is a method established for responding to any expressed dissatisfaction (such as conferences, counseling, arbitration, adjustment of billing, or referral)?

    8. Does the provider maintain financial accountability by keeping accurate records and by having adequate professional liability coverage?

Source: Institute of Medicine: *Primary Care in Medicine.* Washington, D.C., National Academy of Sciences, 1977, p. 8. Reprinted with permission of the National Academy of Sciences.

Accessibility

Ready access to primary care is obviously essential to the first-contact and continuity dimensions of primary care. As noted in the preceding chapter, adequate accessibility includes geographic and around-the-clock availability, as well as reduction of the various barriers to primary care. Thus, concern for the patient and sensitivity to the sociocultural dimensions of illness comprise necessary attributes of availability.

Comprehensiveness

Comprehensiveness relates to the ability, interest, and willingness of the primary-care provider to definitively manage the large majority of health problems occuring in the population served. This is the feature of primary care that most effectively helps to classify health-care services as primary care

Source: The National Ambulatory Medical Care Survey: unpublished data, Rockville, Maryland, National Center for Health Statistics, DHEW, 1974.

TABLE 5-2. PERCENT DISTRIBUTION OF THE MOST FREQUENTLY OCCURRING DIAGNOSIS FOR FOUR SPECIALTIES IN 1974

DIAGNOSIS	PERCENT DISTRIBUTION				Total of Columns 1-4
	General and Family Practice	Internal Medicine	Pediatrics	Obstetrics/ Gynecology	
Medical or special examination	6.7	3.7	29.8	11.5	9.6
Prenatal care	2.6			30.9	5.2
Essential benign hypertension	5.3	9.7			4.8
Acute upper respiratory infection	5.3	1.8	7.3		4.4
Medical and surgical aftercare	2.8	1.4	2.6	5.8	2.9
Chronic ischemic heart disease	2.8	8.0			2.9
Acute pharyngitis	2.4	1.1			2.1
Diabetes mellitus	2.2	4.5	4.2		2.1
Observation without need for medication				7.7	2.0
Obesity	2.5	1.8			1.9
Otitis media			8.4		1.7
Acute tonsillitis			3.7		1.5
Neuroses	1.7	2.5			1.5
Bronchitis, unqualified			2.9		1.4
Inoculations and vaccinations			1.9		1.0
Diarrheal diseases			2.1		1.0
Disorders of menstruation				4.3	0.9
Menopausal symptoms				1.2	0.9
Cystitis				0.8	0.8
Osteoarthritis		1.8			0.8
Infective diseases of uterus, vagina, and vulva				2.6	0.6
Postpartum observation				2.6	0.5
Streptococcal sore throat			1.9		0.4
Diseases of parametrium				1.0	0.3
Total percent	34.3	36.3	64.8	68.4	51.2

or nonprimary care. For example, the psychiatrist may provide readily available first-contact and continuity care for some patients with psychologic problems but does not provide a sufficient range of services to be considered a primary-care physician. Even among the several specialties that are more or less involved in primary care, there is considerable variation in comprehensiveness of services. Table 5-2 shows that family practice and internal medicine provide the broadest range of services, with the ten most commonly reported diagnoses representing only approximately one-third of these practices compared to the top ten diagnoses accounting for about two-thirds of the practices in pediatrics and obstetrics–gynecology.[11]

Coordination

The primary care provider coordinates the patient's total care, including that provided by other specialists. The patient's plan of care is individualized to the patient's family and occupational environment, preferences, way of life, and financial circumstances.[10] The primary-care provider serves as the patient's advocate for care by other specialists or community resources and helps to interpret the patient's needs and options. The importance of well-coordinated care has been documented by many studies. One such study, for example,

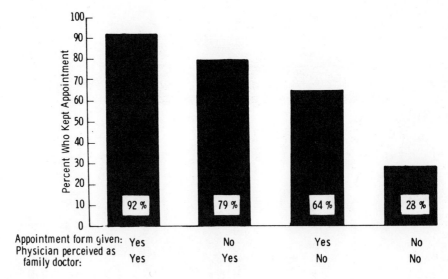

FIGURE 5-3.

Percentage of clinic patients referred to their physicians who kept their appointment, by referral procedure and patient's perception of physician (Chapel Hill, North Carolina, Spring 1967).

Source: Martin DA: The disposition of patients from a consultant general medical clinic: Results of a controlled evaluation of an administrative procedure. *Journal of Chronic Diseases* 17:847, September, 1964. Copyright 1964 by Pergamon Press, Ltd. Reprinted with permission.

showed what one would predict—the greater utilization of laboratory studies and higher cost of care when patients were seen in emergency rooms compared to a comprehensive pediatric care program.[12]

Continuity

Continuity clearly facilitates ongoing personal care with the least fragmentation, and has important implications for acceptability, cost, quality, and even outcome of care. The use of the problem-oriented medical record and well-structured coverage systems within group practice settings allows continuity of care in instances when the individual primary care provider is not available. It has been shown that noncompliance is often a result of disruptions in doctor–patient relationships.[13] It has also been shown that continuity of care is facilitated when patients have a family physician (Figure 5-3).[14]

Accountability

Accountability is not unique to primary care but is essential to it.[10] Accountability calls for a range of activities as shown in Table 5-1. It also requires that the primary-care provider assume moral and legal responsibility for the ongoing care of the patient.

SOME ISSUES IN PRIMARY CARE

As pointed out earlier, the greatly expanded interest in primary care within medicine and in other segments of society during the last decade has raised a number of fundamental issues within primary-care education and practice. Four of the more important issues will be discussed briefly here in an effort to round out a more complete picture of recent developments in primary care.

Who Provides Primary Care?

This question has been somewhat controversial during the past few years, as many disciplines have claimed major interests in primary care. Cynics have been quick to suggest a correlation between these newly discovered interests with changing priorities for federal and state funding toward primary care.

The Millis Commission [4] in 1966 defined the primary care physician as one who

> . . . should usually be primary in the first contact sense. He will serve as the primary medical resource and counselor to an individual or a family. When a patient needs hospitalization, the service of other medical specialists, or other medical or paramedical assistance, the primary physician will see that the necessary arrangements are made, giving such responsibility to others as is appropriate and retaining his own continuing and comprehensive responsibility.

Few hospitals and few existing specialists consider comprehensive and continuing medical care to be their responsibility and within their range of competence.

The definitions of primary care presented earlier, together with the range of indicator activities listed in Table 5-1, demonstrate the wide range of concern and function subsumed by the primary care physician. There is broad agreement that the general/family physician, general internist, and general pediatrician indeed act as primary-care physicians, and those are the only primary-care specialties recognized by the Bureau of Health Manpower for funding purposes. There is considerable controversy as to whether obstetrics–gynecology should be considered a primary-care specialty. Although this specialty is viewed as a primary-care field by the American Medical Association, the relative lack of comprehensiveness of services, combined with a predominantly surgical orientation of the specialty greatly weaken this argument,[15,16] and the field is not considered primary care by the Bureau of Health Manpower. Claims by other specialties for major involvement in primary care clearly fall far short of the mark. Some fields may be heavily involved in first-contact care of limited scope (e.g., dermatology, emergency medicine, and psychiatry) but lack the breadth and continuity required in primary care.

It must be recognized that a number of specialties may devote some proportion of their efforts to incomplete and desultory primary care. In 1975, for example, a survey of physicians by *Medical Economics* showed that 60 percent of physicians surveyed in ten specialties provided some primary care, usually for economic reasons.[17] As Beck and his colleagues[18] point out, however, "although these specialists may be meeting some primary care needs, this informal system of primary care does not provide the patient with either the most appropriate or effective care."

The central role played by general/family physicians in primary care in the United States is well demonstrated by the comparative proportions of office visits to the various specialties as shown in Figure 5-4 and Table 5-3.[19,20]

FIGURE 5-4.
Percentage of office visits to physicians of all specialties— United States, January 1974 through December 1974 (U.S. Department of Health, Education and Welfare).
Source: National Center for Health Statistics, *Monthly Vital Statistics Report* 25:2, 1976.

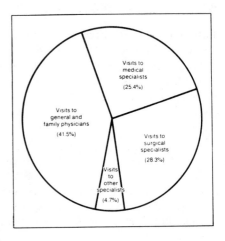

TABLE 5–3. NUMBER AND PERCENT DISTRIBUTIONS OF OFFICE VISITS BY SELECTED PHYSICIAN CHARACTERISTICS—UNITED STATES, JANUARY–DECEMBER 1975

SELECTED PHYSICIAN CHARACTERISTICS	NUMBER OF VISITS (IN THOUSANDS)	PERCENT OF VISITS
All visits	567,600	100.0
Most visited specialties		
General and family practice	234,660	41.3
Internal medicine	62,117	10.9
Obstetrics and gynecology	48,076	8.5
Pediatrics	46,684	8.2
General surgery	41,292	7.3
Ophthalmology	24,667	4.4
Orthopedic surgery	19,316	3.4
Otolaryngology	16,355	2.9
Psychiatry	14,806	2.6
Dermatology	14,094	2.5
Urology	10,832	1.9
Cardiovascular diseases	7,556	1.3
Neurology	2,032	0.4
All other specialties	25,113	4.4
Type of practice		
Solo	339,554	59.8
Other*	228,046	40.2
Location†		
Metropolitan	413,685	72.9
Nonmetropolitan	153,915	27.1

*Includes partnership and group practices.
†Signifies location within or outside the standard metropolitan statistical areas (SMSAs).
Source: Advance Data from Vital and Health Statistics of the National Center for Health Statistics, DHEW (HRA) 12, 6, 1977.

How Comprehensive Is Primary Care?

We have seen that comprehensiveness of care is an essential part of primary care, and we have seen some attempts to define this comprehensiveness, such as by the James' stages outlined in an earlier chapter. While there may be widespread support for this concept today, this support starts to break down into controversy when the real content and scope of comprehensive care are viewed in practical terms.

One basic issue involves the distinction between *medical care* and *health care*. In his excellent book *Ferment in Medicine*, Magraw [21] suggested that "From the standpoint of the doctor's role in society as constituted now and in the future, however, the prevention of disease must be regarded as an extension of his primary function, the care of the sick." But most definitions of comprehensive health care tend to raise more questions than they resolve. The major points of most definitions are reflected in that of Lee,[22] who views comprehensive medicine as:

... the mobilization of all appropriate resources for the care of the patient. It implies a primary concern for the patient (rather than the disease) and a consideration of all significant factors that affect his health. It implies the application of preventive measures to individuals and the employment of all practical means for the early detection of disease.

From the above, comprehensive health care still seems somewhat intangible in practical terms. But it certainly involves expansion of medicine's scope beyond care of the sick to care of the presumably well. Whereas most of our current clinical efforts involve the management of symptomatic disease and are classified as *medical care,* the concept of *health care* is enlarged to also include health education and preventive, rehabilitative, and restorative services.

Many difficult practical questions arise that complicate implementation of comprehensive care. For example, we must ask ourselves: Does our health care system have the capability to render comprehensive medicine to all? Can comprehensive care be afforded (by the patient and his family, private insurance carriers, and government health programs)? What specific programs of preventive medicine are essential? Does the "cost-benefit" justify heavy emphasis on stage I and stage II medicine? How, and by whom, can comprehensive care best be rendered? These questions, and others, are difficult or impossible to answer at this time but must be kept in mind by the medical profession and health planners as future systems of medical practice are developed.

Health maintenance, for example, has already become accepted in many quarters as an unassailable advance in modern medicine, but the research base in this important area is still adequate. Felcher calls for identification of "criteria by which selection of the scope of testing can be made on an individual rather than a mass basis." [23] Sackett has urged that randomized clinical trials of screening and other diagnostic procedures be rapidly expanded to ascertain and document their validity. [24]

We are on more solid ground in looking at the comprehensiveness of what are generally accepted as "medical services." Table 5-4 compares the range of services provided by four specialties in group and nongroup practice with respect to several selected common problems. [25] The comprehensiveness of general/family physicians is demonstrated in these data, as are the relative gaps in comprehensiveness by primary care physicians limiting their practice by age or sex.

Another important dimension of comprehensiveness is by setting (i.e., ambulatory and hospital). Some have suggested that the future primary care physician restrict his/her practice to ambulatory care. [26,27] There are persuasive arguments, however, on the other side of this question. Alpert [8] has this to say on the subject:

> Some would suggest that primary care ought to end when the patient is hospitalized, and that ambulatory care could then be said to equal primary care. Many medical problems that require secondary services are largely treated on an ambulatory basis, however, with only occasional hospitalization. Conversely, the decision to hospitalize

TABLE 5–4.   COMPARATIVE RANGE OF SERVICES AMONG PRIMARY CARE PHYSICIANS IN THE UNITED STATES

PERCENTAGE OF PHYSICIANS OFFERING SERVICE

SERVICE	General Practitioners		Internists		Pediatricians		Obstetricians	
	Nongroup N = 599	Group N = 111	Nongroup N = 231	Group N = 91	Nongroup N = 136	Group N = 43	Nongroup N = 150	Group N = 58
Tape (strap) sprains	86	88	56	42	78	71	16	12
Excise simple cysts	94	90	20	11	28	19	87	93
Suture lacerations	98	95	37	31	85	80	62	65
Do proctoscopic or sigmoidoscopic exam	83	86	89	91	40	39	43	33
Do uncomplicated obstetrics	59	58	—	—	3	—	97	100
Do well-baby care	91	83	7	1	97	100	14	11
Set simple fractures	80	77	6	3	50	32	5	2

Source: Mechanic D: General medical practice: Some comparisons between the work of primary care physicians in the United States and England and Wales. *Medical Care* 10:5, 410, 1972.

a patient may sometimes be based on psychosocial factors in management rather than medical complexity. There is, in addition, strong support for the view that the physician who practices ambulatory and hospital medicine is a better physician than the one who practices only ambulatory medicine. For these reasons, the site of care alone, whether hospital, home, or office, is an insufficient base for a definition of primary care.

In my judgment, the sharp separation of medical careers into community-oriented ambulatory care and hospital-based intensive care of acutely ill patients would involve serious problems both for medical practice and medical education. The creation of a system with built-in discontinuity between ambulatory and hospital patient care could be expected to jeopardize the quality of care, increase its cost, decrease patient compliance, and further depersonalize care. Although it is theoretically possible that the ambulatory-care physician could transmit all necessary medical information to the hospital-based physician regarding each hospitalized patient, it would not be likely to happen in everyday practice. It is more probable that hospital care would be further overutilized, significant medical problems would be overlooked, unnecessary studies and procedures performed, and the patient further confused by relating to an unknown physician at a time of major personal crisis. Although research on the impact of continuity of care is still embryonic, studies have already been reported that indicate that cost of medical care, as well as patient satisfaction and compliance, are adversely affected by lack of physician continuity.[12,28,29]

How Should Primary Care Be Organized?

Private physicians have been and continue to be the foundation on which primary care rests. In 1969, for example, visits to office-based primary-care physicians in private practice constituted about 80 percent of all nonfederal, nonhospital primary-care visits.[30]

Recent years have seen continued attempts by some hospitals to provide primary care through outpatient clinics, as well as the development of newer approaches, such as health maintenance organizations (HMOs) and neighborhood health centers. Federally funded initiatives to establish neighborhood health centers and family health centers in underserved areas, however, have frequently been plagued with problems in physician recruitment and retention, as well as high costs and overhead that have jeopardized their continued economic viability.

Brief discussion of some of the major alternative organizational approaches to the delivery of primary care services illustrates some of the issues involved. Although there are other possible approaches, five basic approaches will be considered here.

SOLO PRACTICE
While this approach offers the primary-care physician maximal autonomy and freedom to practice according to his/her individual style, it presents problems

of coverage, comparative isolation from colleagues, and difficulty in acquiring the equipment, staff, and resources that facilitate optimal primary care. Although coverage problems can often be resolved effectively through call-sharing associations of solo physicians, solo practice is not as attractive to today's young physicians as it was in the past. Among 1977 graduates of family practice residency programs, for example, only 16 percent opted for solo practice, whereas 71 percent opted for partnership or group practice.*

SINGLE-SPECIALTY GROUP PRACTICE
Single-specialty groups of family physicians, internists, or pediatricians have been, and should continue to be, an important and effective approach to providing primary care to families, adults, or children, respectively. Such groups usually include three to five physicians and trade off some of the autonomy of solo practice for a number of advantages of group practice. These advantages include an effective on-call schedule, affording time off for continuing education and vacations, the capability to support the needed resources (physical facilities, equipment, personnel, and methods) for a comprehensive range of primary care services, and the ongoing stimulation of everyday interaction with colleagues through informal consultation and periodic audit of patient care problems.

MULTISPECIALTY GROUP PRACTICE
Most multispecialty groups that are organized for the purpose of primary care inevitably involve much larger groups of physicians. For example, five or more internists are usually found in such groups, as well as four or more pediatricians, several obstetrician–gynecologists, and several surgeons. This is unavoidable, since each specialty is neither qualified nor willing to see patients for problems outside of that specialty or to cover for colleagues in another specialty during nights and weekends. These groups tend to become quite large, since the natural tendency is to add some medical and surgical subspecialists to the group. Although multispecialty groups can provide excellent medical care, they are inherently less effective in their delivery of primary care than are single-specialty primary-care group practices. An individual patient's and family's care is usually fragmented among several physicians. Multispecialty groups are often better suited to referral practice than primary care.

A possible variant of multispecialty groups oriented to primary care is the family practice group including one or more specialists in other fields, such as an internist, pediatrician, obstetrician–gynecologist, and/or general surgeon. Such groups have the advantage of extending the range of services available within the group but may present coverage problems that may or may not be soluble within the group itself.

* Data compiled by Division of Education, American Academy of Family Physicians, Kansas City, Missouri. These data are based on a 68 percent response rate from a survey of 1977 graduates. These results are quite similar to those surveys of 1975 and 1976 residency graduates.

HEALTH MAINTENANCE ORGANIZATIONS (HMOS)

Large prepaid group practices (HMOs) represent a relatively new development in the delivery of health services with considerable potential for effective organization of a broad range of health-care services, particularly in metropolitan areas. A large health maintenance organization with a long experience is represented by the Kaiser system on the West Coast, which utilizes a combination of family physicians, internists, and pediatricians for primary care. A somewhat smaller and extremely effective health maintenance organization developed during the last 25 years in the Pacific Northwest is the Group Health Cooperative of Puget Sound, which bases primary care more solidly on the family physician (goal of 45 percent of the group's physicians in family practice). Health maintenance organizations represent well planned, institutional approaches to providing integrated health care, particularly at primary- and secondary-care levels, with considerable potential for efficiency and cost containment.

HOSPITAL-SPONSORED PRIMARY-CARE GROUP PRACTICE

A recent initiative sponsored by the Robert Wood Johnson Foundation involves the development and evaluation of primary care group practices sponsored by community hospitals. A five-year demonstration project is currently in process throughout the country to determine how and whether hospitals can serve to support satellite primary care groups as part of larger systems of community-based medical practice. It is still too early to assess the potential and problems of this effort, but this initiative represents another dimension of varied approaches being taken to meet the nation's deficits in primary care.

What is the Role of Middle-Level Practitioners in Primary Care?

The last ten years have seen a proliferation of educational programs designed to train "middle-level practitioners" to participate in the delivery of primary care as assistants to the primary care physician. These health professionals, including physicians' assistants and Medex and nurse practitioners, have been viewed by the medical profession as "physician extenders" working under the direct supervision of physicians in order to extend the range and quality of services provided. Considerable emphasis has been placed on the concept of "team practice," and many positive experiences with this approach have been reported across the country. The American Medical Association defines these health professionals as follows[31]:

> The assistant to the primary care physician is a person qualified by academic and clinical training to provide patient care services under the supervision of a licensed physician in a wide variety of medical care settings which are involved in the delivery of primary care. The functions of a primary care physician are interdisciplinary in nature involving medicine, pediatrics, obstetrics, and psychiatry. . . .

The assistant, therefore, is involved in helping the primary care physician provide a variety of personal health services, including but not limited to:

- receiving patients, obtaining case histories, performing an appropriate physical examination, and presenting meaningful resulting data to the physician;
- performing or assisting in laboratory procedures and related studies in the practice setting;
- giving injections and immunizations;
- suturing and caring for wounds;
- providing patient counseling services; referring patients to other health care resources;
- responding to emergency situations which might arise in the physician's absence within the assistant's range of skills and experience; and
- assisting the employing physician in all settings such as the office, hospitals, extended care facilities, nursing homes, and the patient's home.

The ultimate role of the assistant and his functions vary with his individual capabilities and the specific needs of the employing physician, the practice setting in which he works, and the community in which he lives.

Many of the initial issues involved in the delivery of primary care by teams of primary care physicians and these middle-level practitioners have been effectively resolved. A recent national study of 939 physician assistants, for example, demonstrated substantial levels of responsibility in patient care with a wide range of clinical activities, and high levels of physician acceptance of their role.[32] Over 40 percent of these physician assistants were working with general/family physicians. The major potential problem shown by this study with regard to the long-term future role of physician assistants was a common perception of inadequate opportunities for career advancement—one-fifth of the respondents hoped to enter medical school, while another one-fifth had plans to obtain either a master's or a Ph.D. degree.[32]

A more recent issue raised by organized nursing is that of independent practice. The nurse practitioner is not viewed by nursing as a physician extender but as a primary care provider capable of independent practice in a "joint" relationship with the physician. A National Joint Practice Commission was established several years ago, and recently adopted a definition and guidelines for joint practice in primary care. This group views joint practice in these terms[33]:

Neither the nurse nor the physician *alone* is prepared to address adequately the broad range of health, medical and nursing concerns of patients encountered in a primary care setting: each professional has a clear identity, each is licensed in his and her own right, and each is in command of a separate body of knowledge, although there is a shared scientific base of preparation and considerable overlap in many functions. Thus, each professional brings a different approach and additional information and expertise to the setting that the other professional recognizes, values and is unable to provide alone.

There is considerable confusion and controversy today concerning the distinction between expanded "nursing practice" and "medical practice." [34-37] Levinson [36] views the development of markedly expanded clinical roles of nonphysician practitioners as raising "fundamental questions of education, certification, responsibility, organization and remuneration, not only for the new clinicians, but for all practitioners, and for the health-care system. . . . Independent practice is a contemporary, not a future issue. The practice acts of many states are so vague about supervision as to be an endorsement of independent practice. The issue is pivotal and should not be decided without serious debate based on extended evaluation studies."

Despite these issues, much progress has been made during recent years in the delivery of primary care by primary care physicians working with middle-level practitioners. Independent practice by nonphysicians involving medical care is generally not legal without the supervision of physicians. It is both likely and desirable that the future evolution of team practice involving middle-level practitioners will take place under the overall supervision and responsibility of the primary care physician.

COMMENT

Major advances have been made in primary care in the United States during the past ten years. Perhaps the most important products of the 1970s in this regard are the following: (1) general awareness of the dimensions of the nation's deficits in primary health care, (2) recognition that primary care is indeed a legitimate area for various forms of specialized medical practices, and (3) awareness that the delivery of primary health care of high quality requires careful organization, broad clinical content, and excellence of teaching for the various forms of graduate medical education being developed in the primary care specialties.

No one primary care discipline can meet the large and diverse needs for primary care in this country. Family practice has much to contribute to primary care through its broad and personal orientation, breadth of clinical competence, comprehensiveness of services, focus on the family, and flexibility. Internal medicine and pediatrics likewise have much to contribute to primary care, particularly if the trend toward increasing subspecialization can be arrested. A recent study of over 600 physicians trained in primary care fields in Massachusetts between 1967 and 1972, however, showed only 28 percent of former residents in internal medicine and 56 percent of those in pediatrics devoting more than half their time to primary care in 1976.[38] Lee reported in 1976 that almost 40 percent of internists completing training since 1972 had been certified as subspecialists.[39]

There can be no single best way of providing all of the primary care that is needed to meet the needs of a large country with varying local and geographic differences. We can expect to see plural approaches to primary care in coming years. Some will stand the test of time, others will not.

This chapter has raised some of the past and current issues in primary care. While continuing discussion and debate on the issues is healthy and needed, great care must be taken by all involved health care professionals to keep the welfare of the patient at the center of focus, not the special interest of any particular group of health professionals. The collective responsibility of the primary care disciplines is to provide readily accessible health care of the highest possible quality to the entire population with the least possible fragmentation at a cost that can be afforded by an increasingly burdened society.

REFERENCES

1. Somers AR: The missing ingredient. Med Opinion Rev 5:8, 27, 1969
2. Physicians for the Future. Report of the Macy Commission. New York, Josiah Macy Jr. Foundation, 1976, p 9
3. White KL: Primary medical care for families. N Engl J Med 277:847, 1967
4. Report of the Citizens Commission on Graduate Medical Education (Millis Commission). Chicago, AMA, 1966
5. Pellegrino ED: Planning for comprehensive and continuing care of patients through education. J Med Educ 43:751, 1968
6. American Academy of Family Physicians: Education for Family Practice. Kansas City, Missouri, AAFP, 1969
7. Magraw R: Medical education and health services—Implication for family medicine. N Engl J Med 285:1407, 1971
8. Alpert JL: New directions in medical education: Primary care. In Purcell EF (ed): Recent Trends in Medical Education. New York, Josiah Macy Jr. Foundation, 1976, p 166
9. Parker AW: The dimensions of primary care: Blueprints for change. In Andreopoulos S (ed): Primary Care: Where Medicine Fails. New York, Wiley, 1973, p 18
10. Institute of Medicine: Primary Care in Medicine: A Definition. Washington, D.C., National Academy of Sciences, 1977, p 8
11. National Ambulatory Care Survey. National Center for Health Statistics. Rockville, Maryland, DHEW, 1974
12. Heagarty MC, Robertson LS, Kosa J, Alpert JL: Some comparative costs in comprehensive versus fragmented pediatric care. Pediatrics 46:4, 596, 1970
13. Francis V, Korsch BM, and Morris MI: Gaps in doctor–patient communication: Patients' response to medical advice. N Engl J Med 280:535, 1969
14. Martin DA: The disposition of patients from a consultant general medical clinic: Results of a controlled evaluation of an administrative procedure. J Chronic Dis 17:847, September 1964
15. Lee PR: Graduate medical education 1976. Will internal medicine meet the challenge? Ann Intern Med 85:2, 251, 1976

16. Beck JC, Lee PR, LeRoy L, Stalcup J: The primary care problem. Clin Res 24:258, 1976

17. Rosenberg CL: How much general practice by specialists? Med Econ p 131. September 15, 1975

18. Beck JC, Lee PR, LeRoy L, Stalcup J: The primary care problem. Clin Res 24:263, 1976

19. National Center for Health Statistics, Monthly Vital Statistics Report 25:2, 1976

20. Advance Data from Vital and Health Statistics of the National Center for Health Statistics, DHEW (HRA) 12, 6, 1977

21. Magraw RM: Ferment in Medicine. Philadelphia, Saunders, 1966, p 61

22. Lee PV: Medical schools and the changing times. J Med Educ 36:72, 1961

23. Felch WC: Does preventive medicine really work? Prism 1(7):26, 1973

24. Bombardier C, McClaran J, Sackett DC: Medical care policy rounds: Periodic health examinations and multiphasic screening. Can Med Assoc J 109:1123, 1973

25. Mechanic D: General medical practice: Some comparisons between the work of primary care physicians in the United States and England and Wales. Med Care 10:410 1972

26. Proger S: A career in ambulatory medicine. N Engl J Med 292:1318, 1975

27. Petersdorf RG: Internal medicine and family practice: Controversies, conflict and compromise. N Engl J Med 293:331, 1975

28. Alpert J, Kosa J, Haggerty R, et al: Attitudes and satisfaction of families receiving comprehensive pediatric care. Am J Public Health 60:499, 1970

29. Becker M, Drachman R, Kirscht I: A field experiment to evaluate various outcomes of continuity of physician care. Am J Public Health 64:1062, 1974

30. Parker AW: The dimensions of primary care: Blueprints for change. In Andreopoulos S (ed): Primary Care: Where Medicine Fails. New York, Wiley, 1973, p 31

31. Educational Programs for the Physician's Assistant. Chicago, AMA. Department of Allied Medical Professions and Services, Summer 1974, p 3

32. Perry HB: Physician assistants: An overview of an emerging health profession. Med Care 15:982, 1970

33. Joint Practice in Primary Care: Definition and Guidelines. Chicago, Illinois, National Joint Practice Commission, July 1977

34. Breslau N: The role of the nurse–practitioner in a pediatric team: Patient definitions. Med Care 15:1014, 1977

35. Schoen EJ, Erickson RJ, Barr G, Allen H: The role of pediatric nurse practitioners as viewed by California pediatricians. West J Med 118:62, 1973

36. Levinson D: Roles, tasks and practitioners. N Engl J Med 296:1291, 1977

37. Geyman JP: Is there a difference between nursing practice and medical practice? J Fam Pract 5:935, 1977

38. Wechsler H, Dorsey JL, Bovey JD: A follow-up study of residents in internal medicine, pediatrics and obstetrics–gynecology training programs in Massachusetts: Implications for primary care physicians. N Engl J Med 298:15, 1978

39. Lee PR: Graduate medical education 1976. Will internal medicine meet the challenge? Ann Intern Med 85:252, 1976

CHAPTER SIX

Department of Family Medicine (R700)
University of Miami School of Medicine
P. O. Box 016700
Miami, Florida 33101

James M. Gall, M. D., C. C. F. P.
Department of Family Medicine
University of Miami School of Medicine
P. O. Box 016700
Miami, Florida 33101

The Changing Health Care System

Access to health care has become part of the American Dream. The right to care and freedom from disease, disability, and discomfort are part of the endowment of every inhabitant of the richest nation of the world. Equal opportunity to health has joined education as the means whereby all men, created equal, may achieve the promise of a better life.

Charles E. Lewis [1]

For years, as medical care expenditures have risen beyond the rate of inflation, there has been no direct relationship between expense and outcome. Longevity has changed little, and the major illnesses such as malignancy and cardiovascular disease remain unimpeded. Heralded preventive measures, such as multiphasic screening and modification of risk factors for cardiovascular disease yield limited benefit. Illnesses disproportionately affect the poor, major environmental and occupational causes of illness receive little attention and less action, and malpractice charges intensify. Clearly, there is a crisis in health care, both in its effect upon health and in its cost.

Halsted R. Holman [2]

A majority of the people in the United States believe that there is a "crisis" in health care in this country. About three-fifths of the population feel that basic changes are needed in the delivery of medical services.[3] According to a recent Harris poll, the proportion of the public having a "great deal of confidence" in medicine declined from 73 percent in 1966 to 42 percent in 1976.[4] In response to these perceptions, major changes are in process and others are being considered for remodeling the health care system.

Some critics of our present methods of medical practice describe our inadequacies in terms of a "nonsystem." Others believe that what system we do have needs rebuilding. There are many who view the private sector as on trial and under intense pressure to develop improved methods of medical practice as soon as possible. Amid this debate, we are seeing various proposals for new systems, particularly through new financing mechanisms, some envisioning a panacea for today's problems.

The last three chapters have examined three dimensions of the health care system—physician manpower, barriers to health care, and primary health care. This chapter will take a macroview of the changing health care system, with three objectives: (1) to describe briefly the magnitude of the expanding health care industry, (2) to outline four major problems of today's health care system, and (3) to present an overview of past and present approaches to these problems.

THE HEALTH CARE INDUSTRY: A GROWING MONOLITH

The health care industry is one of the largest, most diverse, and fastest growing industries in the country. Over four million people were employed by the industry in 1973 in more than 100 discrete occupations representing over 600 different titles. Approximately three-fourths of this total number were in allied health fields.[5]

National health expenditures have nearly doubled during the last 20 years, and now total almost 9 percent of the Gross National Product (GNP) (Figure 6–1).[6] This accelerating rate of growth reflects inflation in medical care costs, technological and other quality changes, population growth, and increased utilization. Recent estimates project that the nation's expenditures for health care will exceed 10 percent of the GNP by 1981.[7] Comparative expenditures for defense, health and education as a proportion of the GNP are illustrated in Figure 6–2.[8]

The changing patterns of national health expenditures between 1950 and 1976 are illustrated in Figure 6–3. While the proportion spent for physicians' services has remained relatively stable at about one-fifth of total expenditures, expenditures for hospital care have shown a marked increase.[9] Figure 6–4 reflects the accelerated increase in hospital room costs compared to all medical care costs, physicians' fees, and the consumer price index between 1958 and 1976.[10]

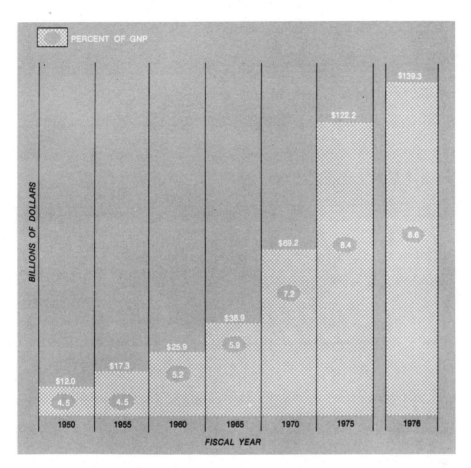

FIGURE 6-1.

National health expenditures as percentage of gross national product,[6] 1950–1976.

Source: *Health 1976–1977. United States Chartbook.* DHEW Publication No. (HRA) 77–1233, 1, 1977.

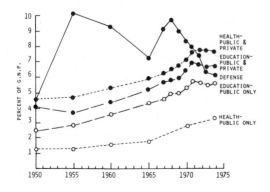

FIGURE 6-2.

Expenditures for defense, health, and education as a percent of gross national product (United States, selected fiscal years, 1950–1974).

Sources: (1) For defense: U.S. Department of Commerce, Bureau of the Census, *Statistical Abstract of the U.S.*, Washington, D.C., U.S. Government Printing Office, 1975, Table 505, p. 314. (2) For Health: Skolnik, AM, and Daces, SR: Social welfare expenditures, fiscal year 1975. *Social Security Bulletin,* Vol. 39, January 1976, Tables 3 and 6, pp. 12 and 15. (3) For Education: Skolnik, AM, and Daces, SR: Social welfare expenditures, fiscal year 1975. *Social Security Bulletin,* Vol. 39, January 1976. Tables 3 and 10, pp. 12 and 19.

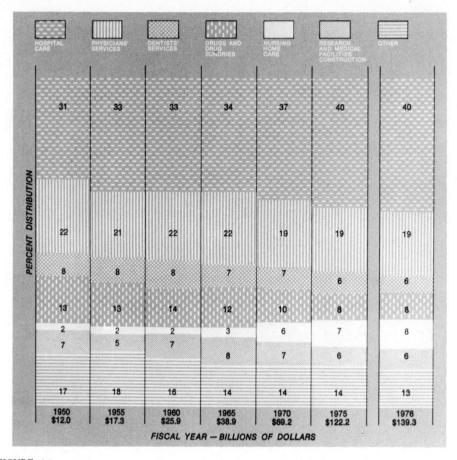

FIGURE 6-3.

Distribution by type of national health expenditures, 1950–1976.

Source: *Health 1976-1977. United States Chartbook. DHEW Publication No. (HRA) 77–1233, 2, 1977.*

Expenditures for personal health care, including hospitalization, physicians' and dentists' services, drugs, and other services and supplies provided to individuals, totaled over 120 billion dollars for fiscal year 1976, representing 86 percent of total health expenditures. Third-party payers, including government and private health insurance, paid for two-thirds of these expenditures. The rapidly increasing role played by third-party payers between 1950 and 1976 in the United States is reflected in Figure 6–5.[11] Figure 6–6 presents a breakdown in the proportion of specific components of private insurance coverage between 1940 and 1973. Although the number of people covered by private health insurance has grown rapidly over this period, it can readily be seen that a large number of people have inadequate coverage for certain kinds of costs, particularly for major medical expenses.[12]

Hospital care represents the largest single part of national health expenditures (about 40 percent of the health care dollar). Although the average length of stay has been reduced in recent years, the numbers of hospital admissions and hospital days per 1000 people per year have continued to rise, as shown in Figure 6–7.[13]

The impressive growth of the health care industry in recent years is not a sign of health, and in fact masks fundamental and severe problems reflecting the paradox of modern medicine in this country. This has been summed up by Somers and Somers in their recent book *Health and Health Care: Policies in Perspective* in the following way [14]:

As America entered the last quarter of the twentieth century, following three decades of unprecedented expansion in medical care services—in volume and technical quality

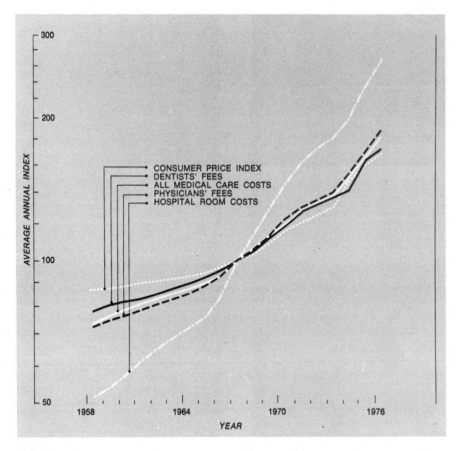

FIGURE 6-4.

Consumer price index and costs of selected components of medical care, 1959–1976.

Source: Health 1976–1977. *United States Chartbook.* DHEW Publication No. (HRA) 77–1233, 6, 1977.

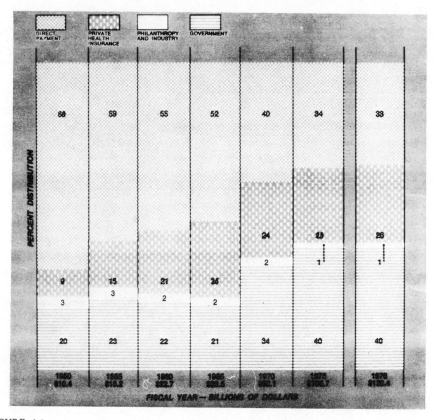

FIGURE 6-5.
Personal health expenditures by source of payment, 1950–1976.
Source: *Health 1976–1977. United States Chartbook.* DHEW Publication No. (HRA) 77–1233, 3, 1977.

of care—many of the premises underlying national health policies were falling under increasing challenge. The major ongoing controversies of past and present—regarding methods of financing, strengthening delivery systems, quality protection, the appropriate role of government, etc.—were rooted in a context of commonly accepted assumptions as to the overriding importance of maximum access to ever-rising levels of scientific medicine and the central place of medical care in individual and national health.

By 1975 the consensus was breaking up. Views were segmenting in various gradations of rejection and defense of traditional assumptions. The conviction was growing that the Western societies' reliance on medical care had become excessive; that it was not, in fact, a primary determinant of health status, and that diversion of resources to more exotic high-technology procedures was socially wasteful.

Starr describes the paradox of today's medicine in these terms [15]:

American medicine today contains a paradox. Outwardly, its institutions, prosperous and authoritative, show imposing strength, yet their social and economic structure

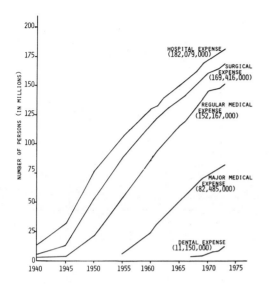

FIGURE 6-6.

Number of persons with private health insurance protection, by type of insurance (United States, 1940–1973).

Source. Health Insurance Institute: *Sourcebook of Health Insurance Data, 1974–75,* New York: The Institute, 1975, p. 20.

is fundamentally unstable, and long-standing assumptions that have governed their operation are in danger of breaking down. A fundamental intellectual reassessment of medicine is taking place; a sense of impending change fills the air. . . . Controlling costs will mean redrawing the "contract," if you will, between the medical profession and the society.

MAJOR PROBLEMS OF THE HEALTH CARE SYSTEM

Although it is somewhat arbitrary and risky to identify any small number of problems as *the* major problems of an organism as complex as the expanding health care system, it is useful in developing an overall perspective within which specific developments, such as changing approaches to primary care, can be better understood. Four major problems will be presented in brief, with full recognition that their interrelatedness prevents sharp dissection from each other, and surely there are other significant problems that will escape mention by this approach.

Limited Access to Health Care

The various barriers to ready access by all to adequate health care in this country were examined in some detail in Chapter 4. It is not productive to recount the dimensions of that problem here, but it is crucial to recognize that major limitations in access to health care do exist for a large part of the population, and this problem must be included in any list of the important problems of the health care system.

With respect to the financial barrier to health care, the Medicare and Medicaid programs have substantially increased access to health care services for

FIGURE 6-7.

Utilization of general hospitals (United States, 1928–1975).

Sources: (1) For 1928–1931: Falk, IS, Klem, MC, and Sinai, N: *The Incidence of Illness and the Receipt and Costs of Medical Care Among Representative Family Groups.* Publications of the Committee on the Costs of Medical Care, No. 26, Chicago, University of Chicago Press, 1933, Appendix Table B-27, p. 283. (2) For 1946–1970. Hospital statistics. *Hospitals*, Guide Issue 45, August 1971, Part 2, Table 1, p. 460. (3) For Population, 1946–1970: U.S. Department of Commerce, Bureau of the Census, *Statistical Abstract of the United States, 1971,* Washington, D.C., U.S. Government Printing Office, 1971, Table 2, p. 5. (4) For 1971–1974: *Hospital Statistics,* 1975 ed., American Hospital Association Annual Survey, Tables 2 and 3, pp. viii.

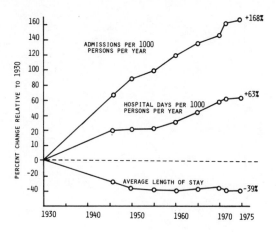

the elderly and the poor since their initiation in 1966. Increased utilization of physician services did not occur during the 1960s, however, for people with annual incomes over 5000 dollars per year. Figure 6–8 shows sharp decreases in the number of physician visits per year for these people in contrast to increasing utilization of physicians' services by low-income groups, suggesting that limited access to health care is a more generalized phenomenon than might be suspected.[16]

Increasing Cost of Health Care

The causes that fuel the spiraling costs of health care as already described are varied and complex. New technology is partly accountable for increased costs through the widespread application of new techniques requiring hospitalization and complicated, expensive equipment. Examples include radiation therapy, renal dialysis, coronary bypass surgery, organ transplants, and advances in various kinds of intensive care. The prevailing attitude that these services are "covered" by third-party payers merely delays full recognition of the cost problem. Many other factors contribute to escalating costs of health care, including inflation, population growth, patient and physician preferences, the potential threat of malpractice claims, and related factors. Table 6–1 reflects the accelerated rise in average cost to hospitals per patient day and stay over the past 30 years.[17] Figure 6–9 shows the relative proportion of several major components in rising health care expenditures between 1950 and 1976.[18]

When health care expenditures are brought down to the level of the individual citizen, the magnitude of the cost problem is further accentuated. Table 6–2 reflects an eightfold increase in per capita expenditures for health care between 1950 and 1976.[18]

Although it is difficult to estimate the extent to which governmental efforts during the last ten years to increase entitlement to health care have contributed to these rising costs, many observers view the Medicare and Medicaid experience

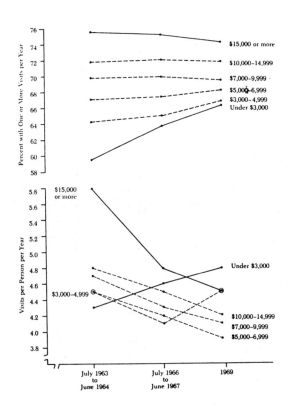

FIGURE 6-8.

Use of physicians' services by income group.
Source: National Center for Health Statistics: *Physician Visits: Volume and Interval Since Last Visit, United States—1969.* Vital and Health Statistics, Series 10, No. 75, Washington, D.C., U.S. Government Printing Office, July 1972, p. 58.

as a warning to future efforts to increase entitlement without attention to the context in which change is introduced.

Duplication and Waste

The competition between hospitals in adding duplicate facilities, equipment, and services without regard to the overall needs of their communities is but

TABLE 6-1.   AVERAGE COST TO HOSPITALS PER PATIENT DAY AND STAY 1946–1976

YEAR	AVERAGE LENGTH OF STAY (DAYS)	AVERAGE COST TO HOSPITAL ($)	
		Per Patient Day	Per Patient Stay
1946	9.1	9.39	85.45
1960	7.6	32.23	244.95
1968	8.4	61.38	515.59
1970	8.2	81.01	664.28
1972	7.9	105.30	831.70
1974	7.8	127.70	996.20
1976*	7.4	158.39	1167.64

*Estimated. Figures are for community hospitals. Sources: American Hospital Association; Health Insurance Institute.

Source: *Medical Economics* July 25, 1977, p. 1.

FIGURE 6-9.

Factors contributing to the increase in personal
health expenditures, fiscal years 1950 and 1976.
Source: *Social Security Bulletin,* U.S. Department of Health,
Education and Welfare, April 1977, p. 16.

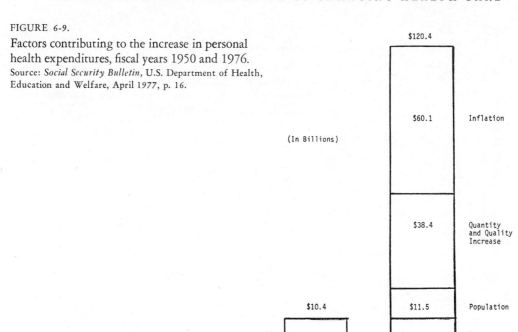

one example of duplication and waste of the health care dollar. The latest in
a long series of examples of this problem is the CT (computerized tomography)
brain and body scanner. The original cost of a CT scanner is about 500,000
dollars, and operating costs average about 370,000 dollars per year.[19] Many
communities have two or three such scanners where one would be adequate,
and many feel that widespread application of this diagnostic tool is premature
and wasteful.[20, 21] Somers and Somers have this to say on the subject.[22]

TABLE 6–2. PER CAPITA NATIONAL HEALTH EXPENDITURES, BY
SOURCE OF FUNDS, 1950–1976

FISCAL YEAR	HEALTH EXPENDITURES (PER CAPITA)		
	Total	*Private*	*Public*
1950	$ 78.35	$ 58.38	$ 19.97
1955	103.76	77.29	26.47
1960	141.63	106.60	35.03
1965	197.75	149.27	48.48
1970	333.57	211.18	122.39
1976	637.97	368.61	269.36

Source: U.S. Department of Health, Education and Welfare: *Social Security
Bulletin,* April 1977.

Granting the scanner's positive potential, the logical first step was not proliferation but controlled clinical trials to determine cost-effectiveness and, insofar as possible, objective technological assessment of the probable social impact. It may now be too late in this case but the lesson should not be lost to public policy. While millions of Americans suffer from neglect in underfinanced and understaffed long-term facilities and others are told there is no money to support such universally essential services as home care and health education, the nation cannot afford to indulge every new technological advance, even though it may prove beneficial to a small number of patients.

Another example of waste that particularly involves physicians is the excess utilization of laboratory tests well beyond their clinical value. Between 1971 and 1975, the number of inpatient laboratory tests increased by almost 60 percent for the average hospitalized patient, while the number of outpatient laboratory tests per patient increased by 122 percent.[23] While the utilization of laboratory tests is increasing, many studies show a low yield of clinically useful results. One such study, for example, showed only 5 percent of laboratory data were actually used in diagnosis and treatment of patients on a general medical service in one teaching hospital.[24]

Marginal Outcomes of Health Care

Quite beyond the problems of limited access, high cost, and excess duplication and waste within the health care system, concern has become more widespread in recent years as to whether the outcomes of health care in this country justify the costs. By such crude measures as life expectancy and mortality statistics, there is ample evidence warranting such concern. During the present age of specialization over the last 25 years, the average life span has increased by only 3 years.[25] By the end of the 1960s, the United States compared poorly with respect to the infant mortality rate among many nations in the world spending smaller portions of their Gross National Product on health care (Figure 6–10). Comparison of the leading causes of death in 1900 and 1974 showed greatly increased mortality rates for three major categories of chronic disease—heart disease, cancer, and cerebrovascular disease—which are far more difficult to control than mortality from infectious diseases of past years (Figure 6–11). Dr. Victor Fuchs, an economist with long interest in health care, sums up the problem in this way [26]:

> . . . health status (as measured by mortality, morbidity, or other indices), depends on many things besides medical care. . . . Current variations in health among individuals and groups are determined largely by genetic factors, environment, and lifestyle (including diet, smoking, stability of family life, and similar variables). To be sure, changes in the health of the population over time are influenced by medical care—but mainly through scientific advances, not through changes in the quantity of care. The most rapid of these gains occurred between 1930 and 1955, largely due to the development of relatively inexpensive, highly effective drugs for the prevention or treatment of influenza and pneumonia, tuberculosis, and other infectious dis-

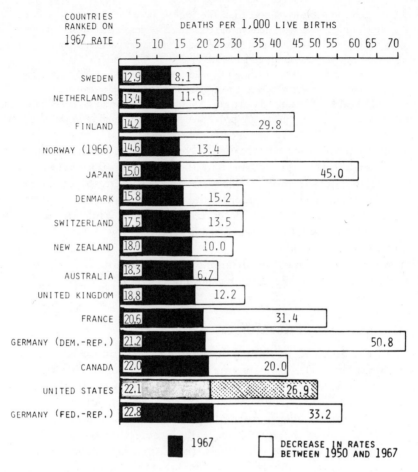

FIGURE 6-10.

Infant mortality rate (selected countries, 1950 and 1967).

Sources: (1) For 1950: United Nations. *Demographic Yearbook, 9th Issue, Special Topic: Mortality Statistics,* New York, 1957, p. 200. (2) For 1967: United Nations. *Demographic Yearbook, 1969, 21st Issue, Special Topic: Mortality Statistics,* New York, 1970, Table 42, p. 575.

eases. The current major health problems—heart disease, cancer, accidents, emotional illness, and viral infections—are more difficult to solve with the available medical technology.

Part of the problem in assessing the impact of medical care is the relative lack of effective measures of health status. As Mechanic observes [27]:

None of the indicators used to measure health status, for example, take into account the essential contribution medical care makes toward relieving worry and uncertainty, alleviating pain and discomfort, providing support and reassurance, and facilitating the ability of individuals to make a better adjustment to their environment.

Although attention to the impact of medical care on illness and death is crucial to an overall evaluation of how best to allocate resources, this perspective should not detract from the caring function of medical service. We must begin to focus more accurately on the extent to which medicine aids a person in using his capacities and fulfilling his aspirations within the limits of physical and psychological handicaps. We must try to ascertain how varying modes of delivering medical services differentially affect the patient who is worried and distressed and to learn the extent to which different models provide support and hope. In short, if medicine exists to enhance the quality of life and to lengthen it, we must examine how successfully its technology and mode of organization fulfill these purposes.

RECENT APPROACHES

It is well beyond the scope of this chapter to discuss in detail any or all of the major responses to the above problems that have been mounted during the past decade. It is, however, useful to outline briefly the effects of some of these approaches in an effort to illustrate some of the issues involved.

In their excellent book *A Right to Health: The Problem of Access to Primary Medical Care*, Lewis, Fein, and Mechanic assess in depth the experience and impact of 11 health care and financing programs intended to increase access to the medical care system and to primary care. Table 6–2 summarizes their perceptions of the impact of six programs designed to affect barriers related to *production* of services, while Table 6–3 deals with the impact of five programs designed to affect barriers to *consumption of services*.[28] Lewis points

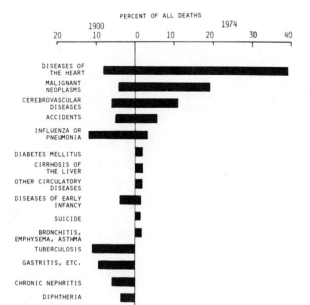

FIGURE 6-11.

Percentage of all deaths by the ten leading causes of death—United States, 1900 (death registration states only) and 1974. Arranged in order of importance in 1974.

Sources: (1) For 1900: U.S. National Office of Vital Statistics: *Vital Statistics of the United States, 1950*, Vol. 1 Washington, D.C., 1950, Table 2.26, p. 170. (2) For 1974: U.S. DHEW. Public Health Service, National Center for Health Statistics. *Monthly Vital Statistics Report*, Vol. 23, No. 13, May 1975, Table C, p. 3.

TABLE 6–3. PROGRAMS DESIGNED TO AFFECT BARRIERS RELATED TO PRODUCTION OF SERVICES

	PRACTICE COMMITMENT/ LOAN FORGIVENESS	RURAL PRECEPTORSHIPS	FAMILY PRACTICE	INCREASED NUMBERS OF PHYSICIANS	NEW HEALTH PRACTITIONERS	NATIONAL HEALTH SERVICE CORPS
Intervention	Loans for tuition; forgiven for practice in areas of physician shortage	Exposure to rural practice (real world)	Boards in family practice Residency training Undergraduate departments of family practice	Increase size of classes Add more schools Shorten curricula	Increase supply and scope of services available	Match physicians to shortage areas
Costs	Most loans: $3000–6000 per borrower over 4–5 years Administrative expense: $300–400 per borrower over 4–5 years (estimated)	Per full-time equivalent student: $12,000–15,000 annually	Residency: $25,000–35,000 per position per year $20 × 10^6 in federal funds since 1971	Construction funds: $186,000 for each new place added Education costs (unknown)	Fiscal year 1969–1974 $39 × 10^6 federal funds Cost per unit of time similar to medical education	$12 per visit
Secondary effects	—	Political pressures to change type of preceptor?	—	—	Increased attention to quality education costs, etc. Increasing conflict among professional organizations	—
Impact on access to primary care	Marginal: Most effective in reinforcing motivations of those with prior decisions to locate in these areas	Marginal: Most effective in reinforcing motivations of those with prior decisions to locate in these areas	Recent efforts probably effective (too early to tell degree of effect) Prior efforts not effective	Minimal, if any: No effects on trends toward specialization and location of practice	Some: Dependent upon location of practice Generally increased access and productivity	None to minimal

Source: Fein R.: Learning from the past. Lewis C.E., Fein R., and Mechanic D. (eds.): In *A Right to Health: The Problem of Access to Primary Medical Care.* New York, John Wiley and Sons, 1976, p. 250.

TABLE 6-4. PROGRAMS DESIGNED TO AFFECT BARRIERS TO CONSUMPTION OF SERVICES

	MEDICARE	MEDICAID	NEIGHBORHOOD HEALTH CENTERS	CHILDREN AND YOUTH PROJECTS	HEALTH MAINTENANCE ORGANIZATIONS
Intervention	Reduced financial barriers for aged	Reduced financial barriers for welfare recipients and medically needy	Reduce financial, geographic, organizational, psychosocial barriers Increase availability of services	Reduce financial, geographic, organizational, psychosocial barriers Increase availability of services	Predictable costs (prepaid) for organized services at fixed locations
Costs	Fiscal year 1967 = 3.4×10^9 Fiscal year 1973 (est.) = 9.5×10^9 Out-of-pocket expenses of those 65 and over 1966 $238 1968 $165 1972 $276	Pre-Title XIX costs for assistance = 1.2×10^9 Fiscal year 1973 (49 programs) = 8.9×10^9	$1.08-7.33 \times 10^6$ per center; $72-$400 per registrant (data incomplete)	Fiscal year 1968: $200 per child Fiscal year 1972: $135 per child	FY 1971–FY 1974: 31.4×10^6 in federal funds for technical assistance and start-up funds; no support for operating expenses No good data on average start-up and operating costs
Secondary effects	Exposed limits of supply Inflated costs Benefits not equitably distributed among those covered	Exposed limits of supply Inflated costs Benefits not equitably distributed among those covered	—	—	Potential development of intra-organizational barriers
Impact on access to primary care	Yes, positive but decreasing with additional barriers of 1970s	Yes, positive but very wide variations in value of benefits and unequitable distribution	Very effective but costs are very high	Very effective on small proportion of target population Moderate costs	? Too early to determine

Source: Fein R.: Learning from the past. In Lewis C.E., Fein R., and Mechanic D. (eds.): A Right to Health: The Problem of Access to Primary Medical Care. New York, John Wiley and Sons, 1976, p. 250.

out the lack of evidence that these 11 programs were planned in a coordinated way as part of a larger strategy for change of the health care system.[29] Fein calls for caution in making assessments of programs such as these that were not designed to build on one another.[30]

Medicare and Medicaid are good examples of programs that failed in large part to achieve their full objectives because of lack of congruency with other elements of the health care system. These programs exposed the nation's serious shortage of primary care providers, with resultant high costs and maldistribution of services.[29]

With regard to these kinds of interventions within the health care system, Lewis sums up the issues in these terms.[29]

> The primary determinants of access to care are the behaviors of consumers and providers, the numbers and locations of primary-care providers and their access to necessary backup resources, and the presence of financial barriers to care. Interventions to date have attempted to deal with only one of these, or else have created artificial microsystems that have dealt with most or all of them at once.
>
> Most of the programs focused on one barrier have either failed to demonstrate the desired impact or else have created secondary, and almost intolerable, side effects. The multibarrier approaches have demonstrated impact but have proved politically and economically unfeasible. As is evident, all of these have been somewhat tangential attempts to deal with primary determinants of access to care.
>
> The natural history of these interventions, as well as their outcome, may be somewhat predictable by an examination of the political forces involved. Three vested-interest groups must be dealt with by anyone who would change the health-care system: consumers, providers, and the organizations producing providers. Consumers cannot tolerate the unavailability of care and also find the costs of care unacceptable. Providers have strongly resisted any attempts to alter the fee-for-service method of payment, as well as attempts to eliminate solo practice in favor of health-care organizations. Providers and the institutions producing providers are opposed to any undemocratic processes that would regulate the numbers of physicians in certain areas and specialties.

and further [29]:

> The only intervention to date that has attempted to deal with the process of producing physicians in the United States has been the legislation creating departments of family practice in medical schools and residency programs for postgraduate training of primary-care specialists. These legislated additions to medical-school curricula provide a means to the end desired, but they will require considerable assistance and reinforcement through funding mechanisms if they are to achieve the results promised.

The failure or limited success of many of the interventions within the health care system in recent years led inevitably by the mid-1970s to a growing sense of disenchantment, frustration, and confusion. Somers and Somers recently described the dimensions of the confusion as follows [31]:

A search for new policies was inevitable. It took many forms. Cost containment was the most frequent demand—with few expressing very clear notions of how it was to be achieved. A growing number saw government itself and public regulation as the principal villains and protested that federal controls had already gone too far, were singularly unproductive, and were at the source of the difficulties. Many still claimed that lack of adequate access remained the major problem and emphasized the unfinished business of national health insurance. Others looked to the delivery system as the major deficiency and advocated reorganization and stronger planning. For some, improvement of quality was the prime consideration; while others saw quality and cost-efficiency as inextricably interrelated.

A small but growing number began to question the heretofore taken-for-granted positive relationship between more health care and better health. They started to look elsewhere—to the environment and particularly to individual life styles—as the more significant determinants of health and more productive per dollar invested. Within the health care field itself there was a heightened groping for forms of health care that were less technology-dependent and more humanistic. More Americans began to look overseas, not to copy but to learn from foreign experience.

CURRENT APPROACHES

Again, it is neither appropriate nor pertinent here to deal with the myriad of approaches currently being mobilized to address today's problems in the health care system. Five selected approaches will be touched on, however, as examples of several important directions toward remodeling the system.

Building the Primary Care Base of Medicine

This approach must be mentioned first, since it represents an essential part of emerging national health policy both within medical education and in the health care delivery system. This approach has already been dealt with in some detail in Chapters 3 and 5, where the present emphasis on resolving specialty and geographic maldistribution among physicians was seen to be replacing previous efforts principally aimed to educate increasing total numbers of physicians.

The fundamental importance of strengthening the primary care base of medicine and of the health care system is well illustrated in the following comments by Fein [32]:

> If access to primary care is to be appreciably increased, it will not be sufficient to dabble at the margin. Primary care cannot be grafted onto the health-care system without affecting the structure and the power relationships of that system. More effective delivery of primary care cannot be attained while leaving all other parts of medicine as they are today. . . . Effective primary care is more than just another specialty, more than just a group of dedicated physicians and other health professionals, more than just another body of knowledge. An effective primary care sector,

linked into the rest of medicine, cannot coexist with the rest of medicine without having its important impact on all that it is linked to and that is linked to it.

Health Systems Agencies

In 1974, Congress passed the National Health Planning and Resources Development Act (P.L. 93–641), which replaced such programs as Regional Medical Programs (RMP), Comprehensive Health Planning (CHP), and the Hill–Burton program. This new law called for the establishment of a national network of over 200 Health Systems Agencies (HSAs), to be set up as independent planning organizations outside of state and local governments. This is an important piece of legislation that deals directly with personal health services and has enlarged functions, authority, and funding compared to its relatively ineffective predecessor, Comprehensive Health Planning (CHP). The law outlines the following purposes for the HSA:

1. To improve the health of residents of the health service area.
2. To increase accessibility, acceptability, continuity and quality of services.
3. To restrain increases in cost of providing services.
4. To prevent unnecessary duplication of health resources.

   The basic population guidelines for each HSA call for 500,000 to 3 million people, with exceptions for metropolitan areas. The formula for HSA representation requires 51 to 60 percent to be consumers (restrictively defined), with the remainder being providers representing physicians and other professionals, health care institutions, insurers, professional schools, and the allied health professions.[33]
   Each HSA is responsible for the following basic functions:

1. Each HSA will assemble and analyze data concerning:
   a. The status of the health of residents in the area.
   b. The status of the health care delivery system in the area and its use.
   c. The effect of the area's health care delivery system on the health of the residents of the area.
   d. The number, type, and location of the area's health resources.
   e. Patterns of utilization of those resources.
   f. Environmental and occupational exposure factors affecting health conditions.
2. Each HSA, acting through its staff, is required to draw up an annual health systems plan (HSP) and an annual implementation plan (AIP).
3. When fully designated, the HSA will set up an Area Health Services Development Fund from which it may make grants and enter into contracts for planning and developing projects and programs that it determines are needed in the area and that advances its plan. Such funds cannot be used to deliver services or to build facilities.

4. When fully designated, the HSA will also review, and approve or disapprove, based on the area's plan, all federal grant money under:
   a. The Public Health Service Act.
   b. The Community Mental Health Centers Act.
   c. The Comprehensive Alcohol Abuse and Alcoholism Prevention, Treatment, and Rehabilitation Act.
5. Among other things, each HSA also will:
   a. Coordinate its activities with PSROs and other appropriate planning and regulatory agencies.
   b. Assist and work with its State Health Planning and Development Agency in the performance of its planning functions, particularly by recommending what is needed in its area.
   c. Recommend to the state annually projects for facility modernization, construction, etc. in its area.
   d. Review at least every five years all institutional health services in the area.

P.L. 93–641 required the states to pass laws obliging hospitals and other institutions to obtain "certificates of need" before undertaking major capital expenditures.[34] The law also established a National Council on Health Planning and Development, which acts in an advisory capacity to develop guidelines for national health planning. As a result of this legislation, the Department of Health, Education, and Welfare in March 1978 issued the guidelines described in Appendix 1. These may well turn out to define a wide range of basic changes in medical education and patterns of medical practice.

Professional Standards Review Organizations

Another piece of landmark legislation of the 1970s was that establishing Professional Standards Review Organizations (PSROs) in 1972. These organizations combine the concept of professional peer review with statutorily defined public accountability. There are now over 200 PSRO areas designated throughout the country, with over one-half of them operational.[35]

PSROs were initially developed as part of an effort to control soaring costs of Medicare and Medicaid by monitoring physicians' treatment of hospitalized patients funded by these programs. PSROs have drawn on the experience of medical foundations, some county medical societies, and federally supported Experimental Medical Care Review Organizations (EMCROs) in developing methods for standard setting and peer review.[35]

As might be expected, PSROs have been controversial and have had major difficulties in establishing effective procedures. The definition of *quality of care* is difficult, as is the correction of deficiencies once identified. Although PSROs have been relatively ineffective to date in controlling costs, they are beginning to develop effective methods for assessing physicians' performance as part of an overall process to define desirable standards of medical care.[34]

Health Maintenance Organizations

Prepaid health care plans represent another approach being encouraged by current national health policy makers. This approach has been popularized under the concept of health maintenance organizations (HMOs), which are of two basic types—prepaid group practice and the medical care foundation, the latter being a loose organizational entity including participating practitioners in otherwise unrelated practices.

Proponents of HMOs believe that such organized systems of care, which emphasize the delivery of a broad range of ambulatory care services, can decrease hospital utilization and costs of health care. In actual fact, the nation's largest HMO, Kaiser Health Plan (2.2 million members, 21 hospitals, and over 2000 physicians),[36] has demonstrated that adequate health care can be provided to its membership with 1.8 hospital beds per 1000 people,[37] compared to the availability of 4.5 beds in the nation's community hospitals per 1000 population in 1975.[38]

The 1973 HMO Bill (P.L. 93–222), as amended in 1976, established the basic requirements for HMOs, which are expected to provide a comprehensive range of health services with high levels of availability, accessibility and continuity. HMOs must assume full financial risk on a prospective basis for provision of basic health services to the enrollee population, must have a quality assurance mechanism, and must enroll broadly representative population groups. Many feel that an enrollment of 30,000 people is needed for a sound and viable plan.[39] The following range of services are provided by HMOs[40]:

BASIC RANGE OF NECESSARY SERVICES

- Physician services, including consultation and referral
- Inpatient and outpatient hospital services
- Medically necessary emergency services, both in and outside service area
- Short-term outpatient mental-health services (20-visit maximum)
- Drug and alcohol abuse treatment and referral services
- Diagnostic laboratory, and diagnostic and therapeutic radiology services
- Home health services
- Preventive health services, including voluntary family planning, infertility studies, preventive dental care for children, and corrective eye examinations for children

SUPPLEMENTAL HEALTH SERVICES (OPTIONAL INCLUSION IN ENROLLEE CONTRACT)

- Intermediate and long-term facilities services
- Vision, dental, and mental health services not included in basic range
- Provision of prescription drugs required in conjunction with services provided under contract

It is still premature to assess the effectiveness of HMOs. Organizational problems include high capital and start-up costs, difficulty in attracting enrollees in sufficient numbers, and problems in physician recruitment and retention. By the end of 1976, only about 6 million people, 3 percent of the population, were yet enrolled.[41] In assessing the impact of HMOs to date, Lewis has this to say[42]:

> As noted at the outset, there is no single HMO formula: characteristics of enrolled populations vary widely. Despite common factors of voluntary enrollment, prepayment, comprehensive coverage, and contractual responsibility for delivering services, the organization of services and the administration of the plan do not fit a single pattern. These differences, indicative of the flexibility of the HMO model, or looseness of the HMO rubric, will certainly increase as development of new HMO's continues under impetus of recent legislation and funding. . . . From the available evidence, there is no suggestion that problems of accessibility, cost containment, and lack of comprehensive services will be completely solved by widespread adoption of HMO-type delivery systems.

National Health Insurance

National health insurance has been a subject of controversy and heated debate for many years in this country. The late 1970s witnessed increasing attention to this issue with the development of numerous alternative proposals, each with an uncertain but large price tag. Although it is beyond the scope of this chapter to discuss any of the specific proposals, some of the major issues are of interest.

In view of the magnitude and diversity of the problems that have been described earlier, it is quite logical that growing interest and study are being directed to fundamental changes of the health care system. Starr suggests that two basic motives now exist for considering national health insurance: (1) to extend insurance protection to those groups not covered by public programs and private health insurance, and (2) to consolidate the financing of health care in the interests of rationalizing its organization.[43]

Many observers have noted the correlation between increased coverage of health care costs by government and third-party payers and the soaring costs of medical care. This has led to a growing realization that cost sharing by consumers will be crucial to any new system of health care financing. As Seidman points out[44]: ". . . our society currently has too little 'major risk' insurance, but far too much 'minor risk' insurance. To advance the goals of equity and efficiency, the strategy for NHI should be to remedy both of these defects."

In an excellent recent paper on the short-range and long-range alternatives to controlling the costs of medical care, Mechanic advocates the appreciation of various types of rationing mechanisms. In his words[45]:

In the forseeable future any system of national health insurance introduced will be a mix of rationing by consumer cost sharing and by implicit and explicit methods. There is relatively little firm knowledge about the effects of different methods of rationing on patients, physicians and the types of relations that evolve between them, and this is a serious question for the near future. The goal is to find a mix of technics that are responsive to patient need, that protect the best aspects of physician discretion and clinical judgment and that protect the public purse.

The choices are not easy, and any serious system of rationing will impose hardships on some. The United States is a wealthy country and is capable of providing a very high level of care. To the extent that opportunities to improve the production of services, and to affect consumer need and desire for them, are taken seriously, they will relieve some of the pressures for more forceful rationing in the future. If rationing is repugnant to health professionals, they must do what they can to contribute to progress on these other fronts.

The subject of national health insurance is clearly an exceedingly complex question made more difficult by lack of research on some crucial issues as well as by the presence of ample room for disagreement on medical, economic, political, and ideologic grounds. At the conclusion of a detailed discussion of national health insurance, Somers and Somers summarize their views as follows[46]:

> The issues we have enumerated are not entirely technical questions that can be resolved by further research and scientific findings. Every possible resolution affects different interests in different ways, and none is equally favorable to all. Each answer is related to certain value judgments, strongly felt and generally not universally shared. The academic assumption that additional knowledge will bring us closer to agreement is not necessarily valid when dealing with divergent ideologies and where the stakes are high for contending parties. The accommodations required in this field will be slow in coming and probably can only be achieved in a step-by-step progression or a gradual phasing-in of programs. . . . It thus appears improbable that any comprehensive NHI program can be enacted in the near future.

At this writing, the Administration subscribes to the following ten basic principles with respect to future legislation for a national health insurance plan [47]:

1. The plan should assure that all Americans have comprehensive health care coverage, including protection against catastrophic medical expenses.
2. The plan should make quality health care available to all Americans. It should seek to eliminate those aspects of the current health system that often cause the poor to receive substandard care.
3. The plan should assure that all Americans have freedom of choice in the selection of physicians, hospitals and health delivery systems.
4. The plan must support our efforts to control inflation in the economy by reducing unnecessary health care spending. The plan should include aggressive cost-containment measures and should also strengthen competitive forces in the health care sector.

5. The plan should be designed so that additional public and private expenditures for improved health benefits and coverage will be substantially offset by savings from greater efficiency in the health care system.

6. The plan will involve no additional federal spending until FY 1983, because of tight fiscal constraints and the need for careful planning and implementation. Thereafter, the plan should be phased in gradually. As the plan moves from phase to phase, consideration should be given to such factors as the economic and administrative experience under prior phases. The experience of other government programs, in which expenditures far exceeded initial projections, must not be repeated.

7. The plan should be financed through multiple sources, including government funding and contributions from employers and employees. Careful consideration should be given to the other demands on government budgets, the existing tax burdens on the American people and the ability of many consumers to share a moderate portion of the cost of their care.

8. The plan should include a significant role for the private insurance industry, with appropriate government regulation.

9. The plan should provide resources and develop payment methods to promote such major reforms in delivering health care services as substantially increasing the availability of ambulatory and preventive services, attracting personnel to underserved rural and urban areas, and encouraging the use of prepaid health plans.

10. The plan should assure consumer representation throughout its operation.

COMMENT

The medical profession shares some responsibility for today's problems in health care and likewise must accept responsibility for sharing in their resolution. As White recently observed [48]:

> We have a society and a medical profession which seem to take for granted that any new form of technical intervention must obviously represent an improvement, and that, because we can invent it, we should apply it to everyone we care to without regard to relative benefits, costs, hazards, or risks. . . . What does it mean to health professions? It means that collectively we seem to be out of step with the anguished cries for help of our patients and unaware of the angry frustrations of society. Our patients have a set of problems, symptoms, and complaints with which they want help—better help and faster help. Society has a limited set of resources, most of them scarce, for which there are multiple competing demands, and we have a vast technological array of pills, potions, and procedures that are occasionally useful, often painful, sometimes hazardous, and nearly always expensive. Most frequently, these procedures remain totally unevaluated with respect to their impact on the resolution of our patients' collective presenting problems.

In order to contribute to future improvements in health care in this country, physicians will have to take off the blinders that may limit their interest to their own specialty and focus their efforts on relating their respective specialties and roles to the real needs of the public. From the vantage point of broad experience in both clinical medicine and government, Roy makes this important point [49]:

> In health care, as in all areas of national endeavors, we cannot do everything for everyone everywhere, and therefore we are now determining, and must in the future in some way determine, what we are going to do where and for whom.

We are now involved in a process of reassessment of priorities at many levels in society with respect to health care. New patterns of health care will undoubtedly emerge that will challenge all physicians to continue to meet the best interests of their patients in an era of limits.

Regardless of the nature of the future health care system, the central importance of the primary care physician is assured. Current directions in national health care policy can be expected to lead toward increased entitlement to health care services, which will further stress the already inadequate system for primary care. As the broadest and most flexible specialty in medicine, and the only one to focus on the family as the object of care, family practice will play a vital role in whatever health care system evolves. Family practice has the responsibility and the capability to limit health care costs while preserving the quality, comprehensiveness, and continuity of personal health care for families.

REFERENCES

1. Lewis CE: Eleven programs for increasing access to primary care. In Lewis CE, Fein R, Mechanic D (eds): A Right to Health: The Problem of Access to Primary Medical Care. New York, Wiley, 1976, p 43
2. Holman HR: The "excellence" deception in medicine. Hosp Pract 11: April 11, 1976
3. Strickland S: U.S. Health Care: What's Wrong and What's Right. New York, Universe, 1972, p 33
4. The Troubled Professions. Business Week, August 16, 1976
5. Stambler HV: Health manpower—The right number. Health Manpower Issues. DHEW Publication No. (HRA) 76–40, 7, 1976
6. Health 1976–1977. United States Chartbook. DHEW Publication No. (HRA) 77–1233, 1, 1977
7. Gibson RM, Mueller MS: National health expenditures, fiscal year 1976. Social Security Bull 40:4, April 1977
8. 1976 Medical Care Chart Book, 6th ed. School of Public Health, Department of Medical Care Organization, University of Michigan, 111, 1976
9. Ibid. #6, p 2, 1977
10. Ibid. #6, p 6, 1977
11. Ibid. #6, p 3, 1977

12. Ibid. #8, p 345, 1976

13. Ibid. #8, p 69, 1976

14. Somers AR, Somers HM: Health and Health Care: Policies in Perspective. Germantown, Maryland, Aspen Systems, 1977, p 1

15. Starr P: Medicine and the waning of professional sovereignty. Daedalus 107:1, 1978

16. National Center for Health Statistics, Physician Visits: Volume and Interval Since Last Visit, United States—1969. Vital and Health Statistics, Series 10, No. 75, Washington, D.C., U.S. Government Printing Office, July 1972, p 58

17. Hospital stays get shorter, more costly. Med Econ p 158, July 25, 1977

18. U.S. Department of Health, Education and Welfare. Social Security Bull 16, April 1977

19. U.S. Congress, Office of Technology Assessment, The Computed Tomography (CT or CAT) Scanner and its Implications for Health Policy. Washington, D.C., U.S. Government Printing Office, September 1976, draft, p 57

20. Shapiro SH, Wyman SM: CAT fever. N Engl Med 294:954, 1976

21. Phillips DF, Lille K: Putting the leash on CAT. Hospitals 50:45, 1976

22. Somers AR, Somers HM: Health and Health Care: Policies in Perspective. Germantown, Maryland, Aspen Systems, 1977, p 445

23. Trends in the volumes of services utilized. Hospitals 50:17, 1976

24. Dixon RH, Laszlo J: Utilization of clinical chemistry services by medical house staff. Arch Intern Med 134:1064, 1974

25. Knouss RF: Health manpower—the right kind. In Health Manpower Issues. DHEW Publication No. (HRA) 76-40, 16, 1976

26. Fuchs VR: Who Shall Live? Health Economics and Social Choice. New York, Basic Books, 1974, p 144

27. Mechanic D: The problem of access to medical care. Lewis CE, Fein R, Mechanic D (eds): A Right to Health: The Problem of Access to Primary Medical Care. New York, Wiley, 1976, p 9

28. Fein R: Learning from the past. In Lewis CE, Fein R, Mechanic, D (eds): A Right to Health: The Problem of Access to Primary Medical Care. New York, Wiley, 1976, p 250

29. Lewis CE: Summary and conclusions. In Lewis CE, Fein R, Mechanic D (eds): A Right to Health: The Problem of Access to Primary Medical Care. New York, Wiley, 1976, p 241

30. Fein R: Learning from the past. In Lewis CE, Fein R, Mechanic D (eds): The Problem of Access to Primary Medical Care. New York, Wiley, 1976, 252

31. Somers AR, Somers HM: Health and Health Care: Policies in Perspective. Germantown, Maryland, Aspen Systems, 1977, p 238

32. Fein R: Some options for the short run. In Lewis CE, Fein R, Mechanic D (eds): A Right to Health: The Problem of Access to Primary Medical Care. New York, Wiley, 1976, p 285

33. Somers AR, Somers HM: Health and Health Care: Policies in Perspective. Germantown, Maryland, Aspen Systems, 1977, p 252

34. Starr P: Medicine and the waning of professional sovereignty. Daedalus 107:189, 1978

35. Somers AR, Somers HM: Health and Health Care: Policies in Perspective. Germantown, Maryland, Aspen Systems, 1977, p 448

36. Somers AR, Somers HM: Health and Health Care: Policies in Perspective. Germantown, Maryland, Aspen Systems, 1977, p 223

37. Boardman JJ: Utilization data and the planning process. In Somers AR (ed): The Kaiser-Permanente Medical Care Program: A Symposium. New York, Commonwealth Fund, 1971, p 65

38. American Hospital Association: Hospital Statistics, 1976 ed, Table 1, p 4, 1976

39. Somers AR, Somers HM: Health and Health Care: Policies in Perspective. Germantown, Maryland, Aspen Systems, 1977, p 259

40. Appendix B, Summary of Main Features of 1973 HMO Bill (P.L. 93–222). In Lewis CE, Fein R, Mechanic D (eds): A Right to Health: The Problem of Access to Primary Medical Care. New York, Wiley, 1976, p 325

41. Somers AR, Somers HM: Health and Health Care: Policies in Perspective. Germantown, Maryland, Aspen Systems, 1977, p 232

42. Lewis CE: Health maintenance organizations: Guarantors of access to medical care? In Lewis CE, Fein R, Mechanic D (eds): A Right to Health: The Problem of Access to Primary Medical Care. New York, Wiley, 1976, p 239

43. Starr P: Medicine and the waning of professional sovereignty. Daedalus 107:187, 1978

44. Seidman LS: A strategy for national health insurance. Inquiry 14:321, 1977

45. Mechanic D: Approaches to controlling the costs of medical care: Short-range and long-range alternatives. N Engl J Med 298:254, 1978

46. Somers AR, Somers HM: Health and Health Care: Policies in Perspective. Germantown, Maryland, Aspen Systems, 1977, p 189

47. President Carter releases NHI principles. Am Family Physician, September 1978

48. White KL: Health problems and priorities and the health professions. Prev Med 6:563, 1977

49. Roy WR: Presentation at the annual meeting of the Society of Teachers of Family Medicine, New Orleans, Louisiana, April 2, 1976

CHAPTER SEVEN

Changing Trends in Medical Education

In 1910, Flexner dealt with the gap between what was then known and what was taught in medical schools. Today, we have a different gap: between what is taught and what is needed for health care to meet public and individual need.

Cecil G. Sheps [1]

The last several chapters have examined some of the major problems and trends in the organization and patterns of medical practice. In shifting the focus to medical education itself, we find an equally dynamic state of affairs, and can anticipate that changing trends in medical education will have an important influence on future medical practice.

The purpose of this chapter is threefold: (1) to summarize briefly some of the important developments in American medical education since 1900, (2) to present an overview of some basic problems in medical education today, and (3) to outline some current trends and future projections for medical education in this country. An understanding of these changing directions is useful in appreciating the milieu in which family practice is developing as the fastest-growing specialty in American medicine.

HISTORICAL PERSPECTIVE

Evolution of the Medical School

The report prepared by Abraham Flexner in 1910 is widely regarded as a milestone in American medical education. Reviewing the standards of medical schools in the United States at that time and comparing them against the high standards of German medical education, he called for adoption of improved standards and goals by all our medical schools.[2] There was great variation among schools as to quality, and many were substandard. He recommended a basic formula whereby medical schools structured the first two years for pre-clinical basic science and the last two years for clinical science, with each department responsible for teaching in its own area of knowledge.[3]

This pattern was held to in a somewhat rigid way until well after World War II. Medical schools became more standardized and of more uniformly high quality. They became university centers for science and learning and escaped the older mold of trade schools.

In the years before World War II, medical schools had limited influence outside of their teaching hospitals, which were oriented primarily toward care of indigent patients. In a book published in 1930 entitled *Universities—American, English and German*, Flexner stressed that the university's main purposes were teaching and research and that large responsibilities for patient care as a service function within the community were to be avoided.[4] During this period, the principle province of medical education was on the undergraduate level, and there were relatively few residencies. A substantial degree of separatism often existed between the practicing physician and the academic physician, resulting commonly in a "town–gown" rivalry. The clinician in the style of Osler was the model around which teaching revolved. Basic sciences were taught in pragmatic terms as required for diagnosis and treatment of patients.[5]

The 25 years since World War II saw a rapid increase in biomedical research. The new academic physician became more the "scientist–physician" than the clinician and often spent more time in research than on patient care.[5] This period witnessed a proliferation of teaching hospitals and residencies, with a new stress on graduate medical education. At the same time, there were increasing expectations by the public and surrounding hospitals and medical communities for support and consultation. Innovative curriculum changes became common since the experiment in interdisciplinary teaching initiated by Western Reserve University School of Medicine in 1952. Medical schools during the 1960s became highly variable in terms of philosophy, goals, and teaching methods.

The complexity of the modern medical school is well illustrated by the following statement made by Anlyan in 1969 [6]:

> Today the dean finds himself at the helm of an academic medical center comprising a complex of undergraduate medical education programs; graduate Ph.D. programs

in the basic sciences; graduate medical education with interns, residents, and fellows equal in number to the number of medical students; continuing education for physicians in the region; a multimillion dollar research program (which in many instances is multidisciplinary and multidepartmental); one or more teaching hospitals which hover on the brink of financial insolvency; a fast-changing and expanding interest of federal and state government in health affairs; expanding needs of society in health care; and, not the least of all, a health manpower shortage combined with a maldistribution of physicians and health personnel. Within the academic medical center, many of the major departments have operational complexities larger than the total medical school of two decades ago.

It has become popular, perhaps to an unfair extent, to hold university medical schools largely responsible for the many deficiencies in our health care system. Medical schools are being looked to for leadership in areas of patient care and methods of health delivery. This creates a difficult dilemma for the medical school: How can it respond to such demands without compromising its primary functions of research, teaching, and advancement of scientific medicine?

Growth of Teaching Programs

In viewing medical education in the United States since 1940, one is immediately struck by the rapid growth in the size and number of teaching programs at all levels. Table 7–1 shows the number of medical schools, enrollment, and graduates over the last 35 years. It can be noted that the number of medical schools has increased by over 50 percent during this period, with a nearly threefold increase in the enrollment and number of graduates.

At the graduate level, an even more remarkable growth has taken place. Figure 7–1 shows a tenfold increase in the number of residency positions offered in the United States since 1940. The number of available residency positions for years has considerably exceeded the needs of graduates of United States medical schools for graduate training. Figure 7–2 displays the increasing proportion of residency positions filled by foreign medical graduates during the last 25 years, as well as a substantial number of vacant positions.

The dramatic growth of residency positions in the United States since 1940 reflects widespread recognition that graduate medical education has become an essential requisite for competent medical practice in all fields. Before 1940, many physicians were adequately prepared for practice by their medical school training and subsequent internship. By 1970, nearly 90 percent of the graduates of United States medical schools entered, and most completed, residency training.[7]

Specialization

The process of specialization in this country over the past 50 years has already been considered in some detail in Chapters 1 and 3. There is no need to

TABLE 7–1.   STUDENTS AND GRADUATES IN MEDICAL AND BASIC SCIENCE SCHOOLS

YEAR	NUMBER OF SCHOOLS*	TOTAL ENROLLMENT	FIRST-YEAR	INTERMEDIATE YEARS	GRADUATES
1940–1941	77	21,379	5,837	10,267	5,275
1945–1946	77	23,216	6,060	11,330	5,826
1950–1951	79	26,186	7,177	12,874	6,135
1955–1956	82	28,639	7,686	14,108	6,845
1956–1957	85	29,130	8,014	14,320	6,796
1957–1958	85	29,473	8,030	14,582	6,861
1958–1959	85	29,614	8,128	14,626	6,860
1959–1960	85	30,084	8,173	14,830	7,081
1960–1961	86	30,288	8,298	14,996	6,994
1961–1962	87	31,078	8,483	15,427	7,168
1962–1963	87	31,491	8,642	15,585	7,264
1963–1964	87	32,001	8,772	15,893	7,336
1964–1965	88	32,428	8,856	16,163	7,409
1965–1966	88	32,835	8,759	16,502	7,574
1966–1967	89	33,423	8,964	16,716	7,743
1967–1968	94	34,538	9,479	17,086	7,973
1968–1969	99	35,833	9,863	17,911	8,059
1969–1970	101	37,669	10,401	18,901	8,367
1970–1971	103	40,487	11,348	20,165	8,974
1971–1972	108	43,650	12,361	21,738	9,551
1972–1973	112	47,546	13,726	23,429	10,391
1973–1974	114	50,886	14,185	25,088	11,613
1974–1975	114	54,074	14,963	26,397	12,714
1975–1976	114	56,244	15,351	27,332	13,561
1976–1977	116	58,266	15,667	28,992	13,607

*Prior to 1956–1957, schools in development were not included.

Source: Medical education in the United States, 1976–1977. *JAMA* 238:26, 1977. Reprinted with permission from the American Medical Association.

recount these developments here, but it is important to recognize this process as a major feature of medical education in this century. The specialty boards have become active parties in the patterns and policies of medical education in this country. Table 7–2 summarizes the current requisites for graduate training in the various specialties.

The 22 specialty boards today confer 32 kinds of general certificates and 33 special certificates in 65 areas of medical practice.[8] The inevitable cycle involved in the process of certification in medicine has been described by Chase as follows[9]:

1. As a result of advances in a field or development of new technology, a new group develops special expertise in this area.
2. An organization or society is formed for an exchange of ideas and to display advances to one another.

3. Membership in the organization becomes a mark of distinction in the field, and in an effort to externalize that recognition, certification of excellence in the field becomes established.
4. Institutions with responsibility for quality of health care soon accept certification as evidence of competence and limit care within the field to those certified.

SOME BASIC PROBLEMS IN MEDICAL EDUCATION

Although it is beyond the scope of this chapter to examine in any depth the many problems in medical education, it is useful to briefly consider four fundamental problems that plague medical education today.

Imbalance between Product and Public Need

There is good reason to credit medical schools with the strengths of American medical education as well as to hold them accountable in large part for the deficiencies of the system. Medical schools today represent a constituency of 117

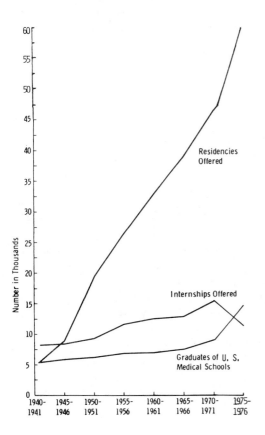

FIGURE 7-1.

Number of residency, internship positions, and graduates of medical schools (United States, selected years, 1940–1975).

Sources: (1) Medical education in the United States, 1970–1971. *JAMA* 218:1221, 1971. (2) Medical education in the United States, 1975–1976. *JAMA* 236:2961, 1976.

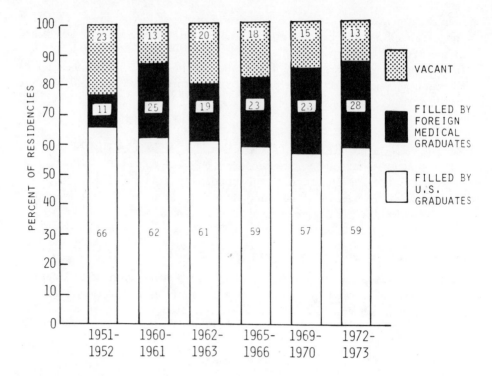

FIGURE 7-2.

Percent distribution of occupancy of residencies (United States, selected years, 1951–1973).

Sources: (1) For 1951–1966: Medical education in the United States, 1965–1966. *JAMA*, 198, 29, 1966, Table 26. (2) For 1970: Ruhe, CAW, et al. *Directory of Approved Internships and Residencies*, Chicago, American Medical Association, 1971, Table 10, p. 9. (3) For 1973: Medical education in the United States, 1973. *JAMA*, 226:938, 1973, Table 25.

schools and over 400 affiliated teaching hospitals whose beds comprise 25 percent of all the hospital beds for acute care in the United States.[10] Their teaching and patient care programs therefore greatly affect the operation of the country's health care system.

Heavy emphasis on biomedical research during the last 25 years has led to a remarkable increase in biomedical knowledge and extensive subspecialization within medical schools. These gains, however, have tended to divert medical schools from other responsibilities, particularly those related to providing leadership toward improving the nation's capacity to apply biomedical advances through a more effective health care delivery system. Wilbur Cohen, as Secretary of the Department of Health, Education and Welfare, in 1969 posed these fundamental questions to medical schools[11]:

Does your responsibility rest only in educating the physician with no obligation to develop new patterns of patient care?

What action do you plan to take in response to the Millis Commission's recommendations dealing with the need for family physicians?

Are you conducting the necessary research to give us answers on how to make the wisest use of the physician's time?

Are you contributing toward analyzing and meeting the health manpower needs of your community, your state, and your region?

Should you extend your efforts to assist the medical education programs of the community hospitals of your region?

Medical schools have shown some concern for some of these larger issues in recent years but have been relatively ineffective in planning and implementing some of the fundamental changes needed. Change of the specialty distribution within graduate medical education is a good example of a pressing issue in the late 1970s that has not yet been adequately approached. The "mix" within today's graduate medical education by specialty clearly is the single most important factor in determining future specialty distribution to and beyond the year 2000. As noted in earlier chapters, there is ample evidence that many specialties are already in surplus, with others projected for surplus numbers by the early 1980s. Yet the number of first-year residency positions in surplus specialties, such as pathology and most of the surgical specialties, has not been reduced, as shown in Table 7–3. It is especially difficult for medical schools to resolve this problem, since most of these surplus residency positions are funded and controlled by hospitals beyond the direct influence of medical schools.

Limited Relevance of Medical Education to Medical Practice

There is growing awareness that undergraduate and graduate medical education could be made more relevant to the needs of society and improved patterns of medical practice. Some feel that medical education is too incomplete. Millis, for instance, argues that though medical education prepares students well for the care of the 10 percent of patients who are critically ill, teaching of common health care of most of the population is largely neglected.[12] Jason addresses the subject of relevance in medical education in these terms[13]:

Clearly, my assumption is that medical education *should* be relevant to medical practice. This presumes that medical school is, in fact, a preparation for medical practice. It is no secret that there are a significant number of schools that adopt the posture that they are not actually preparing students for medical practice but, rather, for careers as instructors and investigators. The facts are, however, that there is no school which has more than 13 percent of its graduates in faculty positions, and only four schools have more than 10 percent of their graduates in academic work. On the other hand, fully 90 percent of all graduates of this country's medical schools are in clinical practice. Indeed, there is no school from which less than 74 percent of the

TABLE 7-2. APPROXIMATE NUMBER OF YEARS OF GRADUATE TRAINING REQUIRED TO COMPLETE TRAINING IN VARIOUS SPECIALTIES

SPECIALTY	PREREQUISITE YEARS BEFORE ENTRY INTO SPECIALTY	MINIMUM YEARS OF TRAINING IN THIS SPECIALTY FIELD	MAXIMUM YEARS OF TRAINING SUBJECT TO APPROVAL IN FIELD
Anesthesiology	1 (clinical base)	2	3
Child psychiatry	2 (general psychiatry)	2	2
Diagnostic radiology	1 (clinical base)	3	3
Dermatology	1 (medicine)	2	3
Family practice	—	3	3
General practice	—	2	3
Surgery	—	4	5–7
Internal medicine	—	3	5
Neurologic surgery	1 (general surgery)	4	4
Neurology	1 (clinical base)	3	5
Nuclear medicine	2 (medicine, pathology, or radiology)	2	2
Obstetrics–gynecology	1 (clinical base)	3	4
Ophthalmology	1 (optional)	3	4
Orthopedic surgery	1 (surgery or others)	3	4
Otolaryngology	1 (general surgery)	3	4
Pathology	—	3	4
Forensic pathology	3 + of pathology	1	2
Neuropathology	4 of pathology	1	2
Pediatrics	—	3	4
Pediatric allergy	3 of pediatrics	1	2
Pediatric cardiology	3 of pediatrics	2	2
Physical medicine	½ + (medicine and surgery)	2	3
Plastic surgery	3 (general surgery)	2	3
Colon and rectal surgery	3 (general surgery)	2	2
Psychiatry	1 (clinical base)	3	3
Radiology	1 (clinical base)	3	3

Therapeutic radiology	1 (clinical base)	3
Thoracic surgery	4 (general surgery)	2
Urology	2 (general surgery)	3
Specialty training in other than hospitals:		
Aerospace medicine	1 (school of public health)	4
General preventive medicine	1 (school of public health)	4
Occupational medicine (academic)	2 (school of public health)	2
Occupational medicine (in-plant)	1 (plus academic)	2 (plus academic)
Public health	3 (school of public health)	4

Source: Medical education in the United States, 1976–1977. *JAMA* 238:26, 1977. Reprinted with permission from the American Medical Association.

TABLE 7–3. TREND IN FIRST-YEAR RESIDENTS, BY SPECIALTY: SELECTED YEARS, SEPTEMBER 1, 1960–1976

SPECIALTY	1960	1967	1970	1973	1976
Total first-year residents	11,070	12,581	14,556	18,076	19,831
General practice	364	265	144	176	196
Medical specialties	3,188	3,706	4,664	6,960	9,602
Dermatology	102	183	205	234	238
Family practice*	—	—	131	766	1,828
Internal medicine	2,193	2,417	3,044	4,139	5,522
Pediatrics†	893	1,106	1,284	1,821	2,014
Surgical specialties	4,274	4,790	5,290	5,820	5,621
General surgery	2,122	2,406	2,514	2,698	2,575
Neurologic surgery	101	116	141	143	121
Obstetrics–gynecology	917	783	857	1,003	1,065
Ophthalmology	288	397	460	495	455
Orthopedic surgery	353	421	528	591	563
Otolaryngology	153	208	234	266	239
Plastic surgery	47	77	120	174	184
Thoracic surgery	89	126	125	130	142
Urology	204	256	311	320	277
Other specialties	3,244	3,820	4,458	5,120	4,384
Anesthesiology	550	612	698	797	570
Child psychiatry	28	147	178	282	268
Neurology	149	233	283	357	329
Psychiatry	1,090	1,246	1,385	1,472	1,292
Pathology	757	704	744	898	778
Physical medicine and rehabilitation	55	109	101	135	161
Radiology ‡	544	755	941	480	209
Miscellaneous §	71	14	135	689	777

*Family Practice residencies not reported before 1970.
†Includes pediatric allergy and pediatric cardiology.
‡Includes therapeutic radiology.
§Includes diagnostic radiology, nuclear medicine, forensic pathology, neuropathology, and colon and rectal surgery.

Sources: (1) Directory of Approved Internships and Residencies, 1974–75. Chicago, American Medical Association, 1975; also prior annual issues. (2). U.S. Department of Health, Education, and Welfare, Bureau of Health Resources Development: The Supply of Health Manpower: 1970 Profiles and Projections to 1900. Publication No. (HRA) 75–38, Washington, D.C., U.S. Government Printing Office, 1974, p. 64. (3) Directory of Approved Residencies, 1977–78. Chicago, American Medical Association, 1977.

graduates are primarily involved in a career of patient care. Our schools obviously have an obligation to provide preparation for the careers their students will in fact pursue. To do otherwise is nothing less than educational malpractice.

and further:

In the absence of systematic data on the demands of current and future practice, and in the absence of appropriate educational planning, medical education has, paradoxically, become less a preparation for becoming a medical practitioner and more a preparation for becoming a medical student.

A considerable part of the problem of relevance in medical education has been due to the setting in which most undergraduate and graduate teaching is carried out—the hospital, which often is heavily oriented to tertiary care. That the student's (resident's) clinical exposure is severely limited by this kind of setting is clearly demonstrated by the classic work of Kerr White, which showed that only one patient out of every 250 adults consulting a physician each month is sent to a university medical center (Figure 7–3).[14]

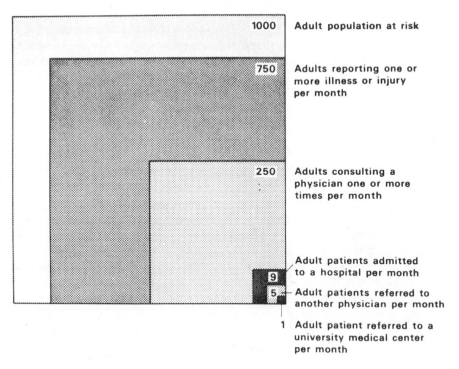

FIGURE 7-3.

Prevalence of illness and utilization of medical care resources among 1000 adults in the United States and Great Britain.

Source: White, KL, Williams TF, Greenberg, BG: The ecology of medical care. *New England Journal of Medicine,* 265:890, 1961. Reprinted by permission of the *New England Journal of Medicine.*

Traditional medical education has neglected, and frequently denigrated, primary medical care as either a productive educational setting or as a worthy career option for medical students and residents. As pointed out by Sheps [1]:

> The overemphasis on tertiary care in the university medical centers distorts their education programs. The fixation on the disease concept of illness in biological terms only is an inadequate, inappropriate, and skewed preparation for the care of most patients in the community.

Lack of a Coordinated Health Manpower Plan

Ineffective past and current efforts to address the problem of maldistribution of physicians by specialty provides clear evidence for the present lack of a coordinated health manpower plan. This is by no means due to lack of previous attempts to resolve this issue.

Rosemary Stevens, a leading expert on the subject of specialization and physician manpower supply in this country, has this to say about the lack of follow-up to a recommendation by the AMA Council of Medical Education 30 years ago to control the number of residency positions and reduce the number of internship positions by 20 to 30 percent [15]:

> There was no incentive for any group to limit the supply of house staff; it was quite the reverse. Attending physicians liked both to teach and to have house staff available; hospitals wanted house staff; specialty boards were, on the whole, interested in expanding the number of diplomates; and medical schools were still reluctant to intervene. There was thus continuing avoidance of the effects of increasing numbers of house staff on the underlying questions of graduate medical education.

Now, 30 years later, with the deficit of primary care physicians severe and the surplus in many limited specialties rapidly increasing, there is still no accepted national plan for distribution of physician manpower that is endorsed by the various organizations and parties needed to implement needed changes. The structure of graduate medical education in the nation's medical schools and teaching hospitals remains a nonsystem featured by uncoordinated local control on a departmental basis. Individual institutions have been unable or unwilling to consider future national, state, or regional needs for physicians by specialty as an important factor in the planning and operation of their residency programs. It is still unclear as to who should formulate and implement policy in this area, but it is increasingly apparent that more direct federal influence will be brought to bear on this problem unless the participatory process becomes more effective than it has to date.

Constraints of Funding

The costs of medical education have increased exponentially during the past 25 years. Tuition in medical schools covers only a fraction of the costs of educating a medical student, and the total cost of residency training is now in excess of 40,000 dollars per resident each year in most fields.

The question of who will pay the costs of medical education has become a critical issue. Reimbursement procedures by third parties for patient care services provided within teaching programs have become more restrictive. Teaching hospitals are faced with growing operational costs and increasing regulation limiting their capacity to recover costs. Governmental agencies at all levels are increasingly hard pressed to maintain past levels of support of medical education programs. At the federal level, for example, the last two years have seen reduction in expenditures by the Bureau of Health Manpower for health manpower programs (Figure 7–4). The proportion of federal expenditures for training and education, research, and construction decreased substantially between 1965 and 1975, as shown in Figure 7–5.

The largest single source of support for medical education is the federal government, which pays, for example, about 40 percent of the costs of medical schools.[10] It can therefore be anticipated that the federal government will exert increasing influence on the size and shape of medical education in coming years.

The Carnegie Council on Policy Studies in Higher Education recently completed an excellent, in-depth report of current problems in medical and dental education in the United States. It is especially noteworthy that two of its five "urgent recommendations" were as follows [16]:

> The nation has a vital stake in maintaining high standards of health among its residents. In recognition of the social benefits flowing from medical and dental education, the federal government should pursue a stable policy of financial support of university health science centers. It should provide a basic floor of support for these centers which can be supplemented by support from state governments and private sources.

And further:

> The federal government should pursue a stable and consistent policy of support of research in the health sciences, increasing its allocations for this purpose along with the rise in real GNP. Federal allocations should cover full research costs and should encourage increased emphasis on ways of achieving greater efficiency in the training of health manpower and in the delivery of health care.

SOME MAJOR TRENDS IN MEDICAL EDUCATION

Stabilization of Growth

One important change being actively proposed and receiving wider acceptance at the close of the 1970s is the need for stabilization of growth of medical education programs at both undergraduate and graduate levels. The previously

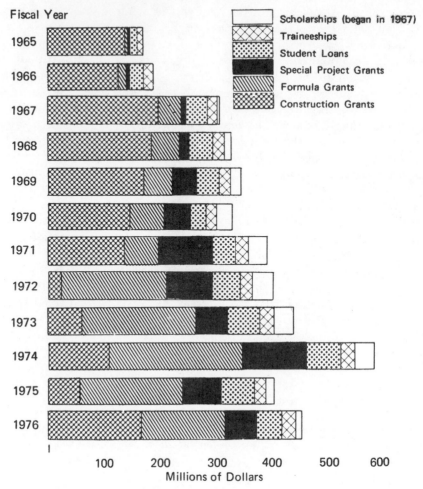

FIGURE 7-4.

Funds awarded by BHM for selected health manpower programs fiscal years 1965–1976. *Note.* Fiscal 1973 data reflect funds actually awarded through June 30, 1973. In a few programs, some fiscal 1973 funds were impounded but released after June 30, 1973, and are included with other data in the fiscal year of the award.

Source: *New Mandate for Manpower, Annual Report Fiscal 1977*, DHEW Publication No. (HRA) 78–41, 36, 1978.

mentioned Carnegie Council on Policy Studies in Higher Education issued this warning [16]:

> We are in serious danger of developing too many new medical schools, and decisive steps need to be taken by both federal and state governments to stop this trend.

This group went further in questioning the desirability of continuing to develop a number of beginning medical schools.

Other national groups have called for limitation of growth of enrollment levels. The Institute of Medicine of the National Academy of Sciences, for example, recommended in 1978 that the number of entrants to medical school remain at current levels.[17]

In 1976, federal legislation recognized for the first time the trend toward surplus in the country's physician supply. In the declaration of policy in the Health Professional Educational Assistance Act of 1976, Congress stated [18] that "there is no longer an insufficient number of physicians and surgeons in the United States such that there is no further need for affording preference to alien physicians and surgeons in admissions to the United States under the Immigration and Nationality Act." That act sharply restricted the entry of foreign medical graduates and shifted the focus from increasing the total number of physicians to specialty and geographic redistribution of physicians.[19]

With regard to limitation of the total number of residency positions, serious consideration is being given to restriction of the annual number of first-year residency positions to a definite number. A figure commonly proposed is 125 percent of the annual number of United States medical graduates, which would still allow some residency positions for a smaller number of foreign medical graduates.[20] Figure 7–6 shows that the total number of first-year

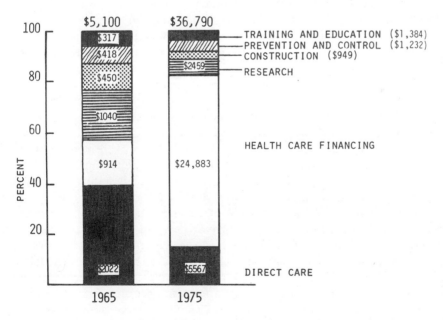

FIGURE 7-5.

Percent distribution of federal health expenditures by type of expenditure (United States, fiscal years 1965 and 1975). (Dollar amounts in millions.)

Source: Office of Management and Budget. *Special Analysis Budget of the United States Government, Fiscal Year 1977. Special Analysis K: Health Special Analysis.* Washington, D.C., U.S. Government Printing Office, 1978, Table K-28, p. 215.

FIGURE 7-6.

Comparison of the number of GME-1 positions offered with the number of graduates of United States medical schools for the years 1952 through 1976.

Source: Graettinger JS: Graduate medical education viewed from the National Intern and Resident Matching Program. *Journal of Medical Education* 51:9, 704, 1976.

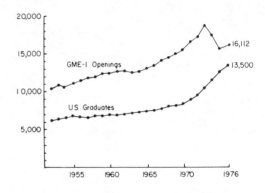

residency positions in the United States has decreased since 1970 and already bears the approximate relationship to the total number of United States medical graduates that is being proposed.

Emphasis on Primary Care

The increasing emphasis on primary care in recent years is a central theme of this book and has been dealt with in some detail in earlier chapters. This direction must certainly be included among the important trends in American medical education today. It involves a redirection in curriculum content, teaching methods, teaching settings, and philosophy and style of practice.

As previously noted, the federal government has recognized three primary care disciplines—family practice, general internal medicine, and general pediatrics. Current federal health manpower policy requires that the percentage of graduates entering primary care residencies in these fields exceed 50 percent in 1980 in order for medical schools to be eligible for capitation grants. At a recent meeting of the Willard Committee on Education for Family Practice, the group recommended that a goal be established for 25 percent of United States medical graduates to enter family practice residency training by 1985.[21]

A survey by the Bureau of Health Manpower has shown that on July 15, 1977, United States medical schools already had 52.8 percent of filled first-year residency positions in the three primary care disciplines, more than enough to meet the 1980 requirement.[22] Of the 7424 residents in first-year primary care residencies at that time, well over one-half were listed in internal medicine. Since it is well known that many first-year residents in internal medicine and pediatrics later subspecialize [23] and that many graduates from general internal medicine and general pediatrics residencies later subspecialize in practice,[24] the 52.8 percent figure in primary care in 1977 should not be cause for optimism in itself. Federal requirements call for monitoring of the number of first-year primary care residents who drop out of primary care residencies and deducting this number from the previous total credited to each medical school seeking capitation funding on this basis.

Family practice teaching programs have enjoyed considerable flexibility in their organizational and curriculum development because of their lack of dependence on past traditions and structures of education. It has been more difficult for residency programs in general internal medicine and general pediatrics to develop in medical schools and teaching hospitals with longstanding commitments to subspecialty training. In an excellent paper dealing with residency training in these two fields, Charney observes that these disciplines have traditionally "focused on the complex rather than the routine, the diagnosis rather than the management, the acute rather than the chronic, the cure rather than the prevention." [25] Fundamental changes of existing residency programs in these fields are therefore required in order to train internists and pediatricians for primary care.

Decentralization and Community Involvement

The trend toward growing numbers of university affiliations with community hospitals represents a major change in medical education. There has been more than a twofold increase in the number of university affiliations with community hospitals during the period from 1966 to 1976, while the number of unaffiliated hospitals declined by over 40 percent (Table 7–4).

This trend does not reflect a "university takeover" of teaching programs in community hospitals, but a genuine interdependence between medical schools and community hospitals with benefits to both parties. The university gains much needed clinical and teaching resources for its medical students and residents, as well as a desirable shift in clinical teaching to less highly selected patients more representative of health problems to be encountered commonly by its graduates later in practice. The involved communities also have much to gain from such affiliations, including enhanced opportunities for continuing medical education for community physicians and a tendency toward improved quality of patient care in their teaching hospitals.

Closely related to the trend of increasing university affiliations with community hospitals is the development of new regional linkages between medical schools and their surrounding areas. There are numerous examples of excellent medical education programs that have been developed on a regional basis by medical schools for both undergraduate and graduate medical education. The University of Washington and Michigan State University are two such examples. The WAMI program is a well-established and viable program with an emphasis on decentralized medical student teaching involving four states in the Pacific Northwest—Washington, Alaska, Montana, and Idaho—in affiliation with the University of Washington.[26] Michigan State University has likewise developed teaching programs linking a substantial area of Michigan with the medical school and has even demonstrated that experimental undergraduate tracks can be conducted in distant rural communities with teaching effective-

TABLE 7-4. HOSPITALS AFFILIATED WITH MEDICAL SCHOOLS

| EDITION OF DIRECTORY | NUMBER OF HOSPITALS BY TYPE OF AFFILIATION | | | | UNAFFILIATED HOSPITALS | TOTAL HOSPITALS WITH PROGRAMS* |
	Major	Limited	Graduate	Total Affiliated		
1966–1967	275	141	101	517	850	1367
1967–1968	339	137	121	597	915	1512
1968–1969	327	174	120	621	791	1412
1969–1970	376	182	141	699	750	1449
1970–1971	516	243	160	919	766	1685
1971–1972	567	288	141	996	696	1692
1972–1973	473	276	134	883	578	1461
1973–1974	694	364	107	1165	546	1711
1974–1975	714	317	105	1136	547	1683
1975–1976	752	301	115	1168	503	1671

*Data included on noninpatient institutions with residencies in preventive medicine.

Source: Medical education in the United States, 1975–1976. JAMA 236:2990, 1976. Reprinted with permission from the American Medical Association.

ness and learning outcomes comparable to those of teaching programs based in metropolitan communities.[27]

Coordination of Undergraduate, Graduate, and Continuing Medical Education

The last ten years have seen increasingly vigorous efforts to achieve some degree of coordination across the continuum of medical education encompassing the needs of medical students, residents, and practicing physicians. Traditionally, undergraduate, graduate, and continuing medical education have been disconnected functionally and conceptually, and the concept of a *continuum of medical education* has until recently been merely a hollow phrase without content.

In 1972, the Coordinating Council on Medical Education (CCME) was organized under the auspices of five parent bodies—the Association of American Medical Colleges (AAMC), the American Board of Medical Specialties (ABMS), the American Hospital Association (AHA), the American Medical Association (AMA), and the Council of Medical Specialty Societies (CMSS). The CCME was established to "coordinate the activities of the various liaison committees that serve as accrediting bodies and to review and recommend policy decisions relating to medical education to the five parent organizations." [28] Initially, the CCME addressed its efforts to the coordination of the activities of the Liaison Committee on Medical Education (LCME), responsible since 1942 for the accreditation of medical schools, and the Liaison Committee for Graduate Medical Education (LCGME), which in 1975 became the official accrediting body for residency training. In 1977, the Liaison Committee for Continuing Medical Education (LCCME) was established as the third group under the LCME, as illustrated in Figure 7–7.

The termination of the free-standing internship during the early 1970s and its integration as the first year of residency training by 1975 represents an important example of more effective coordination within the continuum of medical education. This has undoubtedly been a factor in the rising number of university affiliations with community hospitals. Between 1967 and 1973, the proportion of first-year residents in university-affiliated programs increased from 77 percent to 91 percent.[29] The net result of this change today is to regard residency training as the final phase of the young physician's *basic* medical education.

After six years of operation, the precise roles and authority of the CCME are both uncertain and controversial. Some view CCME as a coordinating organization without authority, while others propose that it become an independent, free-standing commission with authority to regulate all levels of medical education.[28] The CCME has been asked by the federal government to enter into a contract with the Department of Health, Education and Welfare to develop and implement a system designed to assure the training of the

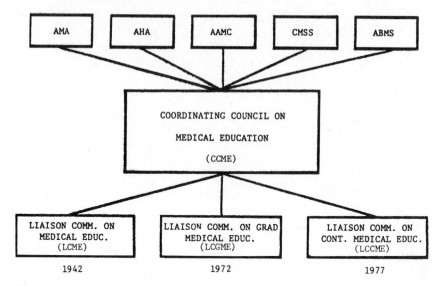

FIGURE 7-7.
Parent bodies and liaison committees of the Coordinating Council on Medical Education.

optimal number and mix of specialists.[30] To date, however, CCME has declined to accept a regulatory function.

It remains to be seen whether efforts by the CCME can be effective in addressing the major problems within their purview. Certainly the track record of voluntary efforts by the medical profession to rebalance medical education in response to public need have been unimpressive to date. Beck and his colleagues seem to be on solid ground in their view[31]:

> Voluntary efforts have stressed quality in individual training programs and the needs of the individual medical specialties. This has not been adequate to address the broader problems of specialty and geographic maldistribution. We do not believe that voluntary action by the medical profession alone will be adequate. We support expanding the federal–academic medicine partnership to certifying and accrediting bodies. Only when the medical profession takes actions which require professional expertise and the federal government assures enforcement of these actions through programs such as capitation payments to medical schools and reimbursement for services will graduate medical education be effectively regulated in the public interest.

Changes in Licensure

Reorganization of graduate medical education and trends in continuing medical education are closely related to some fundamental changes being proposed and studied in the licensure of physicians. Traditionally, medical school graduates have received unlimited licensure for life following satisfactory completion of an internship and passage of one of several licensure examinations. A report in

1973 of The Committee on Goals and Priorities of the National Board of Medical Examiners (the G.A.P. Report) recommended that unlimited licensure be withheld until completion of residency training. Periodic recertification during later practice years was also proposed as shown in Figure 7–8.

Although the G.A.P. Report is currently somewhat controversial in terms of the present applicability of its full recommendations, it represents a direction that is likely to gain momentum in future years. Many states are reassessing their methods for licensing of the professions, and at least eight states have already passed legislation that, in effect, requires periodic relicensure of physicians.[10] Although the American Board of Family Practice is at this writing still the only specialty board requiring periodic recertification (every six years), many other specialty boards already provide opportunities for periodic recertification on a voluntary basis.

The Changing Medical Student

Recent years have seen strong efforts by admissions committees in United States medical schools to select medical students better representing a cross section of the general population. Medical students today represent more diverse cultural, social, and economic groups within our society than at any time in the past, which should increase the capability of medical graduates to meet the diverse health care needs of the nation. Particular progress has taken place in the increasing enrollment of women and minorities in medical schools. The proportion of women enrolled in United States medical schools quadrupled

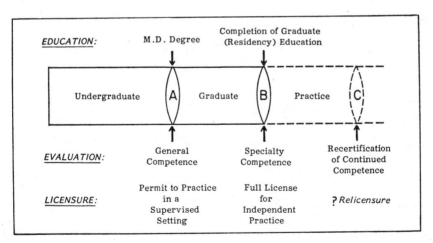

FIGURE 7-8.

A future evaluation system for certification and licensure. The proposed interrelationships of education, evaluation, and licensure in the projected educational continuum.

Source: National Board of Medical Examiners, Committee on Goals and Priorities: *Evaluation in the Continuum of Medical Education.* Philadelphia, National Board of Medical Examiners, June 1973, p. 51.

over the last 25 years from 5 percent in 1959 to 20 percent in 1977. By 1977, the proportion of students from racial minorities totalled 8.3 percent in United States medical schools, including 6.1 percent Afro-American, 1.4 percent Mexican–American, and 0.3 percent American Indian.[32]

The present generation of medical students is quite different in many respects from previous generations. Many medical students today are more interested than their predecessors in the human and social aspects of medicine. Many are more aware, and less accepting of, social injustices and the deficiencies in our health care system. Many are better informed about the world and its problems and better prepared for graduate education.[33]

Medical students today are claiming, and being accorded, a more active role in the planning and evaluation of curricula, teaching methods and other functions within the medical schools. Medical students frequently participate in course planning and review and often serve on admissions committees and other committees.

Shift from Teaching to Learning

An important advance in recent years has been a renewed interest in the learning process itself in medical education and the realization that teaching is not equivalent to learning. The traditional emphasis on didactic teaching by lectures is being supplemented by a variety of other learning modalities, such as seminars, small-group instruction, programmed instruction using audiovisual aids, and the research project instead of the repetitive laboratory experiment.[34]

There is growing awareness that the learning situation should simulate the application situation as closely as possible.[13] Many medical educators are perceiving learning as an active process whereby the teacher leads the student toward discovery through problem-oriented instruction. Increased opportunities are being provided for self instruction through such methods as videotapes and other audiovisual materials.[35, 36]

FUTURE PROJECTIONS FOR MEDICAL EDUCATION

As one looks at the major problems and trends in medical education in the United States, it becomes immediately apparent that the basic educational issues cannot be considered apart from professional, manpower, health planning, and political issues. The problems of medical education are complex and cannot be effectively addressed without some commonly shared view of a future health care system that is realistic, affordable, and responsive to the public interest.

The foregoing discussion demonstrates considerable flux and confusion in the rapidly changing patterns of medical education in this country. Under these circumstances, it is impossible for anyone to forecast with precision the future for medical education. I find the following predictions recently offered by Ruhe, however, to be of particular interest, based as they are on his unique experience in medical education over a period of 20 years with the Council on Medical Education of the American Medical Association [21]:

1. The public perception of the need for more physicians will be satisfied in the early 1980's.
2. Federal capitation support for medical schools will be discontinued about the same time, or even sooner.
3. Although more new medical schools will continue to be established in the next four years, some existing medical schools will be forced to close, primarily because of fiscal problems, in the next decade.
4. Many, if not most, medical schools will reduce the size of their classes during the next decade because of fiscal problems and because of diminished public pressure for large classes.
5. There will be increased external pressure for regulation of the numbers, types and location of residency programs for the next few years, but that pressure will diminish as the public perception of the need for more physician services is satisfied. However, the external pressure will be intermixed with internal pressure from the profession itself which will continue after the public pressure has diminished.
6. Jurisdictional disputes among various medical specialties, and between medicine and various allied health professions (particularly nursing and pharmacy) will become one of the major problems of the medical profession during the 1980's.
7. Jurisdiction disputes will lead to pressures within the profession for regulation and restriction of educational programs.
8. Within the next decade there will be pressures from within and from outside the profession for limited licensure of physicians, i.e. restriction of the type of practice to the specific fields in which the individuals have had residency training or have been board certified. This will inevitably lead to restrictive definitions of the boundaries of permissible practice in the various specialties.
9. Completion of residency training will become a requirement for licensure in most states.
10. Regular participation in continuing medical education will become a *de facto* requirement for all physicians to continue to practice medicine.
11. Universities will exercise greater control over residency training within their jurisdiction, and there will be increasing pressure to bring all graduate medical education under university surveillance.
12. With residency training compulsory, or nearly so, the significance of the M.D. degree will increasingly be called in question. Eventually the M.D. degree may be granted only at the successful completion of residency training and, like the Ph.D. today, may be granted in a specific discipline, e.g., M.D. in Surgery, M.D. in Family Practice, M.D. in Radiology. This in turn will increase the pressures for limited licensure of physicians according to specialty area of practice.
13. Specialty board certification will inevitably change in nature and may even be supplanted by "specialized" M.D. degrees. Specialty boards will come under in-

creasing pressure from the Federal Trade Commission and others as alleged elitist groups in restraint of competition. Board certification may become a prerequisite for licensure limited to a specialty field.

14. Increasing legislation and regulation of the practice of medicine, and increasing demand for public accountability in health care, will lead to a kind of "cookbook" medicine, where almost all procedures and therapy are prescribed by federal agencies or review bodies such as Professional Standards Review Organizations (PSRO's). This will have profound implications for medical education, since it will promote standardized learning rather than independent thinking.

15. The Coordinating Council on Medical Education and its related liaison committees, which serve as the accrediting bodies for the various levels of medical education, are in for some rough years ahead. They will survive because they have been soundly conceived and because there is no viable alternative.

16. The processes of accreditation and certification increasingly will be subject to public scrutiny. Eventually all or portions of the meetings of the various liaison committees will probably be open to the public.

17. The membership of accrediting and certifying bodies will be broadened to include more public members and voting student and resident members.

Although all of Ruhe's predictions may not take place during the next 10 or 20 years, and some may take a somewhat different shape than projected, most are based on currently developing trends and indicate likely directions for the 1980s. Although the inevitable changes during the next decade will require painful adaptation of today's medical education system, fundamental changes are needed in order to correct some of the present deficiencies in medical education and better meet the needs of the public for health care. What is important is that the right questions are being asked, dialogue is well underway among the involved organizations and interest groups, and a new partnership between government and academic medicine is beginning to be formed.

REFERENCES

1. Sheps CG: Education for what? A decalogue for change. JAMA 238:234, 1977
2. Editorial. A new Flexner report? JAMA 290:930, 1969
3. Strassman HD, Taylor DD, Scoles J: A new concept for a core medical curriculum. J Med Educ 44:170, 1969
4. Glaser RJ: The university medical center and its responsibility to the community. J Med Educ 43:793, 1968
5. Funkenstein DH: Implications of the rapid social changes in universities and medical schools for the education of future physicians. J Med Educ 43:443, 1968
6. Anlyan WG: What has happened to the AAMC since the Coggeshall Report of 1965. JAMA 210:1897, 1969
7. Beck JC, Lee PR, LeRoy L, Stalcup J: The primary care problem. Clin Res 24:260, 1976

8. Annual Report, The American Board of Medical Specialties. Evanston, Illinois, 1975, p 3

9. Chase RA: Proliferation of certification in medical specialties; productive or counterproductive. N Engl J Med 294:497, 1976

10. Sheps CG: Education for what? A decalogue for change. JAMA 238:233, 1977

11. Cohen WJ: Medical education and physicians manpower from the national level. J Med Educ 44:15, 1969

12. Editorial. What's wrong with medical education? JAMA 211:1849, 1970

13. Jason H: The relevance of medical education to medical practice. JAMA 212:2093, 1970

14. White KL, Williams TF, Greenberg BG: The ecology of medical care. N Engl J Med 265:890, 1961

15. Stevens RA: Graduate medical education: A continuing history. J Med Educ 53:13, 1978

16. Progress and Problems in Medical and Dental Education: Federal Support versus Federal Control. Report of the Carnegie Council on Policy Studies in Higher Education. San Francisco, Jossey-Bass, 1976, p 1

17. A Manpower Policy for Primary Health Care. Institute of Medicine. National Academy of Sciences, Washington, D.C., 1978, p 6

18. 94th Congress: Health Professions Educational Assistance Act of 1976 (P.L. 94–484). Washington, D.C., U.S. Government Printing Office, 1976

19. Whiteside DF: Training the nation's health manpower—the next 4 years. Public Health Rep 92:99, 1977

20. Beck JC, Lee PR, LeRoy L, Stalcup J: The primary care problem. Clin Res 24:264, 1976

21. Ruhe CHW: Looking ahead in medical education. AHME J 26, Spring 1978

22. New Mandate for Manpower, Annual Report Fiscal 1977, Bureau of Health Manpower. DHEW Publication No. (HRA) 78–41, 10, 1978

23. Marrienfeld RD: Comparison of initial house staff goals with eventual career plans in internal medicine. J Med Educ 52:853, 1977

24. Wechsler H, Dorsey JL, Bovey JD: A follow-up study of residents in internal medicine, pediatrics and obstetrics–gynecology training programs in Massachusetts: Implications for primary care physicians. N Engl J Med 298:15, 1978

25. Charney E: Internal medicine and pediatric residency education for primary care. J Med Educ 130 (suppl.), December 1975

26. Schwarz MR: WAMI—An experiment in regional medical education. West J Med 121:333, 1974

27. Werner PT, Richards RW, Fogle BJ: Ambulatory family practice experience as the primary and integrating clinical concept in a four-year undergraduate curriculum. J Fam Pract 7:325, 1978

28. Medical education in the United States, 1976–1977. JAMA 238:26, 1977

29. McFarland J: The physician's location decision. In Balfe BE, Lorant JH, Todd C (eds): The Profile of Medical Practice. Chicago, AMA, 1973, p 89

30. Editorial: Specialty distribution and the CCME. J Med Educ 52:861, 1977

31. Beck JC, Lee PR, LeRoy L, Stalcup J: The primary care problem. Clin Res 24:266, 1976

32. Medical Education in the United States, 1976–1977. JAMA 238:2771, 1977

33. Davidson CS: Student revolt and our medical schools. In Popper H (ed): Trends in New Medical Schools. New York, Grune and Stratton, 1967, p 124

34. Maloney WF: Problems of new medical schools, here and abroad: Medical education for tomorrow. In Popper H (ed): Trends in New Medical Schools. New York, Grune and Stratton, 1967, p 49
35. Suess JF: Teaching psychodiagnosis and observation by self-instructional programmed videotapes. J Med Educ 48:676, 1973
36. Stenchever MA, Brown TC: A network for the dissemination of teaching materials. J Med Educ 47:702, 1972

CHAPTER EIGHT

Undergraduate Education for Family Practice

Medical schools are owned by their society. The basic unit of society is the family. The history of mankind suggests that as long as there are families there will be a demand for family doctors. In the future our medical schools will produce family doctors in a planned relationship to needs. Public support for medical schools will reflect the adequacy, or inadequacy, of response to needs.
James L. Dennis [1]

Shifting the focus now to education for family practice, this is the first of three chapters that will deal with the continuum of education in the specialty. The first phase in this continuum—the undergraduate phase—has been an area of remarkable development during the last ten years. In 1970, there were just a handful of organized teaching programs in family practice in United States medical schools. At the close of the 1970s, well over 80 percent of medical schools have organized teaching programs in family practice, and they already have made considerable impact on the milieu of undergraduate medical education and on the growth of student interest in family practice as a career.

The purpose of this chapter is fourfold: (1) to discuss briefly some basic issues that underlie the development of undergraduate teaching programs in family practice, (2) to outline the major requisites for these programs, (3) to describe two illustrative programs, and (4) to comment on some of the lessons that have been learned from these efforts during the 1970s.

SOME BASIC ISSUES

At the initial stages of planning for any teaching program in family practice for medical students, a number of fundamental issues present themselves. Five of these merit consideration as a means of better understanding the content, style, and problems of those programs that have developed to date.

Content of Teaching

Two legitimate questions inevitably asked by medical educators and academicians in other disciplines are (1) What is the definition of family medicine? and (2) What can family practice contribute to the medical student's education that is not already being presented by the other departments? The first question has been dealt with in earlier chapters and will not be recounted here. The second question can be answered partly in terms of the content and process of family practice as a delivery mode and partly in terms of gaps in existing undergraduate medical curricula.

The content of undergraduate teaching in family practice can logically be based on the functions of the family physician that have already been described. Thus, as Leaman [2] suggests, the medical student needs exposure and active involvement with the following functional and content areas of family practice:

1. First contact care of clinical problems seen in primary care
2. Comprehensive health care for over 90 percent of the health problems of patients of either sex and any age
3. Health maintenance
4. Intrafamily psychodynamics
5. Community medicine
6. Home care
7. Continuity of care
8. Close doctor–patient relationship

The dimensions of undergraduate teaching in family medicine include the knowledge, skills, and attitudes derived from the role of the family physician. As pointed out by Pellegrino [3]:

Any such curriculum must teach a set of skills—intellectual and practical—that are specific to the clinical function of the generalist and the family practitioner. Defining these skills more precisely, illustrating their use, and demonstrating them clinically in the domain of the family are the special educational assignments of a department of family medicine.

Barnett [4] has taken the additional step of developing some undergraduate courses in family practice oriented to the commonly occurring clinical entities seen in family practice that often represent gaps in the existing curriculum of the medical school. The intent here is to complement, not compete with, the teaching efforts of the other departments.

Site of Teaching

Several basic issues are important with respect to the location of undergraduate teaching in family medicine, such as (1) What should be the relative emphasis between ambulatory and hospital-based teaching? and (2) To what extent should teaching programs be based in the university, in the community, or in a combination of both settings?

Since the predominant focus of family practice, together with the other primary care specialties, is on ambulatory care, it is quite appropriate that the family practice office serve as the principal base of undergraduate teaching in family medicine. However, since the family physician is involved in continuity of care based on the needs of the patient, other ambulatory settings will be involved to a lesser extent (i.e., the emergency room, the nursing home, and the patient's home), and the hospital will likewise be involved for inpatient care provided by the family physician.

There is ample evidence that house staff in the various specialties have provided a substantial part of medical education for many years and that students often learn best from students and residents just two or three years ahead of them in their training. Medical students need to form some impression of the nature of residency training in family practice and to see role models of young physicians in graduate training in this field. For these reasons, it is essential that some portion of undergraduate teaching in family medicine be provided in the context of the family practice residency program.

Since family practice is based in the community as a primary care delivery mode, it is logical that community settings, whether urban, suburban, or rural, be emphasized in the undergraduate teaching of family medicine. There is an important need, however, for university-based teaching of family medicine that affords medical students ready access to family practice faculty and residents as visible role models. There are special problems in developing a teaching practice by family physicians in the university setting. Nevertheless, this has been effectively accomplished by family practice programs in many medical schools, and the maintenance of these teaching practices poses no major obstacles as long as the concepts of family practice remain their orienting focus and excessive involvement in the total needs of the institution for undifferentiated primary care are avoided.

Organization of Curriculum

Another basic issue that immediately surfaces whenever an undergraduate teaching program in family medicine is being considered in any institution is the question of how its curriculum should be organized and integrated within the medical school. This larger question subsumes a number of related questions, such as:

1. To what extent is there consensus within the medical school faculty concerning the desired goals and product of undergraduate medical education?
2. How much of the medical school class should receive exposure to family medicine?
3. Should a family physician "track" or "pathway" be organized within the curriculum?
4. What should be required and/or elective in the family medicine curriculum?
5. To what extent can curriculum time be made available for new courses in another discipline in an already crowded undergraduate curriculum?
6. What is the present and projected capability of the family practice faculty to develop and maintain new undergraduate courses in family medicine?
7. What lead time is needed to implement each increment of family medicine teaching to the overall curriculum?

Assuming that sufficient resources are available to the family practice department and that the institution is committed to the education of future family physicians in substantial numbers, the ideal responses to these questions would clearly involve meaningful exposure of all medical students to family medicine and sufficient flexibility of the overall curriculum to accomplish this aim. Ideal circumstances remain elusive, however, and later sections of this chapter will demonstrate how some of these questions have been addressed to date in actual practice.

Linkage with Graduate Education in Family Practice

Another fundamental question in family practice, as in other clinical disciplines, concerns what should be offered at the undergraduate level as opposed to later residency training in the field. Although there will inevitably be some overlap at each level, the resolution of this issue can be aided by making a distinction between *education* and *training*.

In Britain the Royal Commission on Medical Education [5] has addressed this question in the following terms, which seem equally applicable in the United States:

> We cannot emphasize too strongly that the undergraduate course in medicine should be primarily *educational*. Its object is not to produce a fully qualified doctor, but an educated man who becomes fully qualified in the course of postgraduate training.

Wright elaborates on this point in this way [6]:

> . . . while the hallmark of training is its particularity, the hallmark of education is its universality. Training is predominantly concerned with the preparation of an individual for specific tasks, i.e., with skills (and with knowledge insofar as it is relevant to those skills). Education, by contrast, is not confined to specific tasks, nor to skills and their related knowledge, but is also much concerned with ways of thinking and attitudes. It aims to develop a capacity for "transfer"—the ability to apply the insights of any one discipline to the problems of another and a capacity for intellectual integration and synthesis.

Logistic Problems

It is one matter to identify the needs and develop a plan for an undergraduate teaching program in family medicine, but quite another to implement such a program. One critical dimension in the implementation phase relates to logistic problems, particularly those concerned with the limited resources of most family practice departments in their early years.

As relative newcomers in academic medicine, family practice departments are charged with broad responsibilities simultaneously, including the need to develop their clinical base, organize residency training programs, recruit and develop faculty, and initiate research and other scholarly activities in the discipline. Since these departments usually have limited funding and numbers of faculty to meet all of these goals, priorities need to be established as to what is possible to accomplish within the limits of available resources. Perhaps the most challenging dilemma in this respect is the relative emphasis to be directed to graduate versus undergraduate teaching, since both are essential and interrelated needs.

REQUISITES FOR AN UNDERGRADUATE TEACHING PROGRAM

With this background, it is useful to outline briefly some basic requisites for any developing or projected undergraduate teaching program in family medicine.

Department of Family Practice

Given the scope of the mission of the developing family practice program in the medical school, an academic and administrative unit is clearly needed that can best mobilize and support this effort. A free-standing department is required and is the principal approach being taken in United States medical schools, which by 1978 had organized 88 such departments. As a division of another department, or as a free-standing division responsible to the dean, the capability of the family practice program to develop and flourish in the competitive academic environment is compromised.

The department of family practice (or family medicine) should have its own clinical and teaching service (both ambulatory and inpatient), adequate budget, and full representation as a major clinical department within the medical school. The department should preferably be headed by a family physician with both teaching and practice experience.

Exemplary Clinical Settings

The clinical sites for medical student teaching in family medicine should effectively illustrate the full dimensions of family practice as defined in earlier chapters. These sites will usually include the department's clinical base at the university, but should include an emphasis on community-based practices, whether associated with affiliated family practice residency programs or exemplary group practices of family physicians in the community. The full spectrum of clinical problems seen in the primary care of a diverse patient population should be represented, and ready access to consultants and other community resources should be available.

These clinical settings should be actively involved in the monitoring of quality of care through audit and in the maintenance of modern medical record and data retrieval systems. An atmosphere of critical inquiry is essential to the learning climate for all involved in the teaching program.

Coordinated Four-Year Curriculum

In order to make available to medical students appropriate exposure to the knowledge, skills, and attitudes of the family physician, as well as to provide sufficient experience to allow an informed career decision for their future specialties, family medicine must be offered in each year of the overall curriculum, usually over a four-year period. The curriculum in family medicine should be planned carefully to assure coordination of learning objectives and content. Provisions for progressive levels of responsibility should also be made, as exemplified by the changing role of second-year medical students in the Department of Family Medicine's continuity clerkship at the University of Washington (Table 8–1).[7]

Alfred North Whitehead has divided the process of learning into three phases: (1) romance, (2) precision, and (3) generalization, or synthesis.[8] This concept can serve as a useful framework for progression from a largely passive observational learning experience for first-year medical students (romance); to a more focused, content-based third-year clerkship experience (precision); to a fourth-year advanced clerkship at a subinternship level (synthesis).

In addition to intradepartmental coordination of the undergraduate curriculum in family medicine, further coordination is needed in order to integrate

TABLE 8–1. LEVELS OF PATIENT CARE INVOLVEMENT OVER THREE TERMS FOR 38 CONTINUITY CLERKSHIP STUDENTS

| | PERCENT VISITS | | |
STUDENT LEVELS OF INVOLVEMENT	Fall	Winter	Spring
Observation role	45	27	22
Assistance role	35	39	36
Primary role	20	34	42
Total	100	100	100

Source: Smith, C.K., Gordon, M.J., Leversee, J.H., and Hadac, R.R.: Early ambulatory experience in the undergraduate education of family physicians. *Journal of Family Practice* 5:227, 1977.

the program within the medical school curriculum. An example of the integration of preclinical family medicine electives with the required introduction to clinical medicine courses at the University of Washington is shown in Figure 8–1.[7]

Family Practice Role Models

Perhaps the single most important element in the quality and effectiveness of the undergraduate teaching program in family medicine is the caliber of the family physicians themselves as teachers and role models. Teachers must be

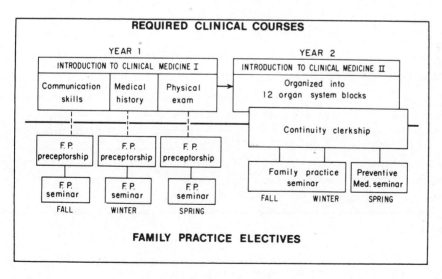

FIGURE 8-1.

Integration of family practice electives into required clinically oriented courses in a preclinical medical school curriculum.

Source: Smith, CK, Gordon, MJ, Leversee, JH, Hadac, RR: Early ambulatory experience in the undergraduate education of family physicians. *Journal of Family Practice* 5:227, 1977.

carefully selected who best demonstrate the attributes of the excellent family physician. As noted by Scherger,[9] when he was a medical student, "The clinical student interested in an alternative to the secondary and tertiary care of the academic center will be taking a very close look at the family physician, his life style, and his practice."

Beyond a high level of clinical competency in dealing with the wide range of clinical problems in family practice, the family physician teacher needs to display a genuine concern for the well being of his/her patients and their families, together with a blending of the art and science of medicine. In addition, the family physician teacher should be comfortable in sharing with students his personal philosophy of practice, including his views of the challenges and satisfactions of everyday practice.

Advising Program

Today's medical student is confronted by a curriculum of increasing complexity and the need to select a field for further training and practice from among a growing number of specialties and subspecialties. This is made more difficult by the elimination in recent years of the internship year, which forces medical students to make what are usually lifetime decisions by the end of the third year or the first part of the fourth year in medical school. The pressure of early career decisions represents a difficult dilemma for many medical students. This can be partly alleviated by an active counseling and advising program by faculty. Family practice faculty need to be fully involved as advisors for students interested in this field, both as role models and for help with selection of courses and options for residency training.

Evaluation System

All parts of the undergraduate teaching program in family medicine require periodic evaluation and revision as needed. The evaluation process includes student and faculty performance, student assessment of courses and faculty, and the content of students' actual learning experiences. Daily student logs have been found useful in the evaluation of a decentralized rural family medicine clerkship for third- and fourth-year medical students at the University of Washington.[10] Tables 8–2 and 8–3, for example, display frequency, level of responsibility and site of experience for diagnoses and procedures, respectively.[10]

TWO ILLUSTRATIVE PROGRAMS

A brief thumbnail sketch of two undergraduate teaching programs in family medicine is of interest in viewing operational curricula and actual progress

TABLE 8-2. DIAGNOSES ENCOUNTERED AT LEAST (A) TWICE PER WEEK, (B) ONCE PER WEEK

DIAGNOSES	FREQUENCY	LEVEL OF RESPONSIBILITY			SITE OF EXPERIENCE					ON-GOING OR NEW	
		Primary	Assisting	Observing	Office	Hospital	House Call	Nursing Home	ER		
A. Twice per week											
Upper respiratory infection	262	239	10	7	196	10	2	1	40	38	193
Otitis media	242	195	24	10	148	4	15	3	45	49	185
Surgical aftercare	219	141	37	35	91	122	3	1	1	164	42
Pre-, post-partum examination	208	165	29	10	167	39	2	0	0	91	110
Pediatric physical	206	184	4	11	139	44	18	0	2	67	131
Fracture	199	103	75	18	56	75	0	1	68	65	119
B. Once per week											
Abdominal pain	188	149	31	3	89	37	1	3	56	66	111
Lacerations	182	161	13	2	54	16	0	0	110	26	138
Hypertension	172	139	22	5	160	4	1	0	3	78	83
Low back pain syndrome	147	128	14	3	68	56	2	1	18	72	67
Sprain	142	119	15	8	68	3	2	0	62	29	109
Medical aftercare	132	109	11	6	34	93	3	0	2	114	12
Adult routine physical	117	101	2	2	90	19	0	1	2	25	79
Drug abuse	99	66	14	11	19	41	3	0	30	30	53
Rash	97	69	20	4	78	1	3	2	8	17	71
Asthma	96	67	17	7	51	16	0	1	24	28	59
Urinary tract infection	96	73	16	4	66	13	2	3	11	29	57
Pneumonia	93	81	8	3	36	46	2	0	10	38	49
Routine delivery	91	28	49	14	0	88	0	0	1	23	60

Source: Zinser, E.A. and Wiegert, H.T.: Describing learning experiences of undergraduate medical students in rural settings. *Journal of Family Practice* 3:287, 1976.

TABLE 8–3. PROCEDURES DONE AT LEAST (A) ONCE PER WEEK, (B) ONCE PER MONTH

PROCEDURES	FREQUENCY	LEVEL OF RESPONSIBILITY			SITE OF EXPERIENCE				
		Primary	Assisting	Observing	Office	Hospital	House Call	Nursing Home	ER
A. Once per week									
Lacerations	278	247	12	7	65	24	0	0	0
Pelvic examination	159	119	20	13	138	13	0	0	6
Pap smear	99	81	7	8	94	5	0	0	0
Cast	96	63	26	9	56	23	3	0	18
Counseling	84	68	9	3	59	20	3	0	1
B. Once per month									
Incision and drainage	50	26	14	9	33	8	0	0	8
Circumcision	42	24	8	10	0	41	0	0	0
Dilatation and curettage	36	11	23	2	1	35	0	0	0
Intrauterine device	34	18	3	13	33	0	0	0	0
Remove foreign body	34	21	8	5	15	3	0	0	16
Remove subcutaneous foreign body	34	23	7	2	16	5	1	0	13
Biopsy excision skin	33	11	17	6	22	11	0	0	0
Exploratory laparotomy	30	0	28	2	0	33	0	0	0
Proctosigmoidoscopy	27	5	13	9	19	7	0	0	1
Hysterectomy	26	0	22	2	0	25	0	0	0
Joint aspiration	25	14	8	4	18	3	0	0	0
Skin lesion cauterization	25	12	6	6	22	1	0	1	2
Tonsillectomy and adenoids	23	5	12	5	0	22	0	0	0
Vasectomy	22	1	14	7	21	1	0	0	0

Source: Zinser, E.A. and Wiegert, H.T.: Describing learning experiences of undergraduate medical students in rural settings. *Journal of Family Practice* 3:287, 1976.

against the general background that has been presented. The two programs are located in different parts of the country and represent a recently established medical school and one that is 30 years old.

Southern Illinois University [11]

The Southern Illinois University School of Medicine was established in the early 1970s with the overall purpose to train the kinds of physicians needed by the state and to improve patient care in its area. The plan from the beginning called for use of existing community facilities, and no new university teaching hospital was built. The first year of medical school is located in Carbondale, Illinois, at the university's main campus, while the rest of the teaching effort in subsequent years of medical school is centered primarily in Springfield in relation to two sizable community hospitals. The charter class of 48 medical students was enrolled in 1973.

In the medical school's formative years, representatives from the community participated in the planning process, and emphasis on family medicine was to be an important part of the school's goals in response to the acute need for primary care physicians in southern Illinois. The chairman of the Department of Family Medicine was the first departmental chairman to be appointed, and other departmental chairmen were partly selected on the basis of their support of family medicine. The medical school's admissions policies favor applicants from central and southern Illinois, and about one-third of the medical students are from communities with populations of less than 10,000. A family medicine curriculum has been developed with exposure to the entire class (48 students) in each year of medical school (Table 8–4).

Sequence I is provided at the Carbondale campus, with active input by family practice faculty into *Introduction to Clinical Medicine I*, a course on interviewing and clinical skills. Sequence II is presented in Springfield, again with the full participation of family practice faculty in *Introduction to Clinical Medicine II*, which includes an "introduction to the clinical clerkship."

TABLE 8–4. SOUTHERN ILLINOIS UNIVERSITY FAMILY
MEDICINE CURRICULUM

Sequence I:	Introduction to Clinical Medicine I
Sequence II:	Introduction to Clinical Medicine II
Sequence III:	Family practice clerkship (26 weeks, part time) Inpatient (4 weeks)
Sequence IV:	Elective preceptorship (2 to 4 weeks) Other electives

Source: Baker, R.M., McWhinney, I., and Brown T.C.: Undergraduate education in family medicine. *Journal of Family Practice* 5:37, 1977.

Sequence III comprises the required clinical clerkships and includes two core experiences in family practice: (1) a longitudinal family practice ambulatory clerkship (one-half day per week for six months in the Family Practice Center); and (2) the family practice hospital clerkship, a one-month rotation on the family practice service in an affiliated community hospital in Springfield. Sequence IV involves an elective preceptorship of two to four weeks' duration in rural or suburban family practices, as well as a number of additional electives including the following:

1. Family practice clinic—6 weeks half time
2. Community service agencies—2 weeks half time
3. Physical medicine and rehabilitation—1 week half time
4. Alcoholism—2 weeks full time
5. Family life enrichment seminar—6 weeks, 1 day per week
6. Preventive and problem-solving counseling—6 weeks, one-half day per week
7. Nutrition—1 week half time
8. Independent research project—4 weeks full or half time

Most of the undergraduate teaching in family medicine is carried out at the medical school, which, as already noted, is community based itself. Medical students on family practice clerkships have ample opportunities to work with family practice residents. There are eight full-time family physicians on the departmental faculty. About two-thirds of the department's efforts are devoted to undergraduate teaching compared to one-third to resident teaching.

Of the class graduating in 1976, 12 went on to family practice residency training, whereas 17 of the 47 graduates in 1977 went into family practice residencies.

University of Washington [11]

The University of Washington School of Medicine was founded in 1946 and during the 1950s and 1960s developed into a nationally recognized academic and biomedical research center. The mission of the medical school was expanded during the late 1960s and 1970s to directly address the needs of the four-state WAMI region (Washington, Alaska, Montana, and Idaho). The class size was increased from 100 to 175, with a total of 60 positions in each class allocated to applicants from Alaska, Montana, and Idaho.

As the only medical school in the WAMI region, the medical school's teaching efforts are decentralized in all four states under the auspices of the WAMI program.[12] Medical students from Alaska, Montana, and Idaho take their entire first year of medical school in these states, and clinical clerkships are offered in all of the major specialties in each of these states.

A major curriculum revision was implemented in 1968 by which four pathways were made available to students during their last two years of medical school—the family physician, the clinical specialist, the behavioral specialist, and the medical scientist pathways. In 1975–1976, these pathways were selected by the entering third-year class as follows: 40 percent, 40 percent, 10 percent and 10 percent, respectively. In 1978, the behavioral specialist pathway was discontinued due to low enrollments. The clinical specialist and family physician pathways drew the largest enrollments throughout the 1970s, with usually about one-half of each class opting for the latter.

The Department of Family Medicine was established in 1971 after one initial organizational year as a division responsible to the dean. Since that time, aided by the solid support of the administration and departments of the medical school, a clinical and teaching base has been established at the University Hospital in Seattle. Heavy emphasis has also been directed to the development of undergraduate and graduate teaching in the community. As part of the WAMI program, eight community clinical units have been established in group family practices in each of the four states in the WAMI region. Six of these units are presently located in rural communities—Anacortes and Omak, Washington; Ketchikan, Alaska; Kalispell and Whitefish, Montana; and Pocatello, Idaho. Two of the units are located in the larger communities of Spokane, Washington, and Anchorage, Alaska.

The current undergraduate curriculum in family medicine is shown in Table 8–5. The Department of Family Medicine has a primary role in the *Introduction to Clinical Medicine* course for first-year medical students. Additional exposure to family practice is provided through the first-year preceptorship with local family physicians as a "romance" experience. More active in-

TABLE 8-5.   UNIVERSITY OF WASHINGTON FAMILY
            MEDICINE CURRICULUM

First year—Basic
    Orientation
    Introduction to clinical medicine
    Introduction to family medicine
       ($\frac{1}{2}$ day per week for 1 quarter)
Second year—Organ systems
    Continuity clerkship and seminar
       ($\frac{1}{2}$ day per week for 3 quarters)
Third year   Advisor
    Basic family medicine clerkship   system
       (4 weeks)
Fourth year—Electives
    Community clinical clerkship in family medicine
       (6 weeks)
    Advanced preceptorship in family medicine

Source: Modified from Baker, R.M., McWhinney, I., and Brown, T.C.: Undergraduate education in family medicine. *Journal of Family Practice* 5:37, 1977.

volvement by students is offered in the second-year continuity clerkship, which again is provided in the practice of family physicians in the Seattle area. A four-week basic family medicine clerkship is now being developed in the setting of the University Hospital Family Medicine Residency Program; this is a structured didactic and experiential clerkship that will be extended during the next two years to eight other family practice residencies within the department's regional network of affiliated residencies. The community clinical clerkship in family medicine is a six-week "synthesis" experience for all medical students in the family physician pathway.[13] It is offered in the eight WAMI community clinical units previously mentioned for medical students in the latter portion of their third or fourth year.

In addition to these courses, the department offers a number of electives, including an advanced preceptorship in family medicine (fourth year) and an independent study/research elective (all years).

The Department of Family Medicine has 11 full-time family physicians on the university-based faculty, and divides its teaching efforts approximately equally between undergraduate teaching and residency training.

The pattern of medical student career choice during the first 10 years after the major curriculum change of 1968 was recently reported by Phillips and his colleagues. Whereas only 5 to 15 percent of each graduating class entered general/family practice before the curriculum change, one-third of graduates have pursued family practice residency training since 1973 (Figure 8-2).[14]

COMMENT

The two programs that have been described have many of the same elements, including active involvement in preclinical teaching (especially through introduction to clinical medicine courses), clerkships, preceptorships, and electives. They differ, however, in the extent to which undergraduate education in family

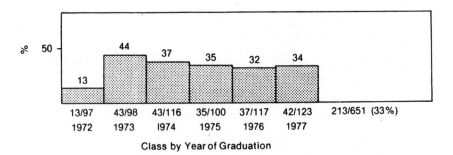

FIGURE 8-2.

Proportion of all graduates entering training for family practice.

Source: Phillips, TJ, Gordon, MJ, Leversee, JH, and Smith, CK: A family physician pathway and medical student career choice. *JAMA* (240:1736), 1978. Copyright 1978 by the American Medical Association.

medicine is decentralized, and in the way the family medicine curriculum is integrated within the overall medical school curriculum. These differences illustrate one point that has been learned during the 1970s—that the organization and conduct of undergraduate teaching in family medicine need to be adapted to the goals, needs, and settings of each individual institution.

Most of the undergraduate teaching programs in family medicine around the country have adopted many of the elements represented by the programs at Southern Illinois University and the University of Washington. Some programs have developed a variety of other approaches to undergraduate teaching, including courses in such areas as geriatrics,[15-17] sexual and marital health,[16] and applied basic science.[18]

A national survey of United States and Canadian undergraduate teaching programs in family practice was conducted in 1975 to study the relationships between administrative structure, size of program, faculty size, and type of undergraduate curriculum and the number of graduates selecting graduate training in family practice. This study involved a response rate of 90 percent

TABLE 8-6. TYPE OF ADMINISTRATIVE UNIT AND PROPORTION OF STUDENTS CHOOSING FAMILY PRACTICE RESIDENCIES

ADMINISTRATIVE UNIT	PROPORTION CHOOSING FAMILY PRACTICE				
	0–10%	11–20%	21–30%	34–40%	N
Department	10.6	51.1	27.7	10.6	47
Division	66.7	22.2	11.1	0.0	9
Other	50.0	50.0	0.0	0.0	6
N	14	29	14	5	62

Source: Beck, J.D., Stewart, W.L., Graham, R., and Stern, T.L.: The effect of the organization and status of family practice undergraduate programs on residency selection. *Journal of Family Practice* 4:663, 1977.

TABLE 8-7. NUMBER OF FULL-TIME SALARIED FAMILY PHYSICIANS AND PROPORTION OF STUDENTS CHOOSING FAMILY PRACTICE RESIDENCIES

NUMBER OF FULL-TIME FAMILY PHYSICIANS	PROPORTION CHOOSING FAMILY PRACTICE				
	0–10%	11–20%	21–30%	31–40%	N
0–2	35.0	40.0	25.0	0.0	20
3–5	20.8	58.3	20.8	0.0	24
6–9	0.0	53.8	15.4	30.8	13
10 +	40.0	0.0	40.0	20.0	5
N	14	29	14	5	62

Source: Beck, J.D., Stewart, W.L., Graham, R., and Stern, T.L.: The effect of the organization and status of family practice undergraduate programs on residency selection. *Journal of Family Practice* 4:663, 1977.

TABLE 8–8.   ASPECTS OF CURRICULUM AND PROPORTION OF STUDENTS CHOOSING FAMILY PRACTICE RESIDENCIES

| | PROPORTION CHOOSING FAMILY PRACTICE | | | | |
	0–10%	11–20%	21–30%	31–40%	N
Clerkship required					
% Yes	20.0	40.0	13.3	26.7	15
% No	22.7	47.7	27.3	2.3	44
N	13	27	14	5	49
Preceptorship required					
% Yes	11.1	44.4	33.3	11.1	9
% No	23.5	47.1	21.6	7.8	51
N	13	28	14	5	60

Source: Beck, J.D., Stewart, W.L., Graham, R., and Stern, T.L.: The effect of the organization and status of family practice undergraduate programs on residency selection. *Journal of Family Practice* 4:663, 1977.

TABLE 8–9.   RELATIONSHIPS BETWEEN TYPE OF ADMINISTRATIVE UNIT AND CURRICULUM

	% Yes	% No	N
Required Preclinical Courses			
Department	82.0	18.0	50
Division	44.4	55.6	9
Other	20.0	80.0	5
N	46	18	64
Required Clerkships			
Department	35.8	64.2	53
Division	23.1	76.9	13
Other	0.0	100.0	6
N	22	50	72
Required Preceptorships			
Department	22.2	77.8	54
Division	15.4	84.6	13
Other	16.7	83.5	6
N	15	58	73

Source: Beck, J.D., Stewart, W.L., Graham, R., and Stern, T.L.: The effect of the organization and status of family practice undergraduate programs on residency selection. *Journal of Family Practice* 4:663, 1977.

and demonstrated a clear relationship between the commitment of the medical school to family practice, the size of the program, and the presence of required courses in the curriculum to the success of the program as reflected by the proportion of graduates choosing family practice residencies.[19] Positive correlations were established between increased numbers of graduates opting for family practice and the presence of a department of family practice (Table 8–6), a larger number of full-time family physicians on the faculty (Table 8–7), and required family practice clerkships and preceptorships (Table 8–8). An organized department of family practice was also found to influence the extent to which preclinical courses, clerkships, and preceptorships in family practice were required in the medical school's curriculum (Table 8–9).

Excellent progress has been made during the 1970s in the undergraduate teaching of family medicine in United States medical schools. These efforts to date have emphasized the romance and synthesis phases of Whitehead's trilogy. Further growth and development of departments of family practice in the 1980s, particularly as the research base expands in the discipline, can be expected to lead to refinement of these undergraduate teaching programs and an increased degree of precision in their courses.

REFERENCES

1. Dennis JL: The future of family practice in our medical schools. J Fam Pract 1:8, 1974
2. Leaman TL: A predoctoral curriculum in family medicine. J Fam Pract 2:107, 1975
3. Pellegrino ED: The academic viability of family medicine: A triad of challenges. JAMA 240:133, 1978
4. Barnett L: Carving an undergraduate curriculum in family practice. J Fam Pract 1:21, 1974
5. Royal Commission on Medical Education: Report. Cmnd. 3569, London, HMSO., 1968
6. Wright HJ: The logic of medicine—the contribution of general practice to the understanding of clinical method. J R Coll Gen Pract 25:531, 1975
7. Smith CK, Gordon MJ, Leversee JH, Hadac RR: Early ambulatory experience in the undergraduate education of family physicians. J Fam Pract 5:227, 1977
8. Miller G: Teaching and Learning in Medical School. Cambridge, Harvard University Press, 1961, p 67
9. Scherger JE: A medical student's perspective on preceptors in family practice. J Fam Pract 2:201, 1975
10. Zinser EA, Wiegert HT: Describing learning experiences of undergraduate medical students in rural settings. J Fam Pract 3:287, 1976
11. Baker RM, McWhinney I, Brown TC: Undergraduate education in family medicine. J Fam Pract 5:37, 1977
12. Schwarz MR: An experiment in regional medical education. West J Med 121:333, 1974

13. Phillips TJ, Swanson AG, Wiegert HT: Community clinical clerkships for educating family medicine students: Process of development (A WAMI progress report). J Fam Pract 1:23, 1974

14. Phillips TJ, Gordon MJ, Leversee JH, Smith CK: A family physician pathway and medical student career choice. JAMA 240:1736, 1978

15. Somers AR, Warburton SW, Moolten S: Teaching geriatric care: Report on an experimental second-year elective. J Fam Pract 6:573, 1978

16. Henderson RA: Elective experiences in family medicine for medical students. J Fam Pract 3:293, 1976

17. Coggan P, Hodgetts PG, Holtzman J, Ryan N, Ham R: A required program in geriatrics for medical students. J Fam Pract 7:735, 1978

18. Davies TC, Barnett BL: Basic science in a predoctoral family practice curriculum. J Fam Pract 6:311, 1978

19. Beck JD, Stewart WL, Graham R, Stern TL: The effect of the organization and status of family practice undergraduate programs on residency selection. J Fam Pract 4:663, 1977

CHAPTER NINE

Department of Family Medicine (R700)
University of Miami School of Medicine
P. O. Box 016700
Miami, Florida 33101

James M. Gall, M.D., C.C.F.P.
Department of Family Medicine
University of Miami School of Medicine
P. O. Box 016700
Miami, Florida 33101

Graduate Education for Family Practice

Given one well-trained physician of the highest type, he will do better work for a thousand people than ten specialists.

William Mayo [1]

Perhaps the single most impressive feature of the progress demonstrated by the new specialty of family practice over the last ten years is the remarkable growth and development of graduate education in the field. Residencies in family practice are carefully designed as coordinated three-year programs, with the first year taking the place of the older rotating internship. Residency development has been based upon the *Essentials for Graduate Training in Family Practice,* a document first prepared through the joint efforts of the American Academy of Family Physicians, the American Board of Family Practice, the Section on General/Family Practice of the American Medical Association, and the AMA Council on Medical Education. This document has been revised and updated during the last two years and is included for reference as Appendix 2.

Family practice residency training represents several important shifts of direction when compared to other kinds of residency programs: from episodic to continuous and comprehensive care, from a disease-oriented emphasis to focus on the whole patient, from the individual to the family as the patient, and from the solo physician to the physician as a member of a group.

By late 1978, there were 358 approved family practice residency programs in operation in the United States, with 6033 residents in training (Appendix 3). The exponential growth in the number of programs and residents in training is reflected in Table 9–1.

TABLE 9–1.   GROWTH OF FAMILY PRACTICE RESIDENCIES*

YEAR	NUMBER OF APPROVED PROGRAMS	NUMBER OF RESIDENTS	AVERAGE NUMBER OF RESIDENTS PER PROGRAM
1970	49	290	5.9
1971	87	534	6.1
1972	133	1015	7.6
1973	191	1771	9.3
1974	233	2671	11.4
1975	259	3720	14.4
1976	272	4675	17.2
1977	325	5421	16.6
1978	358	6033	16.8

* Information for this table was provided by the Division of Education, American Academy of Family Physicians, Kansas City, Missouri.

This chapter will examine the nature of family practice residency training in this country with three purposes in mind: (1) to present some common features of family practice residencies, (2) to briefly describe two illustrative programs, and (3) to provide an overview of the goals, content, types and current directions of family practice residencies in the United States.

COMMON FEATURES OF FAMILY PRACTICE RESIDENCIES

Family Practice Center

The family practice center is the clinical and teaching base of the family practice residency program. It is designed and located so as to maintain the identity and functions of a group practice of family physicians. It may be located within its related hospital or at some distance from its related hospital(s) (usually not over two or three miles away). The family practice center serves as the resident's base for the continuing care of his/her growing practice over a three-year period and is the site for a substantial portion of the resident's training. To the maximal possible extent, the functions of a family practice group in the community are replicated in the family practice center, including its own separate medical record and practice management systems.

The family practice center, even in a smaller residency program, is usually at least 3000 to 5000 square feet in size. It invariably includes a waiting room, business and medical record office, examination rooms, minor surgery room, office laboratory, conference room/library, and faculty/resident offices. X-ray facilities may also be located in the family practice center, although many programs utilize the x-ray facilities of a nearby hospital. There is generally a sufficient number of examination rooms to provide each resident working in the family practice center with two such rooms at any given time.

The patient population served by the family practice center should represent a broad socioeconomic spectrum from the surrounding community with all age groups included. Individuals and their families should be included in the practice who desire continuity and comprehensiveness of care, not just episodic care for acute medical problems. In most programs, the first-year family practice resident is assigned about 25 families for ongoing care, and spends one (sometimes two) half days each week in the family practice center. In the second and third years, the resident becomes responsible for 100 to 150 families and spends more time in the family practice center (up to three or even five half days per week) as the emphasis on hospital training during the first year shifts more toward ambulatory care by the third year. As residents progress through the family practice residency, they are expected to become more proficient in seeing patients expeditiously as will be needed in their future practices. Under normal circumstances, residents see an average of 5, 10, and 10 to 15 patients each half day in the family practice center during their first, second, and third residency years, respectively.

Beyond the usual clerical and clinical support staff required in most family practice offices, many of the residency programs employ other allied health professionals in the family practice center on either a part-time or full-time basis. Thus, medical social workers, clinical psychologists, clinical pharmacists, physician extenders (Medex, physician assistant, and/or nurse practitioner) or others may be involved in the teaching programs. In addition, residency programs are often able to arrange for consultants in other specialties to teach and consult in the family practice center, so that rather extensive teaching resources can be made available to the resident at the program's home base.

Hospital Training

The family practice residency program requires a close linkage to one or more hospitals for the dual purpose of hospital-based teaching services and hospitalization of patients from the family practice center. Under some circumstances the residency program relates to one hospital (usually at least 200 beds), but often two (and occasionally three) hospitals are needed to accommodate all of the required services. If multiple hospitals are involved, care must be taken to avoid undue fractionation of the program's clinical and teaching efforts, but some fractionation may be unavoidable in a community where some hospitals' services have been consolidated. Figure 9–1 shows the current breakdown by type and setting of hospitals in the United States that are involved in family

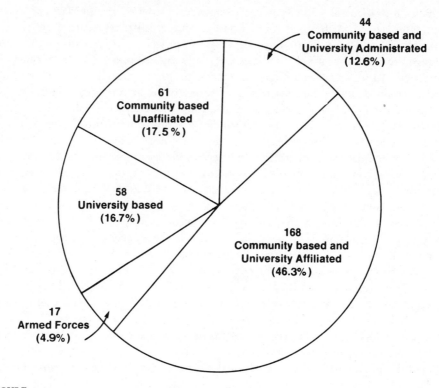

FIGURE 9-1.

Types of family practice residencies (August, 1978). Twelve of the 348 programs utilize one location for the first year and another location for the last two years.

Source: Division of Education, American Academy of Family Physicians, Kansas City, Missouri.

practice residency training. It can be noted that a sizable number of these are university-affiliated community hospitals, and this proportion is increasing.

The great majority of family practice residency programs involve a fixed base over the full three-year period of residency training. A small but growing number of programs, however, are organized on a "one-and-two" basis, with the first year in a larger metropolitan community with its family practice center and large teaching hospital and the final two years of training in a smaller community with the principal family practice center there linked to one or more smaller community hospitals. The "one-and-two" program has several important advantages: (1) it provides family practice residents with a combination of learning experiences in larger and smaller community settings, (2) it affords "reality-based" educational experiences in some smaller community settings without the resources needed for a full three-year program, and (3) it utilizes the potential teaching resources increasingly available in smaller communities in all specialties.[2]

Most programs maintain an active family practice service in a nearby hospital(s) for the care of patients requiring hospitalization from the teaching practice. This assures continuity of care of family practice patients, with consultation requested as needed. Medley and Halstead have reviewed their experience in one family practice residency program, where the family practice service provided care for 631 patients over a one-year period. Consultation was requested in one-third of patients, and in these instances, the family physicians continued to share responsibility for patient care with the consultants. Table 9–2 lists the most common diagnoses encountered during the study.[3]

Hospital teaching rotations are required on all of the major clinical services, including internal medicine, pediatrics, obstetrics–gynecology, and general surgery. The family practice resident also needs inpatient teaching rotations in cardiology and neurology and often takes electives on other services. Emergency room experience and various other specialty experiences add further to the resident's training.

Size of Program

The great majority of family practice residency programs range from 4 residents in each year of the three-year program to 12 residents per year, with the average program having 18 residents (6–6–6). Since the family practice residency is a complex entity requiring continuity of patient care and teaching in the family practice center and its related hospital(s), there must be a sufficient number of residents to meet the program's commitments to patient care, teaching, and related activities. In addition, it is well known that a substantial amount of everyday teaching and learning takes place on a house-staff level between residents one or two years apart in their levels of training. There is now a general consensus that the minimal number or "critical mass" of residents in a family practice residency program should be 12 residents (4–4–4). The optimal size of any one program depends on a number of practical considerations, such as: (1) the extent of educational resources, (2) the need for family physicians in the area served by the program, (3) the availability of funding and other kinds of support for the program, (4) the logistics of inpatient teaching rotations, (5) the logistics of night and weekend coverage, and (6) the size of the teaching practice.[4]

Faculty

The faculty of the typical family practice residency program usually includes three or four full-time family physicians, with the number depending on the size of the program. A common ratio is one full-time family physician teacher for every six residents in the program plus the program director, who also is preferably a family physician with a background in practice and teaching. The full-time family physician faculty is actively involved in the teaching

TABLE 9-2. MOST COMMON DIAGNOSES ON ONE FAMILY PRACTICE RESIDENCY INPATIENT SERVICE

DIAGNOSIS	NUMBER OF CASES
Intrauterine pregnancy (uncomplicated)	96
Newborns (uncomplicated)	90
Newborns (complicated)*	26
Chest pain, possible MI	26
Gastroenteritis	17
Arteriosclerotic heart disease, acute MI	16
Asthma	15
Arteriosclerotic heart disease, not specified	14
Arteriosclerotic heart disease, congestive failure	13
Diabetes mellitus	13
Intrauterine pregnancy (complicated)	13
Low back pain other than herniated nucleus pulposus	13
Pneumonia	12
Overdose	11
Concussion	10
Soft-tissue trauma	10
Abdominal pain	9
Thrombophlebitis	8
Hypertension	8
Urinary tract infection	8
Herniated nucleus pulposus	7
Chronic obstructive pulmonary disease	6
Bronchitis, acute	6
Pelvic inflammatory disease tuboovarian abscess	6
Bony trauma	6
Leg pain	4
Cellulitis	4
Supraventricular tachycardia	4
Seizures	4
Croup	4
Viral illnesses	4
Spontaneous abortion	4
Reflux esophagitis	3
Depression	3
Ureteral colic	3
Excessive weight gain	2
Pyelonephritis	2
Conversion reaction	2
Situational stress reaction	2
Epididymitis	2
Other	126
Total	631

* Includes all newborns with jaundice requiring phototherapy, as well as respiratory distress syndrome, congenital defects, etc.

Source: modified from Medley, E.S., and Halstead, M.L.: A family practice residency inpatient service: A review of 631 admissions. *Journal of Family Practice* 6:817, 1978.

practice in the family practice center, makes daily rounds on the family practice service in the hospital(s), is available to the residents on call during nights and weekends, and participates actively in other parts of the teaching program, such as conferences and didactic sessions.

Other specialties are also involved actively in the teaching program, sometimes on a full-time basis and more often on a part-time basis. The specialties most commonly represented in this capacity include internal medicine, pediatrics, obstetrics–gynecology, and psychiatry. University-based and community hospital programs differ considerably in their arrangements for teaching involvement by other specialties. The larger teaching hospitals tend to have existing full-time and part-time teaching staffs involved in the conduct of their respective teaching services. Family practice residencies in smaller community hospitals often employ part-time consultants in the major specialties to teach in the program as well as to arrange and coordinate the teaching efforts by other consultants in their specialty on a voluntary basis.

Most family practice residencies include a full-time or part-time behavioral science teacher on the regular faculty. Hornsby and Kerr recently studied the patterns of behavioral science teaching in United States family practice residency programs and found that 304 individuals were involved in this kind of teaching in 136 programs, most often on a part-time basis. Of this total, 93 (30 percent) were psychiatrists, 78 (26 percent) psychologists, 42 (14 percent) social workers, and the remainder represented a diversity of backgrounds (Table 9–3).[5]

In addition to the above faculty, the typical family practice residency involves a substantial number of other physicians—in family practice and all of the other specialties—in the teaching program on a voluntary basis. They may participate as attending physicians in the family practice center or on hospital teaching services, present didactic sessions, or contribute to periodic teaching conferences. Thus, the family practice residency, regardless of its setting or size, invariably involves the active participation of a large number of physicians in all of the specialties, as well as nonphysicians in other health professions.

Educational Goals

Goals and objectives for any educational program cannot be developed without understanding the needs for the program, its graduates, and individual residents within the program. Figure 9–2 illustrates what has come to be known as the *process model* of education.

Some of the issues requiring consideration in formulating the goals of a family practice residency program are: (1) What are the needs of the community? (2) What is the community being served (socioeconomically, culturally and geographically)? (3) What kinds of practice settings are likely for program graduates? and (4) How are patterns of health care changing, and how do they influence future needs? Resolution of these issues for any given program clearly

TABLE 9–3.   TEACHERS OF BEHAVIORAL SCIENCE IN 136 FAMILY PRACTICE RESIDENCIES

DISCIPLINE	NUMBER	PERCENT
Medicine	139	46
Psychiatry	93	
Family practice*	37	
Internal medicine	4	
Pediatrics	3	
Neurology	2	
Psychology	78	26
Social work	42	14
Counseling	24	8
Other	21	6
Theology	5	
Sociology	5	
Anthropology	2	
Health education	2	
Media education	2	
Nursing	2	
Management	2	
Hospital administration	1	
Total	304	100

* Family practice and family medicine were combined.

Source: Hornsby, J.L., Kerr, R.M.: Behavioral science and family practice: A status report. *Journal of Family Practice* 8:299, 1978.

relates closely to curriculum, resident selection, design and function of the family practice center, and many other elements of the program.

Three overall goals of a family practice residency program might therefore be formulated as follows:

1. To train family physicians able to respond to changing health care needs of the area/region served by the program.
2. To produce well-trained clinicians capable of providing definitive care of about 95 percent of the health problems of individuals and their families that require physician visits.
3. To encourage group practice by graduate programs involving family practice teams.

FIGURE 9-2.
Process model of education.

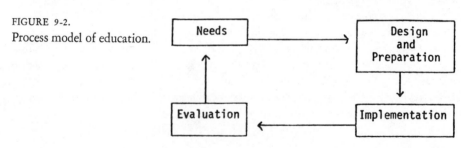

More specific goal statements for family practice residents have recently been developed and endorsed by the Society of Teachers of Family Medicine [6]; the family practice resident shall, after completion of a residency:

1. Demonstrate clinical excellence, utilizing current biomedical knowledge in identifying and managing the medical problems presented by his/her patients.
2. Provide continuing and comprehensive care to individuals and families.
3. Demonstrate the ability to integrate the behavioral, emotional, social, and environmental factors of families in promoting health and managing disease.
4. Recognize the importance of maintaining and developing the knowledge, skills, and attitudes required for the best in modern medical practice in a rapidly changing world and pursue a regular and systematic program of life-long learning.
5. Recognize the need and demonstrate the ability to utilize consultation with other medical specialists while maintaining continuity of care.
6. Share tasks and responsibility with other health professionals.
7. Be aware of the findings of relevant research; understand and critically evaluate this body of research; and apply the results of the research to medical practice.
8. Manage his/her practice in a businesslike, cost-effective manner that will provide professional satisfaction and time for a rewarding personal life.
9. Serve as an advocate for the patient within the health care system.
10. Assess the quality of care that he/she provides and actively pursue measures to correct deficiencies.
11. Recognize community resources as an integral part of the health care system; participate in improving the health of the community.
12. Inform and counsel patients concerning their health problems, recognizing patient and physician backgrounds, beliefs, and expectations.
13. Develop mutually satisfying physician–patient relationships to promote comprehensive problem identification and problem solving.
14. Use current medical knowledge to identify, evaluate, and minimize risks for patient and family.
15. Balance potential benefits, costs, and resources in determining appropriate interventions.

Curriculum

The curricular content of a family practice residency program is described in general terms in the recently revised *Essentials for Graduate Training in Family Practice* (Appendix 2). The curriculum is directed toward three distinct capability levels [7]:

1. *Definitive capability*, including, for example, the management of most common clinical and behavioral problems of families and life-threatening emergencies.

James M. Gall, M.D., C.C.F.P.
Department of Family Medicine
University of Miami School of Medicine
P. O. Box 016700
Miami, Florida 33101

2. *Partial capability*, including the initiation of appropriate diagnostic and/or therapeutic measures for more complex clinical problems requiring consultation and/or referral.
3. *Limited capability*, including the recognition or suspicion of rare or complex problems for referral.

The curriculum is likewise focused on the various stages of comprehensive care—prevention, early diagnosis of asymptomatic disease, care of symptomatic disease, rehabilitation and care of terminal illness.

Although there are some individual program and regional differences in the curricula of family practice residencies in various parts of the country, a basic curriculum has emerged in recent years that meets the current criteria of the Residency Review Committee for Family Practice as well as the recommended guidelines of the Residency Assistance Program,[8] a national program jointly sponsored by the American Board of Family Practice, the American Academy of Family Physicians, and the Society of Teachers of Family Medicine.

The resident's experience and training represents that derived from the care of patients in the family practice center and in the hospital on the family practice service, as well as that derived from other parts of the residency program, such as inpatient rotations on other services and ambulatory experiences in other specialty clinics or community settings. Over a three-year period, the family practice residency program usually involves teaching rotations of about one year in internal medicine (including such medical selectives as cardiology, neurology, and dermatology); six months of pediatrics, three to six months of obstetrics–gynecology, six months of surgery and its subspecialties (including ophthalmology, otolaryngology, orthopedics, and urology), two months of emergency medicine, and one month of psychiatry (together with a strong thread of behavioral science presented longitudinally over the three-year program). Table 9–4 illustrates the curriculum in a "typical" family practice residency today, and Table 9–5 shows generally accepted minimum durations for some of the major curricular areas.

Although there are many practical reasons leading to the common use of this kind of time-based curriculum, it is important to recognize that the amount of time devoted to a specific curricular area does not fully describe the learning experience or level of competency achieved by the resident on completion of this experience. The value of a particular teaching rotation, for example, depends on such variables as the characteristics of the learning setting, clinical volume, level of resident responsibility, and the resident's motivation and capability levels.

More detailed information is still needed to better describe the actual curricular content in currently operational United States family practice residency programs. One area that has received considerable attention, however, is the content of teaching in obstetrics–gynecology. A rather specific core curriculum in this area has been developed jointly by the American Academy of Family

TABLE 9–4. CURRICULUM IN "TYPICAL" FAMILY PRACTICE RESIDENCY

	INPATIENT ROTATIONS	FAMILY PRACTICE CENTER
First year		
Medicine	4 months	
Pediatrics	3 months	
Obstetrics–Gynecology	2 months	1 half-day/week
Surgery	2 months	
Emergency room	1 month	
Second year		
Medicine	4 months	
Pediatrics	3 months	
Obstetrics–Gynecology	2 months	3 half-days/week
Cardiology	1 month	
Psychiatry	1 month	
Emergency room	1 month	
Third year		
Medical selectives	4 months	
Surgical selectives	4 months	4 half-days/week
Electives	4 months	

Source: Geyman, J.P.: Family practice in evolution: Progress, problems and projections. *New England Journal of Medicine* 298:593, 1978.

Physicians and the American College of Obstetricians and Gynecologists (Appendix 4).[9] This core curriculum defines the recommended content of cognitive knowledge and skills at both basic and advanced competency levels for obstetrics–gynecology in family practice. A survey of 190 United States family practice residencies in 1975 revealed the level of experience being obtained in normal and abnormal obstetrics by family practice residents in training (Table 9–6).[10]

TABLE 9–5. MINIMAL DURATION OF CORE CURRICULAR AREAS*

CURRICULAR AREA	DURATION
General medicine	8 months
Cardiology	150 hours
Other medical subspecialties	3 months
Pediatrics	4 months
Obstetrics	2 months
Gynecology	1 month
General surgery	2 months
Orthopedics	200 hours
Ophthalmology	100 hours
Otolaryngology	100 hours

* Behavioral science teaching presented as longitudinal thread during program.

TABLE 9-6. EXTENT OF OBSTETRIC EXPERIENCE

NUMBER OF NORMAL DELIVERIES	NUMBER OF RESIDENCIES	PERCENT
Normal		
0– 49	33	19.0
50– 99	56	32.3
100–149	46	26.4
150–199	28	16.1
200–249	9	5.1
250–299	0	0.0
Total	174	100.0
Complicated		
0	35	20.2
1– 5	20	11.5
6–10	31	17.9
11–15	24	13.9
16–20	19	11.0
21–25	13	7.5
26–50	25	14.5
50	6	3.5
Total	173	100.0

Source: Harris, B.A., and Scutchfield, F.D.: Obstetrical and gynecological teaching in family practice residency programs. *Journal of Family Practice* 4:749, 1977. Data based on a survey of 190 United States family practice residency programs during 1975.

Continuity of Care

Continuity of care is an important element in the design, operation, and accreditation of all family practice residency programs. As stated in the *Essentials for Residency Training in Family Practice* (Appendix 2):

> Experience in the continuity of care offered in the Family Practice Center is essential. Therefore it is imperative that all programs offer three consecutive years of training. . . . However, certain circumstances may permit a resident to enter a program in advanced standing, where the first year of training has been in Family Practice in another location, or where the first year of training has provided educational experience equivalent to that necessary for Family Practice. It is essential that a program provide the second and third years of training in one location, thus assuring the resident the opportunity of providing continuity of care to a given panel of patients.

and further:

> Residents may spend time away from the Family Practice Center if necessary to meet the needs of their training. Such outside rotations which interrupt the continuity of the resident's patient care responsibilities in the Family Practice Center must not exceed a total of two months per year in either of the last two years. After two months of such rotation, the resident must return to the Family Practice Center for a minimum of two months before participating in another outside rotation.

Many pressing and real conflicts arise in all family practice residencies in implementing continuity of care in a complex training program, especially due to the numerous commitments of the residents and the differing expectations of the resident by other faculty members and services. Residents frequently find themselves in a double bind, torn between family practice center responsibilities and inpatient responsibilities, including rounds, ward duties, and night call.

There are a number of practical and effective approaches to this dilemma.[11] One important approach is to organize the residency into resident teams, or modules, preferably involving both staff and physical space units within the residency.[12] An 18-resident program may thereby include three teams of 6 residents (2 in each residency year) facilitating continuity of care on a team basis and fostering the development of attitudes and skills needed by the residents in future group practice. Another useful approach to providing continuity of care in a family practice residency is by pairing of residents on certain hospital services whereby one resident of the pair covers the inpatient service while the other is in the family practice center.[13, 14] Other approaches involve the maintenance of a family practice service by advanced residents, the use of the problem-oriented medical record for improved communication, and the promotion of a group versus solo ethos of patient care by the faculty.[11]

Evaluation

Evaluation is a critical component in all educational programs, and has been viewed by Worthen and Sanders[15] as the "most widely discussed but little used phenomena in today's educational systems." The development, however, of effective and often innovative evaluation systems has received strong emphasis in United States family practice residency programs. Evaluation has been recognized as an essential part of a feedback loop (Figure 9–3) to the resident, to the teacher, and to the program director. As Corley observes[16]: "Formative

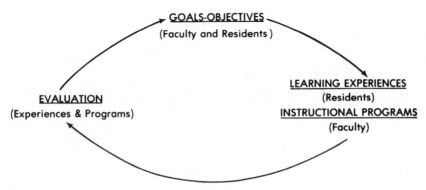

FIGURE 9-3.
The evaluation feedback loop.
Source: Corley, JP: In-training residency evaluation. *Journal of Family Practice*, 3:499, 1976.

in-training evaluation enriches training programs by assessing residents' progressive mastery of professional knowledge, skills and attitudes. It can play a significant role in upgrading a residency."

Evaluation is approached on three levels by most family practice residency programs: (1) at the overall program level, (2) at the level of individual parts of the program (e.g., an inpatient teaching rotation), and (3) at the level of the experience and performance of the individual resident. At the first level, external review by local or national reviewers has been found particularly useful in identifying strengths and weaknesses of programs that might not be readily apparent to those most closely associated with a program. Some departments of family medicine, such as at the University of Iowa and the University of Washington, have instituted a process of internal review within their networks of affiliated residency programs involving site visits by faculty not directly involved with the program being reviewed. On the national level, the Residency Assistance Program provides two-day consultation visits by experienced family practice educators to residency programs requesting assessment and consultation.[9]

The evaluation of individual rotations and individual resident's experience and performance has been addressed in a variety of ways. The experience of family practice residents has been monitored with a problem category index [17] and by practice profiles involving the use of a diagnostic index, the E-book.[18-19] Table 9–7, for example, shows one resident's problem category index profile for a six-month period in the family practice residency program at Lancaster General Hospital, Lancaster, Pennsylvania. Various methods of chart review and patient profiles have been used to evaluate the clinical performance of residents.[20, 21] In-training examinations have been found of value in a number of family practice residencies.[22, 23] Table 9–8 illustrates an example of question-specific feedback from such an examination that affords both feedback and learning to each resident. Another important dimension of evaluation involves periodic assessment by residents of faculty performance, and this, too, is being addressed by some programs.[24]

Costs and Funding

The costs of graduate medical education in any field are substantial. Current estimates for the cost per resident year in family practice are at least 45,000 dollars, including the resident's salary (average 13,000 dollars per year) and prorated costs for faculty, staff, teaching materials, operational costs of the family practice center, and related costs. There are invariably additional start-up costs of the program before the arrival of residents, especially those costs involved by remodeling, or even new construction, of the family practice center. The total cost of a 12-resident family practice residency program can be expected to exceed 540,000 dollars per year.

There are four major sources of funding to offset program costs: (1) patient care revenue, (2) the contributions of the participating hospital(s), (3) state funding, often on a capitation basis, and (4) grants from federal, foundational, or other sources.[5] The last category must be considered "soft," since these funds are often uncertain from year to year and are intended more for start-up needs than ongoing operational needs. Patient care revenue is an important source of support for the program, but should not be expected to cover more than 50 percent of total program costs. The contribution of the program's hospital(s) must therefore provide a solid floor of funding for the residency program. Most hospitals with residency programs include house staff costs in their daily per diem charges. Since the house staff contributes directly to the availability and quality of patient care in the hospital, it is reasonable that a small portion of the patient's daily bill be directed to medical education. State funding has been an essential source of support for many family practice residencies throughout the country and constitutes a wise ongoing investment by the states toward the solution of their common problems of specialty and geographic maldistribution of physicians.

TWO ILLUSTRATIVE PROGRAMS

A brief thumbnail sketch of selected aspects of two graduate education programs in family practice illustrates some commonalities and differences of organizational and operational approaches that have been taken in two regions of the country.

Medical College of Virginia [25]

In 1969, the Virginia State Legislature responded to a documented shortage of family physicians in the state by making specific funds available to Virginia's medical schools to develop family practice training programs. The Medical College of Virginia established the Department of Family Practice in 1970. The first priority identified by the new department was to establish information systems that would provide data in two areas: (1) the supply of primary care physicians throughout the state and (2) the content of primary care.

By 1972, it was demonstrated that 75 additional family physicians would be required each year over the next 20 years, of whom the Medical College of Virginia would accept the responsibility to train between 36 and 42 family physicians each year. At about the same time, a large state-wide study was initiated of the number and kinds of health problems encountered by family physicians in 26 practices representing urban, suburban, and rural sites, as well as both teaching and nonteaching settings.

The department directed most of its resources to residency training and initially decided to establish four affiliated residency programs in shortage areas identified in the physician manpower study—Newport News, Blackstone, Fairfax, and Virginia Beach. An early decision was made to base all residency training in community settings, and a university-based program was not developed.

TABLE 9-7. 42-PROBLEM CATEGORY INDEX FOR 6-MONTH PERIOD ENDING DECEMBER 31, 1974, LANCASTER FACILITY (PHYSICIAN'S NUMBER AND NAME: 48 DR. M. DEE)

DISEASE PROBLEMS	NEW CASES	TOTAL PATIENTS	PATIENT EN-COUNTERS	PERCENTAGE OF ALL PATIENT ENCOUNTERS %	Average of all Physician's Second-year Residents	DISPOSITIONS Rescheduled	Resolved	Hospitalized	Doctor Consultation	Other
++ Anxiety state without somatic symptoms	4	4	4	0.5	1.0	4				
++ Anxiety state with somatic symptoms	19	27	57	7.4	3.0	55	3		2	
Hypertension, benign	9	25	37	4.8	4.1	33	3			
Obesity	8	14	20	2.6	2.1	18	2	1		
** Diabetes mellitus	2	8	14	1.8	2.7	12	2			
** Ischemic heart + myocardial infarction				0	0.4					
** Cardiac failure		2	3	0.4	1.2	3				
** Serum lipid abnormalities				0	0.1					
Pharyngitis	22	22	24	3.1	3.2	22				
Otitis media, acute	13	18	21	2.7	2.9	19	2			
Bronchial asthma	1	4	10	1.3	1.1	6	3		2	
All-vas rhinitis, sinusitis, hay fever	8	9	9	1.2	1.0	6	2	1		
** Chronic pulmonary disease	1	1	1	0.1	1.3	1			1	
Conjunctivitis—ophthalmia	4	4	4	0.5	0.6	2	1			
** Gonorrhea				0	0.1				1	
** Liver, gallbladder, and pancreas disorders				0	0.2					
Intestinal infectious diseases	11	11	11	1.4	1.3	8	2			
++ Peptic ulcer	2	2	2	0.3	0.1	2		1		
** Diverticulitis and diverticulosis				0	0.1					
++ Abdominal pain	20	21	29	3.7	2.1	27				
** Cystitis, acute and chronic	6	6	7	0.9	1.6	6	1			1
++ Menopausal symptoms	2	2	3	0.4	0.1	2	1			

					Your percent	Overall % of all residents					
** Disorders of menstruation	5	5		0.6	1.1	4					1
** Varicose veins	5			0	0.1						
** Vascular lesions of central nervous system				0	0.2			1			
Syncope	1	1		0.1	0.2	1					
++ Iron deficiency anemia	3	4		0.5	0.3	3		1			
** Osteoarthritis	1	1		0.1	0.3	1					
** Cough				0	0.3						
** Malignant neoplasms				0	0.5					1	
Fractures and dislocations	3	4		0.8	0.8	5					
++ Iatrogenic drug reactions	2	2		0.3	0.1	2					
++ Alcoholism	1	2		0.3	0.6	2					
** Situational reactions				0	0.1						
Tension headache	4	4		0.5	0.4	4					
++ Infection of skin + cellular tissue	11	13	14	1.8	3.5	14					
Acne	1	2		0.3	0.3	2	2				
Back pain	7	8		1.2	0.9	7					
++ Well-child examination	71	44	86	11.1	7.7	78	10				
++ Feeding problems + failure to thrive	2	2	3	0.4	0.1	2		1			
** Senility				0	<0.1						
++ Psychosocial and family problems	4	5	5	0.6	0.3	3		2			
Total for 42 index problems	248	277	400	53.8	47.9	354	39	4		7	1
Total for all problems, SLCFHC	408		469	88.5		9.8		1.8		1.0	0.2
Total for all problems, FHS	203		305	88.9		8.1		1.5		0.9	0.6
Combined total for all problems	611		774								

If your disposition average varies by more than 50% from the overall average of all residents, it is circled.

Problem percentages more than 30% below average are preceded by a double asterisk (**)

Problem percentages more than 30% above average are preceded by a double plus sign (++)

Source: Tindall, H.L., Henderson, R.A., and Cole, A.F.: Evaluating family practice residents with a problem category index. *Journal of Family Practice* 2:353, 1975.

TABLE 9–8. QUESTION–SPECIFIC FEEDBACK FOR IN–TRAINING EXAMINATION

QUESTION NUMBER	CONTENT AREA	REFERENCES
6	Immunization procedures in children (especially use of rubeola vaccine)	Krupp MA, Chatten MJ: Current Medical Diagnosis and Treatment. Los Altos, California, Lange, 1974, p 959
19	Treatment of cavernous hemangioma in infant	Sauer GC: Manual of Skin Diseases. Philadelphia, Lippincott, 1973, p 272
20	Diagnosis of aspirated foreign body in lung	Conn HF, Rakel RE, Johnson TW: Family Practice. Philadelphia, Saunders, 1973, p 836
30	Side effects of reserpine	Physicians Desk Reference, 29th ed, Oradell, New Jersey, Medical Economics, 1975, p 1042
71	Diagnosis of perennial vasomotor rhinitis	Ryan RE, et al: Synopsis of Ear, Nose and Throat Diseases. St. Louis, Missouri, Mosby, 1970, p 157
99	Interpretation of T4 column tests	Wallach J: Interpretation of Diagnostic Tests. Boston, Little, Brown, 1974, p 316

Source: Geyman, J.P., and Brown, T.: An in-training examination for residents in family practice. *Journal of Family Practice* 3:409, 1976.

A fifth affiliated residency program was started in Richmond in 1976. Table 9–9 shows the current number of residents in each program within the overall affiliated residency program.

The first year of the curriculum is similar to that of most family practice residencies—hospital-based teaching rotations in internal medicine, pediatrics, obstetrics–gynecology, surgery, and emergency medicine. The curriculum of the second and third years, however, is quite different from most other programs, with only eight additional months of hospital teaching rotations. The emphasis during the last two years is placed on active teaching in the family practice center, with vigorous audit activity directly related to daily teaching by consultants in the various specialties. The department's goal is to develop a curriculum based on practice content, so that the resultant curricular plan involves less inpatient teaching, expanded teaching in the family practice center, and ambulatory psychiatry training. The flow of logic for curriculum development by the department is illustrated in Figure 9–4.

TABLE 9-9.   THE AFFILIATED RESIDENCY PROGRAM,* MEDICAL COLLEGE OF VIRGINIA

PROGRAM SITES	*NUMBER OF RESIDENTS*	*YEAR STARTED*
Blackstone	18	1971
Fairfax (Vienna)	18	1971
Newport News	36	1970
Virginia Beach	18	1973
Chesterfield (Richmond)	18	1976
Total	108	

* There is not a full university-based program (including a family practice center) on the Medical College of Virginia campus. Most of the inpatient clinical rotations for the Blackstone Program are conducted at the university hospital. The family practice centers and their related community hospitals provide the major teaching settings for family practice residents during the entire three-year program.

Source: Leaman, T.L., Geyman, J.P., and Brown, T.C.: Graduate education in family practice. *Journal of Family Practice* 5:56, 1977.

In late 1975, a major practice content study was completed representing the health care problems of about 88,000 patients presented to 118 family physicians (including 82 family practice residents) over a 25-month period. This study was published in 1976 as the *Virginia Study*, and has been an important contribution to the field (Appendix 5).[26] The study revealed that 233 diagnostic entities comprise 95 percent of health care problems encountered in primary care, reported the age–sex incidence of all problems seen, and demonstrated the content of teaching practices to be almost identical to that of nonteaching practices in Virginia (Figure 9–5).[26]

The five affiliated residency programs interact closely as partners within the system. Functionally, the overall program operates through three standing committees—the Records and Research Committee, the Curriculum and Evaluation Committee, and the Practice Organization and Management Committee.

The Department of Family Practice at the Medical College of Virginia is funded by the state on a direct line–item basis at about 1.8 million dollars per year. About 88 percent of these funds are distributed to the affiliated residency programs. These state funds cover a portion of faculty salaries (average of

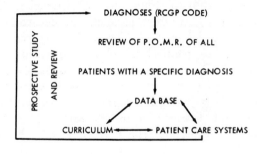

FIGURE 9-4.

Flow of logic for development of curriculum and patient care systems in family practice.

Source: Marsland, DW, Wood, M, Mayo, F: A data bank for patient care, curriculum and research in family practice. Journal of Family Practice, 3:25, 1976.

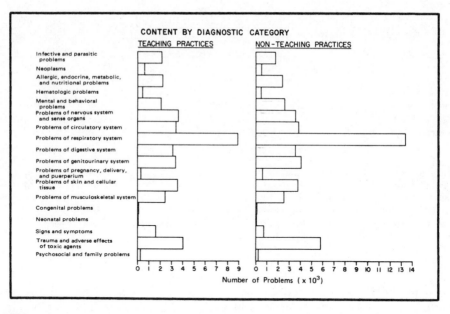

FIGURE 9-5.

Content by diagnostic category of teaching versus nonteaching practices.

Source: Marsland, DW, Wood, M, Mayo, F: A data bank for patient care, curriculum and research in family practice: 526,196 patient problems. *Journal of Family Practice* 3:25, 1976.

three full-time faculty per program), consultants, the salaries of all second- and third-year residents, and full support of all educational and secretarial staff throughout the system.

Follow-up studies have shown that 70 percent of the 133 graduates from the Medical College of Virginia programs through 1978 entered practice in Virginia; 64 percent of these settled in nonmetropolitan areas.

University of Washington

Since its inception in 1971, the Department of Family Medicine at the University of Washington has placed high priority on the development of decentralized family practice residency programs within the four-state WAMI region of Washington, Alaska, Montana, and Idaho. This effort parallels the department's undergraduate teaching program in the WAMI region, which was described in the preceding chapter. As the only medical school serving a geographic area representing one-quarter of the land mass of the United States, decentralization and regionalization comprise an essential part of the medical school's programs, perhaps best illustrated by the WAMI program.[27]

Regional studies of physician supply and distribution in the early 1970s documented a shortage of family physicians throughout the WAMI region.[28, 29] It was estimated that a total of 73 additional family physicians would be needed in the WAMI states each year in order to keep up with an average annual attrition of 4 percent due to death, disability, and retirement. A goal was set to train at least 50 family physicians each year within the region, as well as to monitor the results of annual in-migration of family physicians from other parts of the country, in order to meet the region's deficit of practicing family physicians.

From the outset, it was considered important to establish residency programs in varied settings as well as to decentralize their locations.[30] A university-based program was started at University Hospital in 1972 as a means to establish the department's clinical and teaching base in the medical school itself and to introduce visible family physician role models to medical students on the campus. Three other family practice residencies were started at the same time in Washington—the Group Health Cooperative and Doctors Hospital programs in Seattle and Family Medicine Spokane, which related to three participating hospitals in Spokane. These programs became affiliated with the university in 1972. In 1974, a fifth program was started at Providence Medical Center in Seattle, and in 1975, two additional family practice residencies were established in Yakima, Washington, and Boise, Idaho. This network of affiliated residency programs was further expanded in 1978 with the addition of a new program in Tacoma, Washington, and the affiliation of the previously established family practice residency at Madigan Army Medical Center. Table 9–10 shows the number of residents in training within the network during the 1978–1979 year.

Although there are some variations in the curricula of the various programs within the family practice residency network, they all resemble the "typical" curriculum described earlier as common throughout the country. This involves a balance between hospital-based rotations, the family practice center, and other learning settings. A broad base of hospital-based training is considered necessary preparation for the needs of most practice settings in the region.

TABLE 9–10. THE FAMILY PRACTICE RESIDENCY NETWORK, UNIVERSITY OF WASHINGTON

PROGRAM SITES	NUMBER OF RESIDENTS	YEAR STARTED
University Hospital, Seattle	18	1972
Doctors Hospital, Seattle	18	1972
Group Health Cooperative, Seattle	12	1972
Providence Medical Center, Seattle	12	1974
Family Medicine Spokane	18	1972
Family Medicine Yakima*	12	1975
Family Medicine Tacoma	12	1978
Madigan Army Medical Center, Tacoma	27	1972
Southwest Idaho, Boise	16	1975
Total	145	

* The Yakima program is a "one-and-two" program, with the first year in Spokane hospitals and the subsequent two years based in Yakima.

The now firmly established family practice residency at University Hospital has demonstrated that a clinical and teaching base can be established in an academic medical center more oriented to secondary and tertiary care. A free-standing family medical center is located near the entrance to the medical school, and provides ongoing primary care for approximately 3000 families. An inpatient family medicine service has been established, and the department is responsible for the inpatient care of most obstetric patients, newborns, and most patients admitted with medical problems. Surgical admissions are usually referred to the surgical service.

The nine member programs of the family practice residency network interact closely as a "family" of programs that preserves considerable autonomy for each affiliated program. The network functions through six standing committees with the following areas of responsibility: curriculum, learning resources, faculty development, continuing education, evaluation, and research. Some of the current activities of the network include the development of a common information management and data retrieval system; extension of a basic family medicine clerkship for third-year medical students to all affiliated residency programs; an active evaluation program including the use of resident experience logs, an in-training self-assessment examination, and a process of internal review; and an annual resident research conference.

The four major sources of funding for each residency program within the network are: (1) patient care revenue (covers 40 to 50 percent of most of the individual programs' costs), (2) hospitals' contributions, (3) state capitation funds (about 5000 to 10,000 dollars per resident per year in Washington and Idaho, respectively), and (4) extramural federal or foundation grants. Just over 60 percent of the total budget of the Department of Family Medicine is provided by state funding as a part of the regular university budget.

By the end of 1978, 129 family practice residents had graduated from network programs. Of this number, 107 entered practice within the WAMI region and are evenly distributed in urban, suburban, and rural areas.

COMMENT

Both of the departmental programs represent effective approaches to meeting the needs for well-trained family physicians for their surrounding areas. Both have emphasized teaching settings in the community and have developed strong educational programs. The Medical College of Virginia's program has demonstrated to a remarkable extent a "systems approach" to program and curriculum development. The University of Washington's network program exemplifies a collaborative approach with affiliated residency programs in varied settings within a large geographic region.

The interaction among affiliated residency programs within a network brings important advantages to the participating community hospitals as well as to the university [31]:

Benefits to the community hospital include:

1. Assistance in residency program development through the pooled experience of other affiliated programs.
2. Assistance with the formulation of educational objectives and the evaluation of resident performance.
3. Expansion of teaching resources through visiting professor programs and various teaching materials.
4. Augmented effectiveness of teaching through teacher development programs.
5. Enhanced potential for recruitment of residents of high caliber because of university affiliation and associated medical student clerkship programs.
6. Increased opportunities for resident electives, both at the university and elsewhere within the network.
7. Potential for increased funding through the university and/or grant funds acquired for the network.

Benefits to the university include:

1. Increased opportunity to contribute to the training of the required number of family physicians.
2. Extension of continuing medical education to a larger area beyond the medical school itself.
3. Increased clinical resources and learning opportunities for medical students, residents, and allied health personnel.
4. Opportunities to participate in the development of new models of education and health care delivery.
5. Enhanced potential for collaborative research in family practice.
6. Facilitation of improved linkages between primary, secondary, and tertiary care on a regional basis.
7. Potential for increased utilization of the university for consultation and referral.

The growth and development of graduate education in family practice during the 1970s have been extraordinary in terms of the dimensions that have been discussed. Another important dimension of the quality of this effort relates to student interest in family practice residencies. These programs have been oversubscribed, with more than 2600 graduates of United States medical schools in 1978, for example, applying for the 2200 available first-year positions. Moreover, attrition during family practice residency training has been minimal—13 percent of 1976 first-year residents and only 3 percent of 1976 second-year residents.*

While the principal focus of family practice residency programs is naturally upon resident training, they have much to contribute in other areas—under-

---

* Data provided by the Division of Education, American Academy of Family Physicians, Kansas City, Missouri.

graduate and postgraduate teaching as well as research. At the undergraduate level, family practice residencies provide excellent learning settings for advanced medical students in family practice clerkships. Several kinds of benefits accrue to residency programs involved in such clerkships: (1) expansion of the capacity of teams within the residency, (2) provision of opportunities to residents to teach (and learn through teaching), (3) assistance with special projects within the residency, and (4) assessment of potential future resident applicants through daily contact with medical students during their clerkships.[32]

It is inevitable that family practice residencies will become active sources of continuing medical education in their areas. The residency program of itself is an educational system involving the family practice center, related hospital(s), physicians, and other health professionals within the community. This system usually can accommodate more learners, and the educational needs of practicing family physicians and advanced family practice residents are similar in many respects. Self-assessment and teaching methods that are developed for residents are equally applicable to practicing physicians, and can be made readily available to larger numbers of practicing family physicians because of the wide geographic distribution of these programs.[32]

Family practice residencies likewise have considerable opportunities to become involved in research and innovative demonstration projects whether related to teaching or clinical practice. These residency programs are directly involved in the definition and implementation of modern concepts in family medicine and increasingly have available the necessary tools and resources for substantive research of various types.[33] Some programs have already become involved in research activities. If the teaching practices and family practice centers of family practice residencies are considered laboratories, then the faculty and residents in these programs can contribute immeasurably to research in family medicine.

Much progress has been made during the 1970s in the development of family practice residency programs of high quality throughout the country. Their capacity, however, still falls short of the need. The challenge ahead is to maintain the standards of excellence that have been established and to develop additional programs at a rate that will allow family practice to make an impact on the delivery of health care, which is so urgently needed.

REFERENCES

1. Mayo W: In Strauss MB (ed): Familiar Medical Quotations. Boston, Little, Brown, 1968, p 565
2. Geyman JP: The "one-and-two" program: A new direction in family practice residency training. J Med Educ 52:999, 1977

3. Medley ES, Halstead ML: A family practice residency inpatient service: A review of 631 admissions. J Fam Pract 6:817, 1978

4. Geyman JP: Prevention of complications in initial development of family practice residency programs. J Fam Pract 4:1111, 1977

5. Hornsby JL, Kerr RM: Behavioral science and family practice: A status report. J Fam Pract 8:299, 1979

6. STFM Board approves educational goal statements. Fam Med Times 10:5, 1978

7. Geyman JP: A competency-based curriculum as an organizing framework in family practice residencies. J Fam Pract 1:34, 1974

8. Stern TL, Chaisson GM: The Residency Assistance Program in family practice. J Fam Pract 5:379, 1977

9. Stern TL: A landmark in interspecialty cooperation. J Fam Pract 5:523, 1977

10. Harris BA, Scutchfield FD: Obstetrical and gynecological teaching in family practice residency programs. J Fam Pract 4:749, 1977

11. Geyman JP: Continuity of care in family practice: Implementing continuity in a family practice residency program. J Fam Pract 2:445, 1975

12. Geyman JP: A modular basis of resident training for family practice. J Med Educ 47:292, 1972

13. Phillips TJ, Holler JW: A university family medicine program. J Med Educ 46:821, 1971

14. Lincoln JA: The three-year paired residency program: A solution to a teaching dilemma. J Fam Pract 1:31, 1974

15. Worthen BR, Sanders JR: Educational Evaluation: Theory and Practice. Worthington, Ohio, Charles A. Jones, 1973

16. Corley JB: In-training residency evaluation. J Fam Pract 3:499, 1976

17. Tindall HL, Henderson RA, Cole AF: Evaluating family practice residents with a problem category index. J Fam Pract 2:353, 1975

18. Boisseau V, Froom J: Practice profiles in evaluating the clinical experience of family medicine trainees. J Fam Pract 6:801, 1978

19. Terrell HP: Documentation of resident exposure to disease entities. J Fam Pract 6:317, 1978

20. Kane RL, Leigh EH, Feigel DW, Sundwall DN, Farney MA: A method for evaluating patient care and auditing skills of family practice residents. J Fam Pract 2:205, 1975

21. Given CW, Simoni L, Gallin RS, Sprafka RJ: The use of computer generated patient profiles to evaluate resident performance in patient care. J Fam Pract 5:831, 1977

22. Donnelly JE, Yankaskas B, Gjerde C, Wright JC, Longnecker DP: An in-training assessment examination in family medicine: Report of a pilot project. J Fam Pract 5:987, 1977

23. Geyman JP, Brown T: An in-training examination for residents in family practice. J Fam Pract 3:409, 1976

24. Kelly J, Woiwode D: Faculty evaluation by residents in a family medicine residency program. J Fam Pract 4:693, 1977

25. Leaman TL, Geyman JP, Brown TC: Graduate education in family practice. J Fam Pract 5:56, 1977

26. Marsland DW, Wood M, Mayo F: A data bank for patient care, curriculum and research in family practice: 526,196 patient problems. J Fam Pract 3:25, 1976

27. Schwarz MR: WAMI: An experiment in regional medical education. West J Med 121:333, 1974

28. Lawrence D, Cherkin D: The Physician Manpower Source Book: Washington, Alaska, Montana and Idaho, 1974. Seattle, Washington, University of Washington, 1975

29. Lawrence D, Cherkin D: The Physician Manpower Experience: Washington, Alaska, Montana and Idaho, 1960–1974. Seattle, Washington, University of Washington, 1975

30. Geyman JP: Deisher JB, Gordon MJ: A family practice residency network: Affiliated programs in the Pacific Northwest. JAMA 240:369, 1978

31. Geyman JP, Brown TC: A network model for decentralized family practice residency training. J Fam Pract 3:621, 1976

32. Geyman JP: Family practice residencies and the continuum of medical education. J Fam Pract 5:743, 1977

33. Geyman JP: Research in the family practice residency program. J Fam Pract 5:245, 1977

CHAPTER TEN

Continuing Education in Family Practice

These are days of public accountability for medicine. Among other things the public wants to be assured that every physician is competent and remains competent to do whatever he or she is supposed to be doing in patient care. And for a number of reasons continuing medical education is becoming tied to continuing professional competence. The logic in general appears to be that if education made a physician competent in the first place, then continuing education should make for continuing competence.

Malcolm S. M. Watts [1]

The steady growth of medical knowledge in recent years, together with continuously changing patterns of practice and an increasing emphasis on public accountability in medicine as in other fields, have made continuing medical education an area of major concern in the United States today. Although the concept of lifelong learning in medicine has been endorsed on a voluntary basis for many years, the past ten years have seen a progressive momentum toward mandatory continuing medical education (CME) for all physicians. CME requirements have now been adopted as requisites for membership in many national and state medical societies and hospital medical staffs and as part of recertification requirements by a number of specialty boards. [2]

Continuing medical education has burgeoned to become a large industry in this country. In 1976, it was estimated by the newly formed Alliance for Continuing Medical Education that approximately 2 billion dollars were then being spent each year for CME, including the costs of faculty remuneration, conduct of programs, and accreditation.[3] According to the American Medical Association, the number of CME courses per year more than quintupled between 1961 and 1977, while the number of sponsoring agencies and institutions tripled.[4]

As continuing medical education has become recognized as increasingly important, its goals, content, and methods have been subjected to closer scrutiny. It has become painfully obvious that this is a special kind of education that requires different approaches from those taken in undergraduate and graduate medical education. Each physician's needs for continuing education represent an individual matter, even within the same field. It is difficult for busy physicians to be aware of their individual needs at any given time and to compare their own knowledge and performance with that of their colleagues.

Since continuing medical education must be directed in so many different directions and meet such a diverse range of individualized needs, development of curricula and appropriate methods for such education becomes a formidable task. The task is made even more complex when one realizes that as many as 50 percent of practicing physicians are often said to be poorly motivated to pursue their own continuing education.

Several special features of continuing medical education illustrate the complexities of this area: (1) both students and teachers are usually part time; (2) the classroom model, or even models derived from graduate medical education, are not usually applicable to the purposes of CME; (3) the objectives of CME are more particular and specific than traditional undergraduate and graduate medical education; and (4) CME is inseparable from patient care and ideally should lead to behavioral changes in the physician as relates to the use of new knowledge in patient management, as well as to improved outcomes of patient care.

The purpose of this chapter is to present an overview of continuing medical education as it applies to family practice. Some generic problems of CME will first be considered, together with the basic requisites for effective postgraduate learning. Some current directions of CME in family practice will then be outlined, as well as the developing roles of medical school departments of family practice and some useful approaches for individual family physicians in acquiring more meaningful continuing education.

SOME GENERIC PROBLEMS OF CONTINUING MEDICAL EDUCATION

Brief consideration of various basic problems involved in continuing medical education serves to illustrate the complexities and challenges of this subject.

Expansion of Medical Information

There is no question that the volume of medical information is expanding at an exponential rate in recent years, but the implications of this process are controversial. Some believe that we are involved in a "knowledge explosion." In a paper examining information technologies and health care, for example, Moore has projected a 10 percent annual increment of new medical knowledge and estimated that 5 percent of the physician's total medical knowledge becomes obsolescent each year.[5] That a "publication explosion" has occurred cannot be denied. It can be reasonably assumed that the weight of *Index Medicus* is directly related to the number of publications listed therein, and this weight has shown gigantic growth in the past 100 years (Figure 10–1).[6]

A good case can be made, however, that the amount of clinically applicable medical knowledge has not increased at such a rapid rate. Weiss[7] denies the existence of a true knowledge explosion in this way:

> The semblance of a knowledge explosion has come from using the wrong yardstick. No doubt, there has been a data explosion, liberally equatable with an information explosion, though not all of the collected data are truly informative. Furthermore we are also faced with a publication explosion. But knowledge explosion? Not by criteria of measurement on a scale of relevance.

McWhinney suggests that medical knowledge cannot be viewed simply as information-based, but includes two additional elements: (1) clinical craftsmanship as a skill, and (2) insight and awareness as an integral part of the physician's personality.[8]

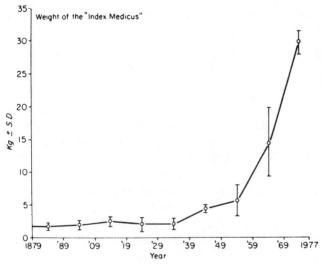

FIGURE 10-1.

Weight of the *Index Medicus* according to ten-year periods from 1879 to 1977. Source: Durack, DT: The weight of medical knowledge. *New England Journal of Medicine* 298:773, 1978. Reprinted by permission of the *New England Journal of Medicine*.

Lack of Correlation between Knowledge and Performance

It is well known that the medical knowledge of physicians often correlates poorly with their clinical performance. A recent report by Ashbaugh and McKean, for example, showed that 94 percent of deficiencies in surgical practice identified by 55 audits of 5499 patient records were in the area of performance, while only 6 percent were on the basis of lack of knowledge.[9]

There are undoubtedly many reasons why physicians' practice behaviors frequently do not change based on newly acquired medical knowledge. These include force of habit, medical fashion, and inadequate effort (i.e., time and priority) in revising one's practice methods. In addition, Scott has pointed out the subtle and easily overlooked biases that any physician may harbor and the need to adopt habits of more critical thought.[10]

Irrelevance of Content

It is likewise readily apparent that the content of most continuing medical education programs as traditionally offered bears little resemblance to the specific learning needs of the individual physician. The dimensions of this problem are graphically stated by Brown[11]:

> The concept of continuing medical education conjures up a roomful of preoccupied but hopeful physicians at a community hospital, anticipating a learned presentation by the medical school faculty either in person or by way of educational television, two-way radio or other media. The members of the audience are caught between the demands of their practices and the hope that such an educational program will somehow be useful in the care of the patients. But such a teacher or planner-oriented approach is both limited and limiting since it may only incidentally or accidentally meet the needs of the learner and possibly less often the needs of the patient. Diagnosis of patient care needs seldom precedes educational therapy.

Logistic Barriers

Physicians often find themselves practicing under circumstances that make further programmed education difficult. Time is short, and the demands of their practices, families, and communities are great. They can leave their practices only occasionally, and coverage of their patients may present a problem. In most cases, physicians must individually schedule their own time off and cease income-producing activities in order to keep up to date with current developments. The demands of solo practice particularly aggravate these kinds of problems. To this extent, therefore, medicine can be said to lack an organizational structure that facilitates the continuing education and retraining of physicians.[12]

Ineffective Teaching Methods

Much of traditional continuing medical education is conducted by the lecture method, an approach that violates classic learning theory as to how adults learn. This method has been demonstrated to be a comparatively ineffective method of teaching, partly due to the lack of active involvement of the learner and partly due to the exclusive focus of this method on information transfer alone. As pointed out by Miller [13]:

> There is ample evidence to support the view that adult learning is not most efficiently achieved through systematic subject instruction. It is accomplished by involving learners in identifying problems and seeking ways to solve them. It does not come in categorical bundles but in a growing need to know. It may initially seem wanting in content that pleases experts, but it ultimately incorporates knowledge in a context that has meaning. It is in short a process model of education.

Lack of Clear Goals and Methods

The accelerating increase in formal continuing medical education courses in recent years is clearly reflected in Table 10–1.[14] This kind of educational activity shows the extent to which the assumption is made that more transfer of new medical information will address the needs of physicians and their patients. It is readily apparent that this confidence is misplaced when one enlarges the scope of desired outcomes of CME to include physician competence, physician performance, and patient health status. Miller succinctly describes this dilemma as follows [15]:

> We are convinced, or so the literature of continuing education would make us seem, that it is our failure to apply new knowledge that represents the weakest link in the chain of assuring that the highest quality of medical care is delivered by the greatest number of physicians to the largest number of patients. While this view may be correct, I am not familiar with any solid data to support it. In fact, the correction of the major health problems in the United States, as in other parts of the world, does not appear to require any substantial body of new knowledge. Rather, it requires that physicians use the knowledge they already have in a different way or more fully exhibit the professional attitudes that have characterized the physician's role for as long as there have been physicians.

By 1978, CME had virtually become mandatory, even though its goals and methods remained unclear and poorly understood. The basic issue was misinterpreted by many as one of adequacy or inadequacy of CME hours and credits. The medical practice acts in at least 19 states by 1978 had given authority to the state licensing boards to require documented CME activity as a condition for relicensure.[16]

TABLE 10–1. CONTINUING MEDICAL EDUCATION COURSES LISTED, 1961–1962 TO 1977–1978

YEAR	TOTAL COURSES REPORTED	NUMBER OF PRIMARY SPONSORS	COURSES OFFERED NUMBER (%)	
			By Medical Schools	By Hospitals
1961–1962	1105	206	—	—
1962–1963	1146	208	626(55)	104(9)
1963–1964	1264*	267*	760(60)*	163(13)*
1964–1965	1569	251	857(55)	265(16)
1965–1966	1641	252	863(53)	351(21)
1966–1967	1608	262	910(57)	338(21)
1967–1968	1830	263	1000(54)	224(12)
1968–1969	1922	300	1024(53)	370(19)
1969–1970	2016	323	886(44)	441(22)
1970–1971	2319	303	813(35)	374(16)
1971–1972	2354	392	895(38)	601(26)
1972–1973†	2082	253	957(46)	343(16)
1973–1974†	2441	287	1061(43)	426(18)
1974–1975†	3677	393	1516(41)	652(18)
1975–1976†	4862	554	1920(40)	919(19)
1976–1977†	5800	660	2338(40)	1327(23)
1977–1978†	7330	918	2945(40)	1875(26)

* Includes courses offered by five Canadian schools not reported in other years.
† Includes only courses offered by accredited institutions or organizations.
Source: Medical education in the United States, 1977–1978. *JAMA* 238:2804, 1977.

The complexities of CME problems and the unanswered challenges in future responses thereto are well summarized by Sanazaro [17]:

> In the absence of alternatives, CME must remain the foundation stone of professional commitment to maintaining competence. But we should face up to some of its serious limitations. Specifically, CME cannot be relied upon to remove deficiencies in performance when the physicians in question already possess the necessary knowledge and simply do not apply it. Also, it is possible that those physicians most in need of CME are not able to attend conferences designed specifically to assist them in better understanding the reasons why a change in their performance is desirable. Then there is the observation that many physicians who are not providing adequate care nonetheless believe they are keeping up with new developments and feel no need for CME.[18] And finally, it is a well documented fact that on the average, with advancing age, physicians devote less effort to CME, demonstrate less cognitive learning and perform at a lower level.[18–23] Physicians under 40 years of age do more in CME and achieve better results on tests and in practice than those past 60, on the average. Taken together, these considerations support the conclusion that CME may well be least effective in those who most need it.

SOME REQUISITES FOR CONTINUING MEDICAL EDUCATION

Brief reference to some well-accepted principles of learning is of interest before focusing on CME in family practice. It is currently believed that five basic conditions must be met for meaningful learning by adults [24]:

1. Students must be adequately motivated to change their behavior.
2. They must be aware of the inadequacy of their present behavior (and the superiority of the behavior they are required to adopt).
3. They must have a clear picture of the new behavior.
4. They must have opportunities to practice the new behavior with a sequence of appropriate materials.
5. They must get continuing reinforcement of the new behavior.

With regard to adult learning as an active process, Miller has this to say [13]:

> . . . men learn what they want to learn. The first step in this long process is not to tell them what they need to know, it is to help them to want what they require. It means involving participants in identifying their own educational needs, in selecting the learning experiences most likely to help them to meet these needs, and assessing whether they have learned what was intended, not merely determining whether they took part in the learning experience, or even whether they liked it.

Two additional points have an important bearing on the learning process. It is well known that there is a forgetting curve—information that is not related to one's continuing practice is easily forgotten. In addition, each of us has his/her own individual style of learning. Some will learn best by reading, others by small-group patient-oriented discussions, and still others by self-instructional media.

These principles can be formulated into four basic requisites for meaningful continuing medical education: (1) a need to know (preferably related to patient care), (2) an active process (preferably problem-oriented instead of subject-oriented), (3) a continuous relevance to everyday medical practice (with the educational experience designed to meet identified learning needs), and (4) a format that fits the individual physician's learning style.

CURRENT APPROACHES TO CONTINUING EDUCATION IN FAMILY PRACTICE

Today's approaches to continuing education in family practice are based on some of the educational principles that have been mentioned and are directly addressing some of the generic problems of CME that were considered earlier.

Profiling and Indexing of Practice Experience

Several methods have been described in recent years whereby the practice experience of family physicians can be readily described in profile form.[25-27] The Illinois Council on Continuing Medical Education, for example, has developed a handbook for physicians describing a profiling method and outlining an approach to developing a personal learning plan based on individual needs.[26] At the University of Wisconsin, a successful program has been developed based on the individual physician profile, which is derived by recording over a four-week period the age and sex of every patient encountered (in the office, hospital, home or by telephone), presenting symptoms, significant findings, major diagnoses, tests ordered, and disposition. Figure 10–2 illustrates a typical profile for a family physician's practice in Wisconsin; this profile is then used as the basis for an individualized self-assessment examination and educational consultation concerning specific learning experiences needed.[27]

Indexing systems have also been developed whereby family physicians can record on simple index cards the names and important clinical information for patients with selected problems.[28] A sample index card is shown in Figure 10–3, and the various advantages of this kind of system are listed in Table 10–2.

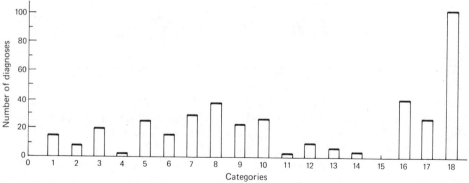

FIGURE 10-2.

Profile of a typical family physician's practice in Wisconsin. The 18 problem categories represent the following areas: (1) infective and parasitic diseases; (2) neoplasms; (3) endocrine, nutritional, and metabolic diseases; (4) diseases of blood and blood-forming organs; (5) mental disorders; (6) diseases of the nervous system and sense organs; (7) diseases of the circulatory system; (8) diseases of the respiratory system; (9) diseases of the digestive system; (10) diseases of the genitourinary system; (11) pregnancy, childbirth, and puerperium; (12) diseases of skin and subcutaneous tissues; (13) diseases of the musculoskeletal system and connective tissue; (14) congenital anomalies; (15) perinatal conditions; (16) physical signs, symptoms, and ill-defined conditions not otherwise specified or not yet diagnosed; (17) accidents, poisonings, and violence; and (18) supplementary classifications (including medical examinations for preventive purposes and various behavioral problems).

Source: Siverston, SE, Meyer, TC, Hansen, R, and Schoenenberger, A: Individual physician profile: Continuing education related to medical practice. *Journal of Medical Education* 48:1006, 1973.

PriCare V. Mental Disorders						
3004 DEPRESSION			RAKEL			
Subcategory			Physician's Name			
Patient Name	Chart Number	Birth Date	Phone	Medication/ Treatment	Date	Comments
Myers, Linda	241-75	11/15/36	351-4634	Elavil	1/19/78	Watch PVC's
Dittoff, Frank	98-76	3/4/31	338-7151	Tofranil	2/7/78	
Kinley, Sharyl	404-76	5/15/36	337-4783	Elavil + EST	2/24/78	Avoid oral contracep.
Morrison, William	11-17	10/30/42	354-2801	Sinequan	3/13/78	Anxiety
Stein, Jeffrey	123-78	1/2/40	351-3842	Lithium	4/5/78	Bipolar

FIGURE 10-3.

Sample problem-indexing card.

Source: Rakel RE: Indexing in office practice: A system for monitoring high-risk patients and filing medical literature. *Continuing Education for the Family Physician* 9:30, 1978. Reprinted by permission.

Increasing Use of the Problem-Oriented Medical Record

The problem-oriented medical record has been widely adopted by family practice teaching programs and has received growing acceptance by many practicing family physicians. The logical format of this record system not only affords improved communication among colleagues and consultants, but also facilitates assessment of quality of care through audit and data retrieval of clinical problems encountered.

TABLE 10–2. ADVANTAGES OF PROBLEM INDEXING

1. Identifies patients with similar problems or medications
2. Simplifies recall when updating of treatment is necessary
3. Identifies patients for whom medications must be changed to avoid newly recognized hazards
4. Simplifies recall for periodic evaluation of chronic problems
5. Assists with self audit by:
   a. assessment of diagnostic accuracy
   b. identification of areas to be stressed in continuing education
   c. identification of conditions rarely encountered (or missed)
6. Provides analysis of practice content for design of teaching objectives
7. Simplifies collection of data for clinical research
8. Identifies new syndromes or unique associations between problems
9. Retrieves cases for recertification

Source: Rakel, R.E.: Indexing in office practice: A system for monitoring high-risk patients and filing medical literature. *Continuing Education for the Family Physician* 9:30, 1978. Reprinted by permission.

Increasing Use of Medical Audit

Audit of medical records both in the office and in the hospital is increasingly emphasized in family practice, and has the potential to close the loop between knowledge and performance. Audit can clearly facilitate the physician's ongoing learning and the improvement of patient care through the basic steps involved in the process: (1) identification of an important problem area for audit, (2) setting of criteria by peers, (3) conduct of the audit, (4) educational response to deficits noted, and (5) reaudit of the problem at a later date to determine if improvements in patient care have actually taken place.

More effective methods are being developed to link CME to learning needs identified by medical audit. One such example is the Quality Assurance-Continuing Education (QACE) Program conducted at The Doctors Hospital in Seattle, Washington, which is organized as shown in Figure 10–4.[29]

Most family practice residency programs stress the use of audit as a means of evaluating the quality of patient care and of learning skills that can facilitate the continuing education of graduates in their future practices. Some programs, such as the Family Medicine Program at the University of Rochester, utilize audit for critical event outcome studies as a teaching tool.[30] One recent study of perceptions of formal in-training evaluation by residents in 20 United States family practice residency programs demonstrated that chart audit and regular chart review were seen by residents as having the greatest educational value of all evaluation methods used.[31]

Self Assessment

Ambulatory and hospital-based audit is an important method of self assessment. Family practice residency programs are developing other approaches to self assessment, including the use of in-training examinations, which are also made available to practicing family physicians. The Connecticut and Ohio Academies of Family Physicians have conducted a successful self-testing and CME program since 1968 known as the Core Content Review of Family Medicine. The most comprehensive self-assessment program in family practice to date is the Home Study Self-Assessment Program developed by the American Academy of Family Physicians. This program consists of multimedia teaching materials; pre- and post-tests; yearly examinations; and booklets providing answers, discussion, and references for each examination question. This program covers 70 subject areas essential to family practice and extends over a six-year period, the interval established by the American Board of Family Practice as a requisite for recertification.

Increased Use of Small-Group Teaching and Self Instruction

The traditional emphasis on the lecture as a primary teaching method has fallen into disrepute in recent years. Lewin, for example, has shown that this method

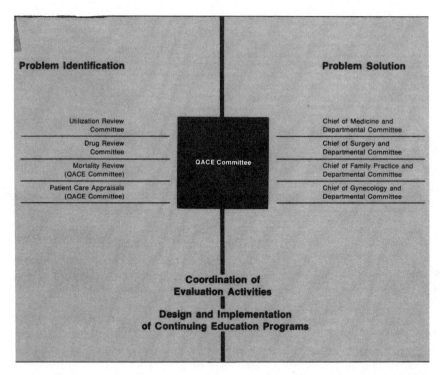

FIGURE 10-4.

Schematic representation of the responsibilities of the committees that make up the Quality Assurance–Continuing Education (QACE) Program at The Doctors Hospital. Problems in patient care are identified by the utilization and drug review committees and by the QACE committee, which conducts mortality review and patient care appraisals (PCAs); the chiefs of service (medicine, surgery, family practice, and gynecology) and their departmental committees solve patient care problems. The QACE committee straddles the line separating problem identification and solution; it not only searches for problems but also coordinates all evaluation activities of the QACE program and conducts continuing education programs, which is one method of corrective action.

Source: Barnes, RH, Hulbert, BL, and Roberts, JG: The case for QACE. *Quality Review Bulletin* 4:16, 1978.

is ineffective in affecting behavioral changes in learners.[32] Many CME programs in family practice today are giving more emphasis to other teaching methods, particularly small-group interactive teaching, multimedia teaching, and programmed learning units for self instruction.

Learning through Reading

Despite the proliferation in recent years of various kinds of teaching modalities, especially involving audiovisual materials, reading remains an essential method of continuing education. A recent survey of directors of medical and continuing education and specialty society officers in California revealed that clinical journals are rated as first choice among all available study methods in enhancing the physician's ability to improve patient care.[33]

Recent years have seen important advances in the types and content of literature in family practice. *The Journal of Family Practice,* for example, represents a major departure from review papers written for the family physician by consultants in the other specialties. Most of the papers in this journal represent original work by family physicians and others involved in the developing discipline of family medicine. The continued expansion of this literature base of original work based on careful studies of the teaching and practice of family medicine should allow family physicians to take a more critical and scholarly approach to patient care.

Learning through Teaching

As more family practice teaching programs have developed in medical schools and community hospitals, opportunities have increased for practicing family physicians to become involved with teaching in various ways.[34] Some serve as preceptors for medical students in their own practices, others participate in resident teaching in nearby family practice residency programs, and still others participate in collaborative research projects involving their practices and teaching programs. As family physicians are exposed to younger, more recently trained students and residents through the teaching process, the interchange is inevitably a learning experience for all involved.

Certification and Recertification by the American Board of Family Practice

The American Board of Family Practice (ABFP) was established in 1969 and is still the only specialty board requiring recertification (at intervals of six years). The ABFP is independent of the American Academy of Family Physicians (AAFP). Although the great majority of board-certified family physicians are Academy members, board certification is not a requirement for AAFP membership.

The ABFP has established the following eligibility requirements to take the certifying examination: (1) completion of an approved three-year family practice residency and (2) completion of at least 300 approved CME credit hours acceptable to the ABFP. * The certifying examination is a two-day examination including multiple choice, pictorial, and patient management problems. The recertification examination may involve a similar two-day cognitive examination, but most candidates opt for a one-day cognitive examination plus review of a total of 20 patient records representing five selected categories.

---

* Prior to 1978, candidates could qualify for the ABFP examination by meeting the CME requirement together with practice eligibility through a minimum of six years of active family practice.

These categories may be selected from any of the 20 categories shown in Table 10–3 and are subject to verification and audit by the ABFP.

TABLE 10–3.   CATEGORIES FOR OFFICE RECORD REVIEW BY THE AMERICAN BOARD OF FAMILY PRACTICE

Abnormal vaginal bleeding
Acute cystitis
Acute duodenal ulcer
Appendicitis
Chronic bronchial asthma
Chronic obstructive pulmonary disease
Colitis
Congestive heart failure
Coronary artery disease
Depression
Diabetes mellitus
Hypertension
Lumbar disk disease
Normal pregnancy through delivery
Obesity
Otitis media
Pediatric patient
Postoperative carcinoma of the breast
Rheumatoid arthritis
Vaginitis

ROLES FOR DEPARTMENTS OF FAMILY PRACTICE

Departments of family practice to date have necessarily given top priority to the development of undergraduate and graduate teaching programs. They have great potential, however, to contribute to continuing medical education through the following kinds of future directions.[34]

1. INCORPORATE CONTINUING EDUCATION INTO THE CONTINUUM OF TEACHING IN FAMILY PRACTICE

As competency-based curricula and more effective teaching methods are developed and refined in family practice residencies, there can be more productive overlap between graduate and postgraduate education in family practice. Departments of family practice have both the opportunity and the responsibility to relate to the surrounding area or region as their "campus," including acceptance of an active role in CME for practicing family physicians. Family practice refresher courses should be more than didactic sessions; they should provide opportunities for self-assessment and problem-oriented small-group interactive learning. Departments of family practice can also serve as an advocate for practicing family physicians in arranging for short-term learning experiences provided by other clinical departments.

2. DECENTRALIZE EDUCATIONAL PROGRAMS ON A REGIONAL BASIS

The development of regional teaching programs on a network basis, especially at the graduate level, allows new relationships to be established with practicing physicians over a wide area. As noted in the last chapter, such networks afford closer communication with medical school and community-based faculty, opportunities to teach in nearby residency programs, and access to clinical methods being developed in teaching programs.

3. DEVELOP SPECIFIC EDUCATIONAL SUPPORT METHODS

Several approaches are of particular value in this respect: (1) a teaching bank for multimedia self-instructional materials, (2) self-assessment materials, and (3) profiling and indexing methods to analyze the practice experience of family physicians. In addition, exchanges can be arranged between third-year family practice residents and individual family physicians in partnership or group practice. These exchanges can allow residents to gain a better perspective of anticipated practice settings (with supervision and teaching provided by the physicians' associates) while providing family physicians coverage of their practices as they pursue selective CME experiences within the residency program.

4. INVOLVE PRACTICING FAMILY PHYSICIANS IN PART-TIME TEACHING

Practicing family physicians have much to offer medical students and residents in training. Students and residents greatly value real-world role models and the teaching input from those engaged in family practice in varied settings. Departments of family practice can augment the teaching skills of part-time teachers and contribute to their satisfaction and learning derived from teaching by conducting periodic teacher development workshops for part-time faculty.

5. CARRY OUT RESEARCH AND EVALUATION OF CME METHODS

There has been comparatively little work done to date on the effectiveness of CME in any field of medicine. It is well known that adult learning is complicated by varied individual learning styles. The practice of family medicine involves a diversity of settings, practice styles, and organizational patterns. The various approaches to CME that are being taken today in family practice require study as to their effectiveness in meeting the three basic goals of CME—increased knowledge and skills, improved clinical performance, and improved outcomes of patient care.

6. ENGAGE IN COLLABORATIVE RESEARCH WITH
   PRACTICING FAMILY PHYSICIANS

Research in family practice is a wide-open field with many areas requiring study. Research efforts are now being facilitated by the establishment of departments of family practice in medical schools, by the development of improved audit and record retrieval systems, and by refinements in disease coding for common clinical problems. Participation in collaborative research projects should be of real educational value to all physicians involved.

IMPLICATIONS FOR THE FAMILY PHYSICIAN

Based on the foregoing, several approaches can be summarized that can help the individual family physician to become involved in meaningful continuing medical education [34]:

1. IDENTIFY YOUR NEEDS

Several approaches have been described for this purpose, including profiling/-indexing of one's practice, the use of the problem-oriented medical record, medical audit, and taking self-assessment examinations.

2. EXPLORE AVAILABLE EDUCATIONAL RESOURCES

This involves looking at resources available within the region, including nearby family practice teaching programs, medical libraries, journals, courses offered, and self-instructional materials.

3. INDIVIDUALIZE YOUR APPROACH TO SPECIFIC NEEDS

A variety of learning options have been mentioned earlier. Family physicians can select their own approach to CME based upon their learning needs and individual learning styles.

4. UTILIZE CONSULTATION AS A LEARNING PROCESS

Consultation affords an important and often neglected avenue for continuing medical education. If consultants are chosen for their competence in dealing with a difficult problem as well as for their willingness and interest in teaching, each consultation can become a valuable learning experience.

5. ESTABLISH A HABIT FOR CONTINUING MEDICAL EDUCATION

This involves organizing one's practice so that time can be allocated to continuing medical education, together with reordering of personal priorities to make this happen. There are more opportunities and options available for CME in family practice than ever before. An active interest in continuing education can lead to improved patient care as well as greater satisfaction and interest in one's practice.

Many years ago Sir William Osler [35] said, "In what may be called the natural method of teaching, the student begins with a patient, continues with a patient, and ends his studies with the patient, using books and lectures as tools, as means to an end." Today, other methods are available in addition to books and lectures, but the essence of this statement is unchanged, and the responsibility for continued education remains with each physician.

REFERENCES

1. Watts MSM: Continuing medical education and continuing professional competence. West J Med 126:220, 1977
2. Richards RK: Past history and future trends in CME. Quality Rev Bull 4:8, 1978
3. Wilbur RS: Mandatory continuing medical education: A liability. Quality Rev Bull 4:12, 1978
4. American Medical Association. Continuing medical education. JAMA 236:2993, 1976
5. Moore FJ: Information technologies and health care. Arch Intern Med 125:504, 1970
6. Durack DT: The weight of medical knowledge. N Engl J Med 298:773, 1978
7. Weiss PA: Living nature and the knowledge gap. Saturday Rev 52:19, 1969
8. McWhinney IR: Family medicine in perspective. N Engl J Med 293:176, 1975
9. Ashbaugh DG, McKean RS: Continuing medical education: The philosophy and use of audit. JAMA 236:1485, 1976
10. Scott AJ: Continuing education: More or better? N Engl J Med 295:444, 1976
11. Brown CR, Uhl HSM: Mandatory continuing education—Sense or nonsense? JAMA 213:1660, 1970
12. Lewis CE, Hassanein RS: Continuing medical education. N Engl J Med 282:258, 1970
13. Miller GE: Continuing education for what? J Med Educ 42:320, 1967
14. Medical Education in the United States, 1977–1978. JAMA 238:2804, 1977
15. Miller GE: Why continuing medical education? Bull NY Acad Med 51:704, 1975
16. Storey PB: Mandatory continuing medical education: One step forward—two steps back. N Engl J Med 298:1416, 1978
17. Sanazaro PJ: Medical audit, continuing medical education and quality assurance. West J Med 125:248, 1976
18. Clute KF: The General Practitioner: A Study of Medical Education and Practice in Ontario and Nova Scotia. Toronto, University of Toronto Press, 1963
19. Peterson OL, Andrews LP, Spain RS, et al: An analytical study of North Carolina general practice 1953–1954. J Med Educ 31:165, part 2, 1956
20. Williamson JW, Alexander M, Miller GE: Continuing education and patient care research: Physician response to screening test results. JAMA 201:938, 1967
21. Meskauskas JA, Webster GD: The American Board of Internal Medicine recertification examination: Process and results. Ann Intern Med 82:577, 1975

22. Youmans JB: Experience with a postgraduate course for practitioners: Evaluation of results. J Assoc Amer Med Coll 10:154, 1975

23. Kotre JN, Mann FC, Morris WC, et al: The Michigan physician's use and evaluation of his medical journal. Mich Med 70:11, 1971

24. Miller HL: Teaching and Learning in Adult Education. New York, MacMillan, 1964, p 33

25. What about your continuing education? Patient Care 5(9):7, 1971

26. Stein LS: Your Personal Learning Plan, A Handbook for Physicians. Chicago, Illinois Council on Continuing Medical Education, 1973

27. Sivertson SE, Meyer TC, Hansen R, Schoenenberger A: Individual physician profile: Continuing education related to medical practice. J Med Educ 48: 1006, 1973

28. Rakel RE: Indexing in office practice: A system for monitoring high-risk patients and filing medical literature. Continuing Educ 9:30, 1978

29. Barnes RH, Hulbert BL, Roberts JG: The case for QACE. Quality Rev Bull 4:16, 1978

30. Metcalfe DHH, Mancini JC: Critical event outcome studies used as a teaching tool. J Med Educ 47:869, 1972

31. Geyman JP, Brown TC, Lee PV: Perceptions of formal in-training evaluation by family practice residents. J Fam Pract 5:869, 1977

32. Libby GN, Weinswig MH, Kirk KW: Help stamp out mandatory continuing education. JAMA 233:797, 1975

33. Soffer A: Are medical journals obsolete? JAMA 238:1402, 1977

34. Geyman JP: A new look at continuing medical education in family practice. J Fam Pract 2:119, 1975

35. Osler W: Aequanimitas, with Other Addresses to Medical Students, Nurses and Practitioners of Medicine, 2nd ed. Philadelphia, Blakiston's, 1932, p 315

CHAPTER ELEVEN

Clinical Content of Family Practice

Those who feel that we should revert to the "jack of all trades" 1930 style general practitioner who does anything and everything he wants to do—and those at the other extreme who would limit the family physician to a role of triage are both quite wrong. Anyone who has been a family physician in a medium to small community knows that sooner or later anything can and will come in through the office door. The family doctor can expect to encounter pathology and emergencies of every description. He must be able to handle prompt decisions, emergency trauma, simple fractures, normal deliveries and the principles of common surgical procedures—but he should be fully responsible to refer that which should and can be referred.

James L. Dennis [1]

The mainspring of family practice is people—well people, sick people, babies, children, adults, and the elderly. The needs of these patients fill the day of the family physician. Most of the people seen by family physicians each day are well known to them, and many of them have become friends. Others present as new patients with acute or chronic complaints, often without previous medical care relative to these complaints. Family physicians are in a unique position to assess their patients as individuals and as members of family units.

This knowledge forms a basis for interpretation of the patient's symptoms and clinical findings as well as for management of the patient's particular illness.

Family practice is thus a field more committed to the continuing needs of individuals and their families for primary health care than to any specific content area per se. At the same time, some basic patterns and variables can be identified to describe the clinical content of family practice and the daily work of family physicians.

Until recent years little was known about the content of the practices of primary care physicians, particularly with respect to ambulatory care. This was partly due to a relative lack of interest in research in primary care in the United States and partly due to a lack of adequate research methods to describe and analyze the content of primary care. Coding systems, for example, were initially designed to describe the clinical problems of hospitalized patients, not the clinical problems encountered by physicians in ambulatory care. The major classification system used in this country until recently was the ICDA (International Classification of Disease Adapted for Use in the United States), which did not afford classification of at least 25 percent of the clinical problems encountered by family physicians in everyday practice. The most widely used classification system today is ICHPPC (International Classification of Health Problems in Primary Care) (Appendix 6), which alleviates many of the earlier coding problems in primary care.

The purpose of this chapter is threefold: (1) to outline some of the variables that influence the clinical content of family practice; (2) to characterize the content of ambulatory and hospital practice of family physicians based on available studies to date in this country, including studies of referral patterns; and (3) to compare the clinical content of family practice with the other primary care specialties. This chapter is focused on the clinical problems of individual patients. The next chapter will examine the clinical problems of families; these two chapters must be considered together in viewing the clinical content of family practice.

SOME VARIABLES AFFECTING
PRACTICE CONTENT

Although there are basic similarities to large portions of the clinical content of family practice throughout the United States, a number of variables may influence the actual practice content of individual family physicians as well as the characteristics of family practice in different regions of the country. Brief consideration of some of these variables illustrates the potential magnitude of these variations.

Some fundamental features of family practice are shown in Table 11–1.[2] Even cursory reflection on these features suggests that the content of family practice in any one setting depends on such factors as the characteristics of

TABLE 11-1. CHARACTERISTICS OF FAMILY PRACTICE

1. The pattern of illness approximates to the pattern of illness in the community; i.e., there is:
    a. A high incidence of transient illness.
    b. A high prevalence of chronic illness.
    c. A high incidence of emotional illness.
2. The illness is undifferentiated; i.e., it has not been previously assessed by any other physician.
3. Illnesses are frequently a complex mixture of physical, emotional, and social elements.
4. Disease is seen early, before the full clinical picture has developed.
5. Relationship with patients is continuous and transcends individual episodes of illness.

Source: McWhinney, I.R.: Problem solving and decision making in primary medical practice. *Canadian Family Physician* 18:11, 1972.

the patient population, environmental factors, physician variables, regional differences in health care delivery, and related factors.

Many features of the practice population directly affect the spectrum of clinical problems seen by the family physician. These include age and other demographic characteristics of the population, socioeconomic factors, mobility of the population, and cultural factors, particularly as they influence health-seeking behavior of the population. Thus, an older, stable population will involve the family physician in the care of an increased proportion of chronic illness and lesser involvement with obstetric and pediatric care as compared with a younger, more mobile population.

Environmental factors likewise may influence the content of family practice in different parts of the country, including geographic, climatic, industrial, occupational, and related factors. Parasitic infestations, for an obvious example, are encountered less often by family physicians in Minnesota than in Louisiana.

Physician variables may produce significant differences in the practices of individual family physicians. The training and experience of family physicians in obstetrics, for example, affects whether or not a given family physician includes obstetrics in his/her practice, which may further influence the age spectrum and proportion of pediatric care in the practice. Another important physician variable relates to the philosophy of the physician concerning the value and need for preventive care. Figure 11-1 illustrates the possible roles of medical intervention over the spectrum of natural history of disease and injury.[3] The practice content of a family physician actively involved in prospective medicine will naturally be quite different from that of a family physician more heavily involved with the care of more advanced stages of disease.

Regional differences in patterns of medical care may alter the practice content of family physicians considerably in some respects. The involvement of family physicians in obstetrics in the northeastern United States, for example, has been relatively limited for some years compared to patterns of family practice elsewhere in the country.

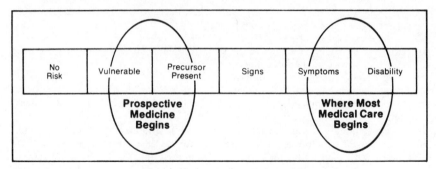

FIGURE 11-1.

Medical care and the natural history of disease.

Source: Robbins, LC: Prospective medicine. *Continuing Education for the Family Physician* 8:24, 1978. Reprinted by permission.

Patients seen by family physicians do not readily lend themselves to precise categorization. As pointed out by Malerich [4]:

> [Family practice] defies categorization or fragmentation because its essence is the care of the whole person in relation to his family and environment. In reality, a patient visit frequently includes more than one aspect of illness or concern.

When patients are seen for multiple problems at a single visit, only some of the problems may be coded for reporting purposes, and some problems (especially behavioral problems) may be underreported for a variety of reasons, as will be seen in the next chapter.

Despite these variables, however, it is still worthwhile to review some attempts to describe the clinical content of family practice, for certain patterns of illness emerge as major components in the practice of any physician providing primary health care to entire families.

SOME STUDIES OF CLINICAL CONTENT

As pointed out in an earlier chapter, the content of medical practice in the community is quite different from that encountered in most teaching settings to which medical students and residents have been exposed. In their studies of the ecology of medical care in the United States, White and his colleagues [5] demonstrated that 750 of 1000 adults at risk during an average month will experience one or more illnesses or injuries. Of these, 250 will consult a physician; of these, 9 will be hospitalized (8 at a community hospital and 1 at a university medical center) and 5 will be referred for consultation to another physician. A similar study in Canada examined the experience of 1000 people over one year. Of these, 800 had some illness and 730 consulted a physician; 590 had some disability during the year, 160 were hospitalized, and only 200 were well throughout the year.[6]

Office Practice

The most comprehensive and definitive study yet conducted of ambulatory care in family practice, as in other specialties, has been the National Ambulatory Medical Care Survey (NAMCS). The most recent data available at this writing are based upon an estimated 234,660,000 visits made to the offices of general practitioners/family physicians during calendar year 1975. These visits accounted for over 41 percent of all office visits to physicians in all fields in the United States in that year.[7]

Table 11–2 presents some physician and patient characteristics of this total experience. It is interesting to note that over 72 percent of these visits were made to physicians in solo practice, a figure that will likely decline in future years as the trend toward group practice increases. It is also of interest that nearly 60 percent of office visits were made by females and that 18 percent of all visits were made by patients over 65 years of age.[7]

The most frequent complaints, symptoms, or other reasons for a patient's visit are shown in Table 11–3. It is estimated that over 6 million visits involved prenatal and postnatal care.[7] The 25 most common principal diagnoses recorded by general/family physicians during 1975 are reflected in Table 11–4, and accounted for approximately one-half of all ambulatory visits.[7]

Table 11–5 represents the number and proportion of office visits by major ICDA diagnostic groupings. It can be noted that four diagnostic groups accounted for over 50 percent of all principal diagnoses made: (1) diseases of the respiratory system, (2) special conditions and examinations without sickness, (3) diseases of the circulatory system, and (4) accidents, poisonings, and violence.[7]

The number and proportion of various diagnostic and therapeutic services performed by general/family physicians during 1975 are listed in Table 11–6. It can be noted that about two-thirds of all visits involved limited or general histories and examinations and that just over one-half of all visits involved the prescription of drug therapy.[7]

Table 11–7 analyzes the office practice experience of general/family physicians during 1975 in terms of prior-visit status, seriousness of problem, disposition, and duration of visit. Strong emphasis on continuity of care is reflected in these figures, with 87 percent of visits involving patients who had been seen previously and 80 percent of visits requested to return as needed or at a specified time. It is of interest that only 1.2 percent of all visits required hospitalization, and that only 3 percent of visits involved referral.[7]

Hospital Practice

In comparison to rather extensive studies of office practice, there have been only limited studies to date of the hospital practice of family physicians in the United States. Three such studies are worthy of note, however, and suggest some general patterns of hospital care by family physicians.

TABLE 11-2. NUMBER, PERCENT DISTRIBUTIONS, AND NUMBER OF VISITS PER 100 PERSONS PER YEAR TO
OFFICE-BASED GENERAL AND FAMILY PRACTITIONERS BY TYPE AND LOCATION OF THE
PHYSICIAN'S PRACTICE AND BY AGE, SEX, AND COLOR OF THE PATIENT—UNITED STATES,
JANUARY–DECEMBER 1975

SELECTED PHYSICIAN AND PATIENT CHARACTERISTICS	NUMBER OF VISITS (THOUSANDS)	PERCENT DISTRIBUTIONS OF VISITS	NUMBER OF VISITS PER 100 PERSONS PER YEAR*
All visits	234,660	100.0	113
Physician Characteristics			
Type of practice			
Solo	171,000	72.9	—
Other†	63,650	27.1	—
Location ‡			
Metropolitan	136,533	58.2	94
Nonmetropolitan	98,127	41.8	146
Patient Characteristics			
Age			
Under 15 years	33,772	14.4	65
15–24 years	37,568	16.0	96
25–44 years	56,476	24.1	108
45–64 years	64,502	27.5	152
65 years and over	42,343	18.0	194
Sex			
Female	138,904	59.2	130
Male	95,756	40.8	95
Color			
White	207,660	88.5	115
Other §	27,000	11.5	99

* Based on population estimates for July 1, 1975, Bureau of the Census, *Current Population Reports*, Series P-25 and P-26.
† Includes partnership and group practices.
‡ Signifies location within or outside the standard metropolitan statistical areas (SMSAs).
§ Of this category, about 81 percent are visits by blacks.

Source: National ambulatory medical care survey of visits to general and family practitioners, January–December 1975. *Advance Data from Vital and Health Statistics of the National Center for Health Statistics*, 15:3. Washington, D.C., U.S. Department of Health, Education and Welfare, 1977.

A study of family physicians in a nonmetropolitan area of southern Illinois showed that they devoted about one-quarter of their time to patient care, with an average of 11 patients seen in the hospital each day. Their hospital care included pediatric, obstetric, general medical and geriatric care, as well as some surgery and surgical assisting.

Garg and his colleagues [8] analyzed the profiles of 4599 hospitalized patients by physician specialty in a study of discharge diagnoses recorded in 1970 in nine general hospitals in Lucas County, Ohio. Family physicians cared for 28 percent of these patients, and averaged 3.1 inpatients per physician each day.

TABLE 11-3. NUMBER, PERCENT, AND CUMULATIVE PERCENT OF VISITS TO OFFICE-BASED GENERAL AND FAMILY PRACTITIONERS, BY THE 25 MOST FREQUENT PATIENT PROBLEMS, COMPLAINTS, OR SYMPTOMS CLASSIFIED BY THE NATIONAL AMBULATORY MEDICAL CARE SURVEY (NAMCS) SYMPTOM CLASSIFICATION CODE—UNITED STATES, JANUARY–DECEMBER 1975

RANK	MOST FREQUENT PATIENT PROBLEM, COMPLAINT, OR SYMPTOM	NAMCS CODE*	NUMBER OF VISITS (THOUSANDS)	PERCENT OF VISITS	CUMULATIVE PERCENT
1	General and required physical examinations	900,901	11,582	4.9	4.9
2	Problems of back	415	9,535	4.1	9.0
3	Throat soreness	520	9,005	3.8	12.8
4	Problems of lower extremity	400	8,847	3.8	16.6
5	Abdominal pain	540	7,279	3.1	19.7
6	Problems of upper extremity	405	7,234	3.1	22.8
7	Cough	311	7,046	3.0	25.8
8	Visit for medication	910	6,436	2.7	28.5
9	Fatigue	004	6,221	2.7	31.2
10	Cold	312	6,077	2.6	33.8
11	Headache	056	5,836	2.5	36.3
12	Pregnancy examination	905	5,709	2.4	38.7
13	Pain in chest	322	4,919	2.1	40.8
14	Allergic skin reaction	112	4,711	2.0	42.8
15	Wounds of skin	116	4,576	2.0	44.8
16	High blood pressure	205	4,432	1.9	46.7
17	Surgical aftercare	986	4,414	1.9	48.6
18	Weight gain	010	3,643	1.6	50.2
19	Vertigo—dizziness	069	3,554	1.5	51.7
20	Problems of face, neck	410	3,161	1.4	53.1
21	Earache	735	3,147	1.3	54.4
22	Fever	002	3,087	1.3	55.7
23	Gynecologic examination	904	2,749	1.2	56.9
24	Shortness of breath	306	2,620	1.1	58.0
25	Flu	313	2,560	1.1	59.1

* Symptomatic groupings and code number inclusions are based on a symptom classification developed for use in the NAMCS.

Source: National ambulatory medical care survey of visits to general and family practitioners, January–December 1975. *Advance Data from Vital and Health Statistics of the National Center for Health Statistics*, 15:5. Washington, D.C., U.S. Department of Health, Education and Welfare, 1977.

TABLE 11-4. NUMBER, PERCENT, AND CUMULATIVE PERCENT OF VISITS TO OFFICE-BASED GENERAL AND FAMILY PRACTITIONERS, BY THE 25 MOST COMMON ICDA-CODED PRINCIPAL DIAGNOSES—UNITED STATES, JANUARY–DECEMBER 1975

RANK	MOST COMMON PRINCIPAL DIAGNOSIS	ICDA CODE*	NUMBER OF VISITS (THOUSANDS)	PERCENT OF VISITS	CUMULATIVE PERCENT
1	Medical or special examination	Y00	14,690	6.3	6.3
2	Essential benign hypertension	401	13,904	5.9	12.2
3	Acute upper respiratory infection, site unspecified	465	8,505	3.6	15.8
4	Diabetes mellitus	250	5,780	2.5	18.3
5	Medical and surgical aftercare	Y10	5,602	2.4	20.7
6	Acute pharyngitis	462	5,204	2.2	22.9
7	Chronic ischemic heart disease	412	5,141	2.2	25.1
8	Other eczema and dermatitis	692	5,075	2.2	27.3
9	Influenza, unqualified	470	4,927	2.1	29.4
10	Obesity	277	4,905	2.1	31.5
11	Neuroses	300	4,126	1.8	33.3
12	Bronchitis, unqualified	490	3,903	1.7	35.0
13	Acute tonsillitis	463	3,884	1.7	36.7
14	Arthritis, unspecified	715	3,457	1.5	38.2
15	Cystitis	595	3,203	1.4	39.6
16	Otitis media	381	3,087	1.3	40.9
17	Osteoarthritis	713	2,895	1.2	42.1
18	Synovitis, bursitis	731	2,868	1.2	43.3
19	Other nonarticular rheumatism	717	2,818	1.2	44.5
20	Diarrheal disease	009	2,709	1.2	45.7
21	Menopausal symptoms	627	2,562	1.1	46.8
22	Chronic sinusitis	503	2,546	1.1	47.9
23	Hay fever	507	2,503	1.1	49.0
24	Sprains, strains of sacroiliac region	846	2,437	1.0	50.0
25	Inoculations and vaccinations	Y02	2,347	1.0	51.0

* Diagnostic groupings and code number inclusions are based on the *Eighth Revision International Classification of Diseases, Adapted for Use in the United States.*

Source: National ambulatory medical care survey of visits to general and family practitioners, January–December 1975. *Advance Data from Vital and Health Statistics of the National Center for Health Statistics,* 15:6. Washington, D.C., U.S. Department of Health, Education and Welfare, 1977.

Department of Family Medicine (R700)
University of Miami School of Medicine
P. O. Box 016700
Miami, Florida 33101

TABLE 11-5. NUMBER AND PERCENT DISTRIBUTION OF VISITS TO OFFICE-BASED GENERAL AND FAMILY PRACTITIONERS BY PRINCIPAL DIAGNOSIS CLASSIFIED BY ICDA GROUP—UNITED STATES, JANUARY–DECEMBER 1975

PRINCIPAL DIAGNOSIS	ICDA CODE*	NUMBER OF VISITS (THOUSANDS)	DISTRIBUTION OF VISITS (%)
All principal diagnoses		234,660	100.0
Infective and parasitic diseases	000–136	10,878	4.6
Neoplasms	140–239	2,795	1.2
Endocrine, nutritional, and metabolic diseases	240–279	13,568	5.8
Diseases of the blood and blood-forming organs	280–289	3,043	1.3
Mental disorders	290–315	7,064	3.0
Diseases of the nervous system and sense organs	320–389	10,906	4.7
Diseases of the circulatory system	390–458	29,005	12.4
Diseases of the respiratory system	460–519	43,304	18.5
Diseases of the digestive system	520–577	9,154	3.9
Diseases of the genitourinary system	580–629	14,946	6.4
Diseases of the skin and subcutaneous tissue	680–709	10,721	4.6
Diseases of the musculoskeletal system	710–738	16,668	7.1
Symptoms and ill-defined conditions	780–796	9,220	3.9
Accidents, poisonings, and violence	800–999	20,168	8.6
Special conditions and examinations without sickness	Y00–Y13	30,188	12.9
Other diagnoses†		544	0.2
Diagnosis "none" or unknown‡		2,486	1.1

* Diagnostic groupings and code number inclusions are based on the *Eighth Revision International Classification of Diseases, Adapted for Use in the United States.*
† Complications of pregnancy, childbirth, and the puerperium (630–678), congenital anomalies (740–759), certain causes of perinatal morbidity and mortality (760–779).
‡ Includes blank, noncodeable, and illegible diagnoses.

Source: National ambulatory medical care survey of visits to general and family practitioners, January–December 1975. *Advance Data from Vital and Health Statistics of the National Center for Health Statistics,* 15:7. Washington, D.C., U.S. Department of Health, Education and Welfare, 1977.

James M. Gall, M.D., C.C.F.P.
Department of Family Medicine
University of Miami School of Medicine
P. O. Box 016700
Miami Florida 33101

TABLE 11-6.   NUMBER AND PERCENT DISTRIBUTION OF VISITS TO OFFICE-BASED GENERAL
AND FAMILY PRACTITIONERS BY DIAGNOSTIC AND THERAPEUTIC SERVICES
ORDERED OR PROVIDED—UNITED STATES, JANUARY–DECEMBER 1975

DIAGNOSTIC AND THERAPEUTIC SERVICE ORDERED OR PROVIDED	NUMBER OF VISITS (THOUSANDS)	PERCENT OF VISITS*
All visits	234,660	100.0
No services provided	4,082	1.7
Diagnostic services		
Limited history/examination	130,516	55.6
General history/examination	29,570	12.6
Clinical lab test	50,618	21.6
X-ray	14,638	6.2
Blood pressure check	94,358	40.2
EKG	5,418	2.3
Hearing test	1,831	0.8
Vision test	3,307	1.4
Endoscopy	1,474	0.6
Therapeutic services		
Drug administered or prescribed†	130,479	55.6
Injection	50,476	21.5
Immunization/desensitization	8,659	3.7
Office surgery	12,113	5.2
Physiotherapy	7,834	3.3
Medical counseling	27,378	11.7
Psychotherapy/therapeutic listening	6,715	2.9
Other services provided	8,451	3.6

* Percents will not add to 100 because most patient visits required the provision of more than one treatment or service.
† Includes prescription and nonprescription drugs.
Source: National ambulatory medical care survey of visits to general and family practitioners, January–December 1975. *Advance Data from Vital and Health Statistics of the National Center for Health Statistics,* 15:8. Washington, D.C., U.S. Department of Health, Education and Welfare, 1977.

The spectrum of primary diagnoses was evenly divided among a variety of diagnostic categories, and the average length of stay was 8.9 days.

Shank[9] studied his inpatient experience over a one-year period, his first year in practice as a family physician in a midwestern community of 15,000. During the study period, 235 patients were hospitalized, with about 20 patients requiring hospital admission each month. The most common principal discharge diagnoses included newborn care, vaginal delivery, congestive heart failure, diabetes mellitus, chronic lung disease, ischemic heart disease, cardiac arrhythmia, urinary tract infection, fractures, hypertension, and pneumonia.

Two other Canadian studies in larger community and hospital settings have shown comparable hospital utilization by family physicians. Tarrant's[10] practice involved 325 hospitalizations per year, while Fowler and Falk's[11] study of family physicians in British Columbia averaged 228 hospitalizations per physician per year, with obstetric care representing the most common reason for hospitalization in both studies.

A Combined Study

The *Virginia Study* mentioned in an earlier chapter represents a statewide study of the practices of 118 family physicians in Virginia over a two-year period between 1973 and 1975. All health care problems were recorded that were encountered during that period in the office, the hospital, the nursing home,

TABLE 11–7. NUMBER AND PERCENT DISTRIBUTIONS OF VISITS TO OFFICE–BASED GENERAL AND FAMILY PRACTITIONERS BY PRIOR–VISIT STATUS, SERIOUSNESS OF PROBLEM, DISPOSITION AND DURATION OF VISIT—UNITED STATES, JANUARY– DECEMBER 1975

SELECTED VISIT CHARACTERISTICS	*NUMBER OF VISITS (THOUSANDS)*	*DISTRIBUTIONS OF VISIT (%)*
All visits	234,660	100.0
Prior-visit status		
Patient seen for the first time	29,847	12.7
Patient seen before		
For another problem	71,446	30.5
For current problem	133,367	56.8
Seriousness of problem		
Serious and very serious	39,941	17.0
Slightly serious	82,440	35.1
Not serious	112,279	47.9
Disposition*		
No follow-up planned	36,326	15.5
Return at specified time	120,379	51.3
Return if needed	68,444	29.2
Telephone follow-up	8,658	3.7
Referred to other physician/agency	6,957	3.0
Admit to hospital	2,861	1.2
Other†	2,276	1.0
Duration of visit‡		
0 minutes	3,885	1.7
1–5 minutes	48,156	20.5
6–10 minutes	79,964	34.1
11–15 minutes	58,478	24.9
16–30 minutes	39,815	17.0
31 minutes or more	4,362	1.9

* Percents will not add to 100 because some patient visits had more than one disposition.
† Includes return to referring physician.
‡ Signifies time spent in face-to-face encounter between physician and patient.
Source: National ambulatory medical care survey of visits to general and family practitioners, January–December 1975. *Advance Data from Vital and Health Statistics of the National Center for Health Statistics,* 15:9. Washington D.C., U.S. Department of Health, Education and Welfare, 1977.

and in the patient's home. A complete listing of the results of this study is provided in Appendix 5, including the rank order of diagnoses by frequency and diagnoses by disease category and age–sex distribution. Of particular interest here is the rather striking similarity between the practice profiles in urban, suburban, and rural settings (Figure 11–2).[12] It can be noted that a somewhat greater frequency of trauma and respiratory illness was cared for in rural practices, but otherwise the profiles are quite comparable. The relatively small proportion of obstetric problems encountered is atypical compared to most parts of the country, since the majority of obstetric care in Virginia is provided by obstetrician–gynecologists.

REFERRAL AND CONSULTATION

As already noted, the average referral rate among general/family physicians across the country has been found to be about 3 percent. Two small but more detailed studies of referral patterns in family practice have shown comparable or lower referral rates. One study of four family physicians in upstate New York during 1973 recorded a referral rate of 2.2 percent of 4604 patient visits.[13] A subsequent study of eight family physicians in northern California

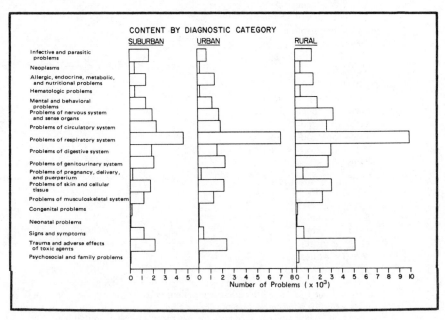

FIGURE 11-2.
Content by diagnostic category in suburban versus rural practices.
Source: Marsland, DW, Wood, M, and Mayo, F: A data bank for patient care, curriculum, and research in family practice: 526,196 patient problems. *Journal of Family Practice* 3:26, 1976.

demonstrated a referral rate of 1.6 percent of a total of 6409 hospital and office visits.[14] Table 11–8 compares the frequency of specialties involved in consultation in both of these studies.[14] The preponderance of referrals in both studies involved the surgical fields, obstetrics–gynecology, and, to a lesser extent, the medical subspecialties. Only occasional consultations were requested from general pediatricians and general internists, which tends to confirm their principal roles as primary care physicians.

Presently available evidence therefore shows that family physicians provide definitive care for at least 97 percent of patient visits in everyday practice. At the same time, consultation and referral represent an essential mechanism for providing the highest quality of patient care and constitute an important method of continuing medical education for family physicians.

COMPARATIVE CONTENT BY SPECIALTY

A number of interesting comparisons can be drawn in several respects between general/family practice and some of the other specialties. First, with regard to the number and proportion of all office visits in the United States during 1975, general/family physicians accounted for over 41 percent of all visits—more than the combined proportions of internal medicine, obstetrics–gynecology, pediatrics, and general surgery (Table 11–9).[7]

General/family physicians in 1975 provided over 41 percent of their office visits in nonmetropolitan areas. Internists, pediatricians, and obstetrician–gynecologists ranged from only 10.9 percent to 18.1 percent of their respective total office visits in nonmetropolitan areas (Table 11–10). What may be surprising to some is that over one-half of all office visits to general/family physicians in 1975 were made in standard metropolitan statistical areas (SMSAs).* Approximately 70 percent of the United States population in 1975 lived within SMSAs, whereas about 65 percent of general/family physicians practiced within SMSAs at that time.[7]

With respect to the number and proportion of office visits to various specialties by patients over and under 65 years of age, Table 11–11 presents some interesting comparisons. The predominant role of general/family physicians in geriatric care is at once evident, with this field accounting for 45 percent of all office visits of patients over 65 years of age. Also of interest is the comparative proportion of geriatric care to nongeriatric care within general/family practice and internal medicine. General/family physicians account for at least 40 percent of all office visits for patients over and less than 65 years of age. The annual rate of office visits to general/family physicians for patients over 65 years of age is almost double the rate of office visits to internists.[15] The

---

* An SMSA was defined by the National Ambulatory Medical Care Survey as a group of contiguous counties containing at least one city of 50,000 people or more or two contiguous cities with a combined population of at least 50,000 people.

TABLE 11–8. A COMPARISON BETWEEN EASTERN AND WESTERN UNITED STATES FAMILY PRACTICE REFERRALS TO SPECIALTIES

SPECIALTY	GEYMAN, ET AL. (1)		METCALFE AND SISCHY (2)		COMBINED DATA	
	Absolute Number	Rank Order	Absolute Number	Rank Order	Absolute Number	Rank Order
General surgery	26	1	26	1	52	1
Orthopedics	20	2	10	3.5	30	2
Obstetrics-gynecology	15	3	11	2	26	3
Opthalmology	14	4	6	8	20	4
Urology	10	5	8	5.5	18	5
Neurology	8	6	8	5.5	16	6
Otolaryngology	3	11	10	3.5	13	7
Internal medicine	7	7.5	3	10	10	8.5
Psychiatry	7	7.5	3	10	10	8.5
Dermatology	0	—	7	7	7	10
Cardiology	4	9.5	1	15	5	11
Acupuncture (MD)	4	9.5	0	—	4	12
Hematology	2	13	1	15	3	13.5
Plastic surgery	0	—	3	10	3	13.5
Endocrinology	1	15.5	1	15	2	15.5
Gastroenterology	2	13	0	—	2	15.5
Allergy	0	—	2	12	2	15.5
Speech therapist	2	13	0	—	2	15.5
Pediatrics	0	—	1	15	1	19
Adolescent behavior clinic	0	—	1	15	1	19
Oncology	1	15.5	0	—	1	19
Totals	126	—	102	—	228	—

Source: (1) Geyman, J.P., Brown, T.C., Rivers, K.: Referrals in family practice: A comparative study by geographic region and practice setting. *Journal of Family Practice* 3:2, 1976.   (2) Metcalfe, D.H.H., Sischy, D.: Patterns of referral from family practice. *Journal of Family Practice* 1:34, 1974.

TABLE 11-9. NUMBER AND PERCENT OF VISITS TO OFFICE-BASED PHYSICIANS BY THE MOST-VISITED SPECIALTIES—UNITED STATES, JANUARY-DECEMBER 1975

MOST-VISITED SPECIALTY	*NUMBER OF VISITS (THOUSANDS)*	*PERCENT OF VISITS*
General and family practice	234,660	41.3
Internal medicine	62,117	10.9
Obstetrics/gynecology	48,076	8.5
Pediatrics	46,684	8.2
General surgery	41,292	7.3

Source: National ambulatory medical care survey of visits to general and family practitioners, January-December 1975. *Advance Data from Vital and Health Statistics of the National Center for Health Statistics,* 15:2. Washington, D.C., U.S. Department of Health, Education and Welfare, 1977.

percent distribution of the most common diagnoses in general/family practice, internal medicine, pediatrics, and obstetrics–gynecology were presented in an earlier chapter (p. 76), together with a comparison of the range of services within these four fields (p. 80). A more specific view of the comparative proportions of office visits by specialty for two diseases–hypertension/hypertensive heart disease and rheumatoid arthritis–is afforded by Tables 11–12 and 11–13, respectively.[16]

Finally, Table 11–14 illustrates the active role played by general/family physicians in inpatient care based upon the results of the previously mentioned study of hospitalized patients in nine Ohio hospitals. This study of over 4500 patients revealed a wide diversity of diagnoses among family physicians, whereas 42 percent of pediatricians' patients were hospitalized for respiratory illnesses and 33 percent of internists' patients were hospitalized for diseases of the circulatory system.[8]

TABLE 11-10. PERCENT DISTRIBUTION OF VISITS TO OFFICE-BASED PHYSICIANS BY LOCATION ACCORDING TO SPECIALTY—UNITED STATES, JANUARY-DECEMBER 1975

LOCATION	*DISTRIBUTION OF VISITS (%)*			
	General and Family Practice	*Internal Medicine*	*Obstetrics-Gynecology*	*Pediatrics*
Total	100.0	100.0	100.0	100.0
Metropolitan	58.2	84.6	81.9	89.1
Nonmetropolitan	41.8	15.4	18.1	10.9

Source: National ambulatory medical care survey of visits to general and family practitioners, January-December 1975. *Advance Data from Vital and Health Statistics of the National Center for Health Statistics,* 15:4. Washington, D.C., U.S. Department of Health, Education and Welfare, 1977

TABLE 11–11. NUMBER AND PERCENT DISTRIBUTION OF OFFICE VISITS BY PERSONS 65 YEARS
AND OVER AND PERCENT DISTRIBUTION OF OFFICE VISITS BY PERSONS UNDER
65 YEARS BY PHYSICIAN SPECIALTY AND TYPE OF PRACTICE—UNITED STATES,
1975

	OFFICE VISITS		
	65 Years and Over		Under 65 Years
PHYSICIAN SPECIALTY AND TYPE OF PRACTICE	Number (thousands)	Percent Distribution	Percent Distribution
All visits	93,061	100.0	100.0*
Physician specialty			
General and family practice	42,343	45.3	40.5
Internal medicine	17,925	19.3	9.3
General surgery	7,335	7.9	7.2
Ophthalmology	6,429	6.9	3.8
Cardiovascular diseases	3,177	3.4	0.9
Urology	3,175	3.4	1.6
Otolaryngology	2,231	2.4	3.0
Dermatology	2,173	2.3	2.5
Orthopedic surgery	1,750	1.9	3.7
Obstetrics–gynecology	1,132	1.2	9.9
Other specialties	5,388	5.8	17.6
Type of practice			
Solo	60,677	65.2	58.8
Other†	32,383	34.8	41.2

* Based on an estimated 474,540,000 visits.
† Includes partnership and group practices.
Source: Office visits by persons aged 65 and over: National ambulatory medical care survey, United States,
1975. *Advance Data from Vital and Health Statistics of the National Center for Health Statistics,* 22:4.
Washington, D.C., U.S. Department of Health, Education and Welfare, 1978.

COMMENT

Several general comments are in order in viewing the aggregate data that have
been presented here to characterize the basic clinical content of general/family
practice in this country during the mid-1970s. Perhaps most important is to
note that all of these practice content studies reflect effective demand, which
does not necessarily correlate well with the needs for primary health care. In
addition, these data represent the field at a time when solo practice was the
most common style of practice, and the overall health care system (including
reimbursement patterns) favored curative medicine and disease care rather
than preventive medicine and health care. It is therefore quite possible that
the future profile of family practice will vary somewhat from existing patterns
as group practice becomes a more common style of practice and as other changes
take place within the health care delivery system.

TABLE 11-12. HYPERTENSION/HYPERTENSIVE HEART DISEASE: VISITS BY SPECIALTY (JULY 1975–JUNE 1976)

SPECIALTY	HYPERTENSION (%)	HYPERTENSIVE HEART DISEASE (%)	ALL HYPERTENSION/ HYPERTENSIVE HEART DISEASE (%)	ALL DIAGNOSES (%)
General/family physician	52	46	51	32
Internist	30	38	31	15
Osteopathic physician	8	6	8	6
Cardiologist	5	8	5	2
All others	5	2	5	45
Total	100	100	100	100
N	61,384	14,477	75,861	1,558,034

Source: *National Disease and Therapeutics Index.* Ambler, Pennsylvania, IMS America Ltd., 1977, p. 3.

TABLE 11–13.   RHEUMATOID ARTHRITIS: VISITS BY SPECIALTY (1976)

SPECIALTY	PERCENT	VISITS/PHYSICIAN/YEAR
Internist	44	85
General/family physician	36	40
Orthopedic surgeon	7	45
Osteopathic physician	7	35
Cardiologist	2	25
General surgeon	1	5
All others	3	
Total	100 (N = 4848)	

Source: *National Disease and Therapeutics Index.* Ambler, Pennsylvania, IMS America Ltd., 1977, p. 15.

Two particular areas warrant further discussion as important determinants of the spectrum of clinical content in family practice—preventive medicine and obstetric care. The role of preventive medicine in family practice, as in other specialties, is receiving increased attention in recent years but remains an area of controversy and confusion. There is some evidence that the public has been oversold on the value of health screening without an adequate research effort to date on the effectiveness or cost-benefit of these efforts. Enthusiasts for health screening point out the high frequency of early diagnosis of treatable problems in screened patients, while skeptics point to the frequently poor cost-benefits of health screening and its lack of impact on mortality and morbidity. Sackett and his colleagues have warned that unless randomized clinical trials of screening and other diagnostic procedures are expanded to determine and document their validity, available resources may be wasted on worthless procedures at the expense of valid clinical efforts.[17] Felcher has suggested that the spectrum of testing should vary with age, sex, genetic, personal, and cultural factors, and that criteria are needed for selection of the scope of testing on an individual rather than a mass basis.[18]

Progress is being made in addressing this dilemma. Breslow and Somers[21] recommend the use of the following eight criteria for the selection of preventive procedures, derived partly from those adopted by the National Conference on Preventive Medicine in 1975[19] and partly from the work of Frame and Carlson in family practice[20]:

1. The procedure is appropriate to the health goals of the relevant age group (or groups) and is acceptable to the relevant population.
2. The procedure is directed to primary or secondary prevention of a clearly identified disease or condition that has a definite effect on the length or quality of life.
3. The natural history of the disease (or diseases) associated with the condition is understood sufficiently to justify the procedure as outweighing any adverse effects of intervention.
4. For purposes of screening, the disease or condition has an asymptomatic period during which detection and treatment can substantially reduce morbidity or mortality or both.

TABLE 11-14. DISTRIBUTION OF PATIENT DISCHARGES BY PHYSICIAN SPECIALTY, MEAN NUMBER OF DAYS HOSPITALIZED, AND MEAN NUMBER OF PATIENTS SEEN PER DAY

SPECIALTY	PHYSICIANS [NUMBER (PERCENT)]	PERCENT OF PHYSICIAN DISCHARGES PER YEAR	MEAN NUMBER OF DISCHARGES PER YEAR PER PHYSICIAN	MEAN NUMBER OF DAYS HOSPITALIZED	MEAN NUMBER OF PATIENTS SEEN PER DAY PER PHYSICIAN
All	532(100)	100	150	8.7	3.6
Primary care	282(53)	45	133	9.6	3.5
Internal medicine	70(13)	13	145	12.1	4.8
General/family practice	185(35)	28	129	8.9	3.1
Pediatrics	27(5)	4	133	6.6	2.4
Other specialties	237(45)	52	168	7.9	3.6
Unspecified and unknown	13(2)	3	202	8.9	4.9

Source: Garg, M.L., Skipper, J.K., McNamera, M.J., and Mulligan, J.L.: Primary care physicians and profiles of their hospitalized patients. *American Journal of Public Health* 66:390, 1976.

5. Acceptable methods of effective treatment are available for conditions discovered.
6. The prevalence and seriousness of the disease or condition justify the cost of intervention.
7. The procedure is relatively easy to administer, preferably by paramedical personnel with guidance and interpretation by physicians, and generally available at reasonable cost.
8. Resources are generally available for follow-up diagnostic or therapeutic intervention if required.

As examples of the application of such criteria, Appendix 7 includes a lifetime health-monitoring program as recommended by Breslow and Somers [21] and a screening flow sheet for health screening of adults as proposed by Frame and Carlson.[20]

The extent of inclusion of obstetric care in family practice also strongly affects the spectrum of the family physician's practice. Although family physicians in some parts of the country have tended to exclude obstetric care from their practices, the growth of group practice among family physicians, together with the widespread inclusion of training in obstetrics–gynecology in United States family practice residencies, can be expected to lead to increasing involvement of future family physicians in obstetric care. One study of four family practices in northern California has shown that practices including obstetrics comprise more pediatrics, gynecology, minor surgery, family counseling, and family care than those excluding obstetrics.[22]

Family practice has much to offer in modern obstetric care. It is both logical and desirable that the family physician continue to provide care for two individual patients—the mother and the newborn infant—as part of the family unit through a major event in the life cycle of the family. Perhaps the most important contribution of family practice to obstetric care is the effort to personalize obstetric delivery and newborn care as a significant human event in the life of the family.

The clinical content of family practice, in summary, is featured by breadth, flexibility, and variations by individual family physicians and by needs of the communities in which they practice. The daily work of the family physician is characterized by variety—variety of clinical problems encountered, variety of stages of care (from health maintenance to terminal care), variety by stages in the life cycle of families, and the endless variety of the needs and responses of people in various stages of health and illness.

REFERENCES

1. Dennis JL: The future of family practice in our medical schools. J Fam Pract 1:6, 1974
2. McWhinney IR: Problem solving and decision making in primary medical practice. Can Fam Physician 18:109, 1972

3. Robbins LC: Prospective medicine. Continuing Educ 8:2, 1978
4. Malerich JA: What constitutes family practice in West St. Paul. GP 40:163, 1969
5. White KL, Williams F, Greenberg B: Ecology of medical care. N Engl J Med 265: 885, 1961
6. Kohn R: The Health of the Canadian People. Ottawa, Queen's Printer, 1965, p 113
7. National Ambulatory Medical Care Survey of Visits to General and Family Practitioners, January–December 1975. Advance Data from Vital and Health Statistics of the National Center for Health Statistics. Washington, D.C., U.S. Department of Health, Education and Welfare 15:1, 1977
8. Garg ML, Skipper JK, McNamera MJ, Mulligan JL: Primary care physicians and profiles of their hospitalized patients. Am J Public Health 66:390, 1976
9. Shank C: Hospital problems cared for by one family physician. J Fam Pract 7:549, 1978
10. Tarrant M: What price admitting privileges? A study of hospital admissions by two family physicians. Can Fam Physician 23:59, 1977
11. Fowler JA, Falk WA: A study of GP hospital admissions in British Columbia. Can Fam Physician 19:56, 1973
12. Marsland DW, Wood M, Mayo F: A data bank for patient care, curriculum, and research in family practice: 526,196 patient problems. J. Fam Pract 3:25, 1976
13. Metcalfe DHH, Sischy D: Patterns of referral from family practice. J Fam Pract 1:34, 1974
14. Geyman JP, Brown TC, Rivers K: Referrals in family practice: A comparative study by geographic region and practice setting. J Fam Pract 3:163, 1976
15. Office Visits by Persons Aged 65 and Over: National Ambulatory Medical Care Survey, United States, 1975. Advance Data from Vital and Health Statistics of the National Center for Health Statistics. Washington, D.C., U.S. Department of Health, Education and Welfare, 22:1, 1978
16. National Disease and Therapeutics Index. Ambler, Pennsylvania, IMS America Ltd., 1977, p 1
17. Bombardier D, McClaran J, Sackett DL: Medical care policy rounds: Periodic health examinations and multiphasic screening. Can Med Assoc J 109:1123, 1973
18. Felcher WC: Does preventive medicine really work? Prism 1:26, 1973
19. Preventive Medicine USA: Theory, practice and application of prevention in personal health services: Quality control and evaluation of preventive health services. New York, Prodist, 1976
20. Frame PS, Carlson SJ: A critical review of periodic health screening using specific screening criteria. J Fam Pract 2:29, 1975
21. Breslow L, Somers AR: The lifetime health-monitoring program: A practical approach to preventive medicine. N Engl J Med 296:601, 1977
22. Mehl LE, Bruce C, Renner JH: Importance of obstetrics in a comprehensive family practice. J Fam Pract 3:385, 1976

CHAPTER TWELVE

The Family in Family Practice

In traditional medical terminology, we have been instructed since medical school days to treat the "whole patient." The general practitioner of the past has modified and enlarged this concept to include the individual's family as the background which, somehow, has a relationship to him and his illness. The new concept which we propose as being an integral one for the practicing family physician is that of viewing the entire family as "the patient," and the individual as merely a symptom-carrier whose behavior, thoughts, physical state, and response to illness are influenced as much by the family with whom he lives as the disease process with which he is burdened.

Martin H. Bauman and Nicholas T. Grace [1]

It is axiomatic that family practice as a specialty is involved with the comprehensive, ongoing care of individual patients and their families over the full course of the family life cycle. It is also axiomatic that the family is the basic unit of care in family practice, but this deceptively simple concept bears further examination. By this, do we mean that the family physician cares for all members of the family as individuals, with due consideration of the family environment as a factor that may modify his/her care of the individual family member? Or does the family physician also care for the family itself as the patient, involving diagnostic and therapeutic efforts oriented to family problems, not just individual problems? Most family physicians accept the first question as a matter of course; but there is less agreement and understanding of the dimensions of the second question.

Although family medicine as a discipline accepts the family as a patient as an article of faith, there is a considerable gap today between this conceptual goal and actual practice. As Carmichael [2] says, "to care for the patient in the context of the family is one thing; to turn the family into the object of care is another."

A common clinical example encountered in everyday practice illustrates this gap. Many family physicians are skilled in recognizing depression as a primary problem or as a problem associated with concurrent organic illness. But how many family physicians take the next step toward diagnosis and management of related, or even causative, problems within the family itself, such as a marital problem, a parent–adolescent relationship problem, or other major dysfunction of the family? In order to accomplish this task, a conceptual shift is needed to perceive the family itself as the patient and to develop and apply a set of clinical strategies that apply to family problems.

Since family physicians have the unique responsibility and opportunity to care for the entire family, they are obliged to know as much as possible about the family as a functional unit and about the patterns of illness in families. The purpose of this chapter is fourfold: (1) to describe briefly the changing roles of the American family, (2) to outline family development in terms of the family life cycle, (3) to discuss the nature of illness within families, and (4) to present diagnostic and management approaches to family problems that are applicable in family practice.

CHANGING ROLES OF THE AMERICAN FAMILY

Behavioral scientists consider that our rapidly moving technologic society has produced changes in the role of the family that engender many family conflicts. What is usually recognized as the traditional model for the modern American family evolved in a predominantly agricultural economy with a majority of the population living in rural or semirural communities. William Ogburn,[3] a sociologist, has enumerated six basic functions of the traditional family which have been essentially lost in recent decades:

1. THE ECONOMIC FUNCTION
Until about 50 years ago, all members of the family shared in producing most of what the family consumed. Today, the husband invariably works outside the home and his role in daily family life is much less dominant. Children usually have little understanding of his working role, and often see him in his nonworking hours in the home as someone too tired to take an active

interest in their activities. In order to contribute to the family's income, today's wife, who works outside the home, often feels conflict between her desire to share in the family's economic life and the inevitable decrease in her involvement with the growth and development of her children.

2. THE PROTECTIVE FUNCTION
Families no longer directly have to protect their own members from bodily harm, but instead rely on police, sheriffs, and others. In times of illness, disability, and unemployment the personal responsibility of the family has been replaced by public mechanisms such as unemployment compensation, social security, health insurance, and other programs. Care of chronic illness, especially in the aged, has often shifted from the home to the convalescent hospital and nursing home.

3. THE RELIGIOUS FUNCTION
Compared with the central role of religious teaching and custom in the earlier traditional family, formal religion plays a much diminished role in the home of today's family. Religious training is more the responsibility of the church, which itself has perhaps a weaker influence on many of the younger generation than in the past.

4. THE RECREATIONAL FUNCTION
The home is no longer the major place for recreation for the entire family. Outside facilities and commercial entertainment are now more likely to attract one or two members of the family than the entire family. Television provides a common entertainment in the home but is usually enjoyed more on an individual than a family basis and competes for time available for intrafamily communication.

5. THE EDUCATIONAL FUNCTION
Children's education has almost entirely shifted from the family to the schools, even including sex education. Family conflicts frequently arise when the standards of behavior and speech learned at school are at variance with those of the family.

6. THE STATUS-CONFERRING FUNCTION
In the past, the family to a large extent determined the individual's socio-economic status. In small communities, families were well known and had a definite place in the social structure. Now the husband's job more often defines the family's status.

Livsey[4] feels that the changes causing increasingly specialized functions of the family parallel the evolutionary changes of society in general at a given time and at a given place. That these changes have resulted in new conflicts, confusion of roles, and personal and family problems cannot be denied.

Though our American society and family structures are admittedly under-going many changes, all evidence leads us to believe that the family is here to stay. There are proportionately more married people in the United States now than at any time in the history of reliable census data. When divorce occurs, there is a strong tendency toward remarriage. Moreover, as reflected by such statistics as suicide rates, it has been amply demonstrated that family life is more directly correlated with satisfactory living adjustments than is the unmarried state. Most behavioral scientists feel the giving and receiving of affection within the family are functions that no other institution can ade-quately perform. Curry [5] takes this one step further in viewing the family as the basic unit of humanity. He sees each person as "a human being because of all the relationships he has about him, all the feelings that exist between others and himself, especially with members of the nuclear family, the simple family, the extended family, and even the community. It is, in the last analysis, our relationships with others which make our lives happy and meaningful, which give us our humanity."

FAMILY LIFE CYCLE

The concept of the family life cycle is based on several basic assumptions: (1) that families within our culture tend to have a beginning and an end, (2) that a number of distinct sequential phases can be recognized, and (3) that various phase-specific tasks can be delineated within each stage.[6]

The family life cycle has been described in a number of ways and has usually been viewed as including five to twelve recognizable stages. Table 12–1 shows five examples of conceptual schemes for the family life cycle that have been proposed during the last 30 years.[6–10]

Regardless of the particular classification of the family life cycle that one finds most useful, they all have in common five basic developmental phases for every elementary family.[11]

1. *Birth of family*—elementary family originates with marriage of couple.
2. *Phase of expansion*—begins with birth of first child and continues until the youngest child reaches adulthood; this phase includes the period of fertility, the period of physical and social maturation of children.
3. *Phase of dispersion*—begins when the first child achieves adult status and continues until all children have grown and left home.
4. *Phase of independence*—begins when all children have reached adulthood and left home so that the parents again live alone.
5. *Phase of replacement*—begins when the parents retire from their major life roles and ends with their death; usually includes a dependency stage of variable length.

Within each stage of the family life cycle, a number of predictable stage-specific tasks occur. As observed by Worby,[6] "these tasks arouse considerable stress within the family system and require of all family members a continuous mutual and reciprocal set of readjustments." Table 12–2 outlines some of the important stage-specific tasks for each stage of the family life cycle as described by Duvall.[12]

Within the family life cycle, some interesting observations have been made of both marital and individual development. Rollins and Feldman,[13] for example, studied levels of marital satisfaction over the family life cycle, and demonstrated similar highs and lows for both wives and husbands, with troughs of lesser satisfaction during the midportion of the cycle (Figure 12–1). They also found remarkably similar changes in individual satisfaction among wives and husbands at different stages of the family life cycle (Figure 12–2).

The family life cycle represents the composite of the individual developmental changes of family members, the evolution of the marital relationship, and the cyclic development of the evolving family as a unit. The life cycle of the family is one of constant change as its individuals grow and develop and as their roles and interrelationships within the family change.

STRESS AND TRANSITIONAL CRISES

The course of the family life cycle involves multiple stress points, particularly associated with major change in the family unit and transition from one stage

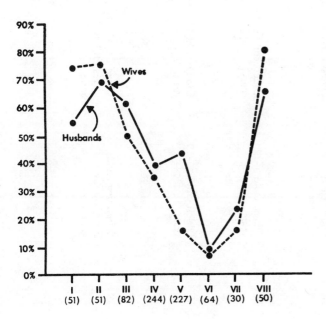

FIGURE 12-1.
Percentage of individuals in each stage of the family life cycle (from Stage I—beginning marriage to Stage VIII—retirement) reporting that their present stage of the family life cycle is very satisfying. Figures in parentheses indicate the number of husbands and also the number of wives in each stage. There was a total of 1598 cases.

Source: Rollins, BC, Feldman, H: Marital satisfaction over the family life cycle. *Journal of Marriage and the Family* 32:25, February 1970. Copyright 1970 by the National Council on Family Relations. Reprinted by permission.

TABLE 12-1.   SEVERAL FAMILY LIFE CYCLE CLASSIFICATIONS

FAMILY LIFE CYCLE STAGE	NATIONAL CONFERENCE ON FAMILY LIFE (7) (1948)	DUVALL (8) (1962)	RODGERS (9) (1960)	WORBY (6) (1971)	SOLOMON (10) (1973)
I	Couple without children	Couple without children	Childless couple	Formation of Family	Marriage
II	Oldest child less than 30 months	Oldest child less than 30 months	All children less than 36 months	First child's birth	Birth of first child and subsequent child bearing
III	Oldest child 2½–5 years	Oldest child 2½–6 years	Preschool family with (a) oldest 3–6 and youngest under 3; (b) all children 3–6	Early individuation of child	—
IV	Oldest child 5–12 years	Oldest child 6–13 years	School-age family with (a) infants, (b) preschoolers, (c) all children 6–13	Child's emerging sexuality	(III) Individuation of family members
V	Oldest child 13–19 years	Oldest child 13–20 years	Teenage family with (a) infants, (b) preschoolers, (c) school-agers, (d) all children 13–20	First child's adolescence	—
VI	When first child leaves till last is gone	When first child leaves till last is gone	Young adult family with (a) infants, (b) preschoolers, (c) school-agers, (d) teenagers, (e) all children over 20	—	(IV) Actual departure of family

	Later years	Empty nest to retirement	Launching family	(VI) Parents alone	(V) Integration of loss
VII	—		Launching family with (a) infants, (b) preschoolers, (c) school-agers, (d) teenagers, (e) youngest child over 20		
VIII	—	—	When all children have been launched until retirement	—	—
IX	—	Retirement to death of one or both spouses	Retirement until death of one spouse	—	—
X	—	—	Death of first spouse to death of the survivor	—	—

Source: Adapted from Rowe, C.P.: The developmental conceptual framework to the study of the family. In Nye, F.I., and Berardo, F.M.: *Emerging Conceptual Framework in Family Analysis.* New York, Macmillan Co., 1966, p. 208.

TABLE 12-2. STAGE-CRITICAL FAMILY DEVELOPMENTAL TASKS THROUGH THE FAMILY LIFE CYCLE

STAGE OF THE FAMILY LIFE CYCLE	POSITIONS IN THE FAMILY	STAGE-CRITICAL FAMILY DEVELOPMENTAL TASKS
1. Married couple	Wife Husband	Establishing a mutually satisfying marriage Adjusting to pregnancy and the promise of parenthood Fitting into the kin network
2. Childbearing	Wife–mother Husband–father Infant daughter or son or both	Having, adjusting to, and encouraging the development of infants Establishing a satisfying home for both parents and infant(s)
3. Preschool-age	Wife–mother Husband–father Daughter–sister Son–brother	Adapting to the critical needs and interests of preschool children in stimulating, growth-promoting ways Coping with energy depletion and lack of privacy as parents
4. School-age	Wife–mother Husband–father Daughter–sister Son–brother	Fitting into the community of school-age families in constructive ways Encouraging children's educational achievement
5. Teenage	Wife–mother Husband–father Daughter–sister Son–brother	Balancing freedom with responsibility as teenagers mature and emancipate themselves Establishing postparental interests and careers as growing parents
6. Launching center	Wife–mother–grandmother Husband–father–grandfather Daughter–sister–aunt Son–brother–uncle	Releasing young adults into work, military service, college, marriage, etc. with appropriate rituals and assistance Maintaining a supportive home base
7. Middle-aged parents	Wife–mother–grandmother Husband–father–grandfather Widow/widower	Rebuilding the marriage relationship Maintaining kin ties with older and younger generations
8. Aging family members	Wife–mother–grandmother Husband–father–grandfather	Coping with bereavement and living alone Closing the family home or adapting it to aging Adjusting to retirement

Source: Duvall, E.M.: Family Development (4th ed.). Philadelphia, J.B. Lippincott Company, 1971. Table 6–5, p. 151. Reprinted by permission of the publisher.

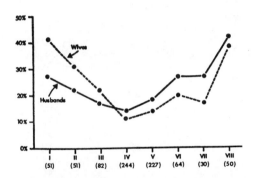

FIGURE 12-2.

Percentage of individuals at each stage of the family life cycle (from Stage I—beginning marriage to Stage VIII—retirement) reporting their marriage was going well "all the time." Figures in parentheses indicate the number of husbands and also the number of wives in each stage. There was a total of 1598 cases.

Source: Rollins, BC, and Feldman, H: Marital satisfaction over the family life cycle. *Journal of Marriage and the Family* 32:25, February 1970. Copyright 1970 by the National Council on Family Relations. Reprinted by permission.

to the next. Critical events such as divorce or death of a spouse precipitate crisis within the family with resultant disequilibrium and need for reorganization. Previous roles and rules of intrafamily relationships frequently fail to maintain satisfactory family organization, and new relationships among family members are often established.

As a result of his work with a social readjustment rating scale, Holmes has concluded that generalizations can be made about the relative stress on family life caused by various life crises. For example, *normative* crises, such as marriage, pregnancy, and retirement, are especially stressful, while divorce, separation, and death are the most stressful among *nonnormative* crises. Table 12–3 shows the relative stress ratings that have been derived from continued research over the years by Holmes and his colleagues for various life events.[14]

The process of family reorganization is often unpredictable and potentially disruptive. While the reorganized family may function as well as or better than before the crisis, the result of reorganization frequently may be increased family dysfunction. Figure 12–3 graphically displays the response of a family to crisis resulting in a new level of family function.[15]

Depending on the outcome of the response of individual family members and the family as a whole, a given "normal" crisis may or may not cause a clinical problem perceived by the individual, the family, or the physician as requiring care. Table 12–4 illustrates various kinds of clinical problems that can occur in response to critical events which commonly occur in the course of a family's life cycle. This kind of conceptual framework can be useful to family physicians in everyday practice by increasing their awareness of potential future crises in the individual patient and his/her family. It is well known that individuals with certain stress problems have a greater likelihood of developing other problems as a result of future crises. Thus, the physician caring for an obstetric patient with postpartum depression would observe her more closely five years later for signs of separation anxiety. This framework also illustrates that two or more individual crises may be concurrent at any given time in a family's development; for example, depression and an "empty nest syndrome" in a

TABLE 12–3.   SOCIAL READJUSTMENT RATING SCALE*

LIFE EVENT	MEAN VALUE
1. Death of spouse	100
2. Divorce	73
3. Marital separation	65
4. Jail term	63
5. Death of close family member	63
6. Personal injury or illness	53
7. Marriage	50
8. Fired at work	47
9. Marital reconciliation	45
10. Retirement	45
11. Change in health of family member	44
12. Pregnancy	40
13. Sex difficulties	39
14. Gain of new family member	39
15. Business readjustment	39
16. Change in financial state	38
17. Death of close friend	37
18. Change to different line of work	36
19. Change in number of arguments with spouse	35
20. Mortgage over $10,000	31
21. Foreclosure of mortgage or loan	30
22. Change in responsibilities at work	29
23. Son or daughter leaving home	29
24. Trouble with in-laws	29
25. Outstanding personal achievement	28
26. Wife begins or stops work	26
27. Begin or end school	26
28. Change in living conditions	25
29. Revision of personal habits	24
30. Trouble with boss	23
31. Change in work hours or conditions	20
32. Change in residence	20
33. Change in schools	20
34. Change in recreation	19
35. Change in church activities	19
36. Change in social activities	18
37. Mortgage or loan less than $10,000	17
38. Change in sleeping habits	16
39. Change in number of family get-togethers	15
40. Change in eating habits	15
41. Vacation	13
42. Christmas	12
43. Minor violations of the law	11

* See Holmes, T.H., and Rahe, R.H.: The social readjustment rating scale. *Journal of Psychosomatic Research* 11:213, 1967, for complete wording of the items.

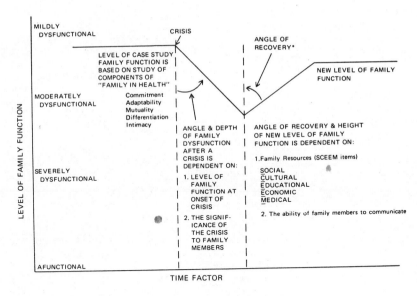

FIGURE 12-3.
Schema for evaluation of family in crisis.
Source: Smilkstein, G: The family in trouble—how to tell. *Journal of Family Practice* 2:19, 1975.

45-year-old wife and mother may coexist with a teenage identity crisis in her 18-year-old son and with postretirement depression in her 66-year-old father.

NATURE OF ILLNESS WITHIN THE FAMILY

General Considerations

Any discussion of the nature of illness within the family is necessarily an extremely complex subject, so that all that will be attempted here is a brief overview of some of the important principles involved in the care of families in health and illness. As already noted, the family is a continuously evolving unit with a life cycle of its own. The occurrence and response of the family to illness are influenced by such diverse factors as the socioeconomic, cultural, environmental, genetic, and educational background of the family; the presence of chronic disease within the family; the level of function of the family as a unit; and previous patterns of health and illness in the family. The family milieu is further complicated by a wide range of complex interactions between the sick family member and the family.

The broad concerns of family physicians bring additional complexity to the subject. They are involved with the full spectrum of health care, including health maintenance, preventive and anticipatory care, recognition and management of acute disease, care of chronic illness, rehabilitation, and, ultimately, care of the terminally ill. Family physicians are also involved with illness in

TABLE 12–4.   EXAMPLES OF MAJOR CRISES

STAGE	"NORMAL" CRISES	CLINICAL PROBLEMS
Birth of family	Early sexual adjustment	Sexual problems
Expansion of family		
Early (preschool)	Birth of child	Postpartum depression
Middle (school)	Separation anxiety	Hyperactive child
Late (adolescence)	"Empty nest" syndrome	Last fling
	Teenage identity crisis	Juvenile delinquency
Dispersion	Career stagnation	Depression
Independence	Menopause	Depression
	Marital readjustment	Alcoholism
	Death of parents	
Replacement	Physical disability	Organic brain syndrome
	Retirement	Depression
	Death of mate	Suicide
	Loneliness	

the family as a unit as well as illness in a family member as an individual. Family physicians therefore must apply their knowledge of the family, understanding of family dynamics, and clinical knowledge and skills in order to recognize and manage the varied problems encountered in everyday practice.

Incidence

The incidence of illness within the family is determined by a number of interrelated factors that may alter considerably the incidence of illness encountered in the individual patient. Some of the more important factors modifying the incidence of illness in the individual include genetic and familial factors, the transmission of infectious disease, and the effect of psychosocial factors.

The occurrence of infectious disease in families has been correlated with several features of family structure and function. Meyer and Haggerty, for example, studied the incidence of streptococcal infections in 16 families over a one-year period. They found that mothers developed streptococcal illness more often than fathers and that the incidence of streptococcal infections was highest between ages 2 and 5 years, in family members sleeping in the same room, and in families with acute or chronic stress. They even demonstrated that the likelihood of developing antistreptolysin-O titer rise depended on the level of stress within the family.[16]

The frequent association of organic and functional problems has been well recognized for years and often clouds the distinction between organic and functional illness. In one study of 141 randomly selected family physicians in

Washington State, 71 percent of the physicians reported between 20 and 30 percent of their patients had "significant mental, psychological, or emotional impairment of some sort." Over one-half of these patients presented with a "physical" complaint but were found to have associated emotional or "psychiatric" problems.[17]

There is abundant evidence that psychosocial factors play a major role in the occurrence of illness within families. Medalie and his colleagues, for example, studied the incidence of angina pectoris among 10,000 men and demonstrated markedly increased incidence of this condition in men with relatively low levels of wives' love and support (Table 12–5) [18] and in men with families with the most family problems (Table 12–6).[19]

TABLE 12-5. EFFECT OF "WIFE'S LOVE AND SUPPORT" ON MALES WITH SAME ANXIETY LEVEL IN RELATIONSHIP TO DEVELOPMENT OF ANGINA PECTORIS IN THE SUBSEQUENT 5 YEARS

ANXIETY LEVEL	WIFE'S LOVE AND SUPPORT	NUMBER OF MEN AT RISK	NUMBER OF A.P. CASES	INCIDENCE RATE/1000
High	High	906	48	53
High	Low	347	31	89

Source: Medalie, J.H.: *Family Medicine—Principles and Applications.* Baltimore, Williams and Wilkins Company, 1978, p. 178.

Although various kinds of family problems, such as marital problems and other family relationship problems, are common in the experience of all family physicians, they tend to be underreported,[20] and their true incidence is not well understood. It has been documented, however, that the sudden increased use of health-care services within families is often a signal to the physician that a family problem exists.[21]

TABLE 12-6. ANGINA PECTORIS INCIDENCE (1963-1968) AS RELATED TO PSYCHOSOCIAL FACTORS IN 1963

PSYCHOSOCIAL AREA	SEVERITY SCORE*	NUMBER OF SUBJECTS	NUMBER OF CASES	AGE–AREA– ADJUSTED RATE PER 1000
Family	0 (least)	1,636	50	31
problems	1	3,972	125	33
	2	1,836	68	38
	3	865	41	49
	4 (most)	219	16	88

* Severity score is a score indicating the number of times a subject reported serious or very serious problems with respect to questions within the psychosocial area (e.g., 0 = no serious problems, 3 = a serious problem in each of the three questions related to the relevant problem area).

Source: Medalie, I.H., Snyder, M., Groen, J.J., et al.: Angina pectoris among 10,000 men: 5-year incidence and univariate analysis: Ann. Int. Med. 55:583, 1973. As adapted by Schmidt, D.D.: The family as the unit of medical care. *Journal of Family Practice* 7:303, 1978.

Presentation of Illness

The presentation of illness in families is also marked by recognizable features and patterns. Figure 12–4 illustrates the variations that often occur within families as a result of a primary nondifferentiated respiratory infection in one family member. Striking variations in symptomatology, timing, and duration of illness are demonstrated among family members.[22]

Peachey has studied the incidence of illness in 25 families of a rural family practice. She has demonstrated four basic patterns of illness—constant illness, regular periodicity, clustering, and simultaneity—and suggests that such patterns may hold predictive value.[23]

The social interactions of a person who is sick or who thinks he/she is sick can be described as *illness behavior*. Such behavior may be appropriate or inappropriate according to the circumstances. Examples of inappropriate illness behavior could take the form of an individual with severe and apparent organic disease refusing to assume the sick role, as well as the other side of the issue whereby an individual without organic disease may acquire a sick role.[11]

Bursten [24] has described this example of the role of family dynamics in affecting illness behavior which involves inappropriate hospitalization of a patient:

We have studied the family of a patient who had a long-standing, mild, chronic bronchitis due to smoking. He had been a mild-mannered husband until his brother had shown a high degree of self-assertiveness in changing his job. Encouraged by his

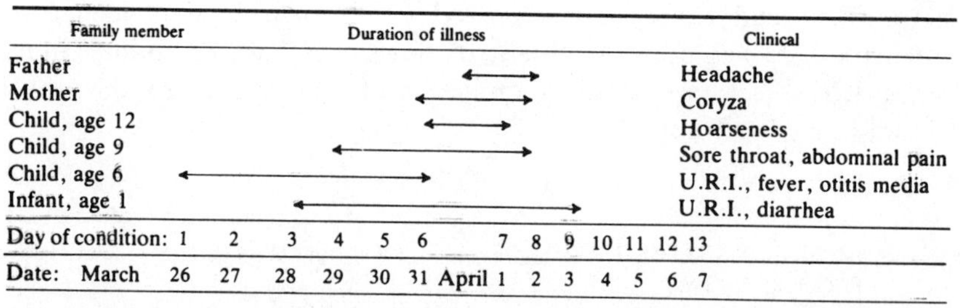

Family member	Duration of illness		Clinical
Father			Headache
Mother			Coryza
Child, age 12			Hoarseness
Child, age 9			Sore throat, abdominal pain
Child, age 6			U.R.I., fever, otitis media
Infant, age 1			U.R.I., diarrhea
Day of condition: 1 2 3 4 5 6 7 8 9 10 11 12 13			
Date: March 26 27 28 29 30 31 April 1 2 3 4 5 6 7			

Comment: This is a very common condition. In this example, the young child aged 6 was the introducer (index or primary case) of the upper respiratory infection (U.R.I.) into the family. On the 3rd and 4th days his siblings, age 1 and 9, became ill (secondary cases) with an added element of diarrhea (in infant) and abdominal pain (child age 9). Two days later, the tertiary cases (sibling age 12 and mother) developed hoarseness and coryza without fever. The father had a headache for 1 day.

This is an example of a common condition in which an undifferentiated respiratory infection affects all members of a family in succession and in varying degrees of severity.

FIGURE 12-4.

Nondifferentiated respiratory infection: primary, secondary, and tertiary cases.

Source: Medalie, JH: *Family Medicine—Principles and Applications.* Baltimore, Williams and Wilkins Company, 1978, p. 86.

brother's success, the patient became more self-assertive in his own family. This assertiveness threatened his wife who "put him in his place" by worrying about his chronic cough. The wife suggested that he go to the hospital for an intensive examination. Feeling defeated by his wife's refusal to allow him his self-assertion, the patient complied. Thus, a family conflict was resolved by the shift in the patient's role from an assertive husband to a sick and compliant patient.

All practicing physicians, particularly those involved in primary care, can recall many patients who presented with a chief complaint that was not the real reason for seeking care but a kind of "ticket" which was felt by the patient to be "legitimate" in medical terms. It takes a perceptive physician to uncover the real problem in these situations, and in many instances it is related to causative or associated family conflicts. In addition, even when the patient's complaints are valid and undisguised, there may be forces within the family that favor the patient's continued sick role and failure to respond to medical management.

Impact of Individual's Illness on Family

As already noted, a major illness in an individual family member usually precipitates crisis within the family with resultant disequilibrium and need for reorganization. Previous patterns of intrafamily relationships are challenged and often break down when a family member is in the hospital, in danger of dying, disabled, or making new demands on the family.

A family's reaction to crisis has been divided by Hill into three basic phases: (1) initial period of stunned denial; (2) period of confusion, anxiety, and frequently resentment toward the sick family member; and (3) period of recovery and reorganization.[25] While the reorganized family may function as well as or better than before the crisis, the result can often be serious emotional pain or functional disability in one or more family members other than the one who is ill. New relationships between family members will have evolved that the physician should understand. In addition to the possible need for treatment of other members of the family, the physician may find that the recovery or rehabilitation of his/her patient may be unfavorably affected by family reorganization. This underscores the importance of considering the entire family when treating an individual patient with a serious disease or disability.

Olsen[26] has observed that "serious illness is a family affair—the family, not just the patient, has the illness." The family is thrown into disequilibrium, acute illness or exacerbations of chronic illness may be precipitated in other family members, and the family will attempt to shift toward a new homeostasis that will be more tolerable. Serious emotional problems or impairment of functional ability may occur in other family members that will call for further intervention beyond the care of the individual patient with the initial illness.

Examples of these concepts are commonly observed. Klein, Dean and Bogdan-off[27] have demonstrated an increase in somatic complaints in the spouse of the sick individual. Downes[28] has shown that some chronic diseases, such as hypertensive vascular disease and arthritis, have appeared in both husband and wife at a rate significantly higher than expected. Family members have even been found to go through stages associated with cancer similar to those the sick family member experiences, including: (1) shock and anger at the diagnosis, (2) guilt for missed past appointments, and (3) a period of anticipatory grief and hope.[29]

Impact of Family on Individual's Illness

Just as illness in the individual can have profound impact on the family, so can the family as a unit have significant influence on the course of illness in the individual family member. This influence can operate in both positive and negative directions in terms of the individual's illness.

On the positive side, the support of other family members (especially the spouse) can greatly improve the outcome of illness in the individual family member. Both patient compliance and control of hypertension have been shown to be enhanced when the spouse participates in the treatment program of patients with hypertension.[30] A strong association has been demonstrated between family reinforcement and the response of patients to rehabilitation programs (Table 12–7).[31] The protective effect of marriage upon the average annual death rates from such diseases as tuberculosis and arteriosclerotic heart disease is shown in Table 12–8.[32]

On the negative side, there are likewise abundant examples of unfavorable impact of the family upon individual illness. One study in North Carolina showed marked increases in morbidity and mortality from cerebrovascular disease in blacks correlated with increased disorganization of the family.[33] Another study has documented increased complication rates during pregnancy in women with the combination of high stress and low family support.[34] The use of illness as a manipulative device has been demonstrated to be commonly

TABLE 12–7.   ASSOCIATION BETWEEN REHABILITATION RESPONSE AS MEASURED BY A
COMPOSITE THERAPEUTIC RATING AND FAMILY'S REACTION TO ILLNESS

FAMILY REACTION	RESPONSE TO REHABILITATION*	
	Good	Poor
Positive reinforcement	51	19
Negative or non-reinforcement	7	23

* $\chi^2 = 21.14$, df = 1, $P < 0.001$, $n = 100$.

Source: Litman, T.J.: The family and physical rehabilitation. *Journal of Chronic Diseases* 19:211, 1966. Copyright 1966 by Pergamon Press, Ltd. Reprinted with permission.

TABLE 12–8.   AVERAGE ANNUAL DEATH RATES FOR SELECTED CASES IN THE MARRIED AND
THE WIDOWED, FOR THE 25 TO 35 AGE GROUP, BY SEX, UNITED STATES 1949–
1951

		DEATH RATE (PER THOUSAND POPULATION)			
CAUSE	*Sex*	*Married*	*Widowed*	*Widowed*	*Married*
Tuberculosis	M	11.2	141.8	12.7	
	F	15.4	76.1	4.9	
Vascular lesions of the	M	3.6	29.3	8.1	
central nervous system	F	4.1	17.4	4.2	
Hypertension with	M	1.7	18.3	10.8	
heart disease	F	2.3	10.9	4.7	
Influenza and pneumonia	M	2.6	20.1	7.7	
	F	2.7	13.4	5.0	
Arteriosclerotic	M	8.6	42.1	4.9	
heart disease	F	2.8	16.5	5.9	

Source: Kraus, A., and Lilienfeld, A.: Some epidemiologic aspects of the high mortality rate in the young
widowed group. *Journal of Chronic Diseases* 10:207, 1959. As modified by Schmidt, D.D.: The family as the
unit of care. *Journal of Family Practice* 7:303, 1978.

used by the family as well as by sick family members. Duff and Hollingshead
studied hospitalized patients on medicine and surgery services, and found both
kinds of negative interactions (Table 12–9). When the individual patient was
being manipulated, the patient was usually male and the manipulator usually
the wife.[35]

The potential influences of a given family on the illness of a family member
depend in large part on the existing level of function of the family as a unit,
whether healthy or dysfunctional. Olsen[36] has noted four features of healthy
families that are adapting well to stress and change:

1. There is a clear separation of the generations so that the parents are satisfying
   each other's emotional needs or, in case of conflict, are able to fight straight.
2. There is a flexibility within and between roles so that shifting can be
   tolerated with relative comfort.

TABLE 12–9.   USE OF ILLNESS AS A MANIPULATIVE DEVICE TO GAIN ENDS WITHIN THE
FAMILY

MANIPULATION OF ILLNESS	*PATIENTS ON MEDICINE SERVICE (%)*	*PATIENTS ON SURGERY SERVICE (%)*	*FEMALE (%)*	*MALE (%)*
By patient on family	35	31	49	16
By family on patient	39	20	16	41
Nonuse by either party	26	49	35	43

Source: Duff, R.S., and Hollingshead, A.B.: *Sickness and Society.* New York, Harper and Row, 1968.

3. There is a tolerance for individuation. The family can accept and enjoy differences and can tolerate the anxiety of disequilibrium in the system as the members grow and change.
4. Communications among the family members are direct and consistent and tend to confirm the self esteem of each.

THE FAMILY AS THE OBJECT OF CARE

Although clinical methods for dealing with the family as the patient in family practice are not yet refined, it is useful to briefly highlight some of the promising approaches to diagnosis and management that are currently being developed.

Diagnostic Approaches

Diagnosis in clinical medicine has traditionally been perceived and carried out on the level of the individual patient (or, in many instances, at the organ system level). Diagnosis in community medicine has been on the community level. There has been little emphasis to date on the use of diagnostic methods at the family level. The importance of all three levels is well illustrated by the coordinated problem list shown in Table 12–10.[37]

In an important paper, "Beyond diagnosis—An approach to the integration of behavioral science and clinical medicine," McWhinney[38] proposes a conceptual foundation that can facilitate the care of the family as a patient. He proposes a taxonomy of patient behavior and of social factors in illness that may be adapted to the problem-oriented medical record and applied by the busy clinician. Thus, for a 28-year-old married woman with blurring of vision secondary to multiple sclerosis and with fear of another pregnancy because her husband refuses to accept birth control, the patient's problems may be described as follows:

- *Clinical*: multiple sclerosis
- *Behavioral*: heterothetic (symptomatic problem of living)
- *Social*: marital maladjustment

Smilkstein has recently described a practical method that appears to be a useful diagnostic approach to assess family function—the family APGAR.[39] This brief screening questionnaire is designed to elicit a data base that assesses the level of family function in terms of five important components—adaptation, partnership, growth, affection, and resolve. A small number of carefully selected open-ended questions can yield basic family function information for each component. The functional elements of family process measured by this method are summarized in Table 12–11. An APGAR scoring system is then applied,

TABLE 12-10.   COORDINATED PROBLEM LIST

PATIENT	FAMILY	COMMUNITY
George Taylor Alcoholic Early death	Members suffer mental, emotional, economic, and physical problems.	Public knowledge that George is an alcoholic. Possibility of community having to support Joan and children following death.
Joan Agitated depression Back injury	Unpleasant family atmosphere. Disruption of family roles.	Any member could become so disabled as to force the community to support him for the rest of his life through insurance or social security.
Laura Meningococcal meningitis	Worry about brain damage or heart problems or death. Others could become infected.	Possibility of others getting meningitis. School may be possible source of bacteria.
Brad Hyperkinetic Dyslexia	Disrupting influence. Source of much frustration— discipline required. Requires additional care and attention.	Source of inferiority complex. Distraction to others in school. Possibility of future member of community with dyslexia (autosomal dominant). Requires special educational program.

Source: Rakel, R.E.: *Principles of Family Medicine.* Philadelphia, W.B. Saunders Company, 1977, p. 515.

which ranges from a highly functional family (APGAR 7 to 10) to a severely dysfunctional family (APGAR 0 to 3) (Table 12–12). Smilkstein suggests that the workup of the dysfunctional family should include, in addition to the family APGAR, two additional diagnostic approaches: (1) identification and evaluation of the family's crises, present and past and (2) assessment of the family's resources.[39]

Arbogast and his colleagues[40] have recently described another method for assessing family function that is presently being used by the Family Medicine Program at the University of Maryland. They have developed a short family interview questionnaire that gathers information on the family life cycle, family process, and the family's social milieu (Table 12–13).

In order to effectively practice family medicine with a focus on the family as patient, a practical method for maintaining a family-oriented medical record is also required. Grace and his colleagues[41] have described such a system, currently in use in their group family practice, which includes a family problem list and family tree data.

TABLE 12-11.   WHAT IS MEASURED BY THE FAMILY APGAR?

Adaptation	How resources are shared, or the degree to which a member is satisfied with the assistance received when family resources are needed
Partnership	How decisions are shared, or the member's satisfaction with mutuality in family communication and problem solving
Growth	How nurturing is shared, or the member's satisfaction with the freedom available within the family to change roles and attain physical and emotional growth or maturation
Affection	How emotional experiences are shared, or the member's satisfaction with the intimacy and emotional interaction that exists in a family
Resolve	How time (and space and money*) is shared, or the member's satisfaction with the time commitment that has been made to the family by its members

* Besides sharing time, family members usually have a commitment to share space and money. Because of its primacy, time was the only item included in the family APGAR; however, the physician who is concerned with family function will enlarge his/her understanding of the family's resolve if he inquires about family member's satisfaction with shared space and money.

Source: Smilkstein, G.: The family APGAR: A proposal for a family function test and its use by physicians. *Journal of Family Practice* 6:1231, 1978.

Management Approaches

Although management approaches to problems of dysfunctional families are not as yet well developed, some broad principles can be briefly outlined that allow for a varied set of treatment options adapted to the particular needs of each family. Crucial to the effectiveness of any approach, however, is the family physician's understanding of the family's problem(s) and the family dynamics in process, together with his/her own skills as a "therapeutic instrument."

The family physician's effectiveness in dealing with family problems is enhanced by the following attributes:

1. Capacity to listen as an active process.
2. Ability to observe and interpret interactions among family members.
3. Knowledge of family dynamics in health and illness.
4. Ability to communicate clearly, to facilitate communication between family members, and to present an empathetic, open self to the family.
5. Ability to be nonjudgmental and to avoid entangling alliances with individual family members.
6. Appreciation of sociocultural and environmental influences on family life styles.
7. Recognition of the family life cycle as the evolving milieu for health and illness in the family.
8. Capacity to integrate behavioral science principles and care of family problems into the traditional medical care of clinical problems of individual patients.

9. Understanding and awareness of oneself as a therapeutic agent.
10. Ability to individualize the care of individual patients and their families based upon the unique circumstances and needs of each family.

Once the family physician has identified a specific family problem, he/she is then faced with the need to select a particular kind and style of intervention. Consideration must be given to frequency and duration of future visits, inclusion of other family members in addition to the identified individual patient(s), and possible participation of other health professionals.

The family physician's interventions will most commonly involve short-term family counseling, including selected family members as appropriate. Ornstein recommends that the family physician develop his/her own personal skills and methods as a therapeutic instrument rather than attempt to apply traditional psychiatric styles of intervention.[42] Cathell echoes this advice, noting that the family physician is more directive, authoritative, problem-oriented, and pragmatic than the psychiatrist and suggesting that the family physician's methods

TABLE 12–12. FAMILY APGAR QUESTIONNAIRE*

	ALMOST ALWAYS	SOME OF THE TIME	HARDLY EVER
I am satisfied with the help that I receive from my family† when something is troubling me.	_____	_____	_____
I am satisfied with the way my family† discusses items of common interest and shares problem solving with me.	_____	_____	_____
I find that my family† accepts my wishes to take on new activities or make changes in my life style.	_____	_____	_____
I am satisfied with the way my family† expresses affection and responds to my feelings such as anger, sorrow, and love.	_____	_____	_____
I am satisfied with the amount of time my family† and I spend together.	_____	_____	_____

* Scoring: The patient checks one of three choices, which are scored as follows: Almost always (2 points), Some of the time (1 point), Hardly ever (0). The scores for each of the five questions are then totaled. A score of 7 to 10 suggests a highly functional family. A score of 4 to 6 suggests a moderately dysfunctional family. A score of 0 to 3 suggests a severely dysfunctional family.
† According to which member of the family is being interviewed the physician may substitute for the word "family" either spouse, significant other, parents, or children.
Source: Smilkstein, G.: The family APGAR: A proposal for a family function test and its use by physicians. *Journal of Family Practice* 6:1231, 1978.

TABLE 12-13.   FAMILY INTERVIEW QUESTIONNAIRE*

Family life cycle
   (I)   1. How many are there in the family?
   (I)   2. Who lives at home?
   (A)   3. In what phase of the family life cycle is this family?
   (I)   4. What problems does this raise for them presently?
   (I)   5. What major problems has this family had in the past (inquire about death, separa-
          tion, major physical or mental illness, financial crisis, etc.)?
   (I)   6. Does this family feel these problems were dealt with satisfactorily?
Family process or psychosocial interior
   (I)   1. Who are the major decision makers in the family?
   (I)   2. Who can each person talk to most easily?
   (I)   3. What are the family members expectations of each other? Are these expectations
          being achieved? (Are they realistic?)
   (I)   4. How does each member of this family get attention?
   (A)   5. How much tolerance for individual difference and self expression is there in the
          family?
Social milieu
   (I)   1. How much contact do you have with relatives? Are they helpful? Do they create
          problems?
   (I)   2. Do the family members have many friends in their neighborhood? To what groups
          or clubs do family members belong?
   (I)   3. What sort of community resources has the family used? Would they use them
          again?
   (I)   4. What is the educational level and the financial status of the parents of the family?

* I = Inquire, A = Assess.

Source: Arbogast, R.C., Scratton, J.M., Krick, J.P.: The family as patient: An assessment schema. *Journal of Family Practice* 7:115, 1978.

should be based on these differences and the particular nature of his practice.[43]

Much can be accomplished by the family physician in the course of office visits linked to other forms of treatment. In the case of a depressed patient being treated for duodenal ulcer, for example, it takes little time to palpate for epigastric tenderness and evaluate response to drug and dietary management. An excellent opportunity is available to uncover sources of stress and related problems in the patient's life and family.

Involvement of other family members may vary from a series of formal counseling sessions for a couple with a marital problem to intermittent visits involving two or more family members, and occasionally a conference of the entire family may be useful. A home visit may frequently provide valuable background and insights to the management of family problems. Counseling visits need not be lengthy—much can be accomplished in a series of visits, each as short as 20 or 30 minutes.

Some recent reports have pointed out the value of family sessions. Liebman, Silbergleit and Farber,[44] for example, have found a family conference of value in the care of the patient with cancer, while Hoebel[45] has found brief family-interactional therapy effective in the management of cardiac-related high-risk behaviors.

Future family practice groups are likely to develop a variety of organizational approaches to deal with family problems. Some may involve other health professionals on either a part-time or full-time basis in the care of these problems within the group setting. Many family practice residency programs are already involving others, such as clinical psychologists and medical social workers, in the management of family problems. Whatever approach family physicians take to these kinds of problems, the overriding requisite is that they perceive the family, not just the individual, as the patient.

REFERENCES

1. Bauman MH, Grace NT: Family process and family practice. J Fam Pract 1:24, 1974
2. Carmichael LP: The family in medicine, process or entity? J Fam Pract 3:562, 1976
3. Ogburn WF: Quoted in: Understanding the changing role of the family today. Patient Care Management Concepts, Vol 3, October 31, 1969, p 22
4. Livsey CG: Family therapy: Role of the practicing physician. Mod Treatment 6:808, 1969
5. Curry HB: The family as our patient. J Fam Pract 1:70, 1974
6. Worby CM: The family life cycle: An orienting concept for the family practice specialist. J Med Educ 46:198, 1971
7. Report of the Committee on the Dynamics of Family Interaction. Report of the National Conference on Family Life. Washington, D.C., 1948
8. Duvall EM: Family Development (Second Edition). Philadelphia, Lippincott, 1962, p.3
9. Rodgers RH: Proposed modification of Duvall family life cycle stages. Paper presented at the American Sociological Association, New York, August 31, 1960
10. Solomon MA: A developmental, conceptual premise for family therapy. Family Process 12:179, 1973
11. Geyman JP: The family as the object of care in family practice. J Fam Pract 5:571, 1977
12. Duvall EM: Family Development, 4th ed. Philadelphia, Lippincott, 1971, p 151
13. Rollins BC, Feldman H: Marital satisfaction over the family life cycle. J Marriage and the Family 32:25, February 1970
14. Holmes TH, Rahe RH: The social readjustment rating scale. J Psychosom Res 11:213, 1967
15. Smilkstein G: The family in trouble—how to tell. J Fam Pract 2:19, 1975
16. Meyer RJ, Haggerty RJ: Streptococcal infections in families: Factors altering individual susceptibility. Pediatrics 29:539, 1962
17. Smith CK, Anderson JC, Masuda M: A survey of psychiatric care in family practice. J Fam Pract 1:39, 1974
18. Medalie JH, Goldbourt U: Angina pectoris among 10,000 men. II. Psychosocial and other risk factors as evidenced by a multivariate analysis of a 5-year incidence study. Am J Med 60:910, 1976
19. Medalie JH, Snyder M, Groen JJ, et al.: Angina pectoris among 10,000 men. Am J Med 55:583, 1973
20. Stewart WL: Clinical implications of the Virginia study. J Fam Pract 3:30, 1976

21. Mechanic D: The influence of mothers on their children's health attitudes and behavior. Pediatrics 33:444, 1964
22. Medalie JH: Family Medicine—Principles and Applications. Baltimore, Williams and Wilkins, 1978, p 86
23. Peachey R: Family patterns of illness. GP 27:82, 1963
24. Bursten B: Family dynamics and illness behavior. GP 50:144, 1964
25. Hill R: Social stresses on the family. Social Case Work 39:139, 1958
26. Olsen EH: The impact of serious illness on the family system. Postgrad Med 47:172, February 1970
27. Klein R, Dean A, Bogdanoff M: The impact of illness upon the spouse. J Chronic Dis 20:241, 1968
28. Downes J: Chronic disease among spouses. Milbank Mem Fund Q 25:334, 1947
29. Bruhn JG: Effects of chronic illness on the family. J Fam Pract 4:1057, 1977
30. Schmidt DD: The family as the unit of care. J Fam Pract 7:303, 1978
31. Litman TJ: The family and physical rehabilitation. J Chronic Dis 19:211, 1966
32. Kraus A, Lilienfeld A: Some epidemiologic aspects of the high mortality rate in the young widowed group. J Chronic Dis 10:207, 1959
33. Smith H: North Carolina Mental Health Planning Staff: A Comprehensive Mental Health Plan for North Carolina, Vol 1, Attach 3, Raleigh, North Carolina: North Carolina Department of Mental Health, 1965, p 35
34. Nuckolls K: Life crises and psychosocial assets: Some clinical implications. In Kaplan BH, Cassel JC (eds): Family and Health. Chapel Hill, North Carolina, Institute for Research in Social Science, University of North Carolina, 1975
35. Duff RS, Hollingshead AB: Sickness and Society. New York, Harper and Row, 1968
36. Olsen EH: The impact of serious illness on the family system. Postgrad Med 47:169, February 1970
37. Rakel RE: Principles of Family Medicine. Philadelphia, Saunders, 1977, p 515
38. McWhinney IR: Beyond diagnosis—An approach to the integration of behavioral science and clinical medicine. N Engl J Med 287:284, 1972
39. Smilkstein G: The family APGAR: A proposal for a family function test and its use by physicians. J Fam Pract 6:1231, 1978
40. Arbogast RC, Scratton JM, Krick JP: The family as patient: An assessment schema. J Fam Pract 17:1151, 1978
41. Grace NT, Neal EM, Wellock CE, Pile DD: The family-oriented medical record. J Fam Pract 4:91, 1977
42. Ornstein PH: The family physician as a "therapeutic instrument." J Fam Pract 4:659, 1977
43. Cathell JL: Somehow, "GP-style" psychotherapy works. Consultant 8:12, 1968
44. Liebman A, Silbergleit I, Farber S: Family conference in the care of the cancer patient. J Fam Pract 2:343, 1975
45. Hoebel FC: Brief family-interactional therapy in the management of cardiac-related high-risk behaviors. J Fam Pract 3:613, 1976

CHAPTER THIRTEEN

Practice Patterns of Family Physicians

The last two chapters have examined the clinical content of family practice from two vantage points—the individual patient and the family as patient. The focus so far has therefore been on *what* is seen in family practice, not *how* this kind of care is actually provided in the community. Against this background, it is now of interest to look at the process of care in family practice.

Before turning to family practice itself, a brief comment is in order concerning some fundamental shifts in medical practice in the United States during the last 50 years. Figure 13–1 illustrates some important changes since 1928 with respect to the volume, type, and location of ambulatory patient visits to physicians in all fields. It can be seen that the number of office visits per person per year has almost doubled during this period. In addition, the proportion of visits in the office has increased by 40 percent and the proportion of home visits has declined precipitously.[1]

The purpose of this chapter is twofold: (1) to describe some basic patterns of family practice in the United States from several perspectives and (2) to compare family practice with other specialties in terms of practice patterns, including workload, problem-solving approaches, and practice satisfaction.

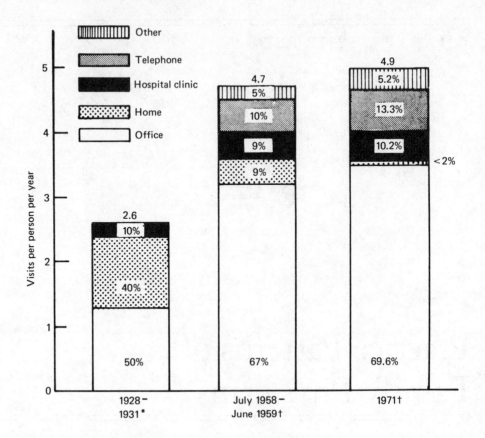

FIGURE 13-1.

Physician visits (excluding visits to patients in hospitals) per person per year by place of visit (United States, specified periods). Number in the bars indicate percentage of all visits.* White families only.† Civilian noninstitutionalized population.

Sources: (1) Kalk, IS, Klem, MC, and Sinai, N. *The Incidence of Illness and the Receipt and Costs of Medical Care Among Representative Family Groups.* Publications of the Committee on Costs of Medical Care, No. 26, Chicago, University of Chicago Press, 1933, Table B-27, p. 283. (2) U.S. National Center for Health Statistics. *Physician Visits—Volume and Interval Since Last Visit: U.S. 1971.* Public Health Service, Series 10, No. 97, Table C,–p. 9, Table B,–p. 5, 1975. From *1976 Medical Care Chart Book* (6th ed.). School of Public Health, Department of Medical Care Organization, University of Michigan, 1976, p. 35.

SOME PATTERNS OF PRACTICE

Organizational Structures

One of the striking features of changing medical practice in most fields of medicine in this country in recent years is the steady growth of group practice. The American Medical Association defines group practice as "the application of medical services by three or more physicians formally organized to provide medical care, consultation, diagnosis and/or treatment through joint use of equipment and personnel, and with the income from medical practice distributed in accordance with methods previously determined by members of the group." The number of groups in the United States doubled between 1965 and 1975, while the proportion of organizational forms represented by partnerships decreased from 77.8 percent in 1965 to 27.7 percent in 1975. During this same ten-year period, the average size of all types of group practice increased—by 1975, family practice groups * averaged 3.5 physicians per group, and multispecialty groups averaged 13 physicians per group.[2]

By 1975, 23.5 percent of all practicing general/family physicians were in group practice, including 9.7 percent in family practice groups and 13.8 percent in multispecialty groups. In 1975, four specialties accounted for 43.3 percent of all practicing physicians in group practice—family practice, general surgery, internal medicine, and radiology.[2] The most common size for family practice groups was three or four physicians (Table 13–1).

TABLE 13–1. FAMILY PRACTICE GROUPS BY AGE AND SIZE OF GROUP

| AGE OF GROUP | NUMBER OF GROUPS BY SIZE | | | | | | |
	Total	3	4	5	6	7	8 or more
Total	798	318	264	105	49	18	44
1 year or less	46	13	19	7	6	1	12
2–3 years	129	59	41	14	2	1	—
4–5 years	148	62	47	18	9	2	10
6–15 years	293	115	95	36	24	7	16
16–25 years	149	62	53	24	6	1	3
26 years or more	33	7	9	6	2	6	3

Source: Goodman, L.J., Bennett, E.H., and Odem, R.J.: *Group Medical Practice in the U.S., 1975.* Chicago, Center for Health Services Research and Development, American Medical Association, 1976, p 103. Reprinted with permission of the American Medical Association.

With the growth of group practice among family physicians, partnership and solo practice have steadily decreased. That this trend will continue unabated is reflected by the choices being made by today's family practice residency graduates—only 16 percent of 1977 graduates, for example, opted for solo practice.

Mechanic's [3] excellent studies of general/family physicians in the early 1970s demonstrated some interesting comparisons of workloads of family physicians in various kinds of practice settings. As shown in Table 13–2, family physicians in prepaid group practice tend to see fewer patients in the office than are seen by family physicians in other group or nongroup practice, while home visits are most common among nongroup family physicians.

* A *family practice group* is defined by the American Medical Association as one composed predominantly of general/family physicians.[2]

TABLE 13-2.   NUMBER OF REPORTED PATIENT VISITS IN OFFICE AND HOME DURING
PREVIOUS DAY

	NUMBER OF REPORTED PATIENT VISITS		
	Group (N = 113) (%)	Nongroup (N = 606) (%)	Prepaid Group (N = 108) (%)
Number of patients seen during previous day at office			
Less than 20	11	16	7
20–29	34	29	35
30–36	20	22	31
37–43	15	14	15
44 or more	20	19	12
X	32.5	32.2	31.5
SD	15.5	14.8	10.3
Number of home visits during previous day			
0	73	50	88
1	19	28	4
2 or more	9	22	8

Source: Adapted from Mechanic, D.: The organization of medical practice and practice orientations among physicians in prepaid and nonprepaid primary care settings. *Medical Care* 13:194, 1975.

There are many advantages to group practice. The group can allow frequent consultation among its members, emergency coverage of nights and weekends on a rotating basis, and many fringe benefits. Vacation and continuing education time can be readily scheduled within the group. Overhead expense can be shared, and more staff and facilities can be afforded than by the individual practitioner. Retirement and pension plans are available, as well as life insurance at a lower cost, and one can enter practice without an initial capital outlay. But there are some disadvantages to group practice, which for some individuals in some communities would make other methods of practice preferable. There may be professional, business, or personality causes of disagreement among physician-members for many reasons. Occasionally older members of larger groups tend to take advantage of their seniority, which becomes a progressive cause of friction and discontent. Income distribution may not correlate well with the productivity of individual members. Group physicians may not set their own pace as easily as if they were in solo or partnership practice. In some multispecialty groups, the family physician may not have the opportunity to practice the full range of his skills and interests.

Partnership with another family physician often affords an excellent method of practice, especially if the two partners have had comparable levels of training and share a similar philosophy of practice. Another common approach is that of expense-sharing agreements, which in a sense are hybrid partnerships/groups. Such arrangements may allow solo practitioners in adjoining offices to share many overhead expenses, as well as provide emergency coverage of each other's practice on nights and weekends. The individual physician can thereby achieve some of the advantages of group practice while alleviating some of the disadvantages of solo practice.

Solo practice allows maximal independence and a full sense of individuality to one's practice. But the increasing need for more complex facilities and staff in family practice, together with the essential need for adequate coverage during time away from the practice, will probably result in a continuing trend away from solo practice for most family physicians.

Although the trend is toward more group practice by family physicians, the variations among individual family physicians and community settings will likely foster the continuation of partnership practice and, to a lesser extent, solo practice.

Practice Settings

As already noted in earlier chapters, family practice is a flexible form of medical practice that directly meets the needs of the community in all types of practice settings, whether urban, suburban, or rural. Family physicians may organize their practices along any of the lines that have just been described and may practice in either the private sector or in a variety of environments within the public sector. The Indian Health Service represents one example of a predominantly rural practice setting in the public sector. The National Health Services Corps represents another practice setting of increasing importance that is presently expanding its focus from rural underserved areas to include urban underserved areas and is likewise placing greater emphasis upon facilitating the retention and continuing practice of NHSC physicians as private physicians in their communities after their obligated practice commitments are met.

A number of recent studies have demonstrated some interesting patterns of choice of specific practice settings by physicians. Cooper and his colleagues [4] studied the factors influencing the location decision of 1161 physicians in the primary care specialties. They found that a wide range of personal and professional considerations are involved in this decision, to the extent that no one factor was ranked as the most important factor by over 50 percent of respondents. Table 13–3 lists the frequency of factors listed first, second, or third in importance in decision making. It can be noted that the opportunity to join a desirable partnership or group practice was the most influential single factor by this group.

A summary of some of the more important dependent and independent variables that have been observed to influence the location of physicians is shown in Table 13–4. Thus, with regard to rural practice, a rural background of the physician and participation in a loan forgiveness program are positively correlated with a decision for rural practice, whereas the relative lack of cultural and recreational resources in the community are negatively correlated with such a decision.[5]

Parker and Sorenson [6] studied the factors influencing physicians to locate their practices in rural communities of upstate New York. Table 13–5 reflects

TABLE 13-3.   FREQUENCY OF FACTORS RANKED FIRST, SECOND, OR THIRD, BY ALL PRIMARY
CARE PHYSICIANS*

FACTOR	NUMBER	PERCENT
Opportunity to join a desirable partnership or group practice	499	43.0
Climate or geographic features of area	402	34.6
Availability of clinical support facilities and personnel	251	21.6
Preference for urban or rural living	250	21.5
Income potential	192	16.5
Opportunity for regular contact with a medical school or medical center	184	15.9
Influence of wife or husband (her/his desires, career, etc.)	181	15.6
Having been brought up in such a community	163	14.0
Having gone through medical school, internship, residency, or military service near area	143	12.3
Recreational and sports facilities	139	12.0
High medical need in area	136	11.7
Quality of educational system for children	119	10.3
Opportunity for regular contact with other physicians	113	9.7
Influence of family or friends	107	9.2
Access to continuing education	103	8.9
Cultural advantages	91	7.8
Opportunity to work with specific institution	68	5.9
Opportunities for social life	40	3.5
Prosperity of community	30	2.6
Organized efforts of community to recruit physicians	22	1.9
Advice of older physician	21	1.8
Prospect of being more influential in community affairs	20	1.7
Influences of preceptorship program	12	1.0
Payment of forgiveness loan	11	1.0
Availability of good social service, welfare, or home care services	11	1.0
Availability of loans for beginning practice	9	0.8

* $N = 1161$

Source: Cooper, J.K., Heald, K.S., and Coleman, S.: Rural or urban practice: Factors influencing the location decisions of primary care physicians. *Inquiry* 12:18, March 1975. Copyright © 1975 by the Blue Cross Association. All rights reserved.

the diversity of significant factors, with seven factors considered important by over 50 percent of the physicians.

Team Practice

Another dimension of changing health care in many fields is the growing emphasis upon team practice. Magraw[7] states the need for this trend in these terms:

Even though we physicians are more nearly self-sufficient than any other group, and in a pinch a physician could set up practice in a barn, we are not actually able to deliver modern medical care by ourselves. Most of these other professions now possess knowledge and skills which physicians, at least in any clinically usable way, do

TABLE 13-4. FACTORS AFFECTING PHYSICIAN LOCATION

DEPENDENT VARIABLE	RELATIONSHIP	INDEPENDENT VARIABLE
Number of physicians	+	Per capita income in state
	+	State education expenditures
	+	Per capita income in county
	+	Construction of hospital in community
	+	Median income in community
	+	Population of area
	+	Physician's price practices, based on per capita income of area
	+	Failure rate of licensing examination
	+	Physician income in state
	−	Lack of recreational facilities
	−	Construction of hospital in rural county
	−	Cyclic variations in income levels in area
Practice in urban areas	+	Graduation from certain medical schools
	+	Graduation from urban medical school
Practice in rural areas	+	Rural background
	+	Participation in loan forgiveness program
Practice in same state	+	Internship and residency training in state
Ability to attract physicians	+	Mobility of community residents
	+	Educational level of population
	−	Percent population in agriculture
Number of primary care physicians	+	Percent population white
	+	Percent population 0–5 years old and 65 + years old
	−	Inadequate cultural and recreational resources in community
Number of specialists	+	Educational level of population
	+	Number of supportive institutions
	+	Number of general hospital beds per 1000 population
	+	Medical school in community
Presence of physician	+	Economic growth rate of town

Source: Cooper, J.K., Heald, K., Samuels, M.: The decision for rural practice. *Journal of Medical Education* 47:939, 1972.

TABLE 13-5.   FACTORS THAT INFLUENCED PHYSICIANS PERSONALLY TO SETTLE IN A SMALL COMMUNITY

PERCENT	ORDER OF IMPORTANCE
84	Appeal of small-community living
82	A good community hospital
82	A medical center in a nearby city
73	Need for physicians in the community
66	A medical community with consultants in various fields available
65	An attractive town in a geographically pleasant part of the country
55	A chance to join a group practice
47	Possibility of having the desired sort of practice, whereas this might not have been possible in a large city
46	A good practice could be built up quickly
42	A prosperous part of the country
27	Spouse had connections in area or was attracted to it
26	Opportunity to return to a familiar part of the country
24	An older established physician needed a partner
22	Came from a small community originally
16	Availability of expert advice on establishing and managing a practice
16	Influence of teachers in medical school or later training
14	Relatives in the community
8	Advertisement in a medical journal

Source: Parker, R.C., and Sorensen, A.A.: The tides of rural physicians: The ebb and flow, or why physicians move out of and into small communities. *Medical Care* 16:152, 1978.

not have. We can be certain that an increasing number of such "paramedical" experts possessed of increasingly specialized skills will play an ever more important part in medical care teamwork.

Currently, about 2.3 allied health personnel are employed per physician.[2] A breakdown of trends for the employment of various types of allied health personnel by physicians in various kinds of group practice is shown in Table 13-6.[2] It can be seen that family practice groups include a larger staff of allied health personnel per physician (2.57) compared to other specialties. This is not surprising in view of the broad range of services and relatively high patient volume characteristic of family practice.

Team practice is not as new a concept as some would have us believe. Certainly it can be argued that physicians working together in a group represent one form of team practice. It is also evident that various kinds of allied health personnel have worked closely with physicians for many years on a teamwork basis. There is, however, a trend toward increased diversity of disciplines contributing to today's patient care, together with greater amounts of responsibility being delegated by physicians to allied health professionals for certain aspects of patient care.

The previously described physician extender (pp. 124–27) represents an important new addition to family practice in many settings. Although functionally

TABLE 13–6. NUMBER AND PER-PHYSICIAN FULL-TIME EQUIVALENT ALLIED HEALTH PERSONNEL BY TYPE OF GROUP

ALLIED HEALTH PERSONNEL	TOTAL GROUPS		SINGLE SPECIALTY		MULTISPECIALITY		FAMILY PRACTICE	
	N	Per M.D.	N	Per M.D.	N	Per M.D.	N	Per M.D.
Total	140527.4	2.10	44699.2	1.90	85673.0	2.18	10155.6	2.57
Secretaries, bookkeepers, receptionists	60191.9	0.90	21163.2	0.90	34554.9	0.88	4473.9	1.13
Total nursing	37077.1	0.55	9029.1	0.38	24373.5	0.61	3674.5	0.93
Registered nurses	18367.7	0.27	5217.5	0.22	11574.6	0.29	1575.6	0.40
Licensed practical nurses	8905.1	0.13	1823.7	0.08	5972.1	0.15	1109.3	0.28
Nurse aides	9804.3	0.15	1987.9	0.08	6826.8	0.17	989.6	0.25
Total technical	28110.6	0.41	11097.1	0.47	15576.4	0.40	1446.1	0.36
Laboratory technicians and assistants	13476.8	0.20	5802.7	0.25	6948.1	0.18	726.0	0.18
X-ray technicians and assistants	9625.9	0.14	3176.1	0.13	5896.3	0.15	553.5	0.14
Medical technicians	5007.9	0.07	2118.3	0.09	2723.0	0.07	166.6	0.04
Pharmacists	1011.0	0.02	187.6	0.01	761.0	0.02	62.4	0.02
Other personnel	14137.1	0.21	3222.2	0.14	10416.2	0.26	498.7	0.13

Source: Goodman, L.J., Bennett, E.H., and Odem, R.J.: *Group Medical Practice in the U.S., 1975.* Chicago, Center for Health Services Research and Development, American Medical Association, 1976, p 45. Reprinted with permission of the American Medical Association.

comparable in terms of training and roles, physician extenders in primary care represent three basic groups—physician's assistant, Medex, and nurse practitioner. As a group, Medex graduates have been most directly involved with family practice and with rural locations. Physicians' assistants and nurse practitioners have gravitated more toward urban and institutional settings, although about one-fifth of them have located in rural areas in association with family physicians.[8] Over 40 percent of all physicians' assistants now in practice are working under the supervision of family physicians.[9]

As shown in Table 13–7, over one-half of Medexes are employed in solo or partnership practices, whereas nurse practitioners and physicians' assistants are most frequently associated with groups or other more organized practice settings.[10] Overall comparisons between the percentage employed and workload of these three groups are shown in Table 13–8.[8]

As physician extenders have become integrated in everyday medical practice, the development of protocols for the care of specific clinical problems has facilitated their active role in patient care. Figure 13–2 illustrates an example of such a protocol for urinary tract infection and vaginitis.[11] The use of this kind of protocol by well-trained physician extenders can save physician time and facilitate the evaluation of medical care without compromising the quality of care (which may be improved in the process). With regard to this particular protocol, the supervising physician is actively involved with the patient's care in the event of associated problems, including pregnancy, diabetes, recurrent urinary tract infection, chronic renal disease, hypertension, incontinence, fever or chills, and severe abdominal pain.

It is likely that other disciplines will in the future contribute more actively, especially on a part-time and consultative basis, to comprehensive care in family practice settings. Blanchard and Kurtz[12] have described the involvement of

TABLE 13–7. PRACTICE ARRANGEMENT BY TYPE OF PHYSICIAN EXTENDER

	NP(%)*	PA(%)†	MX(%)‡	ALL PEs(%)	PHYSICIANS (%)
Solo or partnership	12.3	27.7	53.6	22.8	76.5
Group or other more organized practice	64.1	60.3	38.0	59.9	23.5
Not ascertained	23.6	12.0	8.4	17.3	—
Total	100.0	100.0	100.0	100.0	100.0

* NP = Nurse Practitioner.
† PA = Physician's Assistant.
‡ MX = Medex.

Source: Cantwell, J.R., (ed.): *Profile of Medical Practice*, 1975–1976 ed. Chicago, Center for Health Services Research, American Medical Association, 1976. p. 21. Includes active, nonfederal physicians involved in patient care.   Quoted in Morris, S.B., and Smith, D.B.: The distribution of physician extenders. *Medical Care* 15:1054, 1977.

TABLE 13-8. SELF-REPORTED ACTIVITIES OF GRADUATES*

	PHYSICIAN'S ASSISTANTS	MEDEX	NURSE PRACTITIONER (CERTIFICATE)	NURSE PRACTITIONER (MASTER'S)*
Percentage employed	89	96	90	98
Median number of patients seen daily	24	>25	12	11
Median patient care hours worked per week as NHP	48	48	31	39

* Response rates vary for each item

Source: Adapted from *Nurse Practitioner and Physician Assistant Training-Deployment Study.* Bethesda, Maryland, System Sciences, Inc., Sep 30, 1976. Final Report on Contract No. (HRA) 230–75–0198. Quoted in Kane, R.L., and Wilson, W.M.: The new health practitioner—The past as prologue. *Western Journal of Medicine* 127:258, 1977.

a medical social worker in family practice, with a particular focus on preventive and early interventional services. Clinical psychologists may participate with family physicians in individual and group therapy.[13] Clinical pharmacists may provide drug information, consultation, and related services in family practice groups.[14, 15] Some future family practices may even develop closer working relationships with general dentists, as is already taking place in at least one family practice residency program.[16]

Utilization of Community Resources

Recent years have seen a growing proliferation of health-related community resources at local, state, regional, and national levels. These resources and agencies often have much to contribute to the health care of patients with chronic illness, psychosocial problems, and many other problems. The family physician plays a vital role in linking individuals and families in their practices to appropriate community resources when needed and in coordinating the total health care of their patients. This requires the family physician to be knowledgeable of available resources within the community and to be skilled in the utilization thereof.

A list of community resources that may be available in many communities is provided in Appendix 8, together with a list of selected national voluntary health agencies. Farley and Treat [17] recommend that family physicians develop and maintain an up-to-date index of community resources on the basis of need. They suggest that the following categories be used as the nucleus for an index system:

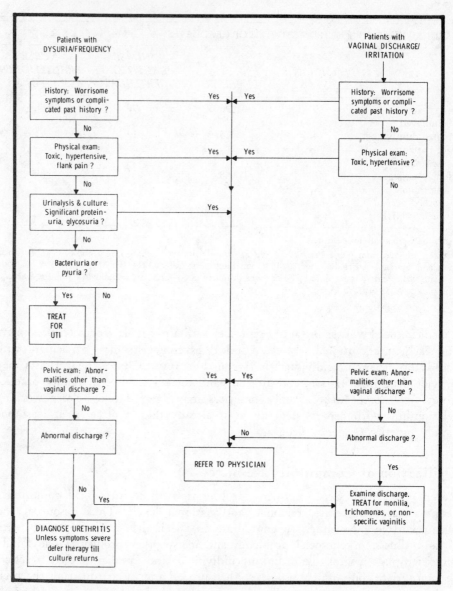

FIGURE 13-2.

Major logic pathways through the urinary tract infection (UTI) and vaginitis protocol. The protocol specifies what is meant by phrases such as *worrisome symptoms* and *toxic*. Beside this logic, the protocol contains many other minor pathways and logic branch points.

Source: Greenfield, S, Friedland, G, Seifers, S, Rhodes, A, Black, WL, and Komaroff, AL: Protocol management of dysuria urinary frequency and vaginal discharge. *Journal of Family Practice* 2:180, 1975.

1. Adoption
2. Aging
3. Alcoholism
4. Birth control
5. Blindness
6. Cancer
7. Chronic illness
8. Communicable disease control
9. Counseling services
10. Drug addiction
11. Handicapped children or adults
12. Mental illness
13. Nursing care
14. Poison control
15. Psychologic testing

The task of identification of community resources is further facilitated by use of a questionnaire for information-gathering purposes (Appendix 8).

Referral of patients to community agencies should involve personal contact by the family physician whenever possible. Werblun and Twersky[18] suggest the following approaches for family physicians making referrals to community agencies:

1. Identify the specific physical and/or psychosocial problem.
2. Identify the patient's (and/or family's) perception of the problem.
   a. What does the patient or family want to do about it?
   b. What has already been done?
   c. What resources have been used in the past?
3. Identify the patient's available resources.
   a. Personal, family, and social support systems.
   b. Financial resources available.
4. Determine community resources available.
   a. Patient's eligibility (e.g., financial, age, geographic location, disability).
   b. Accessibility to the patient.
   c. Patient's ability to meet a "fee for service" requirement.
   d. Waiting period.
   e. Will the services meet the patient's needs?
5. Function as a facilitator in the referral process.
6. Act as the patient's advocate as needed.
7. Evaluate success of referral.
   a. Utilize a "consent for mutual exchange of information" (Appendix 8).
   b. Obtain feedback from patient, family, and agency.

Consultation and Referral

All physicians have their own individual limitations that must be acknowledged and not exceeded. Early in practice, family physicians should become acquainted with physicians in all other specialty fields from whom they can seek advice and help. They will thereby develop patterns of consultation that will depend on their own training and experience, the availability of medical resources within the community, and their proximity to consulting specialists.

There are many methods of consultation used by family physicians. The simplest, and perhaps the most common, is the informal consultation in the hall or doctor's room of the hospital with colleagues in family practice or other fields. Another common form of consultation is by telephone, where the family physician may be advised of further steps in patient care that may or may not involve referral of the patient to the consultant.

Referral of patients can take several forms, and it is important that both the family physician and consultant know what each expects of the other. A referral may be (1) for confirmation of diagnosis, with return of the patient to the family physician for treatment; (2) for a second opinion in any aspect of diagnosis or therapy; and (3) for diagnosis and/or treatment by the consulting physician with return of the patient to the family physician upon conclusion of care for the given clinical problem. Most referrals in family practice are for assistance with treatment rather than for diagnostic opinion. When a patient has been referred to a consultant for a specific problem, the family physician most commonly will continue to play an active role in the care of the patient. Examples of such continued involvement include ongoing management of concurrent medical problems, assisting at surgery, and post-operative care. Figure 13–3 illustrates a consultation request form recommended by the American Academy of Family Physicians for effective communication and clarification of the type of consultation desired.

The process of consultation and referral is a potentially complicated one that requires of the family physician the same level of concern and effort as would be involved in other kinds of prescriptions for the patient. Rudy and Williams [19] have examined the effects of this process on therapeutic outcome and have identified the following pitfalls to be addressed by referring physicians:

1. Resistance to consultation/referral by the referring physician.
2. Resistance to consultation/referral by the patient.
3. Failure to follow through.
4. Failure to adequately interpret the patient/family complex to the consultant.
5. Failure to define for the consultant desired objectives of the consultation.
6. Reticence toward critical evaluation of the consultation by the referring physician.

The family physician's skillful use of consultation not only results in the best possible patient care, but also affords an important avenue of continuing medical education. Good rapport and working relationships based on mutual respect with consultants in all fields enhances the family physician's own enjoyment of the practice of family medicine and is in the best interest of his/her patients.

CONSULTATION AND REFERENCE REQUEST

Introducing:

Referring Physician:

Referred to:

Tentative Diagnosis:

Examination Requested:

Date:

Report requested:

☐ Phone

☐ Letter

☐ Both

Case Work-up Pertaining to This Illness

History:

Pertinent family background:

Physical findings:

Laboratory and X-Ray findings:

Medication or procedures already utilized:

(Use reverse side for further information)

Requested Disposition of Case

Consultation and Report:

  Consult & workup only ☐

  Assume care for this illness only ☐

  Assume future management within your field ☐

Explain to Patient:

  Diagnosis ☐

  Outline treatment ☐

  Refer back for interpretation & treatment ☐

If surgery is indicated:

  Referring physician requests to:

    Assist ☐

    Perform surgery ☐

    Give anesthesia ☐

  Consultant proceed without referring physician's participation ☐

Additional copies of this form may be purchased from the   American Academy of Family Physicians, 1740 West 92nd Street

Kansas City.   Missouri 64114

FIGURE 13-3.

American Academy of Family Physicians consultation request form.

COMPARATIVE PATTERNS AMONG SPECIALTIES

Workload

Several studies during the 1970s of the workloads of various specialties revealed interesting comparisons by field. Mechanic compared the reported time expenditures for a "typical week" among United States primary care physicians [20] (Table 13–9). It can be noted that approximately one-half of general practitioners reported spending at least 50 hours per week seeing patients, a comparable figure to both internists and nongroup pediatricians; by contrast, just over one-third of obstetricians reported this level of activity. All four fields spent substantially more time each week devoted to practice management when in nongroup practice compared to those in group practice. Nongroup physicians in internal medicine, pediatrics, and obstetrics–gynecology likewise reported longer work weeks than group physicians, with the workload in general practice quite comparable between group and nongroup physicians. Nongroup internists in this study were most likely to report a work week in excess of 60 hours.

In this same study, Mechanic examined the number of reported patient visits in the office and patient's home on the previous day for these four fields [20] (Table 13–10). Here it is seen that about one-third of general practitioners reported seeing 37 or more patients on the previous day, comparable to nongroup pediatricians but considerably greater than the number of patients seen by internists and obstetrician–gynecologists. It is also apparent that house calls, though relatively infrequent, were most commonly made by the general practitioners.

The Medical Economics Continuing Survey in 1977 revealed some interesting comparisons in the numbers of total patient visits each week to various specialties (Table 13–11). This survey corroborates the previously described heavier patient volume of general/family physicians and pediatricians compared to the other specialties.

The continuing studies by the American Medical Association of the profile of medical practice in the United States in 1973 compared the numbers of total patient visits per week (Table 13–12) and office visits per week by specialty and location (Table 13–13). Consistent differences were demonstrated among fields for both of these measures, with general practice reporting the largest workload, followed in order by pediatrics, obstetrics–gynecology, and internal medicine. With the exception of psychiatry and radiology, the workload uniformly increased as the size of the community decreased from urban to nonmetropolitan areas.[21]

Age Spectrum of Practice

It is entirely predictable that the age spectrum of the practice population of general/family physicians will necessarily be the most broad of all fields within medicine. The National Ambulatory Medical Care Survey, however, has demon-

TABLE 13–9.   REPORTED TIME EXPENDITURES FOR A "TYPICAL WEEK" AMONG AMERICAN PRIMARY CARE PHYSICIANS

	GENERAL PRACTITIONERS (%)		INTERNISTS (%)		PEDIATRICIANS (%)		OBSTETRICIANS (%)	
	Nongroup N = 599	Group N = 111	Nongroup N = 231	Group N = 91	Nongroup N = 136	Group N = 43	Nongroup N = 150	Group N = 58
Hours spent during a typical week seeing patients								
Less than 40	29	17	17	22	20	24	41	32
40–49	19	33	27	29	27	33	24	32
50–59	24	24	27	33	25	24	15	21
60 or more	29	27	29	16	28	19	20	16
Additional hours during a typical week devoted to practice management (excluding direct patient contact)								
2 or less	29	41	23	46	28	65	35	45
3–5	32	31	35	22	34	21	33	36
6–10	26	21	30	21	28	9	18	14
11 or more	14	6	12	10	9	5	14	5
Additional hours on activities related to practice such as attending meetings, medical reading, etc.								
2 or less	31	35	19	18	19	19	29	28
3–5	35	31	39	31	42	46	37	33
6–10	28	27	28	40	34	28	26	22
11 or more	7	7	13	11	5	7	8	17
Total reported hours spent during a typical week (sum of three above categories)								
Less than 40	10	6	6	9	7	18	25	12
40–49	14	17	11	13	16	14	15	24
50–59	26	28	26	40	27	32	21	29
60–69	22	26	28	20	28	21	14	17
70 or more	28	23	30	18	23	14	26	17

Source: Mechanic, D.: General medical practice: Some comparisons between the work of primary care physicians in the United States and England and Wales. Medical Care 10:402, 1972.

TABLE 13–10. NUMBER OF REPORTED PATIENT VISITS IN OFFICE AND HOME DURING PREVIOUS DAY AMONG VARYING TYPES OF AMERICAN PRIMARY CARE PHYSICIANS*

	GENERAL PRACTITIONERS (%)		INTERNISTS (%)		PEDIATRICIANS (%)		OBSTETRICIANS (%)	
	Nongroup N = 599	Group N = 111	Nongroup N = 231	Group N = 91	Nongroup N = 136	Group N = 43	Nongroup N = 150	Group N = 58
Number of patients seen during previous day at office								
0–10	6	6	21	16	2	5	8	7
11–19	10	5	42	49	9	12	15	12
20–29	27	32	24	29	30	36	42	39
30–36	23	21	9	5	22	21	20	29
37–43	14	16	1	1	13	17	10	7
44–50	8	10	1	—	13	2	3	3
51–64	8	6	1	—	5	7	2	2
65 or more	4	3	—	—	6	—	2	2
Number of home calls during previous day								
None	52	75	70	82	81	95	96	100
1	26	15	18	11	11	3	1	—
2	13	7	8	5	5	3	—	—
3	5	1	3	1	1	—	1	—
4 or more	4	2	1	1	1	—	3	—

* The sample sizes shown here constitute the full sample available in the analysis. Percentages are calculated only for doctors responding to the specific question, and thus sample size may vary slightly from the base and from one question to another. Percentages do not always equal 100 percent due to rounding errors.

Source: Adapted from Mechanic, D.: General medical practice: Some comparisons between the work of primary care physicians in the United States and England and Wales. *Medical Care* 10:402, 1972.

TABLE 13-11. TOTAL NUMBER OF PATIENT VISITS PER WEEK*

	BOARD-CERTIFIED M.D.s	UNCERTIFIED M.D.s
General/family physicians	182	164
Internists	129	126
General surgeons	112	113
Obstetrician–gynecologists	144	124
Pediatricians	151	156
All surgical specialists	113	114
All nonsurgical specialists	121	102
All fields	120	111

* Patient visits include all those during which the doctor personally saw the patient in office, hospital, or other location during a representative full work week in the spring of 1977.
Source: *Medical Economics Continuing Survey, 1977.* Copyright © 1977 by Litton Industries, Inc. Published by Medical Economics Company, a Litton division, at Oradell, New Jersey. Reprinted by permission.

strated some surprising findings with regard to the annual rates of office visits for patients less than 15 years of age and 65 years of age and over. Table 13–14 reveals that this rate for general/family physicians and pediatricians for the younger group is nearly equal, whereas the rate of office visits to general/family physicians by patients in the geriatric age group is almost double the rate of office visits to internists.[22]

Duration of Office Visit

Since general/family practice involves a larger patient volume than other fields, it is not surprising that the average duration of the office visit is somewhat shorter than that of other fields. Table 13–15 shows a wide range in duration

TABLE 13-12. AVERAGE NUMBER OF TOTAL PATIENT VISITS PER WEEK BY SPECIALTY AND LOCATION, 1973

			METROPOLITAN	
SPECIALTY	TOTAL	NON-METROPOLITAN	50,000–999,999 population	1,000,000+ population
Total	137.7	175.9	144.5	118.8
General practice	189.9	212.4	199.3	157.8
Internal medicine	127.2	144.2	141.1	116.0
Obstetrics–gynecology	132.4	154.5	145.6	118.6
Pediatrics	158.1	178.6	168.5	146.3

Source: American Medical Association, Center for Health Services Research and Development: *Profile of Medical Practice '74.* Chicago, American Medical Association, 1974, p. 180. Reprinted with permission of the American Medical Association.

TABLE 13–13.   AVERAGE NUMBER OF OFFICE VISITS PER WEEK BY SPECIALTY AND LOCATION, 1973

| | | | METROPOLITAN | |
SPECIALTY	TOTAL	NON-METROPOLITAN	50,000–999,999 population	1,000,000+ population
Total	97.9	127.5	102.7	84.2
General Practice	145.5	162.8	149.3	125.4
Internal Medicine	79.4	90.0	87.5	73.0
Surgery	81.1	91.5	85.5	74.0
Obstetrics–gynecology	98.4	109.5	106.1	90.8
Pediatrics	134.9	151.3	149.9	121.9
Psychiatry	36.3	29.0	40.6	35.0
Radiology	92.6	84.1	107.0	81.5
Anesthesiology	7.5	18.8	11.1	1.5
Other	95.4	92.5	102.2	91.6

Source: American Medical Association, Center for Health Services Research and Development: *Profile of Medical Practice '74*. Chicago, American Medical Association, 1974, p. 183. Reprinted with permission of the American Medical Association.

of office visits among specialties between dermatology (11.9 minutes) and psychiatry (46.9 minutes). Pediatrics, general/family practice, and obstetrics–gynecology are quite comparable in this regard, with average office visits of 12.1, 12.6, and 13.1 minutes, respectively.[23]

Problem-Solving Approaches

Comparative studies of the problem-solving approaches used by different specialties have been limited to date. McWhinney suggested in 1972 that the problem-solving strategy used in a clinical specialty would depend on four factors: (1) tacit assumptions about the problems likely to be encountered, (2) the general objectives of the specialty, (3) the utility of individual procedures, and (4)

TABLE 13–14.   ANNUAL RATE OF OFFICE VISITS BY PATIENT AGE FOR PRIMARY CARE PHYSICIANS—UNITED STATES, MAY 1973–APRIL 1974

PHYSICIAN SPECIALTY	UNDER 15 YEARS	15–24 YEARS	25–44 YEARS	45–64 YEARS	65 YEARS AND OVER
General/family practice	0.8	1.2	1.2	1.6	2.1
Internal medicine (general)	0.0	0.2	0.3	0.6	1.1
Pediatrics	0.9	0.1	—	—	—

Source: *Preliminary Data from the National Ambulatory Medical Care Survey* (unedited draft, July 15, 1975), p. 34.

TABLE 13–15. DURATION OF OFFICE VISIT BY SPECIALTY *

SPECIALTY	MEAN DURATION (MINUTES)
All specialties	15.0
General and family practice	12.6
Internal medicine	18.2
Obstetrics–gynecology	13.1
Pediatrics	12.1
General surgery	12.7
Ophthalmology	20.3
Orthopedic surgery	14.5
Otolaryngology	13.6
Psychiatry	46.9
Dermatology	11.9
Urology	15.0
Cardiovascular disease	21.5
Neurology	35.5

* Duration of visit is defined to include only the time spent in face-to-face encounter between physician and patient.

Source: *Advance Data from Vital and Health Statistics of the National Center for Health Statistics,* 12:5. Hyattsville, Maryland, U.S. Department of Health, Education and Welfare, October 12, 1977.

tradition.[24] There is some evidence that the problem-solving strategies of family physicians are quite different from those used by other clinical specialties.

Smith and McWhinney studied two groups of physicians—nine family physicians and nine consulting internists—in terms of their diagnostic approaches to three programmed patients simulating three clinical problems: (1) a 32-year-old housewife with fatigue, depression, and mild iron-deficiency anemia; (2) a 19-year-old male presenting with sore throat due to infectious mononucleosis; and (3) a 28-year-old woman presenting with periodic headaches over many years. They found that family physicians asked fewer history questions, requested fewer items of information from the physical examination, and ordered fewer laboratory tests. The family physicians also asked a higher proportion of questions about mental status and life situation in two of the three cases. There were no significant differences in the final diagnoses obtained by the family physicians and internists. Table 13–16 represents the magnitude of these differences.[25]

It is both logical and efficient for the family physician to use time as a diagnostic factor. In contrast to the consultant, who must necessarily emphasize thoroughness and a more extensive diagnostic workup at what may be the only encounter with the patient, the family physician through his/her continuing relationship with the patient can proceed in steps with additional workup for persistent and/or new symptoms or for lack of response to treatment.[26]

TABLE 13–16. COMPARISON BETWEEN INTERVIEWS CONDUCTED ON THREE CLINICAL PROBLEMS BY FAMILY PHYSICIANS AND INTERNISTS

| | ITEMS FROM PHYSICAL EXAMINATION | | | TESTS ORDERED | | |
| | Mean Number | | | Mean Number | | |
PATIENT NUMBER	Family Physicians (N = 9)	Internists (N = 9)	t value	Family Physicians (N = 9)	Internists (N = 9)	t value
1	4.3	12.5	2.814*	1.9	7.2	2.762*
2	6.0	11.5	1.908†	3.2	5.0	2.462‡
3	7.5	11.5	1.817§	1.9	4.1	1.630¶

* $p = <0.02$.
† $p = <0.10, >0.05$.
‡ $p = 0.05$.
§ $p = <0.10$.
¶ $p = 0.20$.

Source: Smith, D.H., McWhinney, I.R.: Comparison of the diagnostic methods of family physicians and internists. *Journal of Medical Education* 50:264, 1975.

Practice Satisfaction

Although satisfaction with medical practice involves innumerable factors and individual variations by specialty and by physician, some patterns emerge from available studies. The Medical Economics Continuing Survey of 1976 showed that greater ease of practice was rated by physicians as the chief practice goal regardless of specialty, as had also been the case in 1965. Table 13–17 reflects comparative rankings of five practice goals for five clinical specialties. These rankings are noteworthy for the commonalities by specialty in most instances. Yet some differences can be noted—pediatricians are least satisfied with their income and general surgeons are most likely to desire more specialization. Within the general/family practice field, it is of interest that three times as many general practitioners wanted smaller practices compared to family physicians in 1976, when national data for family practice showed a weekly average of 190 patient visits in contrast to 163 patient visits per week for general practice.[27]

Mechanic[3] has focused in more detail on a larger number of comparative factors regarding satisfaction in two fields—general practice and pediatrics. Table 13–18 highlights these results, which again are comparable in many respects. Less than 8 percent of respondents in the two fields were dissatisfied in an overall way with their field, although larger numbers were dissatisfied with one or another part of their work. The great majority of general practitioners and pediatricians were very satisfied with their hospital privileges, with the exception of 14 percent of general practitioners in prepaid group practice.

TABLE 13–17.   COMPARATIVE PRACTICE GOALS BY SPECIALTY IN 1976

CHIEF PRACTICE GOAL	G.P.s (%)	F.P.s (%)	INTERNISTS (%)	GENERAL SURGEONS (%)	OBSTETRICIAN-GYNECOLOGISTS (%)	PEDIATRICIANS (%)
Greater ease of practice	41	46	38	44	43	37
More free time	34	37	39	34	40	34
Increased earnings	15	17	17	16	15	28
Reduction in size of practice	22	7	12	7	8	7
More specialization	1	1	3	7	3	3
Other	2	2	2	4	2	2

Source: Owens, A.: What doctors want most from their practices now. *Medical Economics*, March 7, 1977, p. 88. Copyright © 1977 by Litton Industries, Inc. Published by Medical Economics Company, a Litton division, at Oradell, New Jersey. Reprinted by permission.

TABLE 13–18. OVERALL SATISFACTION AND TYPES OF SATISFACTIONS AND DISSATISFACTIONS IN VARYING PRACTICE SETTINGS

	GROUP (%)		NONGROUP (%)		PREPAID GROUP (%)	
	General Practitioners (N = 113)	Pediatricians (N = 43)	General Practitioners (N = 606)	Pediatricians (N = 136)	General Practitioners (N = 108)	Pediatricians (N = 154)
Physician's overall self rating						
Very satisfied	56	47	52	39	42	44
Fairly satisfied	42	49	44	53	51	53
Not very satisfied/dissatisfied	3	5	4	8	7	3
Components of satisfaction:						
With amount of time for each patient						
Very satisfied	19	26	25	18	10	23
Not satisfied	39	23	38	43	49	31
With opportunities for professional contacts						
Very satisfied	50	67	48	48	49	66
Not satisfied	15	5	17	12	14	5
With amount of income						
Very satisfied	47	47	46	37	47	45
Not satisfied	11	12	12	20	10	16
With incentives for high quality in one's practice						
Very satisfied	66	70	70	69	57	64
Not satisfied	2	5	4	7	8	7
With office facilities						
Very satisfied	62	51	55	53	48	36
Not satisfied	11	14	11	17	17	16
With hospital privileges						
Very satisfied	74	77	75	81	56	71
Not satisfied	6	2	7	7	14	5

With amount of time practice requires						
Very satisfied	33	42	35	27	47	52
Not satisfied	28	26	30	35	16	15
With community status and esteem						
Very satisfied	60	60	67	63	54	47
Not satisfied	7	7	6	6	6	12
With amount of leisure time						
Very satisfied	30	35	25	26	41	44
Not satisfied	36	30	47	45	23	26

Source: Mechanic, D.: The organization of medical practice and practice orientation among physicians in prepaid and nonprepaid primary care settings. *Medical Care* 13:189, 1975.

COMMENT

Several aspects of the preceding discussion warrant additional comment. The first is the nature of organizational forms of family practice. In view of the diversity of community needs and environments reflected in different practice settings, from large urban centers on the one hand to isolated rural areas on the other, family practice will necessarily develop varied organizational patterns ranging from large multispecialty groups to solo practice. In my view, however, the relatively small family practice group, including three to five family physicians will emerge as the single most common organizational structure for family practice, particularly in medium and smaller-sized communities. Such a group can adapt well to the needs of a majority of practice settings in the community, and affords the full advantages of group practice to physicians, staff and patients alike without the added complexities of larger organizational structures. It is well known that the potential problems of medical groups increase sharply with the addition of each member beyond this size.

Another area requiring further comment is the projected viability of various types of team practice that are currently being developed and tested. As pointed out in an earlier chapter (p. 86), there is considerable confusion and controversy today surrounding the role of physician extenders in primary care, particularly with regard to their autonomy in patient care and the nature of physician supervision of their activities. These issues are perhaps best illustrated by the emphasis by some in nursing upon joint practice, as opposed to team practice, whereby the nurse practitioner is envisioned as an independent clinician with many of the same roles and skills as the physician. At the conceptual level, the concept of joint practice has blurred the distinctions between medical practice and nursing practice.[28, 29] At the practical level, application of this concept has led some physician extenders to develop "a practice within a practice" in various primary care settings where they function more as physicians and less as team members contributing their special skills to the entire practice.

Although some early results of the deployment of physician extenders are encouraging, it is still too early to extrapolate their widespread utilization in primary care.[30] There are already some disturbing reports that could limit the potential benefits of physician extenders in primary care. In California, for example, a survey of 568 pediatricians showed support of the concept of a pediatric nurse practitioner working as part of a practice team under constant physician surveillance, but not replacing the pediatrician even in well-child care.[31] A more recent study involving a 60 percent response of all pediatricians in Arizona showed that the role of the pediatric nurse practitioner is perceived as competitive rather than collaborative.[32] Another study by Breslau[33] of patient perceptions and evaluations of the role of the pediatric nurse practitioner showed that patients do not perceive the nurse practitioner to have expertise in an exclusive domain of health problems and tended not to consider his/her addition to the office to have improved the physician's services.

A final comment is in order concerning the vital importance of maintaining the highest possible quality of the doctor–patient relationship in family practice regardless of the organizational form or setting of the practice. The doctor–patient relationship today is being affected by such issues as an increasing emphasis on cost-benefit in health care, complexities of third-party billing procedures, questions about confidentiality of records, changing roles of the physician in various forms of team practice, and the threat of malpractice suits for a broader range of results than actual malpractice. Our population is more mobile than in the past, expects more from medicine, and finds health care increasingly fragmented, more costly, and often less accessible and less personal. The primacy of the *person* as the reason for health care needs to be defended and reinforced. The threat of depersonalization of health care poses a critical challenge to the entire medical profession, but is a fundamental concern in family practice as that specialty taking r ;ponsibility for the ongoing care of individuals and their families.

REFERENCES

1. 1976 Medical Care Chart Book, 6th ed. Ann Arbor, Michigan, School of Public Health, Department of Medical Care Organization, University of Michigan, 1976, p 35
2. Goodman LJ, Bennett EH, Odem RJ: Group Medical Practice in the U.S., 1975. Chicago, Center for Health Services Research and Development, AMA, 1976
3. Mechanic D: The organization of medical practice and practice orientations among physicians in prepaid and nonprepaid primary care settings. Med Care 13:189, 1975
4. Cooper JK, Heald K, Samuels M, Coleman S: Rural or urban practice: Factors influencing the location decision of primary care physicians. Inquiry 12:18, 1975
5. Cooper JK, Heald K, Samuels M: The decision for rural practice. J Med Educ 47:939, 1972
6. Parker RC, Sorensen AA: The tides of rural physicians: The ebb and flow, or why physicians move out of and into small communities. Med Care 16:152, 1978
7. Magraw RM: Ferment in Medicine. Philadelphia, Saunders, 1966, p 172
8. Kane RL, Wilson WM: The new health practitioner—The past as prologue. West J Med 127:254, 1977
9. Light JA, Crain MJ, Fisher DW: Physician assistant: A profile of the profession, 1976. PA Journal 7:109, 1977
10. Morris SB, Smith DB: The distribution of physician extenders. Med Care 15:1054, 1977
11. Greenfield S, Friedland G, Seifers S, et al: Protocol management of dysuria, urinary frequency and vaginal discharge. J Fam Pract 2:179, 1975
12. Blanchard LB, Kurtz B: The social worker in a family practice setting. Primary Care 5:173, 1978
13. Friedman WH, Jelly E, Jelly P: Group therapy in family medicine. J Fam Pract 6:1015, 1978

14. Maudlin RK: The clinical pharmacist and the family physician. J Fam Pract 3:667, 1976

15. Davis RE, Crigler WH, Martin H: Pharmacy and family practice: Concept, roles and fees. Drug Intell Clin Pharm 11:616, 1977

16. Layton RH, Schubert MM: Integrated residency training in family medicine and general practice dentistry. J Fam Pract 7:333, 1978

17. Farley ES, Treat DF: Utilization of community resources. In Conn HF, Rakel RE, Johnson TW (eds): Family Practice. Philadelphia, Saunders, 1973, p 118

18. Werblun MN, Twersky RK: Use of community resources. In Rosen G, Geyman JP, Layton RH (eds): Behavioral Science in Family Practice. New York, Appleton, 1980

19. Rudy DR, Williams T: The consultation process and its effects on therapeutic outcome. J Fam Pract 4:361, 1977

20. Mechanic D: General medical practice: Some comparisons between the work of primary care physicians in the United States and England and Wales. Med Care 10:402, 1972

21. Profile of Medical Practice. Chicago, Center for Health Services Research and Development, AMA, 1974, p 180

22. Preliminary Data from the National Ambulatory Medical Care Survey (unedited draft, July 15, 1975), p 34

23. Advance Data from Vital and Health Statistics of the National Center for Health Statistics. Hyattsville, Maryland, U.S. Department of Health, Education and Welfare, 12:5, October 12, 1977

24. McWhinney IR: Problem solving and decision making in primary medical practice. Albert Wander Lecture. Proc R. Soc Med 65:934, 1972

25. Smith DH, McWhinney IR: Comparison of the diagnostic methods of family physicians and internists. J Med Educ 50:264, 1975

26. Curry HB: Phoenix in flight: All systems go! JAMA 222:821, 1972

27. Owens A: What doctors want most from their practices now. Med Econ 54:88, March 7, 1977

28. Geyman JP: Is there a difference between nursing practice and medical practice? J Fam Pract 5:935, 1977

29. Levinson D: Roles, tasks and practitioners. N Engl J Med 296:1291, 1977

30. Glenn JK, Hofmeister RW: Will physicians rush out and get physician extenders? Health Serv Res 11:69, Spring 1976

31. Schoen EJ, Erickson RJ, Barr G, Allen H: The role of pediatric nurse practitioners as viewed by California pediatricians. West J Med 118:62, 1973

32. Bergeson PS, Winchell D: A survey of Arizona physicians' attitudes regarding pediatric nurse practitioners: Rejection of the concept. Clin Pediatr 16:679, 1977

33. Breslau N: The role of the nurse practitioner in a pediatric team: Patient definitions. Med Care 15:1014, 1977

CHAPTER FOURTEEN

Family Practice as a Career Option

What is the most painful and devastating question that can be asked about modern medical practice? It is not whether most doctors are up to date in their knowledge or in their techniques but whether too many of them know more about disease than about the person in whom the disease exists.—The physician celebrates computerized tomography. The patient celebrates the outstretched hand.[1]

Norman Cousins [1]

With the disappearance of the free-standing internship and the continued emergence of more kinds of career options in medicine during recent years, today's medical students are confronted with difficult career decisions at an early stage in their medical education. Because of the lead time requirements of the National Intern and Resident Matching Program (NIRMP) and the need to arrange interview visits to potential residency programs during the preceding three to six months, medical students now find it necessary to make choices among specialties by the end of their third year or start of their fourth year in medical school. For many, this pressure for early career choice may be premature, since it is not possible to experience all, or even most, of the various medical career options by that time.

Over the years, I have been impressed with the frequency of certain misconceptions, concerns, and questions expressed by medical students with respect to family practice as a career option. The purpose of this chapter is therefore fourfold: (1) to clarify some of the common misconceptions, (2) to discuss some of the personal satisfactions in family practice, (3) to outline some of the requisites for prospective family physicians, and (4) to suggest an approach to selection of graduate training in the field.

SOME MISCONCEPTIONS ABOUT FAMILY PRACTICE

Most misconceptions seem to relate to just a few aspects of family practice. Seven of these will be addressed here:

1. PATIENTS USUALLY PREFER A SUBSPECIALIST WHEN THEY ARE SICK

It is a common observation among physicians practicing in most types of communities that patients evaluate their physicians more by their availability and personality than by any certificates on the walls of their consultation rooms. Patients in the general population usually want care for their illnesses by the most direct route and rate highly a physician who is readily accessible and can provide initial and follow-up care for their everyday health problems.

Patients usually want a doctor for the entire family and often become resentful of the expense and inconvenience involved in episodic care of multiple illnesses in family members by many other specialists. As they get to know their family physicians, they tend to consult them initially for virtually all health problems within the family. In fact, it is not uncommon for patients to resist referral to a consultant or to call their family physician from a medical center in a distant city for his/her opinion of recommendations made by a specialist whom they don't know.

That the public's demand for the services of the family physician remains at a high level is reflected by Table 14–1, which shows the experience of the American Medical Association's Physician's Placement Service in 1976.[2] It can be seen that the greatest number of practice opportunities is in general/family practice.

2. FAMILY PRACTICE IS SO INVOLVED WITH MINOR ILLNESS THAT IT LACKS INTELLECTUAL CHALLENGE

The clinical content of family practice was described in some detail in Chapter 11, which provides ample evidence of the breadth and depth of the family physician's everyday practice. It has been shown that family physicians definitively manage about 97 percent of all of their patient visits, including a wide variety of acute and chronic diseases ranging from minor to terminal

TABLE 14–1.   AMA PHYSICIANS' PLACEMENT SERVICE ANNUAL STATISTICAL REPORT FOR
JANUARY–DECEMBER, 1976

SPECIALTY	PHYSICIANS		OPPORTUNITIES	
	Number	%	Number	%
Allergy	10	0.5	6	0.4
Anesthesiology	75	3.6	25	1.5
Dermatology	16	0.8	14	0.8
General/family practice	184	8.7	566	33.0
Internal medicine	548	26.0	399	23.3
Neurology	38	1.8	16	0.9
Neurosurgery	2	0.1	8	0.5
Obstetrics–gynecology	140	6.6	128	7.5
Ophthalmology	79	3.8	40	2.3
Orthopedic surgery	63	3.0	69	4.0
Otolaryngology	34	1.6	37	2.2
Pathology	86	4.1	9	0.5
Pediatrics	190	9.0	103	6.0
Psychiatry	76	3.6	49	2.9
Radiology	54	2.6	27	1.6
Surgery	305	14.5	100	5.8
Urology	104	4.9	24	1.4
Miscellaneous	101	4.8	93	5.4
Totals	2105	100.0	1713	100.0

Source: *Directory of Accredited Residencies.* Chicago, American Medical Association, 1977, p. 13.

illness. Family physicians frequently encounter medical, surgical, and psychiatric emergencies and are constantly challenged by the problems of early diagnosis, the management of multiple-system disease, and the care of patients with various combinations of organic and functional illness.

Family physicians do not equate severe or rare illness with being more "interesting." Instead, their main satisfaction comes from the understanding of patients and their families as people and their ability to manage the great majority of illnesses acquired by these families.

3. FAMILY PHYSICIANS WILL NOT RECEIVE APPROPRIATE HOSPITAL PRIVILEGES

The large majority of hospitals in this country continue to be "open-staff" hospitals. Hospital privileges on the various services are extended on the basis of demonstrated ability, which is as it should be. The extent of hospital privileges for family physicians does vary somewhat from one geographic area to another and by size of the community and reflects the pattern of practice for the involved locale. Only a few hospitals are "closed-staff," limiting privileges on more arbitrary grounds to certain categories of physicians.

As noted in the last chapter, Mechanic's[3] study of over 800 United States general/family physicians during the early 1970s showed the great majority to be quite satisfied with their hospital privileges (p. 270). Two more recent studies in different parts of the country provide further detail concerning current patterns of hospital privileges for family physicians. In 1977, Hansen, Sundwall, and Kane [4] reported the results of a survey of 176 hospitals in the AMA's Region 8 (Arizona, New Mexico, Nevada, Utah, Colorado, Idaho, Wyoming, and Montana). This study showed that 88 percent of the urban and 98 percent of the rural hospitals stated that it would be very likely that a board-certified family physician would obtain full staff privileges. Only a small proportion of hospitals would categorically deny privileges in such areas as surgical obstetrics, the intensive care unit, and the coronary care unit (Table 14–2). In another study in 1978, Warburton and Sadler [5] surveyed 95 hospitals in New Jersey. Figure 14–1 represents the number of hospitals granting privileges to board-certified family physicians in specific areas.

Inappropriate restriction of hospital privileges should not constitute a major problem for future family physicians, who will be well trained in many aspects of hospital care. To an increasing extent, clinical departments of family practice will play an active role, in liaison with the other specialty departments, in the designation of hospital privileges for family physicians and in the monitoring of quality of care and physician performance.

4. FAMILY PRACTICE IS MORE NEEDED IN RURAL THAN METROPOLITAN AREAS

In metropolitan areas and larger communities, the substantial use of hospitals' emergency rooms bears witness to a deficiency of available primary care. Such care as is received by this method is episodic, fragmentary, impersonal, and expensive. As our urban and suburban population grows and as more people demand health care for all four of the James' stages of disease, there will be an increasing need for family physicians in any community regardless of size. A physician entering family practice today has many opportunities to associate

TABLE 14–2.   EXTENT OF PRIVILEGES GRANTED TO FAMILY PHYSICIANS IN SPECIFIC CLINICAL AREAS

| | EXTENT OF PRIVILEGES (%) | | | | | | |
| | Rural Hospitals | | | Urban Hospitals | | | |
	Full	Some	None	Full	Some	None	P VALUE*
General surgery	32	64	4	7	82	11	< 0.005
Nonsurgical obstetrics	76	24	—	24	71	5	< 0.005
Surgical obstetrics	36	52	12	11	60	29	< 0.005
Intensive care unit	54	45	1	30	61	9	< 0.005
Coronary care unit	54	44	2	27	59	14	< 0.005

* Difference between urban and rural hospitals.

Source: Hansen, D.V., Sundwall, D.N., and Kane, R.L.: Hospital privileges for family physicians. *Journal of Family Practice* 7:1019, 1977.

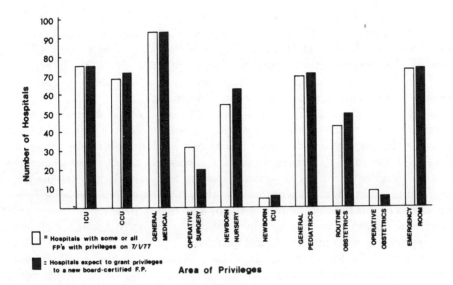

FIGURE 14-1.

Privileges of family physicians in 95 New Jersey hospitals.

Source: Warburton, SW, and Sadler, GR: Family physician hospital privileges in New Jersey. *Journal of Family Practice* 5:114, 1977.

with other family physicians in urban, suburban, and rural communities anywhere in the country. Whether he/she starts practice alone or in association with one or more other physicians, he can expect to be busy within a few months.

As observed in an earlier chapter, two-thirds of United States practicing general/family physicians in 1975 were located in metropolitan areas (p. 79).[6] The latest available data from the American Academy of Family Physicians reveal that about one-half of 1978 graduates of family practice residency programs entered practice in communities with populations of more than 25,000 people.

5. ONE WOULD BE TOO BUSY IN FAMILY PRACTICE

Many physicians are too busy in practice, but this cannot be well correlated with the clinical discipline. Internists, pediatricians, obstetricians, surgeons, and other physicians can all develop uncontrolled practices, which can compromise unduly their own personal and family life.

When physicians get too busy, it is usually due to such factors as inefficient organization of their practices, lack of education of their patients, insufficient coverage by other physicians, or their own masochistic drive to overwork. Many family physicians are able to practice 50 hours a week and share night and weekend calls with other physicians whether they be solo, in an expense-sharing relationship with one or more other physicians, in partnership, or in group practice. A further increase in group and partnership practice can be expected, so that all future family physicians should be able to control their practices.

6. ONE CANNOT POSSIBLY LEARN IT ALL

A common remark expressed by medical students is that family practice is too broad to "learn it all." It is, of course, true that one cannot learn all about each of the component elements of family practice, but this is true to a considerable extent in all clinical disciplines. In the final analysis, one cannot possibly learn all there is to know about any field.

So, in family practice, the goal is not to "learn it all." Rather the goal is to master a specific body of knowledge and acquire a specific range of skills that relate to the prevention, diagnosis, treatment, and rehabilitation of common illnesses of the family. In the course of a three-year family practice residency program, residents cut across territorial lines between all clinical disciplines, developing proficiency as required by their intended location and type of practice. The practice of family medicine becomes a balance of knowing and doing; one maintains competency in many technical skills through their repetitive application to common clinical problems.

As observed by McWhinney,[7] it is quite evident that the family physician caring for 1500 people cannot match the consultant, who selects his/her patients from a population of 50,000 or more, in detailed mastery of one field. But "the deepest and most vital knowledge—the knowledge that determines how information will be used—does not 'explode' or 'have a half-life of five years' as the catchwords have it.—By caring for the whole family, the family physician stands to gain personal knowledge that can be gained in no other way."

Besieged as they are with an overload of information, frequently presented in a context where the relevance to common clinical problems is unclear or lacking, medical students often feel insecure about their capacity to master the knowledge and skills required of a broad specialty. The range, however, of knowledge and skills required by the practicing family physician is not endless, but is finite and allows one to develop and maintain a high level of competence.

7. FAMILY PRACTICE IS MORE SUITED TO MEN THAN WOMEN

There is ample evidence that women physicians traditionally have been unevenly distributed among the various specialties in medicine. In 1971, for example, when women represented 7.1 percent of all active physicians in the United States, they comprised 21.3 percent of the pediatricians, 18.8 percent of the public health physicians, 14.3 percent of the anesthesiologists, and 13.1 percent of the psychiatrists, but only 7.2 percent of the obstetrician–gynecologists, 4.4 percent of the general/family physicians, 1.1 percent of the general surgeons, and 0.5 percent of the orthopedists.[8] There is also evidence of stereotypic thinking among physicians with respect to the believed suitability of medical specialties for women physicians. This has led to attitudes that certain fields are preferable for women in that they (1) involve more limited time commitments (e.g., anesthesiology, dermatology, rehabilitation medicine, and pathology) and (2) call for qualities and aptitudes commonly attributed to women (e.g., pediatrics and psychiatry).[9]

The last decade has seen major changes in the number of women entering medicine and their interest in the various specialties. The proportion of women enrolled in United States medical schools increased from 10.9 percent of the total enrollment in 1972 to 20.5 percent in 1976.[10] The student body of most American medical schools today includes 20 to 30 percent women.

A recent study of male and female medical students in two medical schools showed increased interest by women physicians in nontraditional fields, especially family practice (Table 14–3). Family practice was the only specialty in which men and women selecting the same specialty appeared comparable in personality characteristics.[11] There is no reason to believe that women physicians are categorically less (or more) suited to family practice than to other fields.

By 1976, major shifts had taken place with respect to the relative proportions of women enrolled in various specialty residencies. Table 14–4 shows comparative figures for women residents in training in 1976. Data from the American Academy of Family Physicians in late 1978 showed that 13.9 percent of the 6033 family practice residents then in training were women. That this figure is continuing to increase is reflected by the fact that 16.8 percent of first-year residents enrolled in United States family practice residency programs during the 1978–1979 year were women.

PERSONAL SATISFACTIONS IN FAMILY PRACTICE

Although the practice satisfaction of family physicians is necessarily subject to considerable individual variation, some of the reasons can be sketched

TABLE 14–3. STATISTICALLY SIGNIFICANT DIFFERENCES* BETWEEN MALES' AND FEMALES' FIRST SPECIALTY CHOICES—UNIVERSITY OF COLORADO SCHOOL OF MEDICINE AND UNIVERSITY OF CALIFORNIA, SAN DIEGO, SCHOOL OF MEDICINE, 1974–1975

| | CHOSEN SPECIALTY (IN PERCENTAGES) | | | | | |
SEX	Family Practice†	Internal Medicine	Pediatrics†	Psychology ‡	Surgery†	Total
Male (N = 164)	29	25	14	12	20	100
Female (N = 95)	44	20	25	7	4	100
Total (N = 259)	35	23	18	10	14	100

* χ^2 test.
† $p < 0.01$.
‡ $P < 0.05$.

Source: McGrath, E., and Zimet, C.: Female and male medical students: Differences in specialty choice selection and personality. *Journal of Medical Education* 52:293, 1977.

TABLE 14–4.   WOMEN RESIDENTS BY SPECIALTY—1976*

SPECIALTY	NUMBER	PROPORTION OF WOMEN RESIDENTS (%)
Internal medicine	1298	21.4
Pediatrics	865	16.9
General surgery	528	10.3
Psychiatry	524	10.2
Family practice	432	8.4
Obstetrics–gynecology	272	5.3
Pathology	265	5.1
Anesthesiology	125	2.4
Radiology	118	2.3
Ophthalmology	110	2.1
Other specialties	575	15.6
Total	5112	100.0

* United States and Canadian medical school graduates only.

Source: Adapted from: *Directory of Accredited Residencies.* Chicago, American Medical Association, 1977, Table Q, p. 28.

whereby most family physicians find their practices both interesting and rewarding.

Meeting the Needs

All family physicians can be assured that they are meeting important needs of their patients and families in a direct way. This awareness starts early in the careers of family physicians—when they start looking for locations to start practice. They find a plethora of attractive practice opportunities regardless of the size of community or part of the country. Not only are other physicians seeking their association, but often hospital administrators and other community leaders are searching for new family physicians for their communities.

Medical graduates entering family practice today can do so knowing that they are meeting directly the most pressing challenge in modern health care— the delivery of primary and continuing comprehensive health care to our growing population. In most cases, family physicians find themselves busy in a few short months after starting practice. They do not have to compete with other physicians for patients, and their livelihood is assured by being available for the care of their patients. They can be confident that they will be able to provide more health care to more people during their careers than in any other field of medicine.

A Complete Physician

Family physicians are enabled by good residency training to be soundly competent to function well in all four of James' stages of disease, from prevention and early diagnosis of subclinical disease to treatment and rehabilitation of symptomatic disease. Though they have limitations in all fields of medicine, they will at the same time possess substantial competence across a wide range of the traditional specialties. As observed by Stephens,[12] family physicians "do not have what Harvey Cox called the 'permission to ignore' whatever lies outside their specialty, nor can they participate in what Michael Balint called the 'collusion of anonymity' in which the patient has many doctors but none of them is in charge."

It is deeply satisfying to family physicians to be able to initiate care in virtually any emergency situation. Their capabilities in emergency care usually include such diverse skills as management of cardiac arrest, diagnosis of the surgical abdomen after trauma, tube thoracostomy for a pneumothorax, management of poisoning in a child, or care of a psychiatric emergency in a menopausal patient with depression. Family physicians are trained to evaluate all patients who present to their care, seeking consultation when indicated and after appropriate initial care is rendered. It is likewise rewarding for family physicians to have the opportunity to follow patients and their families where the continuity is measured in years, or even generations.

A Part of People's Lives

Family physicians get close to their patients and their families, and know them better the longer they practice. Many of them become their friends. Family physicians thereby have the privilege of participating in all of the major events of their patients' lives—birth, marriage, serious accidents, and death. They have the opportunity to see them grow and develop as individuals. A preschool examination of a child may recall a breech delivery in the middle of a night six years previously. A woman successfully managed through menopausal symptoms may be followed into years of improved adjustment to her life situation, while her husband's hypertension is found to be more easily controlled with reduced medication. A middle-aged man who was resuscitated in the coronary care unit after a cardiac arrest may be later followed through a program of counseling and exercise and return to work, while anxiety symptoms in his wife are treated concurrently.

A Part of the Community

Family physicians, as other physicians in our society, are usually accorded a high level of respect within their communities. The physician is recognized as a well-educated person and is often expected to be expert in fields outside of medicine. Unfortunately, this is often not the case, and the wise physician is aware of the limitations of his/her expertise. However, by virtue of their broad training, experience, and interests, family physicians have much to contribute to community affairs if they are so inclined.

Natural areas for community involvement include school health, sports medicine, health education, environmental improvement, disaster planning, emergency care services, voluntary health organizations, and health planning. In becoming involved in the community, however, physicians must be as careful to avoid overextension as they are to avoid uncontrolled practices.

A Varied Life

Variety is certainly the spice of the family physician's life. Each day is unpredictable and is a mixture of emergency, acute, chronic, and well-patient care. Each day sees the family physician in the office, in the hospital and its emergency room, and at times in the patient's home. Every day is active and filled with decisions, and family physicians find themselves constantly shifting gears as they adapt to different degrees of urgency and patients with different personalities.

The work of the family physician is concrete, and the results of care are usually apparent. Surprises are not uncommon in family practice. Emergencies have a way of occurring when one is least expecting them. Any given day may include an obstetric delivery, a counseling session for a marital problem, closed reduction of a Colles fracture, management of an acute coronary, and diagnosis of an unsuspected hypertension by a routine physical examination. At the end of a day, family physicians can usually feel that they have made a difference in the lives of their patients.

The Constant Challenge

The scope and variety of family physicians' practices provide continual challenge. They must be able to integrate the unexpected into each busy day, remain cool under stress, and be as therapeutic as possible in dealing with patients and their families. The overall responsibilities of family physicians for the lives and optimal health of all their patients are great. Beyond the wide range of services that they can competently provide, they are responsible for referring their patients to consultants or other community health resources so that any additional problems can be managed appropriately. They must learn the art of timely referral, which maximizes the results of care by the consultant.

Another challenge to family physicians is the need to remain objective. They must develop the art of sorting out the significant from the inconsequential in the large volume of clinical information that confronts them each day. They must become skilled at looking beyond the patient's complaints to detect possible underlying reasons for the patient's visit. At the same time, they must be sufficiently thorough and comprehensive in the approach to each patient so that serious organic disease is not overlooked.

The process of relating meaningfully to a wide variety of patient types and ages is another area that takes years to refine and where improvement is always

possible. The incessant talker with menopausal symptoms may be in one examination room, while in the next is a 16-year-old girl who seems reluctant to give
any kind of history or clue as to what prompted her visit to the office.

REQUISITES FOR THE FAMILY PHYSICIAN

Family practice requires of its practitioners a special combination of abilities
and interests. Other fields, such as radiology, pathology, general surgery, and
psychiatry, have their own special requisites for their practitioners, which in
many ways are different from family practice. An understanding of the particular requisites of any specialty is essential if the medical graduate is to find
satisfaction and be effective in his/her chosen field. A brief review of some of
the requisites important to the family physician is therefore of interest here.

Interest in People

Of top priority for family physicians is a real interest in, and even curiosity
about, people. They should like people and seek close contact with patients. They
should be able to deal with a wide spectrum of personality types. They should
be sufficiently warm with people as to seem approachable with any problem and be nonjudgmental of patients with differing beliefs, behavior, or habits.
They should be able to accept people for what they are, be appreciative of their
potential, and tolerant of their faults.

Good Judgment

Family physicians must be well endowed with common sense and good clinical judgment. They will be confronted daily with a large number of patients
with a larger number of problems. They must be able to sort out effective ave-
nues of management in a level-headed way. They must be adept at recognizing
the relative urgency of situations facing them at a given moment, and be comfortable with dealing with several problems at once, each in a different stage of
resolution. Their good judgment should extend to their communicative skills
with patients, who are often prone to misinterpret a casual remark, making later
management more difficult.

Broad Interests

Family physicians should have more broad interests in clinical medicine than
other specialists. A keen interest in the science of medicine is vital to the quality
of their care of patients and their active participation in continuing medical
education.

Family physicians should enjoy becoming competent in portions of many clinical disciplines and synthesizing information for application to the common illnesses of all members of the family. In order to gain the necessary levels of competence in numerous fields, family physicians need to have high intelligence. They should be as interested in the science of medicine as in people and should be interested in patients in their family context and in families in their community and social context.

Decisiveness

This is an important attribute for family physicians. They see a large number of patients each day (usual average 30 to 40), and many problems encountered require immediate decisions regarding therapy or disposition of the patient. All require some tangible decision as to extent and type of workup and follow-up. This is particularly challenging, since many of the patients seen are unselected and "unlabeled."

A tendency to indecisiveness is incompatible with the role of the family physician. To be effective, family physicians must be able to make frequent decisions throughout a day, based on available information that is often incomplete. As Spooner [13] observes, family physicians need to be comfortable with the uncertainty caused by inadequate data to immediately solve a clinical problem, which is the rule in situations where it is too early in the course of the disease to make a diagnosis.

Assume Responsibility

A hallmark of family practice is the capacity of family physicians to accept total responsibility for patients and their families. Family physicians must feel comfortable with and enjoy this degree of responsibility for the many families in their practice.

The responsibility of family physicians to their patients does not end with referrals they may arrange with consulting specialists. Family physicians usually remain involved in the ongoing care of associated medical problems. In addition, family physicians are responsible for the quality of all requested consultations and for ensuring that further follow-up is continued as needed when the consultants' tasks are completed.

Family physicians must also be ready to accept responsibility for care of both the terminal patient and the chronically ill patient where scientific cure is not possible. Such patients may be difficult to manage, but the family physician is often in the best position to deal with the patient's complaints, if only on a symptomatic and supportive basis. The important thing is that any patient with a debilitating or terminal illness must not be abandoned, and the family physician is best equipped to manage such patients in their family setting.

Of equal importance to the ability to accept responsibility is the ability to share it. Family physicians must disengage themselves from their practices at regular intervals and should have a call system for coverage of their patients by other family physicians during these periods. There are still too many physicians who find it difficult to share responsibility for their patients' care with other physicians. Solo practice without adequate coverage no longer lends itself to good medical care.

Stability

Family physicians are confronted each day with many pressures and with a greater variety of situations than other practitioners. Their busy days are interspersed with difficult decisions and difficult patients. In their close relationship with patients, they will often act as a target for their hostilities. More commonly, they must serve as an "anxiety sponge" for the many patients with acute and chronic anxiety reactions in their practices.

Emotional stability is therefore an essential asset for family physicians. They must continually strive to maintain equanimity, for in this way they will be most effective in treating their patients.

Sensitivity–Objectivity Mix

Family physicians should have another capability with which not everyone is endowed—the ability to be keenly perceptive and receptive to their patients while, at the same time, maintaining sufficient objectivity to manage the problem at hand. Too much empathy without objectivity makes for ineffective and even hazardous patient care. Too little empathy, on the other hand, in the physician–patient relationship carries the risk of overlooking and neglecting underlying functional illness, which often may be the entire basis for the patient's somatic complaints.

The problem of attaining an appropriate balance between sensitivity and objectivity is most marked when the physician is caring for a personal friend. It can become especially difficult for this physician to carry out an emergency procedure, an operative procedure, or family counseling under such circumstances. To a lesser extent, of course, most or all of family physicians' patients may be their friends, so that this is a situation with which they must frequently deal.

Thinker–Doer

Family practice involves an interesting blend of thinking and doing. Family physicians are usually as involved with treatment, often involving manual skills, as with differential diagnosis, history taking, patient education, and counseling.

In their intellectual approach to the science of medicine, they should be as interested in common clinical problems and their variants as in rare and esoteric disease. To the family physician, people themselves are "interesting," as is the care of their everyday illnesses.

Flexibility

Flexibility is another important attribute for family physicians. The need for this quality exists on several levels. Family physicians must remain as open to a new diagnosis as they are to their patients' feelings. This is a particular problem in the primary care role, for they often see an illness at a stage too early for a definitive diagnosis. At a second or third office visit for a new problem, the family physician must be able to reappraise the patient in the light of new history and clinical findings and must not become too committed to an earlier presumptive diagnosis.

There is an additional problem in the long-term patient with one or more chronic illnesses who has become well known to the family physician for many years. Here again, it is quite easy to overlook new problems unless one remains open to new findings.

A distinct facet to each day in family practice is the need to constantly adjust to diverse personalities and family situations. There is also the need to be quickly adaptable to different severities of illness and different clinical disciplines; thus, at any given time in the family physician's office, in three examination rooms, there may be a prenatal patient, a patient terminally ill with carcinoma, and a middle-aged man with a two-hour history of chest pain.

Family physicians must also be able to tailor their treatment to the individual patient, which calls for both flexibility and imagination. From their assessment of the patient's level of intelligence and cooperation, as well as the home setting, they must try to devise a prescription for care that can realistically be followed by the patient. It is well known that many drug prescriptions are either never filled or incompletely taken. Prescriptions for changes in exercise, dietary, or behavior patterns are also not followed unless they are both realistic and understandable to the patient.

Ease with Interpersonal Relationships

Family physicians must be adept at getting along well with their colleagues, office and hospital staffs, and other members of the health team. Many family physicians have come to the view that communicative skills are the key foundation for effective family practice. The role of leadership of the health team itself is becoming an increasingly important task as the care of any patient involves the combined efforts of more allied health workers. New working relationships between the family physician, the nurse, and other paramedical assistants are evolving, and the ability to communicate easily is essential to good patient care.

Comprehensive Approach

Family physicians must be able to "gather up" their patient's history, physical examination, and laboratory findings in a comprehensive way. This skill requires broad training, experience, and practice. Family physicians can often refine an intuitive sense of what is important and what is not. They must be on guard to be sufficiently circumspect to avoid overlooking the subtle diagnosis and the therapeutic procedure that can be performed better by a consultant. They must also think in terms of what aspects of diagnosis, treatment, and rehabilitation should be done by other consultants or community resources.

Other Personal Traits of the Family Physician

In order to be an effective family physician and to practice a high quality of medicine, other traits are desirable: stamina; an ability to pace oneself; and a basic attitude of optimism, tact, and self-confidence. In addition, family physicians must enjoy learning new clinical knowledge and developing new skills. They should approach their residency years with enthusiasm and carry this over later into continuing medical education.

Many of the qualities of the idealized family physician have been outlined toward which most practicing family physicians strive. That this is a big order is acknowledged, but there are many fine physicians in family practice who show that it is possible, and many medical students now in training appear to be well motivated and capable in these directions.

SELECTION OF RESIDENCY TRAINING

Overall Options

Since a substantial part of family practice involves general internal medicine, some medical students wonder whether they should enter a residency in this field. Others wonder whether a primary care residency involving internal medicine and pediatrics might provide a good background. Still others consider the possibility of one year in several specialty fields or a flexible first graduate year followed by continuing medical education in a group practice.

There are significant limitations to all of these approaches. A residency in internal medicine fails to provide exposure and training in many areas integral to family practice, including pediatrics, obstetrics–gynecology, otolaryngology, orthopedics, minor surgery, the behavioral sciences, and family dynamics. The few primary care residencies that have been started concentrate mainly on internal medicine and pediatrics (usually with predominant emphasis on one or the other), still leaving major areas uncovered. It is generally not feasible to take one year of several specialty residencies, and this, too, still leaves out important areas. A flexible first graduate year, equivalent to the old rotating internship, followed by what may be promoted as excellent training in a future group practice, likewise leaves large gap areas. Although the young physician can doubtless learn new knowledge and skills in practice from helpful colleagues, he soon becomes engaged in a practice based largely on existing competencies. It is difficult to pursue a systematic continuing education in a busy practice that can substitute for major deficiencies of graduate training.

Family practice residencies have been designed to provide the knowledge, skills, and attitudes needed to practice good family medicine. Such an approach is now the only way to become board-eligible in family practice. A shorter period of graduate training or more narrow training through an alternative pathway is not likely to prepare one adequately for the demands of modern family practice.

Personal Considerations

One cannot choose among the over 350 United States family practice residency programs without first reflecting upon one's personal goals, interests, and learning style. The general types, structures, and content of family practice residencies have already been outlined in Chapter 9. The available programs represent a wide spectrum from the university-based program in a large academic medical center to a 150-bed community hospital with a family practice residency as the only graduate training program. The patient care and learning environments in these various programs are quite different. The university-based program typically relates closely to highly structured teaching services in the other major specialties, and much of the family practice resident's learning may be derived from other house staff. The family practice residency in a smaller community may involve little or no contact with residents in other specialties, less structured teaching services, and more learning from attending physicians in the community. Family practice residents may acquire the same range of clinical competencies over a three-year program in either setting, but they may be more comfortable in one or the other environment.

Some family practice residencies are designed to prepare their graduates for certain types of future practice settings. A family practice residency located in the inner city, for example, may provide the resident with the experience and background required for urban practice better than a program located in a smaller community. Although a number of family practice residencies in urban areas can adequately prepare graduates for rural practice, a program in a smaller community may provide a more typical patient population and learning environment for residents planning to practice in smaller communities.

In addition to considering their future practice goals, prospective residents need to consider their geographic preferences and related environmental needs. Resident applicants may want to stay in the same community or region where they completed medical school or move to another part of the country for residency training. The desires of one's spouse may be an important factor with respect to occupational or educational needs.

Evaluating Specific Family Practice Residencies

After prospective residents have considered their own personal interests and needs, the next step is to review the current list of approved family practice residencies (Appendix 3).*

This list can be narrowed down to a small number of possible programs by deciding for or against a university- or community hospital-based program and by geographic region. One's list can be further narrowed by talking with a faculty advisor in the department of family practice.

The next *essential* step is planning for interview visits, usually during the summer and fall of senior year. There is no substitute for actually seeing programs. One has an opportunity to talk with faculty and residents, to see the facilities, to learn the philosophy and ethos of the program, and to see if the community is where one would like to live for three years. Such interview visits allow the applicant to ask specific questions about each teaching program and to crystallize feelings about the kind of program that best will meet one's needs. Taking an elective family practice clerkship during the early part of the senior year is another valuable approach to explore a possible program.

Although competition for first-year family practice residency positions has been keen, most applicants have obtained positions. In 1978, there were at least 2665 first-year applicants for family practice, with 2318 obtaining positions (including 1711 matched through the NIRMP). Applicants not using the NIRMP include couples applying together, applicants for military programs, new programs receiving approval too late for participation in the NIRMP, and some programs electing to accept residents outside NIRMP.

Applicants can feel reasonably confident about obtaining a place, particularly if they take the following steps [14]:

1. Plan the senior year carefully to allow interview visits to programs during the summer and fall (many programs terminate interview visits as early as December 1).
2. Consider a family practice clerkship in a hospital in which one has particular interest.
3. Apply to at least ten programs. It also may be prudent to "cover the bases" by applying to some flexible first-graduate-year positions, but one should realize that opportunities for second-year positions in family practice residencies are limited to a small number of developing programs and whatever attrition may occur within existing programs.
4. Apply well in advance of deadlines.

---

* This list is revised every four to six months. An updated list can be obtained by writing to the Division of Education, American Academy of Family Physicians, 1740 West 92 Street, Kansas City, Missouri, 64114.

TEACHING AND RESEARCH

This chapter would not be complete without brief consideration of teaching and research as an important career option in family practice, either on a part-time or full-time basis. As family practice now enters its second decade of development as a clinical specialty and academic discipline, there are well over 400 family physicians involved in full-time teaching in United States medical schools plus a large number of full-time family physicians associated with family practice residency programs in community hospitals. In addition, there are many thousands of family physicians involved on a part-time and voluntary basis in teaching, particularly as attending physicians in family practice residencies or as preceptors for medical students in their practices.

The medical graduate entering family practice today has a wide variety of potential career options within the field. The family physician involved in full-time practice may become involved with part-time teaching in association with a nearby residency program or medical school. He/she may also participate in clinical research, either on an individual or collaborative basis, as will be discussed further in the next chapter. Family physicians engaged in full-time teaching in community hospital-based family practice residencies have an opportunity to combine part-time practice with active teaching and may also become involved with clinical investigative efforts. University-based family physicians may be involved in a diverse mix of activities, including patient care, teaching, research, administration, and university service.

About 5 percent of recent graduates of family practice residency programs are directly entering full-time teaching. There is some debate as to the optimal way to prepare for a career in academic family medicine. Some hold that a preliminary period of three to five years in active practice in the community is an essential prerequisite to full-time teaching/research. Others feel that adequate clinical experience can be obtained within a teaching program as other skills are developed in teaching and/or research. A recent addition to career development options is the small but growing number of fellowship programs in family medicine. There are five currently operational two-year fellowship programs (at Case Western Reserve University, the University of Iowa, the University of Missouri, the University of Utah, and the University of Washington) that offer formal background and experience in teaching and investigative skills.

COMMENT

The choice of a specialty in medicine is probably more difficult for a medical student today than ever before, both because of the large number of options available and the pressure toward early, even premature, decisions about residency training. Each specialty has its own particular challenges, content, and practice style, and each medical student is confronted by the need to match his/her interests, skills, and goals to a compatible, satisfying field.

Pellegrino [15] has discussed the influence of two ideal types on the influence of internal medicine—the German physician–scientist and the Oslerian scholar–consultant. Today, family practice offers medical graduates another kind of model perhaps best described by McWhinney's [7] view of future family physicians:

> They should have a deep commitment to people and obtain their greatest professional fulfillment from their relations with people—to believe, in Lewis Mumford's phrase, in the primacy of the person, to use technology with skill, but to make it always subservient to the interests of the person. . . . [Family practice–educators] want physicians who can think analytically when analysis is required but whose usual mode of thought is multidimensional and holistic. They want them to be concerned with etiology in its broadest sense and to be ever mindful of the need to teach patients how to attain and maintain health. They want people who are not afraid of recognizing and talking about feelings: people who know themselves and can throughout their career recognize their defects, learn from experience and continue to grow as people and as physicians.

REFERENCES

1. Cousins N, Editorial: The doctor as artist and philosopher. Saturday Rev p 56, July 22, 1978
2. Directory of Accredited Residencies. Chicago, AMA, 1977, p 13
3. Mechanic D: The organization of medical practice and practice orientations among physicians in prepaid and nonprepaid primary care settings. Med Care 13:199, 1975
4. Hansen DV, Sundwall DN, Kane RL: Hospital privileges for family physicians. J Fam Pract 5:805, 1977
5. Warburton SW, Sadler GR: Family physician hospital privileges in New Jersey: J Fam Pract 7:1019, 1978
6. National Ambulatory Medical Care Survey of Visits to General and Family Practitioners, January–December 1975. Advance Data from Vital and Health Statistics of the National Center for Health Statistics. Washington, D.C., U.S. Department of Health, Education, and Welfare, 15:1, 1977
7. McWhinney IR: Family medicine in perspective. N Engl J Med 293:176, 1975
8. Pennell MY, Renshaw JE: Distribution of women physicians, 1971. J Am Med Wom Assoc 28:181, 1973
9. Ducker DG: Believed suitability of medical specialties for women physicians. J Am Med Wom Assoc 33:25, 1978
10. Women enrollment and its minority component in U.S. medical schools. J Med Educ 51:692, 1976
11. McGrath E, Zimet C: Female and male medical students: Differences in specialty choice selection and personality. J Med Educ 52:293, 1977

12. Stephens GG: Reform in the United States: Its impact on medicine and education for family practice. J Fam Pract 3:510, 1976
13. Spooner MA: Dealing with uncertainty in family medicine. J Fam Pract 2:471, 1975
14. Geyman JP: Evaluating family practice residencies. New Physician 25:35, 1976
15. Pellegrino ED: The Identity Crisis of an Ideal. Controversy in Internal Medicine. Vol II. Edited by Ingelfinger FJ, Ebert VE, Finland M, et al. Philadelphia, Saunders, 1974, p 41

CHAPTER FIFTEEN

Department of Family Medicine (R700)
University of Miami School of Medicine
P. O. Box 016700
Miami, Florida 33101

James M. Gall, M. D., C.C.F.P.
Department of Family Medicine
University of Miami School of Medicine
P. O. Box 016700
Miami, Florida 33101

Research in Family Practice

The primary care physician has more in common with the naturalist than with the physicist or engineer. In research, the naturalist observes and describes, the naturalist identifies patterns and associations and distributions; less frequently does the naturalist undertake definitive experiments. Although both have their place, medicine urgently needs the wonder, curiosity, and observational powers of the naturalist, as much as, perhaps now more than ever, the mathematical certainty of the physicist or engineer whose methods and concepts have done much to advance the technological side of medicine.

Kerr White [1]

Family practice arose on a different basis from most other clinical specialties in medicine. Most fields have developed to encompass new areas of knowledge and/or technology. A majority of the other specialties developed during the period between 1920 and 1950 when the trend toward biomedical research and specialization was particularly active. Family practice, on the other hand, developed in direct response to a broadly perceived lack of adequate primary care, before an active research base was established.[2]

Family practice originated from the background of general practice, which lacked both commitment and methods for organized research in the field. The teaching and clinical application of general practice was traditionally derivative in nature—its content was derived from portions of all of the other clinical specialties. The emphasis in general practice has been to distill from the other specialties practical approaches to the diagnosis and treatment of common clinical problems that can be applied in a busy practice. Research has been perceived in a negative light by many general practitioners as lacking relevance to their daily work. Such an attitude has often been reinforced by exposure, during their own medical education, to research activities in other disciplines involving "esoteric" conditions and complex pathophysiologic mechanisms not directly applicable to the everyday practice of the general/family physician.

Today's circumstances are quite different. As family practice enters its second decade as a specialty, it is an integral part of the formal system of medical education in the United States. Research is becoming recognized as an essential element in the development of the specialty, and the necessary tools for research are being implanted in many teaching and clinical settings throughout the country.

The developing research efforts in family practice raise a number of basic issues with respect to the process of building an ongoing research effort in a broad clinical specialty. There are questions about the content and focus of research in family practice, and how these relate to teaching and patient care. There are questions about applicable methods for carrying out research in the field, and how teaching programs and practicing family physicians can become involved in research. Additional questions relate to how collaborative and consultative linkages can be established within family practice and with related fields, such as epidemiology and biostatistics. This chapter will present an overview of how these kinds of issues are being addressed through the research efforts that are taking place today in family practice.

BACKGROUND

Medical research has traditionally focused heavily on the study of patients admitted to university medical centers and large teaching hospitals. These patients represent only a minute fraction of the population at risk for disease. Although the large majority of all doctor–patient contacts takes place in the arena of primary and continuing medical care, this area has received little concerted study.[3] It is therefore clear that research in family practice must develop its own traditions and methods in an essentially uncharted area.

The word *research* is still a somewhat misunderstood and charged term to many in family practice. Part of this confusion is due to the yet incomplete definition of the form, content, and methods of research being developed in family practice settings. Traditional biomedical definitions of research in other disciplines cannot be transplanted into family practice, for they were designed for different purposes and conditions. Wood and his colleagues[4] state the situation in this way:

[The term research] still produces an image of a white-coated, bench-bound physician that induces many negative connotations for the problem-solving, decision-making clinician reveling in the cut and thrust of community practice. The former is only one type of research; observing, recording, and analyzing personal or practice experience over a continuum must be considered another type. It qualifies by extending the horizons of knowledge for the individual observer, and doubly so if the data are presented in such a way as to allow comparisons with like situations. The hallmark of research is the representation and applicability of the results to other environments, expanding the body of knowledge available.

Webster defines *research* in a fundamental way: "the diligent and systematic inquiry or investigation into a subject in order to discover or revise facts, theories, and applications." Byrne[5] views *research* as "organized curiosity." Whatever definition for the word one accepts, it is clear that research in family practice must be defined broadly.

Family physicians have a wider perspective and experience with health and disease on the community level than any other field in medicine. Because they deal with the everyday problems of patients and families, family physicians have a number of inherent advantages related to research on a patient-care level, including:

1. Family physicians see all members of the family, of all ages and both sexes.
2. They have direct experience with primary or first contact care of unselected patients.
3. They have the opportunity to follow most of their patients.
4. They bring a multidisciplinary approach to health care.
5. They see patients in any or all of the James' stages[6]:

Stage   I. Foundations of disease
Stage II. Preclinical disease
Stage III. Treatment of symptomatic disease
Stage IV. Rehabilitation and management of medical conditions for which biologic cure is not possible.

McWhinney sees the clinical observation and study of patients in their natural habitat as the center of family practice research. In his words[7]:

Family medicine is, of course, one branch of clinical medicine. Like clinical medicine it has both scientific and technological components. Its scientific subject matter is the phenomena of illness as they present to family physicians; its technological aspect is the development and evaluation of the conceptual, organizational, and material tools used by family physicians. The justification for its independent existence is that the tools are unique to the discipline, not derived from other branches of medicine, and that the phenomena can only be satisfactorily studied from within, rather than outside, the discipline.

SOME BASIC APPROACHES AND METHODS FOR RESEARCH

A Favorable Climate

Perhaps the most important change that has taken place during the last decade in family practice with respect to research is the improving climate within the field concerning investigative work. In nonmeteorological terms, the word *climate* is defined as a particular set of "prevailing attitudes, standards, or environmental conditions of a group, period, or place."[8] There is growing evidence that the necessary attitudes, standards and environmental conditions within family practice are becoming more facilitative of research activity.

There is an increasing number of family physicians who exemplify the attitudes necessary for investigative work. These include the following kinds of attributes[9]:

1. Curiosity
2. Skepticism
3. Intellectual honesty
4. Awareness of limited knowledge
5. Appreciation of the family physician's role in research
6. Valuing of own observations over time
7. Acceptance of responsibility to help advance the field

The standards of "good practice" in general practice in the past have been largely derived from other clinical specialties in the absence of organized study within the primary care environment. As more is learned from research in family practice settings, and as family physicians increasingly take responsibility for peer review and establishing their own criteria for "good practice," research in family practice will be more directly linked to analysis and improvement of clinical practice.

The environmental conditions in a growing number of family practice settings in the United States further facilitate research activities. These particularly include such basic research tools as the use of the problem-oriented medical record, coding and data retrieval methods, and audit.

Some Basic Research Tools

ACCEPTED CLASSIFICATION SYSTEM

Until recently, available classification systems for coding of health problems were based primarily on the diseases of hospitalized patients and were not useful in primary care settings. The last 20 years have seen the development of various classification systems more directly suited to the needs of general/family practice in a number of countries around the world. The International Classification of Health Problems in Primary Care (ICHPPC) has received the most widespread acceptance today and is endorsed by the World Organization of National Colleges and Academies of General Practice/Family Medicine (WONCA).[10] The ICHPPC contains 371 diagnostic titles under 18 categories and permits comparative studies among general/family practice settings around the world. A conversion code has been developed that affords ready conversion from the Royal College of General Practitioners Classification of Diseases (RCGP) to the ICHPPC[11] (Appendix 6).

GLOSSARY OF TERMS

Another basic need for family practice research is the common acceptance of precise and unambiguous terms for use on encounter forms and related medical records. An ad hoc committee of the North American Primary Care Research Group (NAPCRG) has addressed this need and formulated a glossary for primary care that has been generally adopted in this country[12] (Appendix 9).

PROBLEM-ORIENTED MEDICAL RECORD

The problem-oriented medical record, originally developed by Weed, has four basic elements[13,14]:

Defined Data Base. This includes any or all of the following: chief complaint, patient profile and related social data, present illness, past history and systems review, physical examination, and reports of laboratory work and special studies. The extent of the data base that is feasible for a given patient in a given practice depends on the limits of time and cost effectiveness.

Complete Problem List. The problem list (Figure 15–1) displays in the front of the patient's chart a complete list of past and present problems, including dates of resolution of inactive problems. A *problem* is defined by Weed[15] as "anything that requires management or diagnostic workup; this includes social and demographic problems."

Initial Plans. Initial plans are listed for each problem, including further diagnostic studies, therapy and patient education.

Progress Notes. Progress notes are written in a "SOAP" format:

- *Subjective:* presenting, changing, and resolving symptoms
- *Objective:* physical, laboratory, and x-ray findings
- *Assessment:* refinement of diagnosis and assessment of progress
- *Plans:* additional plans for diagnosis and management.

In complicated cases, flow sheets may be used that incorporate frequently monitored observations.

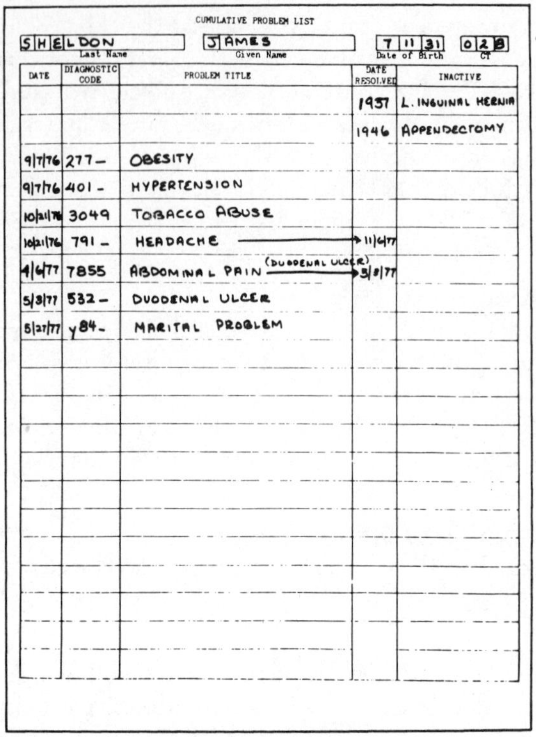
CUMULATIVE PROBLEM LIST

SHELDON (Last Name) JAMES (Given Name) 7 11 31 (Date of Birth) 02B (CT)

DATE	DIAGNOSTIC CODE	PROBLEM TITLE	DATE RESOLVED	INACTIVE
			1957	L. INGUINAL HERNIA
			1946	APPENDECTOMY
9/7/76	277-	OBESITY		
9/7/76	401-	HYPERTENSION		
10/21/76	3049	TOBACCO ABUSE		
10/21/76	791-	HEADACHE →	11/6/77	
4/6/77	7855	ABDOMINAL PAIN (DUODENAL ULCER) →	5/8/77	
5/3/77	532-	DUODENAL ULCER		
5/27/77	Y84-	MARITAL PROBLEM		

FIGURE 15-1.

A sample problem list.

Source: Froom, J: An integrated medical record and data system for primary care. Part 6: A decade of problem-oriented medical records. A reassessment. *Journal of Family Practice,* 5:629, 1977.

AGE–SEX REGISTER

An age–sex register in family practice is an important part of a data system that facilitates clinical research as well as improved office management, outreach, and audit.[16] A sample age–sex index card is shown in Figure 15–2. The use of such cards permits profiling of the practice population by age and sex, an essential part of many comparative clinical studies.

DIAGNOSTIC INDEX

The diagnostic index is a compilation of patients by diagnosis and is synonymous with morbidity index, disease index, and problem index. Various types of diagnostic indexes have been developed for use in primary care. The E-book, perhaps the most widely used method, was first developed by Eimerl in England and introduced into the United States by Wood and Metcalfe.[17] Figure 15–3 shows such an E-book, which is especially useful for audit, outreach, and research purposes.

AGE/SEX INDEX			I.D. #	1 2 3 4 5 - 0 1			
Dr. Code	Surname of Patient		Forename	Date of Birth	S	MS.	Race (circle)
0 1 0	J O R D O N		S A M U E L	05 17 22	M	M	C N. S. O.

DATE OF ENTRY 08 - 16 - 71

Address – Street & City		Zip	C.T.
17 ADELAIDE ST. ROCHESTER		14631	41
315 CONCOURSE ST. ROCHESTER		14620	17

DATE OF REMOVAL _____   CAUSE OF REMOVAL _____

(C) Caucasian   (N) Negro   (S) Spanish, Puerto Rican, Mexican, etc. (O) Other

FIGURE 15-2.

A sample age-sex index card.

Source: Froom, J: An integrated medical record and data system for primary care. Part 1: The age-sex register: Definition of the patient population. *Journal of Family Practice*, 4:953, 1977.

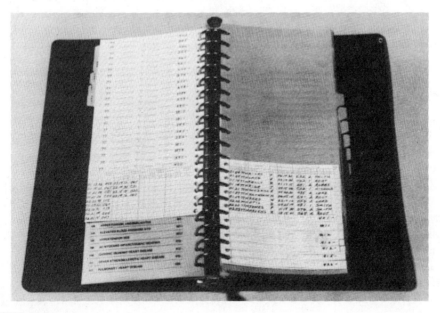

FIGURE 15-3.

The E-book as a diagnostic index.

Source: Froom, J, Culpepper, L, and Boisseau, V: An integrated medical record and data system for primary care. Part 3: The diagnostic index: Manual and computer methods and applications. *Journal of Family Practice* 5:114, 1977.

Department of Family Medicine (R700)
University of Miami School of Medicine
P. O. Box 016700
Miami, Florida 33101

ENCOUNTER FORM

The encounter form provides essential information for each doctor–patient encounter for both practice management and research purposes. Specific kinds of encounter data that are generally required include: (1) facility identification; (2) provider information; (3) person identification; (4) source(s) of payment; (5) date; (6) patient's reason for visit, symptom, or complaint; (7) physician evaluation (diagnosis or problem); (8) diagnostic, therapeutic, or management procedures; and (9) disposition of patient.[18] Figures 15–4 and 15–5 display the encounter form developed and used by the University of Rochester Family Medicine Program. A universal encounter form would be highly desirable for administrative, insurance, and research purposes, and there are some efforts in this direction, but common agreement on a minimal basic data set and a logistic design are first required on the part of all concerned parties.[18]

INDEX OF HEALTH STATUS

Another important need for research in family practice is for methods that can profile a patient's changing health status over time. Such information is vital to the evaluation of different modes of therapy on the duration and severity of clinical problems, identification of high-risk patients, and related research purposes. An example of the definitions of health status for various groups of people is shown in Figure 15–6. These definitions are incorporated into a Health Status Index developed at Michigan State University.[19]

LIBRARY SERVICES

Several recent directions in medical library activities have made literature resources readily accessible to practicing physicians throughout the country. In most states, for example, university medical center libraries have developed excellent interlibrary loan services with libraries in outlying community hospitals.

The National Library of Medicine initiated a new type of monthly bibliography in 1970, the *Abridged Index Medicus*,* which is especially designed for use by individual physicians and libraries of small hospitals and clinics. This publication is based on articles from 100 English-language journals and allows quick review of the literature on clinical subjects.

The National Library of Medicine has also developed a computer-based system for rapid bibliographic access called MEDLINE (MEDICAL LITERATURE ANALYSIS and RETRIEVAL SYSTEM ON-LINE). This system draws on a data base containing references to approximately half a million citations from 3000 biomedical journals. MEDLINE is especially designed to locate specific information rapidly. MEDLINE literature searches are available in about 800 institutions and agencies

---

* The *Abridged Index Medicus* is available on a subscription basis from the United States Government Printing Office, Washington, D.C., 20402; subscription cost in 1978 was $31.35 per year.

(I)

Family Medicine Group
885 South Ave.
Rochester, N.Y. 14620

No. 32193

DATE 7/21/77

NAME Susan Price

FAMILY # 01338-02

DOCTOR Gardner | CODE 313

ADDRESS 436 Pinetree La.

TOWN Rochester

ROOM # 7 | ALSO TO SEE

ZIP 14623 | C.T. 64 | D.O.B. 6-5-21

HEAD OF HOUSEHOLD James Price

APPT. TIME 10:30 | ARRIVAL | DEPART

INSURANCE CO. GVMC | NO. 572436

- [ ] NO SHOW
- [ ] CONFIRMED
- [ ] BILL TO PT
- [ ] BILL TO INS.
- [ ] WORKMENS COMP.
- [ ] CANCELLED
- [ ] WALK IN
- [ ] LEFT
- [ ] RESCHEDULED

MOTOR VEHICLE ACCIDENT YES [ ] NO [X]

(II) I'm tired and my back hurts

- [ ] DOCTOR INITIATED VISIT
- [X] PATIENT INITIATED VISIT
- [ ] 3RD PARTY INITIATED VISIT

REASON FOR VISIT (IN PATIENT'S OWN WORDS)

(III)

SERVICES (100)		CHARGES	LAB (200)		CHARGES	PROCEDURES (300)		CHARGES
101	NEW PT. OR COMPLEX		201 [X] CBC	202 [ ] HCT		301	AUDIOMETRY 302 [ ] VISION	
102 [X]	ROUTINE		203 [ ] WBC	204 [ ] DIFF		303	DPT 304 [ ] OPV	
103	AFTER HRS. 104 [ ] HOME		204 [X] SED. RATE			305	DT 306 [ ] TINE	
105	P.E. INITIAL 106 [ ] ANNUAL		205 [X] U/A 206 [ ] URICULT			307	EAR IRRIGATION	
107	P.E. COLLEGE		207 [ ] CULTURE (SPECIFY)			308	EKG 309 [ ] IUD	
108	P.E. 6-16 YRS.		208 [ ] GRAM STRAIN			310	PROCTO 311 [ ] SIGMOID	
109	P.E. NEWBORN - 5 YRS.		209 [ ] WET MOUNT/KOH PREP			312	TONOMETRY 313 [ ] VITALOR	
110	COUNSELLING PER 1/2 HR.		210 [ ] GUAIAC			314	OTHER (SPECIFY):	
111	OB INITIAL 112 [ ] RECHECK		211 [ ] MONOSPOT 212 [ ] PREG. TEST					
113	WELL CHILD PKG 2 4 6 8 12 18 MOS.		213 [ ] OTHER (SPECIFY):					
114	N.P. NEW PT. OR COMPLEX							
115	N.P. ROUTINE						EQUIPMENT (400)	
116	NURSE VISIT		214 [ ] OUTSIDE LABS (SPECIFY)			401	RENTAL BP CUFF	
117	SURGERY					402	SALE BP CUFF	
118	OTHER (SPECIFY):					403	RENTAL CRUTCHES	
						404	OTHER (SPECIFY):	
							X-RAYS (500)	
						501	CHEST	
	LABS					502 [X]	OTHER (SPECIFY): Spine	
	PROCEDURES							
	TOTAL CHARGE							

- [ ] POSTED BILLED TO INS.

PAYMENT DUE UPON RECEIPT OF BILL

CASH (AMT.) | CHECK (AMT.)

(IV) DISPOSITION	**(V)** WRITTEN DIAGNOSIS FOR INSURANCE	**(VI)** ADDITIONAL INSTRUCTIONS
NEXT APPOINTMENT 10 days	Lumbo-sacral strain, Depression, obesity	1500 calorie/day reduction diet
WITH (F.M. PROVIDER) Gardner		
AMT. OF TIME NEEDED (CIRCLE) 15 (30) 45 60 MIN.		
CONSULTANT/HOSPITAL	SIGNATURE	

BILLING

FIGURE 15-4.

Rochester Family Medicine Program encounter form.

Source: Froom, J, Kirkwood, R, Culpepper, L, and Boisseau, V: An integrated medical record and data system for primary care. Part 7: The encounter form: Problems and prospects for a universal type. *Journal of Family Practice* 5:847, 1977.

DIAGNOSTIC INFORMATION (E-BOOK)

INSTRUCTIONS:
1. Circle N, O, R or F for all conditions considered during each encounter.
   N - New Diagnosis   R - Recheck
   O - Old Diagnosis (not previously recorded)   F - Family History of
2. Use Additional Entries section to note other diagnoses not listed below, and obtain code numbers from ICHPPC booklet.

ICHPPC — COMMONLY USED DIAGNOSTIC CODES

INFECTIVE & PARASITIC DISEASES			RESPIRATORY CONT.			MUSCULOSKELET CONT.		
PRESUMED INFECT. INTEST. DIS.	009-	N O R F	ACUTE TONSILLITIS & QUINSY	463-	N O R F	LOW BACK PAIN WO		
DIARRHEA, CAUSE UNDETERMINED	0091	N O R F	LARYNGITIS & TRACHEITIS, ACUTE	464-	N O R F	RADIATING SYMPTOMS	7289	N O R F
STREP THROAT, SCARLET FEV	034-	N O R F	BRONCHITIS & BRONCHIOLITIS,			SIGN, SYMPTOM, ILL DEFINED COND		
INFECTIOUS MONONUCLEOSIS	075-	N O R F	ACUTE	466-	N O R F	DIZZINESS & GIDDINESS	7805	N O R F
VIRAL CONJUNCTIVITIS	078-	N O R F	INFLUENZA	470-	N O R F	HEADACHE	791-	N O R F
WARTS, ALL SITES	0791	N O R F	PNEUMONIA	486-	N O R F	CHEST PAIN	7820	N O R F
GONORRHEA, ALL SITES	098-	N O R F	BRONCHITIS, CHRONIC	491-	N O R F	EDEMA	7826	N O R F
DERMATOPHYTOSIS & MYCOSIS	110-	N O R F	EMPHYSEMA, BRONCHIECTASIS			ENLARGED LYMPH NODES,		
MONILIASIS, UROGENITAL, PROVEN	1121	N O R F	& COPD	492-	N O R F	NOT INFECTED	7827	N O R F
TRICH, UROGENITAL, PROVEN	131-	N O R F	ASTHMA	493-	N O R F	COUGH	7833	N O R F
ENDOCR, NUTRIT, METABOL DISEAS			HAY FEVER	507-	N O R F	PLEURITIC PAIN	7837	N O R F
NONTOXIC GOITER & NODULE	240-	N O R F	DIGESTIVE SYSTEM DISEASES			NAUSEA/VOMITING	7841	N O R F
HYPOTHYROIDISM	244-	N O R F	TEETH & SUPPORT STRUCTURE			ABDOMINAL PAIN	7855	N O R F
DIABETES MELLITUS	250-	N O R F	DISEASES	520-	N O R F	URINARY SYSTEM OR		
GOUT & HYPERURICEMIA	274-	N O R F	DUOD ULCER W/WO COMPLICATIONS	532-	N O R F	MICTURITION PAIN	7860	N O R F
OBESITY	2772-	N O R F	GASTRITIS/INDIGESTION	536-	N O R F	FREQUENCY OF URINATION	7864	N O R F
LIPID METABOLISM DISORDERS	272-	N O R F	INGUINAL HERNIA W/WO OBSTRUCT	550-	N O R F	PAIN IN LIMB	787-	N O R F
BLOOD DISEASES			HIATUS/DIAPHRAGMATIC HERNIA	551-	N O R F	PAIN IN JOINT	7873	N O R F
MICROCYTIC & IRON DEF ANEMIA	280-	N O R F	IRRIT BOWEL SYNDR/INTEST			FEVER OF UNDETERMINED CAUSE	7888	N O R F
MENTAL DISORDERS			DISOR NEC	564-	N O R F	RASH & OTHER NONSPECIFIC		
SCHIZOPHRENIA, ALL TYPES	295-	N O R F	CONSTIPATION	5640	N O R F	SKIN ERUPT	7882	N O R F
AFFECTIVE PSYCHOSES	296-	N O R F	BLEEDING PER RECTUM NOS	5692	N O R F	WEIGHTLOSS	7884	N O R F
ANXIETY NEUROSIS	3000	N O R F	GENITOURINARY SYSTEM DISEASES			MALAISE, FATIGUE, TIREDNESS	7901	N O R F
HYSTERIC & HYPOCHON NEUROSES	3001	N O R F	CYSTITIS & UTI NOS	595-	N O R F	ABNORMAL URINE TEST FINDING	789-	N O R F
DEPRESSIVE NEUROSIS	3004	N O R F	URETHRITIS NOS, NEC, NONSPEC	597-	N O R F	INJURIES & ADVERSE EFFECTS		
INSOMNIA & OTHER			PROSTATITIS & SEMINAL			FRACTURE RADIUS/ULNA	813-	N O R F
SLEEP DISORDERS	3064	N O R F	VESICULITIS	601-	N O R F	FRACT (META)CARPAL & TARSAL	814-	N O R F
TENSION HEADACHE	3068	N O R F	CHRONIC CYSTIC BREAST DISEASE	610-	N O R F	FRACTURE PHALANGS FOOT/HAND	816-	N O R F
TRANSIEN SITUAT DISTURB,			PELVIC INFLAMMATORY DISEASE	612-	N O R F	SPRAIN/STRAIN WRIST,		
ADJ REACT	307-	N O R F	CERVICITIS & CERVICAL EROSION	620-	N O R F	HAND, FINGERS	842-	N O R F
BEHAVIOR DISORDERS NEC	308-	N O R F	VAGINITIS NOS	6221	N O R F	SPRAIN/STRAIN KNEE &		
ALCOHOL ABUSE	3031	N O R F	MENOPAUSAL SYMPTOMS	627-	N O R F	LOWER LEG	844-	N O R F
TOBACCO ABUSE	3049	N O R F	ABSENT, SCANTY, RARE			SPRAIN/STRAIN ANKLE	8450	N O R F
PERSONALITY & CHAR DISORDERS	301-	N O R F	MENSTRUATION	6260	N O R F	SPRAIN/STRAIN NECK	8470	N O R F
NERV SYSTEM, SENSE ORGAN DISEAS			EXCESSIVE MENSTRUATION	6262	N O R F	CONCUSSION & INTRACRANIAL INJ	850-	N O R F
EPILEPSY, ALL TYPES	345-	N O R F	PAINFUL MENSTRUATION	6263	N O R F	LACERAT/OPEN WOUND/		
MIGRAINE	346-	N O R F	PREMENSTRUAL TENSION	6268	N O R F	TRAUM AMPUTATN	889-	N O R F
CONJUNCTIVITIS & OPHTHALMIA	360-	N O R F	SKIN, SUBCUTANEOUS TISSU DISEAS			INSECT BITES & STINGS	910-	N O R F
OTITIS EXTERNA	380-	N O R F	BOIL & CELLULITIS EXCL			ABRASION, SCRATCH, BLISTER	918-	N O R F
ACUTE OTITIS MEDIA	3810	N O R F	FINGR & TOE	680-	N O R F	BRUISE, CONTUSION, CRUSHING	929-	N O R F
CHRONIC SEROUS & OTITIS MED	3811	N O R F	IMPETIGO	684-	N O R F	BURNS & SCALDS, ALL DEGREES	949-	N O R F
DEAFNESS, PARTIAL OR COMPLETE	386-	N O R F	SEBORRHOEIC DERMATITIS	690-	N O R F	FOREIGN BODY IN TISSUES	888-	N O R F
WAX IN EAR	3871	N O R F	ECZEMA & ALLERGIC DERMATITIS	691-	N O R F	SUPPLEMENTARY CLASSIFICATION		
CIRCULATORY SYSTEM DISEASES			CONTACT & OTHER			MEDICAL EXAM, NO DIS DETECTED	y00-	N O R F
ACUTE MI/SUBAC ISCHEMIA	410-	N O R F	DERMATITIS NEC	692-	N O R F	PROPHYLACTIC IMMUNIZATION	y02-	N O R F
CHRONIC ISCH HRT DIS/ANGINA	412-	N O R F	DIAPER RASH	6929	N O R F	OBSERV/CARE PT ON HI RISK MED	y16-	N O R F
HEART FAILURE	4270	N O R F	PRURITIS & RELATED CONDITIONS	698-	N O R F	OBSERV/CARE OTHER HI RISK PAT	y17-	N O R F
ECTOPIC BEATS, ALL TYPES	4277	N O R F	SEBACEOUS CYST	7062	N O R F	ORAL CONTRACEPTIVES	y41-	N O R F
MURMURS NEC/NYD/FUNCTIONAL	4278	N O R F	INGROWN TOENAIL &			INTRAUTERINE DEVICES	y42-	N O R F
ELEVATED BLOOD PRESSURE NYD	4011	N O R F	NAIL DISEASE NEC	703-	N O R F	OTHER CONTRACEPTIVE METHODS	y43-	N O R F
HYPERTENSION, UNCOMPLICATED	401-	N O R F	URTICARIA, ALLERGIC EDEMA,			GEN CONTRACEPTIVE GUIDANCE	y44-	N O R F
HYPERTENSION INVOLVING			ANGIOEDEMA	708-	N O R F	DIAGNOSING PREGNANCY	y60-	N O R F
TARGET ORGAN	400-	N O R F	MUSCULOSKELET, CONNECTIV TISSU DISEASE			PRENATAL CARE	y61-	N O R F
PHLEBITIS & THROMBOPHLEBITIS	451-	N O R F	RHEUMATOID ARTHRIT &			POSTNATAL CARE	y62-	N O R F
VARICOSE VEINS OF LEGS	454-	N O R F	ALLIED CONDITN	712-	N O R F	ADVICE & HEALTH INSTRUCTION	y71-	N O R F
HEMORRHOIDS	455-	N O R F	OSTEOARTHRITIS & ALLIED COND	713-	N O R F	MARITAL PROBLEM	y84-	N O R F
RESPIRATORY SYSTEM DISEASES			SHOULDER SYNDROMES	717-	N O R F	PARENT & CHILD PROBLEM	y85-	N O R F
ACUTE URI	460-	N O R F	OTHER BURSITIS & SYNOVITIS	731-	N O R F	FAMILY DISRUPTION W/WO		
SINUSITIS, ACUTE & CHRONIC	461-	N O R F	MUSCLE PAIN/MYALGIA	7179	N O R F	DIVORCE	y87-	N O R F

ADDITIONAL ENTRIES:			ABBREVIATIONS	FOR SPECIAL STUDIES
L·S strain	8 4 7 8	N O R F	& and, and/or	
		N O R F	/ and/or	
		N O R F	EXCL excluding	
		N O R F	NEC not elsewhere classified	
			NOS not otherwise specified, unspecified	
			NYD not yet diagnosed	
			WO without	
			W/WO with or without	
			DIS disease	

FIGURE 15-5.

Rochester Family Medicine Program encounter form—reverse side.

Source: Froom, J, Kirkwood, R, Culpepper, L, and Boisseau, V: An integrated medical record and data system for primary care. Part 7: The encounter form: Problems and prospects for a universal type. *Journal of Family Practice* 5:848, 1977.

in North America, and searches for less than 30 citations are usually available in two working days. When information is needed on an emergency basis, a MEDLINE search will be run immediately during hours when the data base is accessible. Specific details concerning the procedures and nominal costs of MEDLINE searches are available through most medical libraries.

Consultation and Collaboration

Consultation is important with colleagues who have done similar kinds of research and with consultants in such fields as epidemiology and biostatistics. Such consultation is more readily available to family physicians than in the past, particularly through linkages established with these disciplines by many family practice teaching programs. It can also be anticipated that collaborative research projects will be carried out with increasing frequency involving departments of family practice in medical schools and practicing family physicians in the community.

Health Status	Definition	Specification of Major Activity				
		Pre-School	School	Housewives	Workers	Retired Persons
Not symptomatic: performs usual major activity	People who are asymptomatic	Takes part in ordinary play with other children	Goes to school	Does housework	Works at any job or business	Performs usual retired activities
Symptomatic: experiences discomfort, performs usual major activity	People in whom symptoms are pronounced (ie, affect comfort) so that person recognizes change in usual health status	Symptomatic, experiences discomfort (same for all categories of persons)				
Activity restricted	People who are unable to engage in major activity, confined to house, almost completely inactive, not bed disabled	Does not take part in play activities other than sedentary, eg, watch TV, look at books	Does not attend school	Does not keep house	Does not attend work or business	Is confined to house
Bed disabled	People who stay in bed all or most of the day — more than 1/2 hours person is usually awake	Stays in bed (same for all categories of persons)				
At risk	People with terminal illness	At risk (same for all categories of persons)				

FIGURE 15-6.

Definition of health status by major activity for preschool and school-age children, housewives, workers, and retired persons.

Source: Given, CW, Simoni, L, and Gallin, RJ: The design and use of a health status index for family physicians. *Journal of Family Practice* 4:289, 1977.

CONTENT AREAS FOR RESEARCH

The spectrum of needed research in family practice is wide. Although incomplete, Table 15–1 presents a simple taxonomy with four major categories of research, together with sample subject areas in each category.[20] Spitzer[21] views the directions for potential research in family practice in these terms:

> The family physician has a distinctive perspective and the obligation to study intact human beings in free-living, non-institutionalized populations over long periods of time, observing transitions from health to disease and back to health, with a unique opportunity to observe, on a firsthand basis, many of the concurrent phenomena that affect health and disease, such as family, employment, housing, and exposure to risk factors.
>
> Some subject areas that deserve high priority in family medicine research are calibrational studies focusing on clinical phenomena such as quantification of pain, quantification of the quality of survival, the development of explicit criteria for adequate clinical management of carefully defined conditions, demarcation of presenting complaints and their combinations as distinct from the demarcation of diagnoses, a taxonomy for behavior associated with disease or perceived disease, prognostic stratification of patients, and the calibration of the clinician himself as a reliable observer.

White[1] goes further in proposing the following kinds of important and researchable problems in primary care and family practice:

- What are the situational circumstances associated with the onset of illness?
- What role does separation play in the genesis of illness?
- What events or changes trigger consultation with a physician?
- What role do environmental factors play in the genesis of illness?
- Does the identification and monitoring of high-risk groups reduce morbidity?
- How valid are probabilistic models in primary care?
- What information does each test or X-ray really contribute to the resolution of the patient's presenting complaint?

These horizons for needed research in family practice are necessarily broad. Although a strong clinical base of research in the field is essential, research in health services and educational dimensions of family practice are also required. Ultimately, the priorities for categories and subjects of research will inevitably be based on local and individual interests and capabilities.

SOME ILLUSTRATIVE STUDIES

Brief presentation of portions of four studies conducted during the last several years in various family practice settings serves to illustrate the diversity of content, methods, and implications of some of the early research efforts in the field.

Patterns of Chest Pain

Blacklock conducted a chart review study of 109 patients presenting with the complaint of chest pain to three family practice groups. The objectives of the study were (1) to establish the incidence of chest pain in the practice population, (2) to determine the age–sex distribution of patients with chest pain of organic and unproven etiology, and (3) to test the hypothesis that certain problems of living will be greater in patients with chest pain than with a group of matched controls.[22] Each control was matched for age group, sex, and practice.

A total of 217 patients with chest pain were identified during the study. Based on a midyear registered population of 4398, this represents a rate of 49.3 chest pain patients per 1000 patients at risk in the three practices over a one-year period. Significant findings included:

- Fifty percent of all chest pain patients were in the unproven category, even after six months' follow-up.
- The rate of unproven chest pain in both males and females was highest in the 45 to 64 age group.
- There were no differences in location of pain between the organic and unproven etiology groups.
- More patients with unproven chest pain described their pain as sharp or pressing than did patients in the organic group.
- There were no statistically significant differences in problems of living between the organic chest pain patients and their controls.
- The rate of anxiety–depression was significantly higher in the unproven chest pain group compared with both matched controls and with the organic chest pain group.

Table 15–2 compares the incidence of problems in living in unproven chest pain patients and controls.

Most review papers and texts on chest pain focus primarily on organic causes, and relatively little is known about nonorganic patterns of chest pain in primary care settings. This study begins to address this problem in a preliminary way.

Susceptibility Patterns of Staphylococcus

Although the incidence of resistant "community" strains of *Staphylococcus aureus* in ambulatory patients has for years tended to be quite low, two recent studies in large, urban centers in the eastern United States had shown over

TABLE 15–1. A TAXONOMY FOR RESEARCH AREAS IN FAMILY PRACTICE

EPIDEMIOLOGICAL AND CLINICAL RESEARCH	HEALTH SERVICES RESEARCH	BEHAVIORAL RESEARCH	EDUCATIONAL RESEARCH

Single illness studies
  Morbidity
  Natural history
  Prevention
  Early diagnosis
  Management
  Case reports
	Consumers
	  Health and illness
	    behavior
	  Needs and demands
	  Consumer participation
	  Patient compliance
	  Effects of health education
		Doctor–patient relationships
		
		Health team and changing
		  roles
		
		Impact of societal changes
		  on primary care
			Medical student interest in family
			  practice
			
			Teaching aids for family
			  practice
			
			Family practice residency
			  programs

Practice studies
  Content
    Common diseases
    Common problems
    Variation with
      geographic setting
  Consultation rates
  Changing patterns
	Providers
	  Numbers and distribution
	  Efficiency (utilization)
	  Physician performance
	  Referral patterns
	  Costs of primary care
	  Solo practice
	  Family practice group
	  Multispecialty group
		Family dynamics
		  Normal
		  Abnormal
		  Changing patterns
		  Developmental aspects of
		    family life cycles
		
		Counseling
		  Methods
			Educational objectives
			Role of problem-oriented
			  record and medical audit
			
			Program costs
			Model family practice
			  clinic costs and
			  revenue

Family studies
Morbidity
Prevention
Role of genetic
   counseling
Crisis intervention

Allied health manpower
   studies
   Task definition
   Health team studies
   Cost and efficiency
      studies
   Drug and laboratory
      procedure studies
   Experimental models for
      delivery of primary care
      (including comparison
      of family practice and
      multispecialty approaches)

Interface
   Patient outcome studies
   Costs and incentives
   Cost-benefit ratios
   Facilities and utilization
   Role of health hazard
      appraisal

Results

Self-assessment methods
   Family practice
      residents
   Practicing family
      physicians

Continuing medical
   education
   Needs of family
      physicians
   Physician performance

Source: Geyman, J.P.: Research in the family practice residency program. *Journal of Family Practice* 5:245, 1977.

TABLE 15-2.   PROBLEMS OF LIVING IN UNPROVEN CHEST PAIN PATIENTS AND CONTROLS

PROBLEM OF LIVING	UNPROVEN CHEST PAIN N = 55	CONTROLS N = 55
Intrapersonal (at least 1)	39	24†
Anxiety–depression	36	15†
Alcohol abuse	3	2
Illicit drug use	0	0
Obesity	12	10
Other*	3	5
Interpersonal (at least 1)	21	15‡
Marital dysfunction	12	11
Family dysfunction	7	4
Chronic illness in family	4	3
Material (at least 1)	10	2
Debt	1	0
Unemployment	2	2
Other*	8	0

* See text for details.
† $P < 0.01$ χ^2 calculation with Yates correction.
‡ Differences not significant using χ^2 calculation with Yates correction.
Source: Blacklock, S.M.: The symptom of chest pain in family practice. *Journal of Family Practice* 4:429, 1977.

80 percent of ambulatory patients with various S. *aureus* infections to be resistant to penicillin G.

There was limited information available on the incidence of resistant strains of S. *aureus* in family practice populations and in other settings. A study was therefore conducted in a family practice residency program in a smaller, midwestern community to determine the incidence of resistant strains of S. *aureus* in a more typical family practice population.

Nasal swabs were obtained from 408 patients, and S. *aureus* was isolated in 109 patients, representing a carrier rate of 26.7 percent. It was found that only 25.7 percent of the isolates were sensitive to penicillin G and ampicillin and that even fewer isolates were sensitive to these drugs in children less than 10 years of age. Table 15–3 shows the susceptibility of S. *aureus* isolates to various antibiotics.[23]

It was concluded that (1) penicillin should not be used in the treatment of S. *aureus* infections, (2) erythromycin should be used for the majority of mild to moderate skin and soft-tissue S. *aureus* infections, and (3) penicillinase-resistant penicillins (e.g., oxacillin) should be used for more serious S. *aureus* infections.

Lead Screening

Frequent reports in recent years of lead poisoning in various settings have led to increased interest in the problem. Since simple screening procedures are available, together with effective methods of therapy and prevention, strategy

TABLE 15–3.   ANTIBIOTIC SUSCEPTIBILITY OF
              109 STAPHYLOCOCCUS AUREUS
              ISOLATES

ANTIBIOTIC	PERCENT SENSITIVE
Ampicillin	25.7
Cephalexin	99.1
Cephalothin	99.1
Chloramphenicol	100
Clindamycin	99.1
Erythromycin	94.5
Oxacillin	99.1
Penicillin G	25.7
Sulfamethoxazole/trimethoprim	99.1
Sulfathiazole	99.1
Tetracycline HCl	94.5

Source: Jones, M.E., Helling, D.K., Rakel, R.E.,
Chamberlain, M.: Susceptibility patterns of staphylo-
coccus in a family practice population. *Journal of
Family Practice* 6:963, 1978.

for screening is needed. This study examined the results of lead screening in a portion of the at-risk population of an urban family practice teaching program.[24]

Of a total of 333 children screened by a micromethod using capillary blood, 18.6 percent had lead levels between 30 and 39 μg/100 ml and 10 percent had lead levels of 40 μg/100 ml or greater. Of the latter group, only 2.7 percent had levels in that range when retested with venous blood samples. Although age and sex were not of predictive value for elevated blood lead levels, socioeconomic status (as determined by census tract residence) was found to have definite predictive value. Table 15–4 shows the range of elevated blood lead levels by socioeconomic class.

Based on these findings, it was decided to selectively screen only those children residing in the lower socioeconomic census tracts, and to advise their parents of the high false positive rate of initial screening and the possible need for retesting with venous blood samples.

Presentation of Illness

Although it is well known that many patients may present with a symptom or illness as a "ticket of admission" for another problem, this kind of "signal behavior" of patients has received limited study and is poorly understood by physicians. A study was done involving 389 visits of randomly selected women presenting to five family physicians over a six-month period. The patients' behaviors were classified by seven categories.[25] The major findings included:

TABLE 15–4.   CHILDREN WITH CONFIRMED
LEVELS OF 40 μg/100 ml OR
GREATER AND UNCONFIRMED
LEVELS OF 30 TO 39 μg/100 ml

	NUMBER	PERCENT OF EACH TESTED GROUP
Sex		
Male	49	26.1
Female	34	23.4
Age		
1	17	30.4
2	16	33.3
3	14	25.9
4	16	22.2
5	11	21.6
6	9	17.3
Socioeconomic status (I is highest)		
I	1	3.4
II	3	6.8
III	38	21.0
IV	32	50.0
V	9	60.0

Source: Froom, J.: Lead screening by family physicians. *Journal of Family Practice* 4:631, 1977.

- Signal behavior was observed in 14 percent of visits, and psychosocial problems were presented frankly in another 22 percent.
- The distribution of patient behaviors differed for patient- and doctor-initiated visits and differed among the five family physicians.
- No significant differences were noted by age, social class, or educational level as to whether problems of living were presented frankly or as signals.
- Characteristics of the physician, rather than those of the patient, had greater influence on the extent to which patients used signal behavior or frank presentation of psychosocial problems.

Table 15–5 compares frank presentation and signal behavior for the five participating physicians.

As a result of this study, two major conclusions were drawn: (1) patient-initiated visits (especially those for minor illnesses) are likely to mask or signal other problems, and (2) the interest of the physician in psychosocial problems, together with his/her willingness to listen to the patient, results in increased frank presentation of psychosocial problems and decreased signal behavior.

TABLE 15-5.   FRANK VERSUS SIGNAL BEHAVIOR SHOWN FOR EACH PARTICIPATING
PHYSICIAN

PHYSICIAN	*PERCENTAGE DISTRIBUTIONS OF FRANK AND SIGNAL BEHAVIOR**			
	Signal	*Frank Psychosocial Problem*	*Total*	*N*
1	50.0	50.0	100.0	6
2	36.1	63.9	100.0	61
3	21.3	78.7	100.0	47
4	88.2	11.8	100.0	17
5	66.7	33.3	100.0	6
Total	39.4	60.6	100.0	137

* χ^2 = 25.8 on 4 df, $p < 0.001$

Source: Stewart, M.A., McWhinney, I.R., and Buck, C.W.: How illness presents: A study of patient behavior. *Journal of Family Practice* 2:411, 1975.

OPPORTUNITIES FOR INVOLVEMENT IN RESEARCH

Any research project inevitably must begin with a question asked by an individual. We have seen that the potential range of researchable questions in family practice is extremely wide. What the curious individual does next with respect to ways and means of planning and conducting a research project depends on such variables as the nature of the study, the numbers of subjects required for meaningful results, the availability of time and resources, the need for specialized assistance from other disciplines, and the experience and skills of the prospective researcher.

In an excellent paper on these kinds of issues, Phillips proposes a spectrum of involvement styles by which interested family physicians may participate in research studies. Figure 15-7 illustrates a three-dimensional view of this spectrum incorporating three parameters—relevant disciplines, type of research, and level of involvement by the researcher.[26] By means of this grid, one can describe a particular study and level of involvement; for example, a clinical strategy study may draw especially from epidemiology and involve the family physician as a volunteer observer, as the principal investigator, in a collaborative way with peers, or as part of a multicenter regional or national study.

The planning of any research project is a critical and demanding process that involves progressive refining of the research question before the project itself can be designed and carried out. A useful, stepwise process for planning clinical, social, and behavioral research projects has been developed by Gordon and is included as Appendix 10.[27]

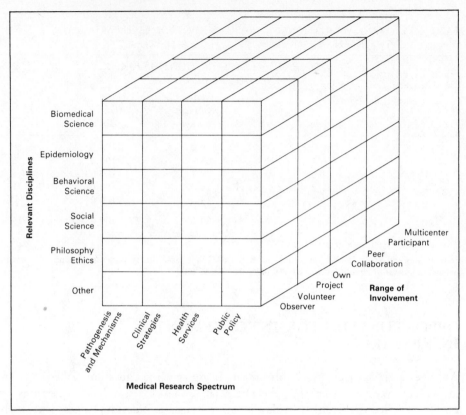

FIGURE 15-7.

Spectrum of involvement styles.

Source: Phillips, TJ: Research considerations for the family physician. *Journal of Family Practice* 7:127, 1978.

Collaborative studies offer ideal opportunities for interested family physicians without research experience to become involved with research. The previously mentioned *Virginia Study* (p. 213) is a good example of a statewide collaborative study involving 82 family practice residents and 36 practicing family physicians in a number of urban, suburban and rural communities in Virginia.[28] Another example of a collaborative research project has been developed at the University of Pennsylvania linking the medical school's Department of Psychiatry with practicing family physicians in the surrounding area for the study of selected psychotropic drugs.[29] Participating physicians in this project gain some experience in the techniques and process of research as well as a focused continuing education experience. Figure 15–8 represents the functional inter-relationships between the family physicians and the medical school's research unit.

Departments of family practice in medical schools have both the opportunity and responsibility to develop active research programs involving their own faculty, residents, and students, as well as faculty from other disciplines and interested family physicians in the surrounding area. Active collaboration between academic centers and practicing family physicians is a vital linkage in the development of a sound foundation of empirical and experimental research in family practice.

COMMENT

Family practice is in the process of redefining traditional connotations of medical research as various kinds of research questions are being addressed in the clinical environment of the family physician. This process involves the development of some new investigative techniques, the modification of other established research methods to adapt to the family practice environment, and the potential collaboration of a wide range of related disciplines. The ultimate

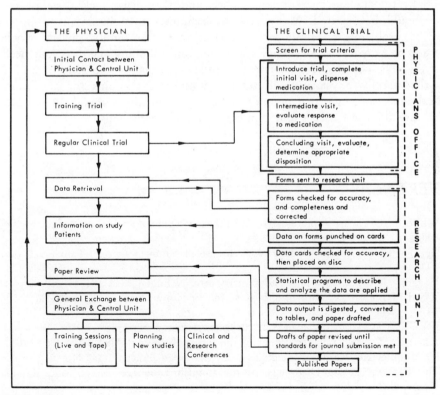

FIGURE 15-8.

Private practice research group operation.

Source: Hesbacher, P, Rickels, K, Zamostein, B, Perloff, M, and Jenkins, W: A collaborative research model in family practice. *Journal of Family Practice* 1:54, 1977.

result of this process will be to convert family practice from an applied derivative field drawing entirely from other disciplines to a clinical discipline basing its approaches to patient care and teaching more directly on the results of examined clinical experience in its own environment.

Research in family practice has a good start but is still in a relatively early phase involving primarily *descriptive* studies. It can be anticipated that future research in the field will also move into *experimental* studies. As pointed out by Wood and his colleagues [4]:

> Unasked and unanswered questions abound in family practice. Observation, recording, analysis, reflection, and discussion among peers are the basic tools. They must be used and will eventually serve as referent points for research that uses experimental design methodologies.

Basic to the progress of research in family practice is an attitude of critical inquiry among family physicians. Questions need to be asked about the effectiveness of current clinical approaches in family practice. Documentation should be sought to validate current approaches, and those that lack demonstrated value should be rejected. Many related disciplines may be involved in the study of problems in family practice, but it is the family physician who must accept primary responsibility for asking and pursuing the questions needing study. The benefits of this process include expansion of the body of knowledge that family physicians will teach, an ongoing stimulus for continuing medical education, increased practice satisfaction, and most importantly, better health care for the patients and families of family physicians.[30]

REFERENCES

1. White KL: Primary care research and the new epidemiology. J Fam Pract 3:579, 1976
2. Geyman JP: On the developing research base in family practice. J Fam Pract 7:51, 1978
3. Haggerty RJ: The university and primary care. N Engl J Med 281:416, 1969
4. Wood M, Stewart W, Brown TC: Research in family medicine. J Fam Pract 5:64, 1977
5. Byrne PS: Why not organize your curiosity? J Fam Pract 5:188, 1977
6. James G: The general practitioner of the future. N Engl J Med 270:1286, 1963
7. McWhinney IR: Family medicine as a science. J Fam Pract 7:54, 1978
8. The Random House Dictionary of the English Language. New York, Random House, 1967, p 277
9. Geyman JP: Climate for research in family practice. J Fam Pract 7:69, 1978
10. Froom J: An integrated medical record and data system for primary care. Part 2: Classifications of health problems for use by family physicians. J Fam Pract 4:1149, 1977

11. Schneeweiss R, Stuart HW Jr, Froom J, et al.: A conversion code from the RCGP to the ICHPPC classification system. J Fam Pract 5:415, 1977

12. Glossary for Primary Care. Report of the North American Primary Care Research Group (NAPCRG) Committee on Standard Terminology. J Fam Pract 5:633, 1977

13. Weed LL: Medical Records, Medical Education, and Patient Care. Cleveland, Ohio, The Press of Case Western Reserve University, 1970, p 13

14. Froom J: An integrated medical record and data system for primary care. Part 6: A decade of problem-oriented medical records: A reassessment. J Fam Pract 5:627, 1977

15. Hurst JW, Walker HK, eds: The Problem-Oriented System. New York, Medcom, 1972, p 23

16. Froom J: An integrated medical record and data system for primary care. Part 1: The age–sex register: Definition of the patient population. J Fam Pract 4:951, 1977

17. Froom J, Culpepper L, Boisseau V: An integrated medical record and data system for primary care. Part 3: The diagnostic index: Manual and computer methods and applications. J Fam Pract 5:855, 1977

18. Froom J, Kirkwood R, Culpepper L, Boisseau V: An integrated medical record and data system for primary care. Part 7: The encounter form: Problems and prospects for a universal type. J Fam Pract 5:845, 1977

19. Given CW, Simoni L, Gallin RJ: The design and use of a health status index for family physicians. J Fam Pract 4:289, 1977

20. Geyman JP: Research in the family practice residency program. J Fam Pract 5:245, 1977

21. Spitzer WO: The intellectual worthiness of family medicine. Pharos Alpha Omega Alpha 40:2, July 1977

22. Blacklock SM: The symptom of chest pain in family practice. J Fam Pract 4:429, 1977

23. Jones ME, Helling DK, Rakel RE, Chamberlain M: Susceptibility patterns of staphylococcus in a family practice population. J Fam Pract 6:963, 1978

24. Froom J: Lead screening by family physicians. J Fam Pract 4:631, 1977

25. Stewart MA, McWhinney IR, Buck CW: How illness presents: A study of patient behavior. J Fam Pract 2:411, 1975

26. Phillips TJ: Research considerations for the family physician. J Fam Pract 7:121, 1978

27. Gordon MJ: Research Workbook: A guide for initial planning of clinical, social and behavioral research projects. J Fam Pract 7:145, 1978

28. Marsland DW, Wood M, Mayo F: A data bank for patient care, curriculum and research in family practice: 526,196 patient problems. J Fam Pract 3:25, 1976

29. Hesbacher P, Rickels K, Zamostien B, Perloff M, Jenkins W: A collaborative research model in family practice. J Fam Pract 1:52, 1974

30. Geyman JP: On the need for critical inquiry in family medicine. J Fam Pract 4:195, 1977

Further Reading

Anderson JE, Lees REM: Optional hierarchy as a means of increasing the flexibility of a morbidity classification system. J Fam Pract 6:1271, 1978

Department of Family Medicine (R700)
University of Miami School of Medicine
P. O. Box 016700
Miami, Florida 33101

Bass MJ: Approaches to the denominator problem in primary care research. J Fam Pract 3:193, 1976

————, Newell JP, Dickie GL: An information system for family practice. Part 2: The value of defining a practice population. J Fam Pract 3:525, 1976

Boyle RM, Rockhold FW, Mitchell GS, Van Horn S: The age–sex register: Estimation of the practice population. J Fam Pract 5:999, 1977

Dickie GL, Newell JP, Bass MJ: An information system for family practice. Part 4: Encounter data and their uses. J Fam Pract 3:639, 1976

Eimerl TS, Laidlaw AJ: A Handbook for Research in General Practice. Edinburgh, Livingstone, 1969, p 1

Friedman GD: Primer of Epidemiology. New York, McGraw-Hill, 1974, p 1

Froom J, Culpepper L, Becker L, Boisseau V: Research design in family medicine. J Fam Pract 7:75, 1978

Fry J: On the natural history of some common diseases. J Fam Pract 2:327, 1975

————: The contribution of research to improving a family practice. In Medalie JH, ed: Family Medicine—Principles and Applications. Baltimore, Williams and Wilkins, 1978, p 269

Geyman JP, Bass MJ: Communication of results of research. J Fam Pract 7:113, 1978

Gordon MJ: Research traditions available to family medicine. J Fam Pract 7:59, 1978

Jones FS: How to read a research article. Res Staff Physician 21:101, July 1975

Keller K, Podell RN: The survey in family practice research. J Fam Pract 2:449, 1975

Kilpatrick SJ, Wood M: Analysis and interpretation of data. J Fam Pract 7:101, 1978

Newell JP, Bass MJ, Dickie GL: An information system for family practice. Part 1: Defining the patient population. J Fam Pract 3:517, 1976

————, Dickie GL, Bass MJ: An information system for family practice. Part 3: Gathering encounter data. J Fam Pract 3:633, 1976

Scherger JE: The use of epidemiologic methods in family practice. J Fam Pract 6:849, 1978

Smith SR: Application of the tracer technique in studying quality of care. J Fam Pract 4:505, 1977

Spitzer WO, Feinstein AR, Sackett DL: What is a health care trial? JAMA 233:2, 1975

Wood M: Collection of data. J Fam Pract 7:91, 1978

CHAPTER SIXTEEN

Progress in the 1970s

Since family practice had no formal place in medical education in the United States before 1969, a number of basic questions were understandably raised as the new specialty took root. Some of the more important questions were the following: Can viable teaching programs be organized and maintained at a high level of quality? Can faculty be recruited to teach in developing programs? Can interest among medical students in this emerging specialty be developed and sustained? Will graduates of family practice residencies locate in areas of need? Can the academic discipline of family medicine be defined and nurtured through ongoing research efforts?

Previous chapters have examined various aspects of these questions and documented substantial progress in all of these areas. A brief overview of several dimensions of the specialty's first decade of development is now of interest in order to measure the field's overall progress and principal needs as family practice enters its second decade of further development.

SOME MEASURES OF PROGRESS

Organization of Teaching Programs

The development of teaching programs in family practice, at both under-graduate and graduate levels, was the central concern of the specialty during the 1970s. The magnitude of this effort in just one decade is indeed remarkable. Table 16–1 and Figures 16–1 and 16–2 reflect impressive growth of under-graduate and graduate programs, respectively.

TABLE 16–1.   ORGANIZATIONAL UNITS FOR FAMILY PRACTICE IN MEDICAL SCHOOLS*

	NUMBER	PERCENT
Departments	88	67.1
Divisions	14	10.7
Other programs	4	3.0
Departments under development	5	4.0
Schools without activity	20	15.2
Total	131	100

* Data compiled by Division of Education, American Academy of Family Physicians, Kansas City, Missouri. These data represent all medical schools in the United States, including branch campuses and medical schools not yet fully accredited but in an advanced stage of development.

As noted in the first chapter, the number of general/family physicians in the United States has been steadily declining for about 50 years. In 1976, this trend was reversed, with an increase in the number of general/family physicians in active practice observed for the first time over that period.[1] Gratifying as this progress is, the graduates of family practice residency programs have not yet increased sufficiently to make a major impact on the needs for primary care physicans in this country, and expansion of the capacity of residency programs will continue as an important need well into the 1980s. The propor-tion of American medical school graduates entering family practice residency training was 12.7 percent, 13.7 percent, and 15.0 percent, respectively, in 1975, 1976, and 1977.[1] It is currently projected that the graduating class will reach 16,000 by the early 1980s. Since it is generally accepted that family practice residencies should be able to accommodate at least 25 percent of United States medical graduates, considerable expansion will be required beyond today's level of 2500 first-year family practice residency positions.

The development of teaching programs in family practice to date has like-wise been impressive in qualitative terms. As described in Chapters 8 and 9, excellent progress has been made in curriculum design, teaching techniques, and evaluation methods at both undergraduate and graduate levels. That family practice residencies have been found attractive by American medical graduates is reflected by fill rates of first-year family practice residencies of 94 percent and 96.3 percent, respectively, in 1977 and 1978, when the proportion of

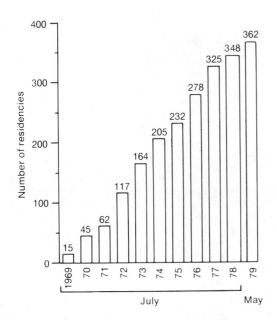

FIGURE 16-1.

Approved family practice residencies in the United States.

foreign medical graduates in these programs was only 5.9 and 5.2 percent, respectively.* The attrition rate from family practice residency programs has been quite low (Table 16–2), and the great majority of vacated positions have been promptly filled. Many of the residents dropping out of family practice residencies have entered another residency in this specialty, as shown in Table 16–3. In 1978, there was an overall attrition rate of only 2.9 percent of the 5421 family practice residents then in training.

Especially noteworthy in terms of quality control in family practice teaching is the previously mentioned Residency Assistance Program (p. 172).[2] A panel of over 30 experienced family practice educators has developed guidelines for quality graduate education in family practice that address such issues as curriculum content, teaching facilities, and faculty supervision.† Consultations are provided to family practice residency programs on a voluntary basis and are intended to facilitate information sharing, identification of problems, and collaborative problem solving.

Faculty Recruitment

The recruitment of faculty for family practice teaching programs has been a challenging process because of the previous lack of an established teaching

---

* Data provided by the Division of Education, American Academy of Family Physicians, Kansas City, Missouri. Fill rates above 90 percent are generally considered complete filling, due to unavoidable logistical problems involved in the matching process.[1]

† Copies of these guidelines are available by writing to the Project Director, Residency Assistance Program, 1740 West 92 Street, Kansas City, Missouri 64114.

FIGURE 16-2.

Family practice residents in the
United States.

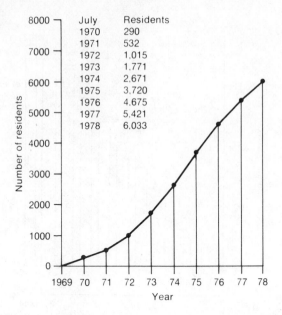

July	Residents
1970	290
1971	532
1972	1,015
1973	1,771
1974	2,671
1975	3,720
1976	4,675
1977	5,421
1978	6,033

tradition in family medicine. The critical need has been to attract excellent
clinicians from active family practice in the community with interest and
skills in teaching and the capacity to serve as role models for students and
residents. Many of these individuals have also been called upon to organize and
administer teaching programs and contribute to the developing academic
discipline of family medicine.

Significant progress has been made in faculty recruitment. In the five-year
period between 1971–1972 and 1976–1977, the number of full-time faculty

TABLE 16-2.   ATTRITION IN UNITED STATES FAMILY PRACTICE RESIDENCY PROGRAMS—
FIRST- AND SECOND-YEAR RESIDENTS, 1977

	NUMBER	PERCENTAGE OF 1977 FIRST-YEAR RESIDENTS	NUMBER	PERCENTAGE OF 1977 SECOND-YEAR RESIDENTS
Research	1	0.1	0	0.0
Teaching	0	0.0	0	0.0
Administration	0	0.0	0	0.0
Further training*	96	5.2	18	1.1
Practice	69	3.7	20	1.3
Other	80	4.3	21	1.3
Total	246	13.2	59	3.7

* Other than family practice

Source: Division of Education, American Academy of Family Physicians, Kansas City, Missouri.

TABLE 16–3.   SPECIALTIES FOR FURTHER TRAINING—1977 RESIDENTS

	NUMBER	PERCENTAGE OF 1977 FIRST-YEAR RESIDENTS	NUMBER	PERCENTAGE OF 1977 SECOND-YEAR RESIDENTS
Family practice	42	2.3	7	0.4
Nonbedded	32	1.7	6	0.4
Other primary care	44	2.4	7	0.4
Miscellaneous	20	1.1	5	0.3
Total	138	7.5	25	1.5

Source: Division of Education, American Academy of Family Physicians, Kansas City, Missouri.

in family practice in United States medical schools increased from 82 to 396.[3] A much larger number of full-time family practice faculty are now teaching in community-based teaching programs, but accurate estimates of this number are not yet available. Many thousands of additional family physicians have become involved in part-time teaching, often on a volunteer basis, in connection with residency teaching and student preceptorship programs.

A national study conducted in 1975 of 240 full-time family practice faculty characterized this group in terms of practice experience, previous training, and board certification. The average age of these family practice teachers was 45 years, and about two-thirds had at least ten years of practice experience. A similar proportion had completed two or more years of graduate training, usually in general/family practice residencies. Table 16–4 shows the types of board certification in this group.[4]

TABLE 16–4.   BOARD CERTIFICATION BY FULL-TIME FAMILY MEDICINE EDUCATORS

CERTIFICATION	NUMBER OF PHYSICIANS
Family practice	197
Internal medicine	16
Pediatrics	8
Surgery	2
Other (pathology, preventive medicine neurology, etc)	11

Source: *Description of Salaried Medical School Faculty, 1971-72 and 1976-77.* Washington, D.C., Association of American Medical Colleges, 1977, p. 26.

The development of teaching and research skills is by no means a spontaneous process, as is sometimes assumed in medical education. Considerable emphasis has been placed on faculty development programs to augment teaching skills of family practice faculty, and more recently, some programs have been initiated for the purpose of developing research skills. The Society of Teachers of Family Medicine and the American Academy of Family Physicians have sponsored a number of national and regional faculty development workshops. Currently there are at least 30 federally-funded faculty development programs in the country ranging from short-term learning experiences to formal, one-year fellowship programs. The Robert Wood Johnson Foundation has provided funds to establish two-year fellowship programs in five medical school departments of family medicine (at Case Western Reserve University, the University of Iowa, the University of Missouri, the University of Utah, and the University of Washington). These programs often lead to a Master of Public Health degree, and emphasize the development of research skills as well as teaching skills.

Despite this progress, the recruitment of well qualified family practice faculty to the expanding number of teaching programs remains a pressing need. It can be anticipated, however, that this problem will be relieved somewhat during the next five years as the ranks of graduates of family practice residencies continue to grow and as more of these young physicians opt for careers in teaching and research.

Student Interest

A question raised by some in the late 1960s, as family practice was first developing, was whether substantial student interest could be developed and sustained in this new specialty. At the start of the 1980s this question can be answered strongly in the affirmative. Many medical schools report 15 to 35 percent of their graduates entering graduate training in family practice. State medical schools report higher proportions of their graduating classes opting for family practice than private medical schools, as is also the case of medical schools with departments or divisions of family practice compared to institutions without established undergraduate teaching programs in family medicine.

Since there are not yet enough family practice residencies available to adequately meet student demand, a sizable number of medical school graduates are entering flexible first-graduate year programs with the hope of obtaining a second-year position in a family practice residency thereafter. This creates a difficult problem that can only be resolved by expanding the capacity of family practice residency programs, since the total number of available second-year positions in family practice residencies is very small.

There is considerable evidence documenting the high caliber of young physicians opting for family practice in recent years. A study was done in one medical school, for example, comparing family practice residents with residents in four other major specialties on the basis of both cognitive and noncognitive measures. It was found that family practice residents equalled the highest scoring group on cognitive tests and scored higher on affiliation need and lower on aggression and materialism than the other groups.[5]

Distribution of Graduates

The shortage of primary care physicians, especially of those trained in breadth to care for the everyday problems of families, is a generalized phenomenon throughout the country in urban, suburban, and rural locations. About 5000 family physicians have already graduated from United States family practice residency programs, and the record to date shows that these graduates are entering practice in communities of all sizes and types. Table 16–5 shows the distribution of practice locations of family practice residents graduating in 1977 and 1978. It can be noted that 11.1 percent and 8.4 percent of respondents, respectively, entered practice in rural communities of less than 2500 population more than 25 miles from large cities in 1977 and 1978. It can also be seen that over one-half of 1977 and 1978 surveyed graduates established practice in communities smaller than 25,000 population, whereas 27.6 percent and 27.1 percent of these groups in 1977 and 1978 entered practice in large communities with populations more than 100,000 people. There is evidence, however, that the impact of family practice upon low income, inner city communities with populations over 500,000 people has been relatively minimal, with only about 3 percent of graduates selecting practice sites in these settings.

Patient Care

A number of important changes took place during the 1970s in family practice with respect to patient care. Earlier chapters have described refinements in medical record systems, the increasing use of audit (including office-based audit as part of recertification requirements by the American Board of Family Practice), and the evolution of various kinds of team practice. The strong trend to partnership and group practice is another significant change evident in the last decade, particularly among recent graduates of family practice residency programs. Studies conducted by the American Academy of Family Physicians have shown that about 60 percent of surveyed 1977 and 1978 residency graduates entered partnership or group practice (Table 16–6).

Several studies have been undertaken comparing the quality of patient care in family practice with that of other specialties. Garg and his colleagues,[6] for example, found no significant difference in the quality of care provided by family physicians, internists, and cardiologists in the care of patients with congestive heart failure, transient ischemic attack, or recent stroke. They likewise found that the quality of care was comparable among family physicians and urologists in the care of patients with acute and chronic urinary tract

TABLE 16–5. DISTRIBUTION OF GRADUATING RESIDENTS BY COMMUNITY SIZE—1977–1978

CHARACTER AND POPULATION OF COMMUNITY	1977 GRADUATING RESIDENTS			1978 GRADUATING RESIDENTS		
	Number Reporting	Percentage of Total Reporting	Cumulative Percentage of Total Reporting	Number Reporting	Percentage of Total Reporting	Cumulative Percentage of Total Reporting
Rural area or town (less than 2500) not within 25 miles of large cities	81	11.1	11.1	91	8.4	8.4
Rural area or town (less than 2500) within 25 miles of large city	20	2.7	13.8	34	3.1	11.5
Small town (2500–25,000) not within 25 miles of large city	180	24.7	38.5	257	23.8	35.3
Small town (2500–25,000) within 25 miles of large city	107	14.7	53.2	183	16.9	52.2
Small city (25,000–100,000)	127	17.4	70.6	186	17.2	69.4
Suburb of small metropolitan area	14	1.8	72.4	38	3.5	72.9
Small metropolitan area (100,000–500,000)	78	10.7	83.1	90	8.3	81.2
Suburb of large metropolitan area	55	7.5	90.6	103	9.5	90.7
Large metropolitan area (500,000 or more)	45	6.2	96.8	72	6.7	97.4
Inner city/low income area (500,000 or more)	23	3.2	100.0	28	2.6	100.0
Total	730	100.0%		1082	100.0	

Source: Division of Education, American Academy of Family Physicians, Kansas City, Missouri. These data are based on response rates of 68 percent and 89.5 percent, respectively, for 1977 and 1978 graduating residents.

TABLE 16–6. PRACTICE ARRANGEMENTS OF GRADUATING RESIDENTS—1977–1978

TYPE OF PRACTICE ARRANGEMENT	1977 GRADUATING RESIDENTS		1978 GRADUATING RESIDENTS	
	Number Reporting	*Percentage of Total Reporting*	*Number Reporting*	*Percentage of Total Reporting*
Family practice group	268	33.2	411	30.2
Multispecialty group	80	9.9	138	10.2
Two-person family practice group (partnership)	146	18.1	262	19.3
Solo	117	14.5	185	13.6
Military	56	6.9	130	9.6
Teaching	40	5.0	70	5.1
USPHS	27	3.3	61	4.5
Emergency room	32	4.0	12	0.9
Hospital staff (F–T)	30	3.7	51	3.8
None of the above	11	1.4	39	2.8
Total	807	100.0	1359	100.0

Source: Division of Education, American Academy of Family Physicians, Kansas City, Missouri.

infections. Other studies have demonstrated comparable quality of obstetric care provided by family physicians and obstetrician–gynecologists.[7,8]

Another recent trend is the development of growing numbers of clinical departments of family practice in community hospitals. Guidelines have been developed by the American Academy of Family Physicians for the organization and operation of these departments, including an active role in the monitoring of quality of care by family physicians and the delineation of their hospital privileges conjointly with other departments.[9]

Academic Discipline and Research

An early chapter alluded to the evolution of family medicine as the academic discipline of family practice during the 1970s (pp. 19–20). What has evolved is a functional definition of family medicine based on the focus of the specialty's concerns in providing continuing, comprehensive care to patients and their families over time. This focus departs from the traditional reductionist view of disease of the biomedical model and subscribes to the psychobiomedical model proposed by Engel [10] as applied to families, not just to individual patients.

With respect to the definition of family medicine as an academic discipline, some have looked for the unique aspects of the specialty not shared by the traditional specialties. That this is an unrealistic and illusionary approach is suggested by the following view of specialties expressed by Draper and Smits [11]:

> In fact there is nothing intrinsically rational or permanent about the way in which medical specialties are currently defined; all are more or less arbitrary. The first

modern specialties, surgery and obstetrics–gynecology, were based on technic. Subsequent fields depended for their definition on particular organs or systems, such as endocrinology or neurology, on the age of the patient, such as pediatrics or geriatrics, or on a specific aspect of medical technology, such as radiology. A specialty is essentially a social definition rather than a scientific or logical one; it is simply a social recognition of a grouping of practitioners who are carrying out similar work. Furthermore, the definitions of specialties are constantly changing, and the boundaries of few specialties are hard and fast: the nephrologist will need to be able to read kidney biopsies as well as or better than his colleague in pathology; specialists in respiratory diseases would not consider it appropriate to ask a radiologist to interpret chest X-ray films for them. Any clinical specialty is in fact a mixture of fields such as pathology, anatomy, physiology, biochemistry, pharmacology, and psychology; what defines the specialty is its focus rather than a unique kind of knowledge or skill.

Thus, family medicine subsumes a range of content areas and an orientation distinctively different from those of the other specialties because of its functional role in medical practice. The last ten years have described this range of content and orientation with some degree of specificity, as noted in the chapters outlining undergraduate and graduate teaching programs. In fact, family practice has already developed more specific educational objectives than exist in many specialties. That there is overlap of content with many other specialties is undeniable, but substantial overlap exists among most specialties in medicine.

As summarized in the preceding chapter, considerable progress has been made during the last decade in the definition of research goals and content areas, as well as in the development of research methods applicable in family practice. This progress can be measured in several ways, such as (1) the initiation of fellowship programs for faculty development of research skills, (2) the increasing participation of family physicians in the North American Primary Care Research Group, (3) the creation of a scientific journal in the specialty fostering a growing literature base of original work in the field (Figure 16–3), and (4) the growing awareness within the field that an active research base is the life blood of the specialty's clinical and teaching functions.

Organizational Development

Excellent progress was made by several kinds of organizations during the 1970s in support of the developing specialty of family practice. Perhaps most noteworthy is the American Board of Family Practice (ABFP), which with more than 19,000 diplomates has already become one of the largest American specialty boards. In the last five years, only the American Board of Internal Medicine has certified more diplomates than the ABFP.[1] Figure 16–4 illustrates the growth in numbers of family physicians certified by the ABFP, and Table 16–7 presents a profile of the characteristics of these diplomates.

The American Board of Family Practice has developed several innovative approaches that are likely to have considerable influence on the process of

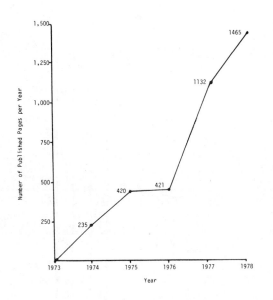

FIGURE 16-3.
Published pages in the *Journal of Family Practice* (1973–1978).

specialty certification in the United States. The ABFP was the first among American specialty boards to require all diplomates to pass the certification examination (no "grandfathering") and to impose compulsory periodic re-certification (every six years).[1] The ABFP has also taken a leadership role by including a practice-audit component in the recertification process.

The American Academy of Family Physicians (AAFP) has played a principal role in the initiation and subsequent nurturing of family practice as a specialty. Second in size only to the American Medical Association among medical organizations in the United States, the AAFP has been involved in a wide range of activities, including faculty development; consultation to teaching programs; continuing medical education; liaison with other medical organizations and government and other groups; and related organizational functions.

The Society of Teachers of Family Medicine (STFM) was established in 1968 as an academic organization concerned primarily with the development of the educational content of family medicine and the improvement of teaching skills among family practice faculty. This organization has grown to a membership of over 1400, including not only family physicians but also others involved in the teaching of family medicine, such as behavioral scientists, social workers, and other health care professionals. The STFM is represented on the Council of Academic Societies of the Association of American Medical Colleges and functions in a liaison capacity with a variety of academic, professional, and government organizations. The major activities of the STFM include faculty development, curriculum development, evaluation, and to a lesser extent, research.

The most recent family practice organization to develop is the Association of Chairmen of Departments of Family Medicine. This group provides a forum

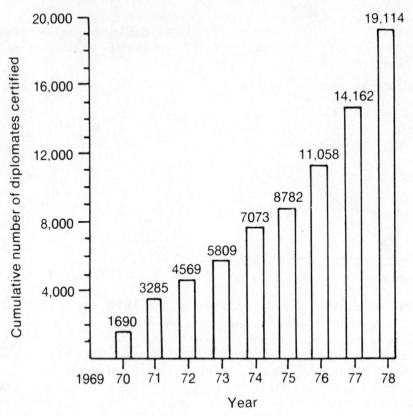

FIGURE 16-4.

Diplomates certified by the American Board of Family Practice.

TABLE 16-7.   PROFILE OF DIPLOMATES OF THE AMERICAN BOARD OF FAMILY PRACTICE—
1970–1978

80.0% were members of the American Academy of Family Physicians
47.5% were located in communities of less than 100,000 in population
52.5% were located in communities of over 100,000 population
35.0% were in partnership or group family practice
35.0% were in solo family practice
24.0% were less than 34 years of age
23.0% had completed full three-year family practice residency programs
 8.0% were over 60 years of age
 7.0% were involved in full-time teaching
 2.0% were also board-certified in another specialty (most commonly internal medicine and
       pediatrics)

Data provided by Nicholas Pisacano, M.D., Secretary, American Board of Family Practice, University of Kentucky, Lexington, Kentucky. This information is based on surveys of 19,114 diplomates of the ABFP certified between 1970 and 1978.

for chairmen of medical school departments of family medicine to share information and address common issues and problems related to the academic and organizational development of the field in medical schools and affiliated community settings.

Although not exclusively a family practice organization, the North American Primary Care Research Group, established in the mid-1970s, is playing an increasingly important role in the promotion of research in family practice. The annual meetings of this informal, apolitical organization are devoted to the presentation and critique of original work in the primary care disciplines, and provide meaningful faculty development experiences in terms of research methods and skills.

COMMENT

Excellent progress has been made during the first ten years of the development of family practice. Most of the initial organizational issues have been successfully addressed, and there is now general consensus that family practice is not only viable as a specialty but as an essential part of the changing health care system.

At the same time, however, it is clear that the development of any specialty is a long-term evolutionary process and that some of its important needs cannot be approached or met until the more pressing initial organizational efforts have been completed.[12] This is quite true of family practice, which has now embarked upon a second phase of further development and maturation.[4]

The issues today are quite different than those encountered by the emerging specialty in the late 1960s and early 1970s. The most urgent needs today can be summarized as follows:

INCREASED NUMBERS OF FAMILY PRACTICE FACULTY

Many of the family practice teaching programs in operation today are still short of qualified faculty, and this shortage is exacerbated by the need to further expand the capacity of these programs at both undergraduate and graduate levels. It can be anticipated, however, that a variety of faculty development efforts now underway, combined with a steadily growing pool of potential teachers trained in family practice residencies, will gradually alleviate this problem in the next few years.

EXPANSION OF FAMILY PRACTICE TEACHING PROGRAMS

As previously discussed, the present national goal calls for expansion of the capacity of family practice residencies to accommodate 25 percent of United States medical graduates by 1985. Even this goal may ultimately fall short of the public's need for primary care services by broadly trained family physicians. It is likely that some form of National Health Insurance (NHI) will be enacted during the next few years. Table 16–8 shows current federal projections for demand-based requirements for primary care physicians in the United States to 1990 based upon three estimated rates of utilization of services, any one of which will require a major increase in the number of practicing family physicians.[13] More family practice teaching programs are still needed together with the expansion of many existing programs.

STRENGTHENING OF THE FAMILY PRACTICE BASE
IN MEDICAL SCHOOLS
Although some of the departments of family practice are already quite well established, many are still short of faculty, funding, space, and curriculum time. The development of a strong base in medical schools will invariably call for additional resources as are essential to the mission of these departments and to their effective interface with other departments and with affiliated programs in the community.

REFINEMENT OF QUALITY-CONTROL MECHANISMS
IN TEACHING PROGRAMS
A good start has been made in the development of useful evaluation and monitoring techniques to assess the quality of individual student/resident learning experiences and the various elements of the teaching program. Further refinement of these approaches is a high priority as the capacity of these programs is expanded.

INCREASED FUNDING
Present funding of family practice programs is a somewhat unstable combination of federal, state, and local support together with revenue from patient care. Since the clinical income of family practice programs is relatively low compared to the more procedure-oriented specialties, and because the teaching commitments of these programs are quite high, there is an urgent need to stabilize their funding. This will require ongoing state and federal support, as well as a revision of reimbursement policies to more adequately cover the range of services provided by family physicians.

DEVELOPMENT OF RESEARCH BASE
Although some progress has been made in the definition of research goals and the development of research methods applicable to family practice, visible and respected examples of research programs and researchers have not yet emerged in most family practice settings in the United States. This deficit has been partly due to the overriding initial priority of organizational and teaching efforts in developing programs and partly due to the lack of experience and skills in research among most family practice faculty and practitioners. As stressed in the preceding chapter, the development of a vigorous research base in family practice is absolutely essential to the future of this specialty and to the quality of its teaching and patient care functions.

TABLE 16–8. DEMAND–BASED REQUIREMENTS FOR PRIMARY CARE PHYSICIANS UNDER NATIONAL HEALTH INSURANCE*

PRIMARY CARE PHYSICIANS	1975			1980			1990		
	1975 Utilization Rate	30 Percent Increase	75 Percent Increase	1975 Utilization Rate	30 Percent Increase	75 Percent Increase	1975 Utilization Rate	30 Percent Increase	75 Percent Increase
Total	93,780	121,910	164,120	97,990	127,390	171,480	107,910	140,280	188,840
General and family practice	61,570	80,040	107,750	64,900	84,370	113,580	71,400	92,820	124,950
Pediatrics	15,000	19,500	26,250	14,300	18,590	25,030	15,910	20,680	27,840
Internal medicine	17,210	22,370	30,120	18,790	24,430	32,880	20,600	26,780	36,050

* Calculations based on 1975 utilization rates and specified increases in those rates.

Sources: (1) National Center for Health Statistics: *Current Estimates from the Health Interview Survey*, United States, 1975, DHEW Publication No. (HRA) 77–1543, plus unpublished tabulations. (2) Bureau of the Census, projections of the population of the United States, 1975–2050, *Current Population Reports*, Series P–25, No. 601, October, 1975 and No. 643, January, 1977. (3) C.E. Phelps and J.P. Newhouse, Coinsurance, the price of time and demand for medical source. *Review of Economics and Statistics* 56:334, August, 1974. Quoted in *Physician Manpower Requirements*. GMENAC Staff Papers. Washington, D.C., DHEW Publication No. (HRA) 78–10, 1978. p. 34.

As mentioned in an earlier chapter, the 1966 report of the Ad Hoc Committee for Family Practice, established by the American Medical Association, was instrumental in the genesis and early development of family practice as a specialty. Eleven years later, this group met again in 1977 to reconsider the progress, problems, and needs of the specialty. All of the initial recommendations were reviewed, and new recommendations were made for the specialty's further development. Table 16–9 lists both the original and new recommendations of this group.[1]

In summary, the progress made by family practice during the 1970s has been quite remarkable. Family practice has already demonstrated its viability as an essential and major specialty in medicine, and its future is one of promise and further maturation.

TABLE 16–9. RECOMMENDATIONS OF THE AD HOC COMMITTEE FOR FAMILY PRACTICE (WILLARD COMMITTEE)

ORIGINAL RECOMMENDATION	NEW RECOMMENDATION
1. Major efforts should be instituted promptly to encourage the development of new programs for the education of large numbers of family physicians for the future, as described in the body of this report. The educational programs should relate to all levels of medical education, including premedical preparation, medical school education, internship and residency training, and continuing medical education. Keynotes should be excellence comparable with programs in other specialties and flexibility to permit the design of programs that will meet the needs and interests of individual physicians.	Major efforts should continue to increase the number and size of modern educational programs for family practice at all levels of medical education. It is particularly important to develop strong family practice programs in medical schools, because medical school experience usually exerts a strong influence on the career choices of medical students. Without a strong department, many students may fail to consider family practice as a career choice because they know nothing about it. The keynotes for such programs should continue to be excellence and flexibility. A goal should be established to have 25 percent of the graduates of United States medical schools enter residency training in family practice by 1985.
2. Medical schools and teaching hospitals should be urged to explore the possibility of developing models of family practice, in cooperation with the practicing profession.	Every family practice program, whether in an urban or a rural setting, should provide the opportunity for experience in a model of family practice. The model of family practice continues to be an absolute essential for a family practice program; without a satisfactory model, the family practice program is not worthy of the name. Flexibility in the design of the model should be permitted, provided that the essential characteristics of the model are maintained, as described in the original Ad Hoc Committee report.

TABLE 16–9.   Continued

ORIGINAL RECOMMENDATION	*NEW RECOMMENDATION*
3. New sources of financial assistance should be developed for the support of family practice teaching programs. Substantial funds should be made available for all aspects of the programs, including the conduct of the educational program, the recruitment and training of full-time faculty, the development of facilities and models of family practice, and the conduct of research in patient care and community medicine.	Adequate, sustained financial support should be provided for the development of new programs and for the maintenance and expansion of existing educational programs in family practice. The financial support is necessary at both undergraduate and graduate levels, for the development of facilities and models of family practice, for the stipends of residents, for the recruitment and training of faculty, and for the conduct of appropriate research. The sources of financial support should be diversified, and the use of the funds should be as unrestricted as possible to permit flexibility and originality in the design of educational programs. Reimbursement policies of third-party payers should be modified to permit full funding of health care services in ambulatory settings and particularly in models of family practice.
4. Recognition and status equivalent to other medical specialties should be given to family practice. An appropriate system of specialty certification should be provided for those who have completed approved educational programs and have demonstrated their competence as family physicians. The graduate program, i.e., internship–residency program, should be an integrated whole and evaluated for accreditation by one body rather than two.	The Committee believes that the ABFP satisfies the need for recognition of those who take specialty training in family practice and that the board has achieved status comparable with that of other specialty boards. The committee has no new recommendation to offer in this area.
5. Careful attention should be given to other factors that should make the environment for family practice more favorable and serve as incentives to medical students and young physicians to enter this field.	Continued attention should be given to factors that will make the environment for family practice more favorable and increase the attractiveness of the field to medical students, residents, and faculty members. The AMA, the American Hospital Association, and the Joint Commission on Accreditation of Hospitals should take steps to ensure that family physicians can obtain practice privileges commensurate with their education and demonstrated competence and without arbitrary restrictions. There should be further study of the use of physician extenders by family physicians and of the function of family physicians with other allied health personnel, with particular reference to compensation for services provided and the possibility of

TABLE 16–9   Continued

ORIGINAL RECOMMENDATION	*NEW RECOMMENDATION*
	reduction in the cost of medical care. Improvement of the academic environment for family practice will require that the status and recognition of family practice faculty be enhanced through the development of appropriate areas for scholarly investigation, probably in the social and behavioral sciences. Assistance should be provided to family practice faculty with limited teaching and research experience to develop competence and confidence in these important activities.
6. Careful study should be made of the effect of premedical programs and the admission procedures, curricula, and student evaluation policies of medical schools upon the production of family physicians.	No additional recommendation

ADDITIONAL RECOMMENDATIONS

Preceptorships	—Further emphasis should be given to the development of well-planned and well-conducted preceptorship programs in family practice at both undergraduate and graduate levels of medical education. The possibility should be explored of developing residency programs that make extensive use of preceptorships with group practices of good quality and with highly qualified individual physicians, as a basic part of the educational experience.
Regulation of residencies	—There should be full and free access to residency training in all specialty fields of medicine. It would not be in the public interest or in the interest of the field of family practice to restrict entrance to residency training or to have regulation of the number, type, and location of residency programs or positions, either by a federal agency or by an agency in the private sector.
Geographic distribution of physicians	—The Committee commends the AAFP for carrying out careful studies of the distribution and function of graduates of family practice residency programs and recommends that such studies be continued and expanded in the future to provide an evaluation of the impact of the family practice movement.

REFERENCES

1. Willard WA, Ruhe CHW: The challenge of family practice reconsidered. JAMA 240:454, 1978
2. Stern TL, Chaisson GM: The Residency Assistance Program in family practice. J Fam Pract 5:379, 1977
3. Description of salaried medical school faculty, 1971–72 and 1976–77. Washington, D.C., Association of American Medical Colleges, 1977, p 26
4. Longenecker DP, Wright JC, Gillen JC: Profile of full-time family practice educators. J Fam Pract 4:111, 1977
5. Collins F, Roessler R: Intellectual and attitudinal characteristics of medical students selecting family practice. J Fam Pract 2:431, 1975
6. Garg ML, Mulligan JL, Gliebe WA, Parekh RR: Physician specialty, quality and cost of inpatient care. Soc Sci Med (to be published)
7. Ely JW, Ueland K, Gordon MJ: An audit of obstetric care in a university family medicine department and an obstetrics–gynecology department. J Fam Pract 3:397, 1976
8. Phillips WR, Rice GA, Layton RH: Audit of obstetrical care and outcome in family medicine, obstetrics and general practice. J Fam Pract 6:1209, 1978
9. Family Practice in Hospitals. Kansas City, Missouri, American Academy of Family Physicians, 1977
10. Engel GL: The need for a new medical model: A challenge for biomedicine. Science 196:129, 1977
11. Draper P, Smits HL: The primary-care practitioner—specialist or jack-of-all trades. N Engl J Med 293:904, 1975
12. Geyman JP: Family practice in evolution: Progress, problems and projections. N Engl J Med 298:593, 1978
13. Physician Manpower Requirements. GMENAC Staff Papers. Washington, D.C. DHEW Publication No. (HRA) 78–10, 1978, p 34

Epilogue

Human ills are too personalized and individualized to fit the tight frame of any specialty for long. The more technically confined the specialty, the more it needs the generalist, since the patient's problems can extend so readily beyond its categorical perimeters.

Edmund D. Pellegrino [1]

This book has sketched some of the major problems of today's health care system in the United States (many prefer to call it a nonsystem). Within this context, the first decade of development of family practice has been examined, for this phenomenon can only be understood by reference to the specialty's larger environment. It is now useful to further broaden our view in order to gain perspective of the anticipated future role of family practice in a changing health care system.

Medical education in the United States is over 200 years old. Since the first medical graduate in 1770, the medical profession in this country has grown to over 400,000 physicians. Specialism is little more than 60 years old, and family practice as a primary care specialty is only about 10 years old.

The last 40 years have seen a rapid and vast development of medical technology. Increasing specialization has not only evolved from biomedical advances, but also in large part has been responsible for them. However, a paradoxical situation has developed. Despite the potential availability of a remarkable level of technical excellence and a high quality of medical care, such care cannot be provided to all of the country's expanding population. The process of health care is proceeding rapidly in the direction of fragmentation and de-personalization. With the decline of the general practitioner, as Freidson[2] has observed:

> . . . the layman has had less and less chance to gain responsiveness from professionals to his own views. And as the state comes to intervene more and more—a state which has become so large and formal as to be rather distant from the lives of its citizens, and whose notions of public good are guided largely by professionals—the individual has even less opportunity to express and gain his own ends. Some way of redressing the balance must be found.

It is now apparent that this country is at an important turning point in the development of medicine. At many levels, both within and outside of the medical profession, serious reevaluation is taking place in an effort to devise a health care system that can better cope with the exponential increase in need and demand for health care services. Although the shape and function of the future health care system in the United States is inevitably unclear due to the large number of variables involved, it is germane to list some of the lessons of the last 30 years about which there can be little disagreement.

It is clear that today's health care system needs reorganization. The cost of health care is rapidly approaching the limits of what can be afforded, and there is much duplication in the present system. It is difficult to demonstrate the cost-benefit of many procedures and approaches in today's medical practice. There are many existing barriers to health care that preclude even basic medical care for many people.

It is clear that simply increasing the total number of physicians available for patient care is not enough. An oversupply of physicians exists in many fields, yet there are acute shortages in other fields. The more specialized in a narrow field that physicians become, the less productive they are in terms of patient care. As Millis[3] has observed, "The more sophisticated, the higher the level of competence of anyone of us, the less productive we are. . . . The fact is that medicine year-by-year becomes less productive."

It is likewise clear that the most critical shortage of physicians is in the area of primary care. It is here where the greatest opportunity lies to improve the state of health in the general population. Health care is now more diverse and complex, and coordination of care on an individual and family basis becomes more vital each year.

The shift of emphasis to primary care in recent years has posed a vexing conceptual and educational problem to a number of the traditional specialties, particularly internal medicine, pediatrics, and obstetrics–gynecology. These specialties have faced the dilemma of clarifying their present and future roles as consultants or generalists. This is a somewhat schizoid task, for excellence in both roles simultaneously is a conflictual goal. This situation has led to some degree of competition between these specialties and family practice. Territorial disputes of this nature, however, will inevitably turn, as they should, on the capacity of each discipline to meet societal needs, not on the vested interest of any of the specialties themselves.

As a specialty in breadth, family practice is neither encumbered by the generalist–consultant dilemma nor limited by age or sex with respect to its patient population. Earlier chapters have documented the extent to which family practice is meeting the needs of the public for primary health care.

It is likely that much of the present debate about primary care will resolve in the next few years as the interests and needs of each specialty become clarified and tested against societal needs. The Ad Hoc Committee for Family Practice of the American Medical Association currently views this issue as follows [4]:

> The Committee is aware that efforts are being made to emphasize residency education in general internal medicine, general pediatrics, and general obstetrics and gynecology, in preference to subspecialty education in those disciplines, in the hope that this will meet the need for more physicians prepared specifically to provide primary care. While these efforts are commendable, the Committee believes that there is a greater probability that the graduates of family practice residencies will function as family physicians providing primary care than that this function will be assumed by the graduates of other kinds of residency programs. Consequently, the Committee believes that the needs of the public for more family physicians are most likely to be met by increasing the number of residents in family practice.

Pellegrino [5] sees the evolution of primary care in similar terms:

> General internal medicine itself has a problematic future. I believe it has a unique and legitimate role in secondary and tertiary care under special circumstances.[6] The general internist certainly can also function as a personal physician for adults, and the general pediatrician can do so for children. But if the general internist and the pediatrician intend to assume the care of the family, they must augment their skills as generalists with special knowledge of the care of the family and the age groups each now excludes. Under these circumstances, they become de facto family physicians. It is more likely that general internal medicine and pediatrics will merge gradually with family medicine, and that much of the current stress among them will be slowly dissipated.

Public expectations of medicine may well be unrealistic in many respects, but the pressures to change the system in an attempt to better meet the perceived needs of the public have become strong. Though the challenges facing medicine today are great, there is much room for optimism. From our present acute sense of awareness of our deficiencies and the active reappraisal of our resources and methods of practice will come a better health care system. In 1964, Lester

James M. Gall, M.D., C.C.F.P.
Department of Family Medicine
University of Miami School of Medicine
P. O. Box 016700
Miami, Florida 33101

Evans[7] called for rediscovery of the medical student as the reason for medical education and the patient as the reason for medicine. This is now starting to take place.

The challenge now before medicine is to participate constructively in the reassessment and remodeling of the health care system to extend the highest possible quality of care to the entire population at a cost that can be afforded in a society approaching the limits of what can be allocated from its gross national product to health care. Although by no means a panacea for all the problems of this country's health care system, the continued successful development of family practice as the foundation of primary care in the United States is an important part of this remodeling process and represents an effective response to existing and projected deficits in primary health care.

REFERENCES

1. Pellegrino ED: The academic viability of family medicine: A triad of challenges. JAMA 240:132, 1978
2. Freidson E: Profession of Medicine: A Study of the Sociology of Applied Knowledge. New York, Dodd, Mead, 1970, p 352
3. Millis JS: The future of medicine. JAMA 210:500, 1969
4. Willard WR, Ruhe CHW: The challenge of family practice reconsidered. JAMA 240:455, 1978
5. Pellegrino ED: The academic viability of family medicine: A triad of challenges. JAMA 240:135, 1978
6. Pellegrino ED: Internal medicine and the functions of the generalist: Some notes on a new synergy. Clin Res 24:252, 1976
7. Evans LJ: The crisis in medical education. Ann Arbor, Michigan, University of Michigan Press, 1964

National Health Planning Guidelines*

PART 121—NATIONAL GUIDELINES FOR HEALTH PLANNING

Subpart A—General Provisions

Sec.
121.1   Definitions.
121.2   Purpose and scope.
121.3   Applicability of national guidelines to Health Systems Plans.
121.4   Applicability of national guidelines to State health plans.
121.5   Responsibility of health systems agencies.
121.6   Adjustment of standards for particular Health Systems Plans.

---

* From: Department of Health, Education, and Welfare, Public Health Service: Health planning—National guidelines. *Federal Register* 43:13044, 1978.

Subpart B—National Health Planning Goals

[Reserved]

Subpart C—Standards Respecting the Appropriate Supply, Distribution, and Organization of Health Resources

121.201   General hospitals—Supply.
121.202   General hospitals—Occupancy rate.
121.203   Obstetrical services.
121.204   Neonatal special care units.
121.205   Pediatric inpatient services—Number of beds.
121.206   Pediatric inpatient services—Occupancy rates.
121.207   Open heart surgery.
121.208   Cardiac catheterization.
121.209   Radiation therapy.
121.210   Computed tomographic scanners.
121.211   End-stage renal disease (ESRD).

AUTHORITY: Sec. 1501 of the Public Health Service Act, 88 Stat. 2227 (41 U.S.C. 300k-1).

§ 121.1   DEFINITIONS.
Terms used herein shall have the meanings given them in 42 CFR 122.1.

§ 121.2   PURPOSE AND SCOPE.
Section 1501 of the Public Health Service Act requires the Secretary to issue, by regulation, national guidelines for health planning. The guidelines are to include national health planning goals (section 1501 (b) (2)) and standards respecting the supply, distribution, and organization of health resources (section 1501 (b) (1)). This subpart includes general provisions applicable to such goals and standards; subpart B of this part sets forth specific national health planning goals; and subpart C sets forth specific standards respecting the supply, distribution, and organization of health resources.

§ 121.3   APPLICABILITY OF NATIONAL GUIDELINES TO
          HEALTH SYSTEMS PLANS.
Section 1513 (b) (2) of the Act requires health systems agencies, in the development of their Health Systems Plans, to give "appropriate consideration" to the national guidelines for health planning. Health Systems Plans must also "take into account" and be "consistent with" the standards respecting the supply, distribution, and organization of health resources set forth in subpart C.
  (a) *Meaning of "consistent with."* A Health Systems Plan will be considered

"consistent with" a standard set forth in subpart C where it (1) establishes a target level which is not in excess of the level set forth in the standard where that level is stated as a maximum, or not less than the level set forth in the standard where that level is stated as a minimum, except where a specific adjustment is justified in accordance with subpart C or § 121.6 of this subpart, and (2) includes plans which, if implemented, are reasonably calculated to achieve that target level within five years.

(b) *Effective date.* Health Systems Plans established after December 31, 1978, must be "consistent with" each standard set forth in subpart C.

§ 121.4   APPLICABILITY OF NATIONAL GUIDELINES TO
STATE HEALTH PLANS.

Each State's State health plan developed under Title XV of the act must be "made up of" the Health Systems Plans of the health systems agencies within the state, revised as found necessary by the Statewide Health Coordinating Council to achieve their appropriate coordination with each other or to deal more effectively with Statewide health needs. (Section 1524(c)(2)(A) of the Act.) Since Health Systems Plans must individually give appropriate consideration to the national guidelines for health planning and take into account and be consistent with the standards respecting the supply, distribution, and organization of health resources, the State health plan will accordingly reflect the guidelines.

§ 121.5   RESPONSIBILITY OF HEALTH SYSTEMS AGENCIES.

Subject to the authority of the Statewide Health Coordinating Council to require the revision of Health Systems Plans under section 1524(c)(2)(A) of the Act, each health systems agency is responsible for analyzing the needs and conditions in its health service area and applying the national guidelines for health planning in the development of its Health Systems Plan, including the need for adjustments.

§ 121.6   ADJUSTMENTS OF STANDARDS FOR PARTICULAR
HEALTH SYSTEMS PLANS.

Subpart C of this part includes provisions for adjustment of individual standards. In addition:

(a) Health systems agencies must make such adjustments as may be necessary:

(1) To take into account special needs and circumstances of Health Maintenance Organizations;

(2) To take into account services available to local residents from Federal health care facilities; and

(3) To take into account higher minimum target levels and lower maximum levels that are established for State Certificate-of-Need and related programs.

(b) Whenever a health systems agency concludes, on the basis of a detailed analysis, that development of a Health Systems Plan consistent with one or more of the standards set forth in subpart C would result in:

(1) Residents of the health service area not having access to necessary health services;

(2) Significantly increased costs of care for a substantial number of patients in the area; or

(3) The denial of care to persons with special needs resulting from moral and ethical values; and that result cannot be avoided through use of the adjustments specifically provided for in the standard or in paragraph (a) of this section. The agency may include in the Health Systems Plan a special adjustment of the standard or standards which will avoid this result. Whenever a special adjustment is so included, the plan must also contain a detailed justification for the adjustment and documentation of the circumstances that are the basis of the justification. In the case of an adjustment included on the basis of (1) or (2) above, the plan must further include an analysis indicating whether the need for such an adjustment is permanent. If it is, the supporting rationale must be documented and if it is not, an estimate must be included of how long inclusion of the adjustment will be required along with a detailed justification for that length of time.

(c) Any proposed adjustment under this section and the analyses supporting it must be reviewed by the State health planning and development agency in its preparation or review of the preliminary State health plan under section 1523 (a) (2) of the Act and by the Statewide Health Coordinating Council in its preparation or review of the State health plan under section 1524 (c) (2) of the Act. On the basis of that review, and consistent with Statewide health needs and the need to coordinate Health Systems Plans as determined by the Statewide Health Coordinating Council, the adjustment may be made part of the State health plan. The Statewide Health Coordinating Council shall report its comments on and disposition of the proposed adjustments to the Secretary under section 1524 (c) (1) of the Act.

§ 121.201   GENERAL HOSPITALS—BED SUPPLY.

(a) *Standard*. There should be less than four non-Federal, short-stay hospital beds for each 1,000 persons in a health service area except under extraordinary circumstances. For purposes of this section, short-stay hospital beds include all non-federal short-stay hospital beds (including general medical/surgical, children's, obstetric, psychiatric, and other short-stay specialized beds). Conditions which may justify adjustments to this ratio for a health service area include:

(1) *Age*. Individuals 65 years of age and older have a higher hospital utilization rate—up to four times that of the general population—than any other age group. Bed-population ratios for health service areas in which the percentage of elderly people is significantly higher (more than 12 percent of the population) than the national average may be planned at a higher ratio, based on analyses by the HSA.

(2) *Seasonal population fluctuations*. Large seasonal variations in hospital utilization may justify higher ratios. Plans should reflect vacation and recreation

patterns as well as the needs of migrant workers and other factors causing unusual seasonal variations.

(3) *Rural areas.* Hospital care should be accessible within a reasonable period of time. For example, in rural areas in which a majority of the residents would otherwise be more than 30 minutes travel time from a hospital, the HSA may determine, based on analyses, that a bed-population ratio of greater than 4 per 1,000 persons may be justified.

(4) *Urban areas.* Large numbers of beds in one part of a Standard Metropolitan Statistical Area (SMSA) may be compensated for by fewer beds in other parts of the SMSA. Health service areas which include a part of an SMSA may plan for bed-population ratios higher than 4 per 1,000 persons reflecting existing patterns if there is a joint plan among all HSAs serving the SMSA which provides for less than 4 beds per 1,000 persons in the SMSA as a whole.

(5) *Areas with referral hospitals.* In the case of referral institutions which provide a substantial portion of specialty services to individuals not residing in the area, the HSA may exclude from its computation of bed-population ratio the beds utilized by referred patients who reside outside both the SMSA and the HSA in which the facility is located.

(b) *Discussion.* There is general agreement that the number of general hospital beds in the United States is significantly in excess of what is needed and that utilization of acute in-patient care resources is often higher than necessary. Excess bed capacity and use contribute to the high cost of hospital care with little or no health benefits. Empty beds are often filled by patients who could be cared for as well or better in less expensive ways, such as ambulatory care or home care.

The Institute of Medicine's Report on "Controlling the Supply of Hospital Beds" in 1976 recommended that the nation should achieve at least a 10 percent reduction in the bed population ratio in the next five years and further significant reductions thereafter. The Institute statement noted: "This would mean a reduction from the current national average of approximately 4.4 non-Federal short-term general hospital beds per 1,000 population to a national average of approximately 4 in five years and well below that in the years to follow." Similarly a study reported by Inter-Study of Minneapolis, Minn., the same year concluded that a 10 percent reduction in hospital bed supply would be a desirable and reasonable first step toward reducing excess hospital capacity. As part of the process for determining this standard, the Department reviewed projections in State health facilities planning plans. Such plans have set targets for future hospital bed supply that, on an aggregate nationwide basis, project just under 4 beds per thousand. Many States set lower targets. Health Maintenance Organizations and similar groups have shown that high quality care can be provided with less than 3 beds per 1,000 population. Thus, 4 beds per 1,000 population is a ceiling, not an ideal situation. HSAs are expected to identify the desirable local ratio, working closely with the State Health Planning and development Agency and the Statewide Health Coordinating Council. It is anticipated that in subsequent plans HSAs will be required to indicate how they will reach a bed-population ratio of less than 3.7 per 1,000 population except under extraordinary circumstances. HSAs whose areas are now below the 4 per 1,000 level are urged to attempt to decrease bed-population ratios below 3.7 per 1,000 population. In areas where Federal medical facilities and Health Maintenance Organizations provide substantial services to local residents, lower ratios should be readily achieveable. Population growth must be carefully analyzed; in many cases, this factor alone will bring the area below the target level if no unnecessary additional beds are built. Under some conditions, a higher target ceiling may be justified by the HSA. Travel distance to the nearest hospital is one of the most important factors to be analyzed, especially in rural areas. A planning criteria of 30 minutes has been set, in line with the policies of many local and State health planning agencies around the country. In analyzing ways of reducing bed supply, it should be recognized that greater savings will be achieved when entire facilities are considered. In developing such plans, priority consideration should be given to maintaining and strengthening resources that are emphasizing activities identified as national health priorities in section 1502 of the Act.

§ 121.202   GENERAL HOSPITALS—OCCUPANCY RATE.

(a)   *Standard.* There should be an average annual occupancy rate for medically necessary hospital care of at least 80 percent for all non-Federal, short-stay hospital beds considered together in a health service area, except under extraordinary circumstances. Conditions which may justify an adjustment to this standard for a health service area include:

(1) *Seasonal population fluctuations.* In some areas, the influx of people for vacation or other purposes may require a greater supply of hospital beds than would otherwise be needed. Large seasonal variations in hospital utilization which can be predicted through hospital and health insurance records may justify an average annual occupancy rate lower than 80 percent based on analyses by the HSA.

(2) *Rural areas.* Lower average annual occupancy rates are usually required by small hospitals to maintain empty beds to accommodate normal fluctuations of admissions. In rural areas with significant numbers of small (fewer than 4,000 admissions per year) hospitals, an average occupancy rate of less than 80 percent may be justified, based on analyses by the HSA.

(b) *Discussion.* There is substantial evidence that excess capacity and use contribute significantly to high hospital costs. The 1976 report by the Institute of Medicine, for example, found that "there is a growing concern that the surpluses of hospital beds are contributing significantly to the recent rise of health care costs at a rate well beyond that of general inflation. This concern has not only to do with the cost of maintaining unused hospital bed capacity, but also with the unnecessary and inappropriate uses of hospital beds, especially those in the short-term care category." Occupancy rates currently average about 75 percent nationwide. Many hospital capacity studies, including those by

InterStudy and the Bureau of Hospital Administration of the University of Michigan, indicate that an average hospital occupancy rate exceeding 80 percent is a reasonable target. In addition, many State and local health planning agencies have established higher occupancy targets. For example, health planning agencies in Illinois, New Jersey, New York, Massachusetts, Michigan, and Wisconsin have recommended occupancy rates higher than 80 percent for larger hospitals. Higher averages have been advocated, especially for medical-surgical units. While past studies typically apply these rates to individual institutions, the Department, in line with the objectives of community-wide planning, has extended this concept to apply on an area-wide basis. Within local health service areas, hospitals of varying size and circumstances will have varying occupancy rates; a collective rate exceeding 80 percent on an area-wide basis is a reasonable, achievable goal except in rural areas and when situations present extraordinary circumstances. Increases are to be attained through constrained capacity growth and improved planning and management. It is not, of course, intended that increased rates be achieved through unnecessary hospital admissions or stays.

§ 121.203   OBSTETRICAL SERVICES.
(a) *Standard* (1) Obstetrical services should be planned on a regional basis with linkages among all obstetrical services and with neonatal services.

(2) Hospitals providing care for complicated obstetrical problems (Levels II and III) should have at least 1,500 births annually.

(3) There should be an average annual occupancy rate of at least 75 percent in each unit with more than 1,500 births per year.

(b) *Discussion.* The importance of developing regional systems of care for maternal and perinatal health services has been broadly recognized. The Committee on Perinatal Health, representing the American Academy of Family Physicians, American Academy of Pediatrics, American College of Obstetricians and Gynecologists, and the American Medical Association issued a report in 1976, "Toward Improving the Outcome of Pregnancy." The report identified opportunities to reduce rates of maternal, fetal and neonatal mortality as well as to improve deployment of scarce resources, especially those needed to provide comprehensive services for high-risk patients. The impact on quality of care of both under-utilization and over-utilization was emphasized.

The report states: "A systematized, cohesive regional network including a number of differentiated resources is the approach most likely to achieve the objective. Each component of the regional system must provide the highest quality care, but the degree of complexity of patient needs determines where, and by whom, the care should be provided." Level I hospitals provide services primarily for uncomplicated maternity and newborn cases. Level II hospitals provide services for uncomplicated cases and for the majority of complicated problems, and certain specialized neonatal services. Level II hospitals are able also to handle all the serious types of illness and abnormalities. Established arrangements should provide for early access of high-risk pregnant women and prompt referrals among levels of care as appropriate. Regional planning should include a cooperative, coordinated network of hospitals, physicians and other health care professionals, providing: (1) Expert consultation and referral, (2) basic and continuing education for health professionals and consumers, (3) transport of selected patients to facilities possessing more specialized maternal and neonatal services, (4) a continuing evaluation of the effectiveness and costs of regionalized programs. In 1972 the American College of Obstetrics and Gynecology identified a minimal target of 1,500 births per year for facilities in communities of 100,000 population or more to provide a full range of obstetrical services in an efficient manner. In 1974, this figure was revised: "The experience of many obstetric departments indicate that the size, equipment, services and personnel adequate to maintain a consistently high standard of ordinary obstetrical care and a reasonably economic operation generally require more than 2,000 deliveries." (Standards for Obstetrical and Gynecological Services, Committee on Professional Standards of the American College of Obstetricians and Gynecologists, 1974.) The Committee on Perinatal Health also identified the 2,000 minimum figure for facilities identified as Level II facilities. In determining the 1,500 target, the Department took into consideration these reports as well as the comments received from the public and from members of the expert advisory panel, particularly the criticism that a 2,000 target was too high. The 1,500 level is in line with the policies of many local and State health planning agencies and can help assure more economic use of specialized resources while avoiding inappropriate utilization of such facilities. The Department also recognizes that there are substantial differences among facilities which provide different ranges of services, and there are circumstances, such as those involving special moral and ethical preferences, which may necessitate the HSA providing an adjustment to this standard. In addition, in order to promote more economical use of resources the Department has established the 75 percent minimum occupancy rate in Level II and III facilities. The 75 percent figure was derived from an analysis of various occupancy rate figures in a number of source documents, whose recommendations range from 50 percent to over 80 percent. The Hill-Burton program recommended an occupancy level for obstetrical units of at least 75 percent. The Department anticipates that institutions operating at Levels II and III will usually be able to exceed this level.

In keeping with the national priority set forth in Section 1502 of the Act for the consolidation and coordination of institutional health services, the consolidation of multiple, small obstetrical units with low occupancy rates should be undertaken unless such action is undesirable because of needs to assure ready access and sensitive care.

§ 121.204   NEONATAL SPECIAL CARE UNITS.
(a) *Standard*. (1) Neonatal services should be planned on a regional basis with linkages with obstetrical services.

(2) The total number of neonatal intensive and intermediate care beds should

not exceed 4 per 1,000 live births per year in a defined neonatal service area. An adjustment upward may be justified when the rate of high-risk pregnancies is unusually high, based on analyses by the HSA.

(3) A single neonatal special care unit (Level II or III) should contain a minimum of 15 beds. An adjustment downward may be justified for a Level II unit when travel time to an alternate unit is a serious hardship due to geographic remoteness, based on analyses by the HSA.

(b) *Discussion.* For this standard, the Department has adopted the widely endorsed concept of regionalization, involving various levels of care. Under this concept, Level III units are staffed and equipped for the intensive care of newborns as well as intermediate and recovery care. Level II units provide intermediate and recovery care as well as some specialized services. Level I units provide recovery care. Neonatal special care is a highly specialized service required by only a very small percentage of infants. The Department believes that four neonatal special care beds for intensive and intermediate care per 1,000 live births will usually be adequate to meet the needs, taking into account the incidence of high risk pregnancies, the percentage of live births requiring intensive care, and the average length of stay. ("Bed" includes incubators or other heated units for specialized care and bassinettes.) In addition, the Department has established a minimum of 15 beds per unit for Levels II and III as the minimum number necessary to support economical operation for these services. Both standards are supported and recommended by the American Academy of Pediatrics. The American Academy of Pediatrics has noted that "the best care will be given to high-risk and seriously ill neonates if intensive care units are developed in a few adequately qualified institutions within a community rather than within many hospitals. Properly conducted, early transfer of these infants to a qualified unit provides better care than do attempts to maintain them in inadequate units." This regionalized approach is reflected in the minimum size standard which is designed to foster the location of specialized units in medical centers which have available special staff, equipment, and consultative services and facilities. Since perinatal centers, which include neonatal units will serve the patient load resulting from a representative population of more than one million, a defined neonatal service area should be identified by the relevant HSAs in conjunction with the State Agency. Special attention should also be given to ensure adequate communication and transportation systems, including joint transfers of mother and child and maintenance of family contact. Hospitals with such units should have agreements with other facilities to serve referred patients. The regional plan should include a structured ongoing system of review, including assessment of changes in health status indicators.

§ 121.205   PEDIATRIC INPATIENT SERVICES—NUMBER OF BEDS.

(a) *Standard.* There should be a minimum of 20 beds in a pediatric unit in urbanized areas. An adjustment downward may be justified when travel time to an alternate unit exceeds 30 minutes for 10 percent or more of the population, based on analyses by the HSA.

(b) *Discussion.* Pediatric services should be planned on a regionalized basis with linkages among hospitals and other health agencies to provide comprehensive care. The 1977 report of the Committee on Implications of Declining Pediatric Hospitalization Rates for the National Research Council states that "for a policy of housing children separately to be effective, certain minimum services and facilities are needed, thus requiring bed capacity utilization to make provision for these services and facilities economically feasible." This standard was developed by the Department in this context.

A number of sources support a minimum unit size of 20 pediatric beds, including planning agencies in California, Massachusetts, Ohio, Pennsylvania, and Wisconsin. Consolidation of pediatric care in units of at least 20 beds in urbanized areas will promote the concentration of nursing and support staff with special pediatric knowledge and skills, the increased training of staff, and the provision of special treatment and other ancillary facilities which meet the special needs of children. (A pediatric inpatient unit is a specific section, ward, wing, hospital or unit devoted primarily to the care of medical and surgical patients usually less than 18 years old, not including special care for infants.)

The criteria of 30 minutes travel time reflects interest in ensuring that children remain close to their homes, family and friends. Frequent visits to hospitalized children are highly desirable and can be an aid to improvement and recovery. The American Academy of Pediatrics has recommended to its State Chapters that child health plans should provide that primary care for children should be available within 30 minutes. This access standard is consistent with those of many local and State planning agencies such as those in Massachusetts, New York, Pennsylvania, and Wisconsin.

§ 121.206   PEDIATRIC INPATIENT SERVICES—OCCUPANCY RATES.

(a) *Standard.* Pediatric units should maintain average annual occupancy rates related to the number of pediatric beds (exclusive of neonatal special care units) in the facility. For a facility with 20–39 pediatric beds, the average annual occupancy rate should be at least 65 percent; for a facility with 40–79 pediatric beds, the rate should be at least 70 percent; for facilities with 80 or more pediatric beds, the rate should be at least 75 percent.

(b) *Discussion.* Variable occupancy rates are designed to reflect the need for smaller units to maintain the capacity to accommodate normal day-to-day fluctuations in admissions and to set aside pediatric beds for particular ages and types of cases. Such scheduling problems are less severe in pediatric units of a greater capacity. Moreover, large units are able to sustain higher occupancy rates because they are frequently associated with regional centers which serve patients needing types of care that can be scheduled on a more flexible basis. It is not intended, of course, to encourage unnecessary admissions or stays to achieve these levels. This standard is identical to that recommended by the American Academy of Pediatrics.

§ 121.207   OPEN HEART SURGERY.
(a) *Standard.* (1) There should be a minimum of 200 open heart procedures performed annually, within three years after initiation, in any institution in which open heart surgery is performed for adults.

(2) There should be a minimum of 100 pediatric heart operations annually, within three years after initiation, in any institution in which pediatric open heart surgery is performed, of which at least 75 should be open heart surgery.

(3) There should be no additional open heart units initiated unless each existing unit in the health service area(s) is operating and is expected to continue to operate at a minimum of 350 open heart surgery cases per year in adult services or 130 pediatric open heart cases in pediatric services.

(b) *Discussion.* Open heart surgery for congenital and acquired heart and coronary artery disease represents a marked advance in patient care. Highly specialized open heart procedures require very costly, highly specialized man-power and facility resources. Thus, every effort should be made to limit dupli-cation and unnecessary resources related to the performance of open heart procedures, while maintaining high quality care. Minimum case loads are essential to maintain and strengthen skills. (Open heart surgery procedures are defined as procedures which use a heart-lung by-pass machine to perform the functions of circulation during surgery.) A minimum of 200 adult open heart surgery procedures should be performed annually within an institution to main-tain quality of patient care and make most efficient use of resources. This standard is based on recommendations of the Inter-Society Commission on Heart Disease Resources. In order to prevent duplication of costly resources which are not fully utilized, the opening of new units should be contingent upon existing units operating, and continuing to operate, at a level of at least 350 procedures per year. The 350 level assumes an average of 7 operations a week, a schedule that in the Department's judgement is feasible in most institutions providing these services to children, lower targets are indicated because of the special needs involved. The established level for pediatric units is consistent with the recom-mendation of the Pediatric Cardiology Section of the American Academy of Pediatrics. In determining the utilization target of 130 pediatric open heart cases, the Department used the same ratio as for adult units. In the case of units that provide services to both adults and children, at least 200 open heart procedures should be performed, including 75 for children. In some areas, open heart surgical teams, including surgeons and specialized technologists, are utilizing more than one institution. For these institutions, the guidelines may be applied to the combined number of open heart procedures performed by the surgical team where and adjustment is justifiable in line with Section 121.6(B) and promotes more cost effective use of available facilities and support personnel. In such cases, in order to maintain quality care a minimum of 75 open heart procedures in any institution is advisable, which is consistent with recommendations of the American College of Surgeons. Data collection and quality assessment and control activities should be part of all open heart surgery programs.

§ 121.208   CARDIAC CATHETERIZATION.

(a) *Standard.* (1) There should be a minimum of 300 cardiac catheterizations, of which at least 200 should be intracardiac or coronary artery catheterizations, performed annually in any adult cardiac catheterization unit within three years after initiation.

(2) There should be a minimum of 150 pediatric cardiac catheterizations performed annually in any unit performing pediatric cardiac catheterizations within three years after initiation.

(3) There should be no new cardiac catheterization unit opened in any facility not performing open heart surgery.

(4) There should be no additional adult cardiac catheterization unit opened unless the number of studies per year in each existing unit in the health service area(s) is greater than 560 and no additional pediatric unit opened unless the number of studies per year in each existing unit is greater than 250.

(b) *Discussion.* The modern cardiac catheterization unit requires a highly skilled staff and expensive equipment. Safety and efficacy of laboratory performance requires a case load of adequate size to maintain the skill and efficiency of the staff. In addition, the underutilized unit represents a less efficient use of an expensive resource and frequently reflects unnecessary duplication. Based on recommendations from the Inter-Society Commission on Heart Disease Resources, the Department believes that a minimum level of 300 catheterizations per year is indicated to achieve economic use of resources. Several State health planning agencies, such as New Jersey, suggested a higher minimum level and the Department will be considering whether a higher level should be established in the future. The Department has also determined the existing units should be performing more than 500 cardiac catheterizations or 250 pediatric cardiac catheterizations before a new unit is opened. The 500 level is based on an average of two catheterizations a day, a rate that is in the Department's judgement readily achievable in most institutions providing these services and that will foster more effective use of current resources prior to the development of additional resources. More than 600 procedures are performed annually in some institutions. Pediatric cardiac catheterizations require special facilities and support services. Lower target numbers are presented in these cases because of the special conditions and needs of children. The established levels are consistent with the recommendations of the Section on Cardiology of the American Academy of Pediatrics and the Inter-Society Commission on Heart Disease Resources. The patient studied in the cardiac catheterization unit is frequently recommended for open heart surgery. While acceptable inter-institutional referral patterns exist in some areas, cardiac catheterization units should optimally be located within a facility in which cardiac surgery is performed.

§ 121.209   RADIATION THERAPY.

(a) *Standard.* (1) A megavoltage radiation therapy unit should serve a population of at least 150,000 persons and treat at least 300 cancer cases annually, within three years after initiation.

(2) There should be no additional megavoltage units opened unless each existing megavoltage unit in the health service area(s) is performing at least 6,000 treatments per year.

(3) Adjustments downward may be justified when travel time to an alternate unit is a serious hardship due to geographic remoteness, based on analyses by the HSA.

(b) *Discussion.* While various types of radiation are indicated and used for tumors with different characteristics, megavoltage equipment is accepted as the most efficacious for treatment of deep-seated tumors. Megavoltage equipment is expensive to purchase, install, and support on a continuing basis. Every effort should thus be made to avoid unnecessary duplication of this costly resource. Established standards should provide needed treatment capabilities while preventing unnecessary duplication of radiation therapy units and under-utilization of existing capacity. A unit refers to a single megavoltage machine or energy source. The most common types of units to deliver megavoltage therapy are cobalt 60 and linear accelerators. Treatments are meant to be the same as patient visits. A treatment or visit averages 2.2 fields, according to reports from the American College of Radiology. It also reports that about half of new cancer patients require megavoltage radiation therapy, and that many require subsequent courses of treatment. The American College of Radiology has indicated that at least 300 cancer cases annually are a reasonable minimum load for a megavoltage radiation therapy unit in order to maintain an efficient high quality operation. Based on the information and recommendations of the College, as well as comments received from the public and from members of the expert advisory panel which reviewed the standard, the Department has set a minimum standard of at least 300 cancer cases per unit per year. In 1974, the Department commissioned a study of the use of radiation therapy units. A committee appointed by the American College of Radiology and the American Society of Therapeutic Radiology to review that study suggested that economical operation of radiation units would call for existing units to do 5,000–8,700 treatments per year. The 7,500 level was included in the September 23, 1977 NPRM. This target would have required units to treat an average of 30 patients per day. Based on comments received from the profession and the general public, the Department has adjusted the standard downwards to 6,000 treatments per year, an average of about 25 patients per day, to take into account variations in patient mix and work schedules. Since many institutions meet and exceed these targets, this standard in the Department's judgement represents an attainable, efficient level of operation. The indicated target levels are minimal and should generally be exceeded.

Dedicated special purpose and extra high energy machines which have limited but important applications may not perform 6,000 treatments per year and should be evaluated individually by HSAs in the development of Health Systems Plans.

§ 121.210   COMPUTED TOMOGRAPHIC SCANNERS.

(a) *Standard.* (1) A Computed Tomographic Scanner (head and body) should operate at a minimum of 2,500 medically necessary patient procedures per year, for the second year of its operation and thereafter.

(2) There should be no additional scanners approved unless each existing scanner in the health service area is performing at a rate greater than 2,500 medically necessary patient procedures per year.

(3) There should be no additional scanners approved unless the operators of the proposed equipment will set in place data collection and utilization review systems.

(b) *Discussion.* Because CT scanners are expensive to purchase, maintain and staff, every effort must be made to contain costs while providing an acceptable level of service. Intensive utilization of existing units, regardless of location, will prevent needless duplication and limit unnecessary health care costs. Estimates and surveys for efficient utilization of CT scanners range from 1,800 to over 4,000 patient procedures a year. (One patient procedure includes, during a single visit, the initial scan plus any necessary additional scans of the same anatomic area of diagnostic interest.)

The Institute of Medicine, the Office of Technology Assessment and others have carefully reviewed these data and the capabilities of various available units. The Department has reviewed these analyses as well as the extensive literature that has been developed on CT scanners. In arriving at a standard for the use of these machines, the Department has considered a variety of factors, including the difference in time required for head scans and body scans, the need for multiple scans in some patient examinations, variations in patient mix, the special needs of children, time required for maintenance, and staffing requirements. Moreover, the Department considered the actual operating experience of hospitals and institutions reflected in reports on the use of CT scanners.

The standard set in the Department's guidelines is intended to assure effective utilization and reasonable cost for CT scanning. These machines are expensive, and therefore must be used at levels of high efficiency if excessive costs are to be limited. The Department recognizes that the cost of some machines is declining, particularly those that perform only head scans which require less time. For machines that do predominantly head scans, the standard represents an efficient but more easily attainable level of utilization. For scanners capable of performing both head and body scans, it is imperative that they be effectively used in order to spread the high capital expenditures over as much operating time as possible. As the Institute of Medicine report stated. "The high fixed costs of operating a scanner argue for as high a volume of use as the equipment allows without jeopardizing the quality of care."

The Department believes that a 50–55 hour operating week is both consistent with the actual operating experience of many hospitals and a reasonable target.

Based on reported experience for the time required for both head scans and body scans, the Department estimated that a patient mix of about 60 percent head scans and about 40 percent body scans, making allowance for the other factors identified above, would allow a CT scanner to perform about 2,500 patient procedures per year if it is efficiently used about 50–55 hours per week. This estimate assumes a higher percent of body scans than is currently being performed. If fewer than 40 percent body scans are performed, then 2,500 patient procedures would involve even less than 50–55 hours per week. Basing the standard on a higher percentage of body scans also takes account of current trends toward increased proportions of such scans.

The Department believes that sharing arrangements in the use of CT scanners is desirable, in line with the national health priorities of section 1502. Individual institutions or providers should not acquire new machines until existing capacity. is being well utilized.

In planning for CT scanners, the HSA should take into consideration special circumstances such as: 1) an institution with more than one scanner where the combined average annual number of procedures is greater than 2,500 per scanner although the unit doing primarily body scans is operating at less than 2,500 patient procedures per year; 2) units which are, or will be, devoting a significant portion of time to fixed protocol institutionally approved research projects and 3) units which are, or will be, servicing predominantly seriously sick or pediatric patients. A summary of the data collected on CT scanners should be submitted by the operators to the appropriate HSA to enable it to adequately plan the distribution and use of CT scanners in the area. The data to be collected should include information on utilization and a description of the operations of a utilization review program.

§ 121.211   END-STAGE RENAL DISEASE (ESRD).

(a) *Standard.* The Health Systems Plans established by HSAs should be consistent with standards and procedures contained in the DHEW regulations governing conditions for coverage of suppliers of end-stage renal disease services, 20 CFR Part 405, Subpart U.

(b) *Discussion.* The ESRD Program was created pursuant to section 2991 of the Social Security Amendments of 1972 (Pub. L. 92–603), which extends Medicare benefits to any individual who has end-stage renal disease requiring dialysis or transplantation, provided that such individual: (1) is fully or currently insured or entitled to monthly benefits under Title II of the Social Security Act; or (2) is the spouse or dependent child of an individual so insured or entitled to such monthly benefits. In order for an ESRD facility to qualify for reimbursement under the program, the facility must meet the conditions for coverage of suppliers of end-stage renal disease services as established by regulation. These conditions incorporate standards which relate to supply, distribution, and organization of ESRD facilities. The standards were developed by the Department of Health, Education, and Welfare and were based on extensive consultation with professionals and other persons knowledgeable in the areas of nephrology and transplant surgery. Because these standards are already published as regulations, they are not republished here. The regulations do not try to encourage any particular type of dialysis setting. It is widely recognized that self-care dialysis can significantly contain costs without impairing the quality of care of the suitably chosen patient. The organization of resources to support self-care dialysis is therefore encouraged to the maximum extent practicable.

Essentials for Family Practice Residencies[*]

SPECIAL REQUIREMENTS FOR RESIDENCY TRAINING IN FAMILY PRACTICE

Residencies in Family Practice [1] should be specifically designed to meet the educational needs of medical school graduates intending to become Family Physicians.[2]

ORGANIZATION OF TRAINING

The Family Practice Residency is three years in duration after graduation from medical school and must be planned in a way that assures an integrated, meaningful, and coherent educational program.

Applicants who have had other types of previous training may be considered for admission to the Family Practice program. Credit for this previous training may be given only in the amount that is compatible with the "Essentials" of

---

[*] This document was approved by the Residency Review Committee for Family Practice at its meeting of September 18, 1977, held in Denver, Colorado, for transmittal to the three parent organizations.

training in Family Practice. In these situations, the Director of the Family Practice Residency shall be responsible for insuring that each resident who completes the program shall have met the training requirements of the "Essentials" of an accredited program.

Experience in the continuity of care offered in the Family Practice Center is essential. Therefore, it is imperative that all programs offer three consecutive years of training. It is highly desirable that all residents have three consecutive years of training in a Family Practice Center of one institution.

However, certain circumstances may permit a resident to enter a program in advanced standing where the first year of training has been in Family Practice in another location, or where the first year of training has provided educational experience equivalent to that necessary for Family Practice. It is essential that a program provide the second and third years of training in one location, thus assuring the resident the opportunity of providing continuity of care to a given panel of patients. It is imperative that the Program Director encourage the resident to take the final two years in the same location.

As stated in the "General Requirements" of the "Essentials of Approved Residencies," it is not necessary, or even desirable, that all residencies adopt exactly the same program, nor that they offer a rigidly uniform sequence of experience. Programs may be developed which can be regarded as experimental or pilot in nature. It is necessary, however, that all programs for graduate training in Family Practice be able to meet the minimal requirements of an accredited program. However, as stated in the "Essentials," programs may vary.

Family Practice residency programs must provide for experience and responsibility for each resident in those areas of medicine which will be of importance to the resident's future practice. Since Family Practice programs are in part dependent upon other specialties for the training of their residents, it is essential that the ability and commitment of the institution to fulfill these requirements be assured. Specifically, the sponsoring institution must assure the existence and availability of those basic educational and patient care resources necessary to provide the Family Practice resident meaningful involvement and responsibility in the other major clinical specialties. Further, there must be agreement regarding the resident's need to maintain concurrent commitment to his patients in the Family Practice Center.

It is necessary that the Family Practice resident's identity be maintained throughout graduate training while learning the appropriate skills, techniques, and procedures of other specialties. Instruction in the other specialties must be arranged and conducted by faculty with expertise in these fields. Curriculum and plans for such rotations should be developed in concert with the Family Practice faculty. Participation in other services should be jointly planned when the resident is serving on other specialty services so as to keep in view the principles and philosophical attitudes associated with Family Practice.

If a resident desires to emphasize one of the other specialties in his future

Family Practice, he should obtain necessary additional training in those areas beyond that provided in his training for Family Practice.

Clearly formulated educational objectives must be delineated in addition to the time frames concerned with the different subjects. The achievement of a high level of competence by all residents must be the principal goal.

CONTENT

The following covers the general content of training in Family Practice and, as such, should be available to the resident, although certain portions may be emphasized, depending upon the knowledge and skill of the resident, his interests, and the character of his anticipated practice. In all cases, continuing emphasis of the basic clinical sciences must be maintained. The "General Requirements" as outlined for all residency programs should be met as well as the special requirements that apply to Family Practice.

Family Medicine

The teaching of Family Practice takes place in the ambulatory facilities of the Family Practice Center and on the hospital inpatient services. The experience should be designed so that the resident maintains continuing patient responsibility when his patients from the Family Practice Center require hospitalization.

The patient composition of the whole Family Practice service should be a stable one in order to insure continuity of experience for the resident. A patient population seeking only episodic care does not meet this requirement. Patients who provide a broad spectrum of problems and represent varied income levels should be included, attended, and managed either in the hospital, the Family Practice Center, at home, or in institutions for long-term care or rehabilitation. Training also must include emergency room care as well as a large component devoted to health maintenance and preventive health care in order to provide for the entire range of needs of the patient and the family.

A major requirement for the training of Family Practice residents is a Family Practice Center. This should be designed in a way that will clearly identify and keep separate the special features of a family physician's office.

Residents may spend time away from the Family Practice Center if necessary to meet the needs of their training. Such outside rotations which interrupt the continuity of the resident's patient care responsibilities in the Family Practice Center must not exceed a total of two months per year in either of the last two years. After two months of such rotation, the resident must return to the Family Practice Center for a minimum of two months before participating in another outside rotation. The educational value of these rotations must be clearly documented. The availability of constant on-site supervision is required.

Internal Medicine

Internal medicine is a major component of programs in Family Practice. The resident must receive sufficient instruction and experience in this field that he can exercise sound judgment in assessing the condition of the patient, in the use and interpretation of laboratory and other special studies, and in differential diagnosis.

Emphasis should be placed upon the basic mechanisms of disease, and the resident must have the opportunity to become competent in the management of the major disorders he is apt to encounter in this field.

Pediatrics

The special contributions of pediatrics are needed, and relate to understanding the growth and development of the newborn through adolescence, to emotional problems and their management, and to training of the resident in the recognition and management of behavioral, medical, and surgical problems of children and adolescents in home, ambulatory, and hospital settings. Modern pediatrics includes a large component of preventive medicine and emphasizes the care of ambulatory patients and of patients in their homes.

Psychiatry and Behavioral Sciences

The behavioral sciences and psychiatry are essential components of a Family Practice education program and must be available in a continuum throughout the training years. The behavioral aspects of patients with disease, medical practice relationships, and community life shall be emphasized in all phases of the training program. The diagnosis and management of behavioral and emotional disorders must be taught as well as counseling techniques and the principles of their treatment. The Family Practice resident must understand the importance of communication and interaction within the families under his care.

The resident is expected to develop competence in the management of common psychological and behavioral problems and must have enough exposure to recognize stages of stress in the family life cycle.

In Family Practice training, most of this knowledge and skill is best acquired through a program in which psychiatry and behavioral sciences are integrated with medicine, pediatrics, and the other disciplines throughout the resident's entire educational experience.

The resident must have an opportunity to work in a psychiatric service or treatment center where patients with acute problems are treated. Limitation of the resident's experience in psychiatry to chronic, long-term psychotic patients is not acceptable, although experience with such patients is desirable to enable the resident to appreciate and recognize major psychoses.

Obstetrics and Gynecology

The resident shall be provided the instruction necessary to understand the biological and psychological impact of pregnancy, delivery, and care of the newborn upon a woman and her family. The resident shall acquire technical skills in the provision of antepartum and postpartum care and the normal delivery process. The resident should also have an understanding of the complications of pregnancy and their management. The resident shall be taught certain operative skills in obstetrical and gynecological procedures as a part of a broadly-based curriculum. To obtain such skills requires a structured obstetrics–gynecologic educational program.

Marriage counseling, sex education and family planning are important areas of responsibility for the Family Physician, and the training program should afford an opportunity for the acquisition of skills in these areas. Additional training in the management of the more complicated high-risk obstetrical patients should be arranged for those residents who wish to assume this kind of responsibility in the future.

Surgery

The resident should acquire competence in the recognition and management of surgical emergencies and when referral of them for specialized care is appropriate. He should also be able to recognize conditions that preferably may be managed on an elective basis.

It is important for him to appreciate the kinds of surgical treatments that might be employed for his patients as well as the problems that might arise from them. Knowledge of these matters enables him to give proper advice, explanation, and emotional support to his patients.

He should be trained in basic surgical principles, and acquire the technical proficiency required for those surgical procedures a Family Physician may be called upon to perform. If he expects to include surgery as a major aspect of his regular practice, he must obtain additional training.

Community Medicine

Community medicine is one of the important components of Family Practice. The teaching of this subject should be integrated throughout the entire program and not necessarily be given separate block time. The resident should understand the principles of epidemiology, environmental health, and the health resources of the community and its organization for health. He should understand the roles and interrelationships of persons in various professional and technical disciplines which provide health services.

The resident should be provided with an understanding of community medicine resources with an approach to the evaluation of health problems and needs of a community. The experience should help the resident to understand the role of private enterprise, voluntary organizations, and government in modern health care.

Other Disciplines

All Family Practice residents must obtain a useful experience in dermatology, neurology, ophthalmology, otolaryngology, and orthopedics. Training in these disciplines is advised for the second and third years. Experience in urology and diagnostic radiology is strongly recommended. Training in cardiopulmonary resuscitation, emergency airway procedures, and other emergency lifesaving procedures is required. Training in the administration of anesthetics may be desirable for some residents.

Electives

Electives which are well constructed, purposeful, and effective learning experiences are an essential part of a Family Practice residency program. Most electives will be concerned with subspecialized areas of the major primary specialties and may be obtained in various ways.

Research

The participation of the resident in an active research program should be encouraged. Generally, this activity should be concurrent with other assignments, provided the responsibilities of the resident are adjusted in a way to permit a reasonable time for research activity. Studies relating to the problems of delivery of health care relevant to Family Practice may be included as an integral part of the regular assignments. Independent research by the resident should be in addition to, rather than in lieu of, clinical instructions.

For those residents desirous of additional skills in one or more particular fields, training beyond the third year is encouraged.

Notes

1. The official definition of *Family Practice* adopted by the American Academy of Family Physicians Board of Directors and the American Board of Family Practice Board of Directors follows:

   Family Practice is comprehensive medical care with particular emphasis on the family unit, in which the physician's continuing responsibility for health care is not limited by the patient's age or sex nor by a particular organ system or disease entity.

Family Practice is the specialty in breadth which builds upon a core of knowledge derived from other disciplines—drawing most heavily on internal medicine, pediatrics, obstetrics and gynecology, surgery and psychiatry—and which establishes a cohesive unit combining the behavioral sciences with the traditional biological and clinical sciences. The core of knowledge encompassed by the discipline of Family Practice prepares the Family Physician for a unique role in patient management, problem solving, counseling and as a personal physician who coordinates total health care delivery.

2. The official definition of *Family Physician* adopted by the American Academy of Family Physicians Board of Directors follows:

The Family Physician provides health care in the discipline of Family Practice. His training and experience qualify him to practice in the several fields of medicine and surgery.

The Family Physician is educated and trained to develop and bring to bear in practice unique attitudes and skills which qualify him or her to provide continuing, comprehensive health maintenance and medical care to the entire family regardless of sex, age, or type of problem, be it biological, behavioral or social. This physician serves as the patient's or family's advocate in all health-related matters, including the appropriate use of consultants and community resources.

Family Practice Teaching Programs

FAMILY PRACTICE TEACHING PROGRAMS (AS OF JANUARY 10, 1979)

SPONSORING INSTITUTION	CHAIRMAN OF MEDICAL SCHOOL DEPARTMENT (IF APPLICABLE)	DIRECTOR OF RESIDENCY PROGRAM AND FAMILY PRACTICE CENTER ADDRESS AND PHONE NUMBER
Alabama		
University of Alabama—Birmingham School of Medicine 1016 South 18th Street University Station Birmingham, Alabama 35294	G. Gayle Stephens, M.D. Professor and Chairman Dept. of Family Practice (205) 934–5320	
University of Alabama—Huntsville School of Primary Medical Care 101 Governors Drive Southeast Huntsville, Alabama 35801	Herbert T. Smith, M.D. Chairman Dept. of Family Practice (205) 536–5511	

FAMILY PRACTICE TEACHING PROGRAMS—CONTINUED

SPONSORING INSTITUTION	CHAIRMAN OF MEDICAL SCHOOL DEPARTMENT (IF APPLICABLE)	DIRECTOR OF RESIDENCY PROGRAM AND FAMILY PRACTICE CENTER ADDRESS AND PHONE NUMBER
University of South Alabama College of Medicine 307 University Boulevard Mobile, Alabama 36688	Henry C. Mullins, Jr., M.D. Chairman Dept. of Family Practice (205) 476–3930	
University of Alabama— Tuscaloosa College of Community Health Sciences P.O. Box 6291 Tuscaloosa, Alabama 35486	William F. DeShazo, III, M.D. Chairman Dept. of Family and Community Medicine (205) 349–1770	
Northeast Alabama Regional Medical Center 901 Leighton Avenue P.O. Box 2208 Anniston, Alabama 36201 2/A (University of Alabama)		C. Neal Canup, M.D. Anniston Family Practice Center 901 Leighton Avenue P.O. Box 2208 Anniston, Alabama 36201 (205) 237–8527
Carraway Methodist Medical Center 1615–25th Street North Birmingham, Alabama 35234 1/A		Robert Whitter, M.D. Family Practice Residency 2714–31st Avenue North Birmingham, Alabama 35234 (205) 323–2526
East End Memorial Hospital 7916 Second Avenue South Birmingham, Alabama 35206 2/A (University of Alabama— Birmingham)		John A. Maloof, M.D. Family Practice Residency 7916 Second Avenue South Birmingham, Alabama 35206 (205) 838–1611 Ext. 636
University of Alabama Medical Center Department of Family Practice University of Alabama— Birmingham University Station Birmingham, Alabama 35294 4A (University of Alabama— Birmingham)		G. Gayle Stephens, M.D. Family Practice Residency Program 1016 South 18th Street Birmingham, Alabama 35294 (205) 934–5320
Baptist Memorial Hospital 1007 Goodyear Avenue Gadsden, Alabama 35903 2A (University of Alabama— Birmingham)		Arnold C. Williams, M.D. Family Practice Residency Program 1007 Goodyear Avenue Gadsden, Alabama 35903 (205) 492–1240

FAMILY PRACTICE TEACHING PROGRAMS—CONTINUED

SPONSORING INSTITUTION	*CHAIRMAN OF MEDICAL SCHOOL DEPARTMENT (IF APPLICABLE)*	*DIRECTOR OF RESIDENCY PROGRAM AND FAMILY PRACTICE CENTER ADDRESS AND PHONE NUMBER*
Huntsville Hospital Ambulatory Care Center 201 Governors Drive Southeast Huntsville, Alabama 35801 3/A (University of Alabama— Huntsville)		Charles T. Moss, Jr., M.D. Family Practice Residency 201 Governors Drive, Southeast Huntsville, Alabama 35801 (205) 536-5511
University of South Alabama Medical Center 2451 Fillingim Street Mobile, Alabama 36617 4/A (University of South Alabama)		H.C. Mullins, Jr., M.D. Family Practice Residency 2451 Fillingim Street Mobile, Alabama 36617 (205) 476-3930
Jackson Hospital and Clinic, Inc. 1235 Forest Avenue Montgomery, Alabama 36106 3/A (University of Alabama— Birmingham)		William East Lotterhos, M.D. Montgomery Family Practice Program P.O. Box 4897 Montgomery, Alabama 36111 (205) 832-4935
Selma Medical Center 1015 Medical Center Parkway Selma, Alabama 36701 2/A (University of Alabama— Tuscaloosa)		Donald C. Overstreet, M.D. Selma/Dallas County Family Practice Residency 429 Lauderdale Street Selma, Alabama 36701 (205) 875-4184
College of Community Health Sciences University of Alabama 700 University Boulevard East Tuscaloosa, Alabama 35401 3/A (University of Alabama— Tuscaloosa)		Russell L. Anderson, M.D. University of Alabama— College of Community Health Science Family Practice Residency Program 700 University Boulevard East Tuscaloosa, Alabama 35401 (205) 349-1770

Arizona

University of Arizona College of Medicine Health Sciences Center Tucson, Arizona 85724	Jesse W. Tapp, M.D. Acting Chairman Dept. of Family and Community Medicine (602) 626-6244	

FAMILY PRACTICE TEACHING PROGRAMS—CONTINUED

SPONSORING INSTITUTION	CHAIRMAN OF MEDICAL SCHOOL DEPARTMENT (IF APPLICABLE)	DIRECTOR OF RESIDENCY PROGRAM AND FAMILY PRACTICE CENTER ADDRESS AND PHONE NUMBER
Good Samaritan Hospital 1130 East McDowell Road Phoenix, Arizona 85006 1/A		Robert A. Price, M.D. Family Practice Center 1010 East McDowell Road Suite 102 Phoenix, Arizona 85006 (602) 254–7017
Phoenix Baptist Hospital and Medical Center 6025 North 20th Avenue Phoenix, Arizona 85015 1A		James L. Grobe, M.D. Family Practice Residency Program 6025 North 20th Avenue Phoenix, Arizona 85015 (602) 249–0059
Saint Joseph's Hospital and Medical Center 350 West Thomas Road Phoenix, Arizona 85013 1/A		Donald McHard, M.D. 521 West Thomas Road Phoenix, Arizona 85013 (602) 279–9301
Scottsdale Memorial Hospital 7301 East Fourth Street Suite 22 Scottsdale, Arizona 85251 1/A		Jack E. Cook, M.D. Family Practice Residency 7301 East Fourth Street Suite 22 Scottsdale, Arizona 85251 (602) 947–8026
University Hospital 1501 North Campbell Street Tucson, Arizona 85724 4/A (University of Arizona— Tucson)		Arnold Greensher, M.D. Family Practice Office Arizona Health Sciences Center 1450 North Cherry Avenue Tucson, Arizona 85719 (602) 882–6709

Arkansas

| University of Arkansas College of Medicine 1700 West 13th Street Little Rock, Arkansas 77202 | Benjamin N. Saltzman, M.D. Coordinator Dept. of Family and Community Medicine (501) 661–5371 | |
| Northwest Arkansas Area Health Center 241 West Spring Street Fayetteville, Arkansas 72701 3/A (University of Arkansas— Little Rock) | | James K. Patrick, M.D. Family Practice Residency 241 West Spring Street Fayetteville, Arkansas 72701 (501) 521–8269 |

FAMILY PRACTICE TEACHING PROGRAMS—CONTINUED

SPONSORING INSTITUTION	CHAIRMAN OF MEDICAL SCHOOL DEPARTMENT (IF APPLICABLE)	DIRECTOR OF RESIDENCY PROGRAM AND FAMILY PRACTICE CENTER ADDRESS AND PHONE NUMBER
Area Health Education Center 100 South 14th Street Fort Smith, Arkansas 72901 3/A (University of Arkansas— Little Rock)		John R. Williams, M.D. Family Practice Residency 100 South 14th Street Fort Smith, Arkansas 72901 (501) 785–2431
University of Arkansas for Medical Sciences 4301 West Markham Little Rock, Arkansas 72201 4/A (University of Arkansas— Little Rock)		Kenneth G. Goss, M.D. Family Medical Center 1700 West 13th Street Little Rock, Arkansas 72202 (501) 661–6300
University of Arkansas for Medical Sciences Area Health Education Center—Pine Bluff 1515 West 42nd Avenue Pine Bluff, Arkansas 71603 3/A (University of Arkansas— Little Rock)		James A. Lindsey, M.D. Family Practice Center 1310 Cherry Pine Bluff, Arkansas 71601 (501) 541–0770

California

SPONSORING INSTITUTION	CHAIRMAN OF MEDICAL SCHOOL DEPARTMENT (IF APPLICABLE)	DIRECTOR OF RESIDENCY PROGRAM AND FAMILY PRACTICE CENTER ADDRESS AND PHONE NUMBER
University of California— Davis School of Medicine Davis, California 95616	George Snively, M.D. Acting Chairman Dept. of Family Practice (916) 453–2748	
University of California— San Diego School of Medicine P.O. Box 109 La Jolla, California 92093	Doris A. Howell, M.D. Chairman Division of Family Practice	
Loma Linda University School of Medicine Loma Linda, California 92354	W.P. Ordelheide, M.D. Chairman Dept. of Family Medicine (714) 785–7484	
Charles R. Drew Post Graduate Medical School 1621 East 120th Street Los Angeles, California 90059	David Satcher, M.D. Chairman Dept. of Family Medicine (213) 603–4965	
University of California School of Medicine Center for Health Sciences, 50–078 Los Angeles, California 90024	Ralph Berggren, M.D. Acting Chief Division of Family Practice (213) 825–5532	

FAMILY PRACTICE TEACHING PROGRAMS—CONTINUED

SPONSORING INSTITUTION	CHAIRMAN OF MEDICAL SCHOOL DEPARTMENT (IF APPLICABLE)	DIRECTOR OF RESIDENCY PROGRAM AND FAMILY PRACTICE CENTER ADDRESS AND PHONE NUMBER
University of California— Irvine School of Medicine 101 City Drive, South Orange, California 92668	Raymond C. Anderson, M.D. Chairman Department of Family Practice	
University of California 513 Parnassus Avenue San Francisco, California 94143	Jonathan Rodnick, M.D. Chief of the Section of Family Medical in the Division of Ambulatory and Community Medicine (707) 527-2826	
University of Southern California School of Medicine #205 Raulston Building 2025 Zonal Avenue Los Angeles, California 90033	Samuel C. Matheny, M.D. Director Division of Family Medicine (213) 226-2215	
Stanford University School of Medicine 300 Pasteur Drive Stanford, California 94305	Count D. Gibson, Jr., M.D. Head Division of Family and Community Medicine	
Kern Medical Center 1830 Flower Street Bakersfield, California 93305 2/A (University of California—Los Angeles)		Ramon H. Neufeld, M.D., M.P.H. Family Practice Residency 1830 Flower Street Bakersfield, California 93305 (805) 323-7651
Naval Regional Medical Center Camp Pendleton, California 92055 5/A		CDR Robert W. Higgins, M.C., U.S.N. Family Practice Residency Program Naval Regional Medical Center Camp Pendleton, California 92055 (714) 725-1398
Kaiser Foundation Hospital 9961 Sierra Avenue Fontana, California 92335 1/A		Raymond W. Pickering, M.D. Family Practice Residency Program—Kaiser Foundation Hospital 9961 Sierra Avenue Fontana, California 92335 (714) 829-5582

FAMILY PRACTICE TEACHING PROGRAMS—CONTINUED

SPONSORING INSTITUTION	*CHAIRMAN OF MEDICAL SCHOOL DEPARTMENT (IF APPLICABLE)*	*DIRECTOR OF RESIDENCY PROGRAM AND FAMILY PRACTICE CENTER ADDRESS AND PHONE NUMBER*
Silas B. Hays Army Hospital Fort Ord, California 93941 5/A		Major William J. Meinert, M.C., U.S.A. Family Practice Residency Fort Ord, California 93941 (408) 242-7626
Antelope Valley Medical Center 1600 West Avenue J. Lancaster, California 93534 2/B (University of California—Los Angeles; first year spent at U.C.L.A.)		William Walsh, M.D. Antelope Valley Hospital Medical Center Family Practice Residency Program 1620 West Avenue J Lancaster, California 93534 (805) 948-5971
Valley Medical Center 445 South Cedar Avenue Fresno, California 93702 2/A (University of California—San Francisco)		H. John Blossom, M.D., Acting Chief Family Practice Residency 445 South Cedar Avenue Fresno, California 93702 (209) 453-4000 Ext. 2537
Glendale Adventist Hospital 1509 Wilson Terrace Drive Glendale, California 91206 2/A (Loma Linda University)		William D. Putnam, M.D. Family Practice Center 1560 East Chevy Chase Drive—Suite 260 Glendale, California 91206 (213) 247-5733
Memorial Hospital Medical Center 2801 Atlantic Avenue Long Beach, California 90801 2/A (University of California—Irvine)		Edson DeLong Beebe, M.D. Memorial Family Practice Res. 2701 Atlantic Avenue Long Beach, California 90806 (213) 595-5255
King–Drew Medical Center 1621 East 120th Street Los Angeles, California 90059 4/A (Charles R. Drew Postgraduate Medical School)		David Satcher, M.D. Family Practice Residency 1621 East 120th Street, Trailer # 1 Los Angeles, California 90059 (213) 603-4965
University of California Center for Health Sciences Los Angeles, California 90024 4/A (University of California—Los Angeles)		Mary Elizabeth Roth, M.D. Family Practice Center 1072 Galey Avenue Los Angeles, California 90024 (213) 825-8942

FAMILY PRACTICE TEACHING PROGRAMS—CONTINUED

SPONSORING INSTITUTION	CHAIRMAN OF MEDICAL SCHOOL DEPARTMENT (IF APPLICABLE)	DIRECTOR OF RESIDENCY PROGRAM AND FAMILY PRACTICE CENTER ADDRESS AND PHONE NUMBER
Kaiser Foundation Hospital 1526 North Edgement Street Los Angeles, California 90027 1/A		Irving M. Rasgon, M.D. Family Practice Residency 1526 North Edgement Street Los Angeles, California 90027 (213) 667-5484
Contra Costa County Medical Services 2600 Alhambra Avenue Martinez, California 94553 2/A (University of California—Davis)		J.L. Aiken, M.D. Family Practice Residency 2600 Alhambra Avenue Martinez, California 94553 (415) 372-4200
Merced Community Medical Center P.O. Box 231 290 East 15th Street Merced, California 95340 2/B (University of California—Davis; first year at Sacramento Medical Center)		J. Edward Hughell, M.D. Family Practice Residency P.O. Box 231 290 East 15th Street Merced, California 95340 (209) 723-3941
Scenic General Hospital 830 Scenic Drive Modesto, California 95350 1/A		Fred Fowler, M.D. Family Practice Residency 830 Scenic Drive Modesto, California 95350 (209) 526-6160
Northridge Hospital Foundation 18300 Roscoe Boulevard Northridge, California 91328 2/A (University of California—Los Angeles)		Myron C. Greengold, M.D. Family Practice Residency 18406 Roscoe Boulevard Northridge, California 91325 (213) 885-1261
University of California, Irvine—Medical Center 101 City Drive South Orange, California 92668 4/A (University of California—Irvine)		J. Dennis Mull, M.D. Family Practice Residency 101 City Drive South Orange, California 92668 (714) 634-5171
Shasta General Hospital 2630 Hospital Lane Redding, California 96001 2/B (University of California—Davis; first year at Sacramento Medical Center)		Norman T. Woolf, M.D. Shasta–Cascade Family Practice Residency 2630 Hospital Lane Redding, California 96001 (916) 246-7800

FAMILY PRACTICE TEACHING PROGRAMS—CONTINUED

SPONSORING INSTITUTION	CHAIRMAN OF MEDICAL SCHOOL DEPARTMENT (IF APPLICABLE)	DIRECTOR OF RESIDENCY PROGRAM AND FAMILY PRACTICE CENTER ADDRESS AND PHONE NUMBER
Riverside General Hospital 9851 Magnolia Avenue Riverside, California 92503 2/A (Loma Linda University School of Medicine)		Perry Pugno, M.D. Family Practice Residency 9851 Magnolia Avenue Riverside, California 92503 (714) 785-7484
Sacramento Medical Center 2315 Stockton Blvd. Sacramento, California 95817 4/A (University of California—Davis)		Robert C. Davidson, M.D. Dept. of Family Practice 2221 Stockton Boulevard, Room 13 Sacramento, California 95817 (916) 453-2818
Natividad Medical Center of Monterey County 1330 Natividad Road P.O. Box 1611 Salinas, California 93901 2/A (University of California—San Francisco)		B. Clair Eliason, M.D. Natividad Medical Center Family Practice Residency P.O. Box 1611 Salinas, California 93902 (408) 424-2541 Ext. 297
San Bernardino County Medical Center 780 East Gilbert Street San Bernardino, California 92404 2/A (University of California—Los Angeles)		David Mark Hess, M.D., Acting Director Family Practice Residency San Bernardino County Medical Center 780 East Gilbert Street San Bernardino, California 92404 (714) 383-3077
University Hospital— San Diego 225 Dickinson Street San Diego, California 92103 4-A (University of California—San Diego)		George R. Simms, M.D. Family Practice Residency 225 Dickinson St. H-809 San Diego, California 92103 (714) 294-5776
San Francisco General Hospital 1001 Potrero Avenue San Francisco, California 94110 3/A (University of California—San Francisco)		Peter Sommers, M.D. Family Practice Residency 1001 Potrero Avenue, Building 90, Room 109 San Francisco, California 94110 (415) 282-0677

FAMILY PRACTICE TEACHING PROGRAMS—CONTINUED

SPONSORING INSTITUTION	CHAIRMAN OF MEDICAL SCHOOL DEPARTMENT (IF APPLICABLE)	DIRECTOR OF RESIDENCY PROGRAM AND FAMILY PRACTICE CENTER ADDRESS AND PHONE NUMBER
San José Hospital and Health Center 675 East Santa Clara Street San José, California 95112 1/A		William Fowkes, M.D. Family Practice Center 25 North 14th San José, California 95112 (408) 998–3212
Santa Ana—Tustin Community Hospital 1001 North Tustin Avenue Santa Ana, California 92705 1/A		J. Blair Pace, M.D. Family Practice Residency Program Santa Ana—Tustin Community Hospital 1001 North Tustin Avenue Santa Ana, California 92705 (714) 835–3555
Santa Monica Hospital and Medical Center 1225 15th Street Santa Monica, California 90404 2/A (University of California—Los Angeles)		Sanford Bloom, M.D. Family Practice Residency 1225 15th Street Santa Monica, California 90404 (213) 451–1511
San Pedro and Peninsula Hospital 1300 West Seventh Street San Pedro, California 90732 1–A		Lawrence R. Leiter, M.D. Acting Director San Pedro and Peninsula Hospital 1300 West Seventh Street San Pedro, California 90732 (213) 832–3311
Community Hospital of Sonoma County 3325 Chanate Road Santa Rosa, California 95402 2/A (University of California—San Francisco)		Richard C. Barnett, M.D. Family Practice Residency 3325 Chanate Road Santa Rosa, California 95402 (707) 527–2907
San Joaquin County Health Care Services Box 1020 Stockton, California 95201 2/A (University of California—Davis)		Bruce S. Nickols, M.D. Family Practice Residency Box 1020 Stockton, California 95201 (209) 982–1800

FAMILY PRACTICE TEACHING PROGRAMS—CONTINUED

SPONSORING INSTITUTION	CHAIRMAN OF MEDICAL SCHOOL DEPARTMENT (IF APPLICABLE)	DIRECTOR OF RESIDENCY PROGRAM AND FAMILY PRACTICE CENTER ADDRESS AND PHONE NUMBER
Los Angeles County Harbor General Hospital 1000 West Carson Street Torrance, California 90509 2/A (University of California—Los Angeles)		Norman J. Diamond, M.D. Harbor General Family Planning Center 1000 W. Carson Street Torrance, California 90509 (213) 328–2380 Ext. 1963
David Grant U.S. Air Force Medical Center/SGHF Travis Air Force Base, California 94535 5/A		Lt. Col. John T. Reppart, M.C., U.S.A.F. Dept. of Family Practice David Grant U.S. Air Force Medical Center Travis Air Force Base, California 94535 (707) 438–2578
Ventura County General Hospital 3291 Loma Vista Ventura, California 93003 2/A (University of California—Los Angeles)		David C. Fainer, M.D. General Hospital of Ventura City Family Practice Residency Program 3291 Loma Vista Ventura, California 93003 (805) 654–3131
Presbyterian Intercommunity Hospital* 12401 East Washington Boulevard Whittier, California 90602 3/B (first year at Los Angeles County University of Southern California)		Donald G. Hogan, M.D. Family Practice Center 12401 East Washington Boulevard Whittier, California 90602 (213) 698–0811

Colorado

University of Colorado School of Medicine 4200 East Ninth Avenue Denver, Colorado 80220	Eugene S. Farley, M.D. Chairman Dept. of Family Medicine (303) 394–5191	
Mercy Hospital 1619 Milwaukee Street Denver, Colorado 80206 1/A		Carl Flaxer, M.D. Mercy Hospital Family Care Center 2901 East 16th Avenue Denver, Colorado 80206 (303) 321–8851

FAMILY PRACTICE TEACHING PROGRAMS—CONTINUED

SPONSORING INSTITUTION	CHAIRMAN OF MEDICAL SCHOOL DEPARTMENT (IF APPLICABLE)	DIRECTOR OF RESIDENCY PROGRAM AND FAMILY PRACTICE CENTER ADDRESS AND PHONE NUMBER
St. Joseph Hospital 1835 Franklin Street Denver, Colorado 80218 1/A		Mary Jean Berg, M.D. Family Practice Center 1570 Humboldt Denver, Colorado 80218 (303) 832-5781
University of Colorado Affiliated Hospitals A.F. Williams Family Medicine Center 1180 Clermont Street Denver, Colorado 80220 4/A (University of Colorado—Denver)		Eugene S. Farley, M.D. A.F. Williams Family Medicine Center 1180 Clermont Street Denver, Colorado 80220 (303) 394-5191
Poudre Valley Memorial Hospital 1024 Lemay Avenue Fort Collins, Colorado 80521 2/B (University of Colorado; first year spent at University of Colorado)		C.E. Basye, M.D. Family Practice Residency 1224 Doctors Lane Fort Collins, Colorado 80521 (303) 221-5770
St. Mary's Hospital and Medical Center 2333 North 6th St. Grand Junction, Colorado 81501 2/B (University of Colorado; first year spent at University of Colorado)		L.E. Ellinwood, M.D. A.H. Gould Family Practice Residency 2333 N. 6th Street Grand Junction, Colorado 81501 (303) 245-1198
Weld County General Hospital 16th Street at 17th Avenue Greeley, Colorado 80631 2/A (University of Colorado—Denver)		David E. Bates, M.D. Family Practice Residency 1661 18th Avenue Greeley, Colorado 80631 (303) 356-2424
Southern Colorado Family Medicine 1600 West 24th Street Pueblo, Colorado 81003 2/A (University of Colorado—Denver)		F. William Barrows, M.D. Family Practice Residency 1600 West 24th Street Pueblo, Colorado 81003 (303) 544-5202

FAMILY PRACTICE TEACHING PROGRAMS—CONTINUED

SPONSORING INSTITUTION	*CHAIRMAN OF MEDICAL SCHOOL DEPARTMENT (IF APPLICABLE)*	*DIRECTOR OF RESIDENCY PROGRAM AND FAMILY PRACTICE CENTER ADDRESS AND PHONE NUMBER*
Connecticut		
University of Connecticut School of Medicine 1280 Asylun Avenue Farmington, Connecticut 06032	Alexander Berger, M.D. Chairman Dept. of Family Medicine (203) 674–2928	
University of Connecticut Health Center Room 4073 Farmington, Connecticut 06032 4/A (University of Connecticut)		John E. Donnelly, M.D. Family Practice Residency University of Connecticut— Health Center Room 4073 Farmington, Connecticut 06032 (203) 674–2928
Middlesex Memorial Hospital 77 Crescent Street Middletown, Connecticut 06457 2/A (University of Connecticut)		Dewees H. Brown, M.D. Family Practice Residency 77 Crescent Street Middletown, Connecticut 06457 (203) 347–4288
St. Joseph Hospital 128 Strawberry Hill Avenue Stamford, Connecticut 06904 2/A (New York Medical College)		William I. Gefter, M.D. St. Joseph Hospital Family Practice Residency 128 Strawberry Hill Avenue Stamford, Connecticut 06904 (203) 327–3500
Delaware		
Wilmington Medical Center P.O. Box 785 Wilmington, Delaware 19899 1/A		Dene T. Walters, M.D. Family Practice Residency Program Wilmington Medical Center 1401 Washington Street, Box 785 Wilmington, Delaware 19899 (302) 428–2928
District of Columbia		
Georgetown University School of Medicine 3900 Reservoir Road, N.W. Washington, D.C. 20007	Francis L. Land, M.D. Professor and Director of the Division of Family Practice (202) 625–2025	

FAMILY PRACTICE TEACHING PROGRAMS—CONTINUED

SPONSORING INSTITUTION	CHAIRMAN OF MEDICAL SCHOOL DEPARTMENT (IF APPLICABLE)	DIRECTOR OF RESIDENCY PROGRAM AND FAMILY PRACTICE CENTER ADDRESS AND PHONE NUMBER
Howard University College of Medicine 520 "W" Street, Northwest Washington, D.C. 20001	Gertrude Hunter, M.D. Chairman Dept. of Community Health and Family Practice (202) 636–6300	
Howard University Hospital 2041 Georgia Avenue, Northwest Washington, D.C. 20060 4/A (Howard University)		Genevieve Jones, M.D., Acting Director Dept. of Family Practice 2041 Georgia Avenue, Northwest 2B58 Washington, D.C. 20060 (202) 745–1451
Malcolm Grow Hospital Andrews Air Force Base Washington, D.C. 20331 5-2/A (Uniformed Services— Bethesda, Maryland)		Major Louis R. Royal, M.C., U.S.A.F. Family Practice Residency Andrews Air Force Base Washington, D.C. 20331 (301) 981–3786
Georgetown University School of Medicine 3900 Reservoir Road, Northwest Washington, D.C. 20007 4/A (Georgetown University)		Francis L. Land, M.D. Georgetown Providence Family Practice Residency 3900 Reservoir Road, Northwest Washington, D.C. 20007 (202) 625–2025

Florida

SPONSORING INSTITUTION	CHAIRMAN OF MEDICAL SCHOOL DEPARTMENT (IF APPLICABLE)	DIRECTOR OF RESIDENCY PROGRAM AND FAMILY PRACTICE CENTER ADDRESS AND PHONE NUMBER
University of Florida College of Medicine Box J 222 J. Hillis Miller Health Center Gainesville, Florida 32610	J. Russell Green, Jr., M.D. Acting Director Dept. of Community Health and Family Medicine (904) 392–2787	
University of Miami School of Medicine P.O. Box 520875 Biscayne Annex Miami, Florida 33152	Lynn P. Carmichael, M.D. Chairman Dept. of Family Medicine (305) 547–6604	
University of South Florida College of Medicine 12901 North 30th Street Tampa, Florida 33612	Ronald G. Blankenbaker, M.D. Chairman Dept. of Family Medicine (813) 974–2309	

FAMILY PRACTICE TEACHING PROGRAMS—CONTINUED

SPONSORING INSTITUTION	*CHAIRMAN OF MEDICAL SCHOOL DEPARTMENT (IF APPLICABLE)*	*DIRECTOR OF RESIDENCY PROGRAM AND FAMILY PRACTICE CENTER ADDRESS AND PHONE NUMBER*
Polk General Hospital 2010 East Georgia Street P.O. Box 816 Bartow, Florida 33830 2/A (University of Southern Florida)		Bernard Breiter, M.D. Family Practice Residency 2010 East Georgia Street, Box 816 Bartow, Florida 33830 (813) 533-1111
Halifax Hospital and Medical Center P.O. Box 1990 303 Clyde Morris Boulevard Daytona Beach, Florida 32015 2/A (University of Southern Florida)		Richard W. Dodd, M.D. Family Practice Residency 303 Clyde Morris Boulevard, Box 1990 Daytona, Florida 32015 (904) 258-1584
U.S.A.F. Regional Hospital Eglin Air Force Base, Florida 32542 5/A		Col. Larry J. Ehemann, M.C., U.S.A.F. Family Practice Residency Program U.S. Air Force Regional Hospital Eglin Air Force Base, Florida 32542 (904) 885-3288
Alachua General Hospital 801 Southwest Second Avenue Gainesville, Florida 32601 3/A (University of Florida— Gainesville)		J. Russell Green, Jr., M.D. Acting Director 625 Southwest Fourth Avenue Gainesville, Florida 32601 (904) 392-4321
Naval Regional Medical Center Jacksonville, Florida 32214 5/A		C.D.R. James N. McLamb, M.C., U.S.N. Family Practice Residency Box 227, Naval Regulation Medical Center Jacksonville, Florida 32214 (904) 772-2216
St. Vincent's Medical Center Barrs Street and St. John's Avenue Jacksonville, Florida 32204 2/A (University of Florida— Gainesville)		Cranford O. Plyler, Jr., M.D. Family Practice Residency Program 1851 King Street Jacksonville, Florida 32204 (904) 384-5267

FAMILY PRACTICE TEACHING PROGRAMS—CONTINUED

SPONSORING INSTITUTION	CHAIRMAN OF MEDICAL SCHOOL DEPARTMENT (IF APPLICABLE)	DIRECTOR OF RESIDENCY PROGRAM AND FAMILY PRACTICE CENTER ADDRESS AND PHONE NUMBER
University of Miami School of Medicine P.O. Box 016700 Miami, Florida 33101 4/A (University of Miami)		Irving Vinger, M.D. Department of Family Medicine University of Miami—School of Medicine P.O. Box 016700 Miami, Florida 33101 (305) 547-6415
Florida Hospital 601 East Rollins Orlando, Florida 32803 2/A (University of Southern Florida and Loma Linda— California)		Julius M. Garner, M.D. Florida Hospital—Family Practice Residency 601 East Rollins Orlando, Florida 32803 (305) 896-6611
Naval Aerospace and Regulation Medical Center Naval Air Station—Box 11265 Pensacola, Florida 32512 5/A		C.D.R., R.A. Weaver, M.C., U.S.N. Family Practice Residency Naval Air Station—Box 11265 Pensacola, Florida 32512 (904) 452-6672
Pensacola Educational Program 5151 North 9th Avenue Pensacola, Florida 32501 2/A (University of Florida— Gainesville)		Joseph Howard, M.D. Family Practice Residency Program 1000 West Moreno Street Pensacola, Florida 32501 (904) 434-4904
Bayfront Medical Center 701 Sixth Street South St. Petersburg, Florida 33701 2/A (University of Southern Florida)		Charles E. Aucremann, M.D. Family Practice Residency 701 Sixth Street South St. Petersburg, Florida 33701 (813) 823-1234
Tallahassee Memorial Hospital Miccosukee and Centerville Roads Tallahassee, Florida 32303 1/A		Harry Barrick, Jr., M.D. Tallahassee Memorial Hospital 1301 Hodges Drive Tallahassee, Florida 32303 (904) 599-5430

Georgia

Medical College of Georgia School of Medicine 1120 Fifteenth Street Augusta, Georgia 30902	Jon C. Calvert, M.D., Ph.D. Chairman Dept. of Family Practice (404) 828-3245	

FAMILY PRACTICE TEACHING PROGRAMS—CONTINUED

SPONSORING INSTITUTION	CHAIRMAN OF MEDICAL SCHOOL DEPARTMENT (IF APPLICABLE)	DIRECTOR OF RESIDENCY PROGRAM AND FAMILY PRACTICE CENTER ADDRESS AND PHONE NUMBER
Medical College of Georgia 1459 Gwinnett Street Augusta, Georgia 30902 4/A (Medical College of Georgia)		Jon C. Calvert, M.D., Ph.D. Dept. of Family Practice 1120 Fifteenth Street Augusta, Georgia 30902 (404) 828-3245
The Medical Center 1936 8th Avenue P.O. Box 951 Columbus, Georgia 31902 1/A		Howard G. Vigrass, M.D. Family Practice Residency 1936 8th Avenue, P.O. Box 951 Columbus, Georgia 31902 (404) 324-4711
Martin Army Hospital Fort Benning, Georgia 31905 5/A		Col. Jimmie W. Varnado, M.C., U.S.A.F. Family Practice Center Martin Army Hospital Fort Benning, Georgia 31905 (404) 544-4750
Dwight David Eisenhower Army Medical Center Fort Gordon, Georgia 30905 5/A		Lt. Col. John B. Baxley, III, M.C., U.S.A. D.D.E.A.M.C.—Family Practice Fort Gordon, Georgia 30905 (404) 791-5368
Medical Center of Central Georgia 784 Spring Street Macon, Georgia 31201 1/A		Don D. Purdy, M.D. Family Practice Residency 784 Spring Street Macon, Georgia 31201 (912) 745-5464
Floyd Hospital Turner McCall Boulevard Rome, Georgia 30161 1/A		M.C. Adair, M.D. Family Practice Residency— Floyd Hospital Turner-McCall Boulevard Rome, Georgia 30161 (404) 234-8211
Memorial Medical Center P.O. Box 6688 Station C Savannah, Georgia 31405 1/A		Irwin Streiff, M.D. Family Practice Center 4700 Waters Avenue Savannah, Georgia 31405 (912) 354-1500

FAMILY PRACTICE TEACHING PROGRAMS—CONTINUED

SPONSORING INSTITUTION	CHAIRMAN OF MEDICAL SCHOOL DEPARTMENT (IF APPLICABLE)	DIRECTOR OF RESIDENCY PROGRAM AND FAMILY PRACTICE CENTER ADDRESS AND PHONE NUMBER
Hawaii		
University of Hawaii John A. Burns School of Medicine 1960 East–West Road Honolulu, Hawaii 96822	Donald L. Farrell, M.D. Chairman Dept. of Family Practice and Community Health (808) 949–5811	
Kaiser Foundation Hospital 1697 Ala Moana Boulevard Honolulu, Hawaii 96815 2/A (University of Hawaii)		Donald L. Farrell, M.D. Family Practice Residency 1697 Ala Moana Boulevard Honolulu, Hawaii 96815 (808) 949–5811
Tripler Army Medical Center Jarrett White Road Honolulu, Hawaii 96438 5–2/A (University of Hawaii)		Commander Tripler Army Medical Center Family Practice Residency Program Tripler Army Medical Center, Hawaii 96859 (808) 433–6886
Idaho		
Family Practice Residency of Southwest Idaho 414 North First Street Boise, Idaho 83702 2/A (University of Washington—Seattle)		Robert W. Matthies, M.D. Family Practice Residency of Southwestern Idaho, Inc. 414 North First Street Boise, Idaho 83702 (208) 345–3404
Illinois		
Rush Medical College 1725 West Harrison Street Chicago, Illinois 60612	Erich E. Brueschke, M.D. Chairman Dept. of Family Practice (312) 942–7083	
University of Illinois Abraham Lincoln School of Medicine 1919 West Taylor Chicago, Illinois 60612	D. Dettore, M.D. Acting Chairman Dept. of Family Practice (312) 996–2901	

FAMILY PRACTICE TEACHING PROGRAMS—CONTINUED

SPONSORING INSTITUTION	CHAIRMAN OF MEDICAL SCHOOL DEPARTMENT (IF APPLICABLE)	DIRECTOR OF RESIDENCY PROGRAM AND FAMILY PRACTICE CENTER ADDRESS AND PHONE NUMBER
Loyola University of Chicago Stritch School of Medicine 2160 School First Avenue Maywood, Illinois 60153	Walter S. Wood, M.D. Chairman Dept. of Community and Family Medicine	
Chicago Medical School North Chicago, Illinois 60064	Lawrence L. Hirsch, M.D. Chairman Dept. of Family Medicine (312) 473-9200	
University of Illinois Peoria School of Medicine 123 Southwest Glendale Peoria, Illinois 61605	Noel Guillozet, M.D. Chairman Dept. of Family Practice (309) 671-3090	
University of Illinois Rockford School of Medicine 1601 Parkview Avenue Rockford, Illinois 61101	L.P. Johnson, M.D. Chairman Dept. of Family Practice (815) 987-7075	
Southern Illinois University School of Medicine P.O. Box 3926 Springfield, Illinois 62708	William L. Stewart, M.D. Chairman Dept. of Family Practice (217) 782-5872	
University of Illinois School of Clinical Medicine Urbana, Illinois 61801	L.W. Tanner, M.D. Professor of Clinical Science (Family Practice) (217) 443-6891	
MacNeal Memorial Hospital 3249 South Oak Park Avenue Berwyn, Illinois 60402 2/A (Abraham Lincoln School of Medicine)		Kenneth F. Kessel, M.D. Professional Services Building, Family Practice Center 3231 South Euclid Ave. Brewyn, Illinois 60402 (312) 795-7800
Doctor's Memorial Hospital 404 West Main Street Carbondale, Illinois 62901 3/A (Southern Illinois University)		Kevin K. Mooney, M.D. Family Practice Residency 404 West Main Street Carbondale, Illinois 62901 (618) 536-6621
Columbus Hospital 2520 North Lakeview Avenue Chicago, Illinois 60614 2/A (Northwestern University)		Ronald A. Ferguson, M.D. Family Practice Residency Program Columbus–Cuneo–Cabrini Medical Center Columbus Hospital 2520 North Lakeview Avenue Chicago, Illinois 60614 (312) 883-7300

FAMILY PRACTICE TEACHING PROGRAMS—CONTINUED

SPONSORING INSTITUTION	CHAIRMAN OF MEDICAL SCHOOL DEPARTMENT (IF APPLICABLE)	DIRECTOR OF RESIDENCY PROGRAM AND FAMILY PRACTICE CENTER ADDRESS AND PHONE NUMBER
Cook County Hospital 1824 West Harrison Chicago, Illinois 60612 2/A (Chicago Medical School)		Jorge Prieto, M.D. Family Practice Residency 720 South Wolcott Chicago, Illinois 60612 (312) 633-8587
Illinois Masonic Medical Center 923 West Wellington Chicago, Illinois 60657 2/A (Abraham Lincoln School of Medicine)		Norman N. Monitz, M.D. Family Practice Residency 923 West Wellington Chicago, Illinois 60657 (312) 525-2300 Ext. 748
Resurrection Hospital 7435 West Talcott Avenue Chicago, Illinois 60631 2/A (Loyola University)		Thomas C. Tomasik, M.D. Resurrection Hospital Family Practice Center 7447 West Talcott Chicago, Illinois 60631 (312) 774-9144
Rush University Rush Medical College 600 South Paulina Chicago, Illinois 60612 4/A		Erich F. Brueschke, M.D. Rush-Christ Family Residency Program Christ Hospital 4440 West 95th Street Oak Lawn, Illinois 60453 (312) 942-7083
Saint Joseph Hospital 2900 North Lake Shore Drive Chicago, Illinois 60657 2/A (Northwestern Medical School)		Roger A. Nosal, M.D., Ph.D. Chairman Family Practice Residency 2900 North Lake Shore Drive Chicago, Illinois 60657 (312) 975-3454
South Chicago Community Hospital 2320 East 93rd Chicago, Illinois 60617 1/A		Clement R. Brown, M.D. Family Practice Center 17225 South Paxton South Holland, Illinois 60473 (312) 895-4400
St. Mary of Nazareth Hospital Center 2233 West Division Street Chicago, Illinois 60622 1/A		Robert T. Swastek, M.D. Ruth and Frank Korte Family Practice Center 2238 West Thomas Street Chicago, Illinois 60622 (312) 770-2000

FAMILY PRACTICE TEACHING PROGRAMS—CONTINUED

SPONSORING INSTITUTION	*CHAIRMAN OF MEDICAL SCHOOL DEPARTMENT (IF APPLICABLE)*	*DIRECTOR OF RESIDENCY PROGRAM AND FAMILY PRACTICE CENTER ADDRESS AND PHONE NUMBER*
Swedish Covenant Hospital 5145 North California Ave. Chicago, Illinois 60625 2/A (Rush Medical College)		Philip D. Anderson, M.D. Family Practice Residency 5145 North California Ave. Chicago, Illinois 60625 (312) 878–8200 Ext. 444
East Central Illinois Medical Education Foundation 103 North Robinson Danville, Illinois 61832 2/A (University of Illinois, School of Basic Medical Sciences—Urbana)		L. William Tanner, M.D. Danville Family Practice Residency 103 North Robinson Danville, Illinois 61832 (217) 443–6891
St. Mary's and Decatur Memorial Hospital* 155 West King Street Decatur, Illinois 62521 3/A (Southern Illinois University)		David Ouchterlony, M.D. Family Practice Residency Program 155 West King Street Decatur, Illinois 62521 (217) 423–9000
Hinsdale Sanitarium and Hospital 120 North Oak Hinsdale, Illinois 60521 2/A (Loma Linda— California)		W. Duane Dodd, M.D. Hinsdale Family Medicine Center 135 North Oak Hinsdale, Illinois 60521 (312) 887–2935
Community Memorial General Hospital 1323 Community Memorial Drive LaGrange, Illinois 60525 2/A (Rush Medical College)		Russell W. Zitek, M.D. Community Family Practice Center 1323 Community Memorial Drive LaGrange, Illinois 60525 (312) 352–7470
West Suburban Hospital 518 North Austin Boulevard Oak Park, Illinois 60302 2/A (Rush Medical College)		A.L. Burdick, Jr., M.D. Family Practice Center 10 West Ontario Street Oak Park, Illinois 60302 (312) 383–8045
Lutheran General Hospital 1775 Dempster Street Park Ridge, Illinois 60068 2/A (Abraham Lincoln School of Medicine)		Leighton B. Smith, M.D. Family Practice Residency Room 415—South Lutheran General Hospital 1775 Dempster Street Park Ridge, Illinois 60068 (312) 696–7969

FAMILY PRACTICE TEACHING PROGRAMS—CONTINUED

SPONSORING INSTITUTION	CHAIRMAN OF MEDICAL SCHOOL DEPARTMENT (IF APPLICABLE)	DIRECTOR OF RESIDENCY PROGRAM AND FAMILY PRACTICE CENTER ADDRESS AND PHONE NUMBER
Methodist Medical Center of Illinois 221 Northeast Glen Oak Peoria, Illinois 61636 2/A (Peoria School of Medicine)		Dean R. Bordeaux, M.D. Family Practice Residency 221 Northeast Glen Oak Peoria, Illinois 61603 (309) 672–4985
Saint Francis Hospital— Medical Center 530 Northeast Glen Oak Avenue Peoria, Illinois 61637 1/A		Carl F. Neuhoff, M.D., Chairman Family Practice Residency 530 Northeast Glen Oak Avenue Peoria, Illinois 61637 (309) 672–2003
Rockford Medical Education Foundation and Affiliated Hospitals 1601 Parkview Avenue Rockford, Illinois 61101 3/A (Rockford School of Medicine)		L.P. Johnson, M.D. Family Practice Residency 1601 Parkview Avenue Rockford, Illinois 61101 (815) 987–7075
U.S. Air Force Medical Center Scott Air Force Base, Illinois 62225 5/A		Lt. Colonel Reed C. Rasmussen, M.C., U.S.A.F. Family Practice Residency Scott Air Force Base, Illinois 62225 (618) 256–7312
St. John's Hospital 419 North 7th Street Springfield, Illinois 62708 3/A (Southern Illinois University)		Peter G. Coggan, M.D. Family Practice Residency 421 North 9th Street Springfield, Illinois 62702 (217) 782–0220
Carle Foundation 611 West Park Street Urbana, Illinois 61801 2/A (University of Illinois, School of Basic Medical Science—Urbana)		Paul W. Yardy, M.D. Carle Foundation Family Practice Residence 611 East Park Street Urbana, Illinois 61801 (217) 337–3311

Indiana

Indiana University School of Medicine 1100 West Michigan Street Indianapolis, Indiana 46202	A. Alan Fischer, M.D. Chairman Dept. of Family Medicine (317) 264–4971	

FAMILY PRACTICE TEACHING PROGRAMS—CONTINUED

SPONSORING INSTITUTION	*CHAIRMAN OF MEDICAL SCHOOL DEPARTMENT (IF APPLICABLE)*	*DIRECTOR OF RESIDENCY PROGRAM AND FAMILY PRACTICE CENTER ADDRESS AND PHONE NUMBER*
St. Francis Hospital Center 1600 Albany Street Beech Grove, Indiana 46107 2/A (Indiana University)		Robert B. Chevalier, M.D. St. Francis Hospital, Family Practice Residency 1600 Albany Street Beech Grove, Indiana 46107 (317) 783–8136
Deaconess Hospital 600 Mary Street Evansville, Indiana 47747 2/A (Indiana University)		Wallace M. Adye, M.D. Family Practice Residency 611 Harriet Street, Suite L–100 Evansville, Indiana 47747 (812) 426–3363
St. Mary's Hospital 3700 Washington Avenue Evansville, Indiana 47750 2/A (Indiana University)		Raymond W. Nicholson, M.D. Family Practice Residency 801 St. Mary's Drive Evansville, Indiana 47715 (812) 479–4455
Methodist Hospital of Gary 2318 West Fifth Avenue Gary, Indiana 46402 2/A (Chicago Medical School and University of Indiana)		David E. Ross, M.D. Methodist Family Health Center 2318 West 5th Gary, Indiana 46404 (219) 944–9713
Fort Wayne Medical Education Program 2101 Coliseum Boulevard East Fort Wayne, Indiana 46805 2/A (Indiana University)		Alvin J. Haley, M.D. Family Practice Unit 3217 Lake Avenue Fort Wayne, Indiana 46805 (219) 422–1541
Community Hospital of Indianapolis 5626 East 16th Street Indianapolis, Indiana 46218 2/A (Indiana University)		William E. Kelley, M.D. Family Practice Residency 5626 East 16th Street Indianapolis, Indiana 42618 (317) 359–7740
Indiana University School of Medicine Long Hospital 1100 West Michigan Street Indianapolis, Indiana 46202 4/A (Indiana University)		Thomas A. Jones, M.D. Family Practice Residency Long Hospital 1100 West Michigan Street Indianapolis, Indiana 46202 (317) 264–4971

FAMILY PRACTICE TEACHING PROGRAMS—CONTINUED

SPONSORING INSTITUTION	CHAIRMAN OF MEDICAL SCHOOL DEPARTMENT (IF APPLICABLE)	DIRECTOR OF RESIDENCY PROGRAM AND FAMILY PRACTICE CENTER ADDRESS AND PHONE NUMBER
Methodist Hospital Graduate Medical Center 1604 North Capitol Avenue Indianapolis, Indiana 46202 2/A (Indiana University)		Kenneth L. Gray, M.D. Family Practice Education— Methodist Hospital Graduate Medical Center 1604 North Capitol Indianapolis, Indiana 46202 (317) 924-8425
St. Vincent Hospital 2001 West 86th Street Indianapolis, Indiana 46260 2/A (Indiana University)		Fred M. Blix, M.D. St. Vincent Family Practice Residency 8402 Harcourt Road, Suite 501 Indianapolis, Indiana 46260 (317) 871-2420
Ball Memorial Hospital 2401 University Avenue Muncie, Indiana 47303 1/A		Ross L. Egger, M.D. Family Practice Residency 2300 West Gilbert Muncie, Indiana 47303 (317) 747-3376
Memorial Hospital of South Bend 615 North Michigan Street South Bend, Indiana 46601 2/A (Indiana University)		L. Louis Frank, Jr., M.D. Family Practice Residency 615 North Michigan Street South Bend, Indiana 46601 (219) 284-7353
Saint Joseph's Hospital 811 East Madison Street South Bend, Indiana 46600 2/A (Indiana University)		H.R. Stimson, M.D. and D.G. White, M.D. Family Practice Residency 811 East Madison Street South Bend, Indiana 46600 (219) 237-7256
Union Hospital 1606 North 7th Street Terre Haute, Indiana 47804 1/A		James R. Buechler, M.D. Union Hospital Family Practice Residency 1513 North $6\frac{1}{2}$ Street Terre Haute, Indiana 47807 (812) 232-6400
Iowa		
University of Iowa College of Medicine 100 College of Medical Administration Building Iowa City, Iowa 52242	Robert F. Rakel, M.D. Chairman Dept. of Family Practice (319) 356-2975	

FAMILY PRACTICE TEACHING PROGRAMS—CONTINUED

SPONSORING INSTITUTION	CHAIRMAN OF MEDICAL SCHOOL DEPARTMENT (IF APPLICABLE)	DIRECTOR OF RESIDENCY PROGRAM AND FAMILY PRACTICE CENTER ADDRESS AND PHONE NUMBER
Mercy Hospital 701 Tenth Street Southeast Cedar Rapids, Iowa 52402 1/A and St. Luke's Methodist 1026 A Avenue, Northeast Cedar Rapids, Iowa 52402		Carl R. Aschoff, M.D. Cedar Rapids Family Practice Residency 1026 A Avenue, Northeast Cedar Rapids, Iowa 52402 (319) 398-7393
Mercy Hospital and St. Luke's 1326 West Lombard Street Davenport, Iowa 52804 2/A (University of Iowa— Iowa City)		Forrest W. Smith, M.D. Family Medical Center 516 West 35th Street Davenport, Iowa 52806 (319) 386-3700
Broadlawns Polk County Hospital 18th and Hickman Road Des Moines, Iowa 50314 2/A (University of Iowa— Iowa City)		Loran F. Parker, M.D. Family Practice Residency 18th and Hickman Road Des Moines, Iowa 50314 (515) 282-2275
Iowa Lutheran Hospital University at Pennsylvania Ave. Des Moines, Iowa 50316 2/A (University of Iowa— Iowa City)		Arnold T. Nielson, M.D., Acting Director Iowa Lutheran Hospital University at Pennsylvania Avenue Des Moines, Iowa 50316 (515) 283-5674
University of Iowa Hospital and Clinics Family Practice Center Iowa City, Iowa 52242 4/A (University of Iowa— Iowa City)		Robert E. Rakel, M.D. University of Iowa Hospital and Clinics Iowa City, Iowa 52242 (319) 356-2975
St. Joseph Mercy Hospital 84 Beaumont Drive Mason City, Iowa 50401 2/B (University of Iowa; first year spent at University of Iowa—Iowa City)		Richard E. Munns, M.D. Family Practice Residency 101 South Taylor Mason City, Iowa 50401 (515) 423-9200
Siouxland Medical Education Foundation 2417 Pierce Sioux City, Iowa 51104 2/A (University of Iowa— Iowa City)		Gerald J. McGowan, M.D. Siouxland Medical Education Foundation 2417 Pierce Sioux City, Iowa 51104 (712) 252-3886

FAMILY PRACTICE TEACHING PROGRAMS—CONTINUED

SPONSORING INSTITUTION	CHAIRMAN OF MEDICAL SCHOOL DEPARTMENT (IF APPLICABLE)	DIRECTOR OF RESIDENCY PROGRAM AND FAMILY PRACTICE CENTER ADDRESS AND PHONE NUMBER
Black Hawk Area Medical Education Foundation 441 East San Marnan Drive Waterloo, Iowa 50702 2/A (University of Iowa— Iowa City)		C.A. Waterbury, M.D. Black Hawk Area Family Practice Center 441 East San Marnan Drive Waterloo, Iowa 50702 (319) 234-4419

Kansas

SPONSORING INSTITUTION	CHAIRMAN OF MEDICAL SCHOOL DEPARTMENT (IF APPLICABLE)	DIRECTOR OF RESIDENCY PROGRAM AND FAMILY PRACTICE CENTER ADDRESS AND PHONE NUMBER
University of Kansas School of Medicine 39th and Rainbow Boulevard Kansas City, Kansas 66103	Jack D. Walker, M.D. Chairman Dept. of Family Practice (913) 588-6510	
University of Kansas Wichita State University Branch 1001 North Minneapolis Wichita, Kansas 67214	Donald J. Gessler, M.D. Acting Chairman Dept. of Family and Community Medicine (316) 268-8221	
University of Kansas Medical School 4125 Rainbow Boulevard Kansas City, Kansas 66103 4/A (University of Kansas— Kansas City)		Jack D. Walker, M.D. Family Practice Residency 4125 Rainbow Boulevard Kansas City, Kansas 66103 (913) 588-6510
Saint Francis Hospital 929 North St. Francis Street Wichita, Kansas 67214 2/A (University of Kansas— Wichita)		Donald J. Gessler, M.D. St. Francis Family Practice Center 1122 North Topeka Wichita, Kansas 67214 (316) 265-2876
Saint Joseph Medical Center Clifton at Harry Wichita, Kansas 67218 2/A (University of Kansas— Wichita)		Lawrence H. Miller, M.D. Family Practice Center 3400 Grand Avenue Wichita, Kansas 67278 (316) 685-4354
Wesley Medical Center 550 North Hillside Wichita, Kansas 67214 2/A (University of Kansas— Wichita)		Stanley Mosier, M.D. and Victor Vorhees, M.D. Family Practice Residency— Wesley Medical Center 550 North Hillside Wichita, Kansas 67214 (316) 685-2151

FAMILY PRACTICE TEACHING PROGRAMS—CONTINUED

SPONSORING INSTITUTION	CHAIRMAN OF MEDICAL SCHOOL DEPARTMENT (IF APPLICABLE)	DIRECTOR OF RESIDENCY PROGRAM AND FAMILY PRACTICE CENTER ADDRESS AND PHONE NUMBER
Kentucky		
University of Kentucky College of Medicine 800 Rose Street Lexington, Kentucky 40506	H. Thomas Wiegert, M.D. Chairman Dept. of Family Practice (606) 233–6418	
University of Louisville School of Medicine 801 Barret Avenue Louisville, Kentucky 40204	John C. Wright, II, M.D. Chairman Dept. of.Family Medicine (502) 588–5201	
St. Elizabeth Hospital 21st and Eastern Avenue Covington, Kentucky 41014 2/A (University of Kentucky—Lexington)		Richard Allnutt, M.D. Family Practice Residency Family Medicine Unit 400 Dudley Road Edgewood, Kentucky 41017 (606) 331–8333
University of Kentucky Medical Center Annex 2, Room 1 Lexington, Kentucky 40506 4/A (University of Kentucky—Lexington)		E.C. Seeley, M.D. Dept. of Family Practice 913 South Limestone Lexington, Kentucky 40503 (606) 233–6371
University of Louisville 801 Barret Avenue Louisville, Kentucky 40204 3/A (University of Louisville)		Daniel Dill, M.D. University of Louisville Family Practice Department 801 Barret Louisville, Kentucky 40204 (502) 588–5203
Trover Clinic Foundation Hopkins County Hospital 237 Waddell Avenue Madisonville, Kentucky 42431 2/A (University of Louisville)		Dan A. Martin, M.D. Family Practice Residency 237 Waddell Avenue Madisonville, Kentucky 42431 (502) 821–7171 Ext. 271
Louisiana		
Louisiana State University School of Medicine 1542 Tulane Avenue New Orleans, Louisiana 70112	Gerald R. Gehringer, M.D. Chairman Dept. of Family Medicine (504) 568–4570	

FAMILY PRACTICE TEACHING PROGRAMS—CONTINUED

SPONSORING INSTITUTION	CHAIRMAN OF MEDICAL SCHOOL DEPARTMENT (IF APPLICABLE)	DIRECTOR OF RESIDENCY PROGRAM AND FAMILY PRACTICE CENTER ADDRESS AND PHONE NUMBER
Louisiana State University School of Medicine in Shreveport P.O. Box 33932 Shreveport, Louisiana 71130	Rozelle Hahn, M.D. Chairman Dept. of Family Medicine and Comprehensive Care (318) 226–3230	
Earl K. Long Memorial Hospital 5825 Airline Highway Baton Rouge, Louisiana 70805 2/A (Louisiana State University—New Orleans)		Vance G. Byars, Jr., M.D. Family Practice Residency 5825 Airline Highway Baton Rouge, Louisiana 70805 (504) 356–3361 Ext. 411
Bogalusa Community Medical Center 433 Plaza Bogalusa, Louisiana 70427 3/B (First year at Louisiana State University—New Orleans) and Washington—St. Tammany Charity Hospital Bogalusa, Louisiana 70427		Rafael C. Sanchez, M.D. P.O. Box 459 Bogalusa, Louisiana 70427 (504) 732–7107
Lake Charles Charity Hospital 1000 Walters Street Lake Charles, Louisiana 70601 3/A (Louisiana State University—New Orleans)		Eli Sorkow, M.D. Family Practice Residency 1000 Walters Street Lake Charles, Louisiana 70601 (318) 478–6346
Louisiana State University School of Medicine Department of Family Medicine 1542 Tulane Avenue New Orleans, Louisiana 70112 4/A		Francis I. Nicolle, M.D. Family Practice Residency Program Louisiana State University 1825 Cleveland Avenue New Orleans, Louisiana 70112 (504) 568–4570
Louisiana State University Medical Center P.O. Box 33932 Shreveport, Louisiana 71130 3/4 (Louisiana State University—Shreveport)		Charles R. Sias, M.D. Louisiana State University Medical Center—Shreveport P.O. Box 33932 Shreveport, Louisiana 71130 (318) 226–3230

FAMILY PRACTICE TEACHING PROGRAMS—CONTINUED

SPONSORING INSTITUTION	CHAIRMAN OF MEDICAL SCHOOL DEPARTMENT (IF APPLICABLE)	DIRECTOR OF RESIDENCY PROGRAM AND FAMILY PRACTICE CENTER ADDRESS AND PHONE NUMBER

Maine

Central Maine Family Practice
  Residency
12 East Chestnut Street
Augusta, Maine 04330
1/A

H. Douglas Collins, M.D.
Central Maine Family Practice
  Residency
12 East Chestnut Street
Augusta, Maine 04330
(207) 622-9361

Eastern Maine Medical Center
489 State Street
Bangor, Maine 04401
1/A

A. Dewey Richards, M.D.
Eastern Maine Medical
  Center—Family Practice
  Residency
Family Practice Center
417 State Street
Bangor, Maine 04401
(207) 947-3341

Central Maine Medical Center
76 High Street
Lewiston, Maine 04240
2/A (Boston University School
  of Medicine)

David D. Smith, M.D.
Family Practice Residency
  Program
P.O. Box 4500
Lewiston, Maine 04240
(207) 795-2286

Maine Medical Center
Department of Family
  Practice
22 Bramhall Street
Portland, Maine 04102
2/A (Tufts University School
  of Medicine)

Ian MacInnes, M.D., Chief
Family Practice Unit
272-274 Congress Street
Portland, Maine 04102
(207) 871-2781

Maryland

University of Maryland
School of Medicine
522 West Lombard Street
Baltimore, Maryland 21201

Edward Kowalewski, M.D.
Chairman
Dept. of Family Practice
(301) 528-5688

Uniformed Services
University of Health Sciences
6917 Arlington Road
Bethesda, Maryland 20014

Lt. Col. Chris Marquart,
  M.C., U.S.A.F.
Chairman
Dept. of Family Practice
(301) 981-3786

FAMILY PRACTICE TEACHING PROGRAMS—CONTINUED

SPONSORING INSTITUTION	CHAIRMAN OF MEDICAL SCHOOL DEPARTMENT (IF APPLICABLE)	DIRECTOR OF RESIDENCY PROGRAM AND FAMILY PRACTICE CENTER ADDRESS AND PHONE NUMBER
Franklin Square Hospital 9000 Franklin Square Drive Baltimore, Maryland 21237 1/A		William Reichel, M.D. Department of Family Practice Franklin Square Hospital 9000 Franklin Square Drive Baltimore, Maryland 21237 (301) 391–4453
University of Maryland Hospital 22 South Greene Street Baltimore, Maryland 21201 4/A (University of Maryland)		C. Earl Hill, M.D. Family Practice Program 22 South Greene Street Baltimore, Maryland 21201 (301) 528–5012
Prince George's General Hospital Hospital Drive Cheverly, Maryland 20785 2/A (University of Maryland)		Albert Roth, M.D. Family Practice Residency Hospital Drive Cheverly, Maryland 20785 (301) 341–6444
Washington Adventist Hospital 7600 Carroll Avenue Takoma Park, Maryland 20012 2/A (Loma Linda— California)		Morrill C. Quinnam, Jr., M.D. Family Practice Residency 7600 Carroll Avenue Takoma Park, Maryland 20012 (301) 891–7662

Massachusetts

University of Massachusetts Coordinated Medical School 55 Lake Avenue, North Worcester, Massachusetts 01605	Robin J.O. Catlin, M.D. Chairman Dept. of Family Practice and Community Medicine (617) 856–2246	
University of Massachusetts Coordinated Program 2 Burbank Hospital Nicholas Road Fitchburg, Massachusetts 01420 2/B (First year at University of Massachusetts Hospital)		Robert A. Babineau, M.D. Fitchburg Family Practice Residency University of Massachusetts Hospital Medical Center 47 Ashby State Road Fitchburg, Massachusetts 01420 (617) 343–3022

FAMILY PRACTICE TEACHING PROGRAMS—CONTINUED

SPONSORING INSTITUTION	CHAIRMAN OF MEDICAL SCHOOL DEPARTMENT (IF APPLICABLE)	DIRECTOR OF RESIDENCY PROGRAM AND FAMILY PRACTICE CENTER ADDRESS AND PHONE NUMBER
University of Massachusetts Coordinated Program 1 Department of Family Practice 55 Lake Avenue, North Worcester, Massachusetts 01605 4/A (University of Massachusetts)		Paul Hart, M.D. Acting Director Family Practice Residency Program 55 Lake Avenue North Worcester, Massachusetts 01605 (617) 856–3025

Michigan

University of Michigan Medical School 1335 Catherine Street Ann Arbor, Michigan 48109	Terence Davies, M.D. Chairman Dept. of Family Practice (313) 764–8010	
Wayne State University School of Medicine 540 East Canfield Detroit, Michigan 48201	Joseph W. Hess, M.D. Chairman Dept. of Family Medicine (313) 577–0882	
Michigan State University College of Human Medicine B–100 Clinical Center East Lansing, Michigan 48824	Roy J. Gerard, M.D. Chairman Dept. of Family Practice (517) 353–0850	
Oakwood Hospital 18101 Oakwood Boulevard Dearborn, Michigan 48124 2/A (Wayne State University)		Everal M. Wakeman, M.D. Family Medical Center 19130 Sumpter Road Bellville, Michigan 48111 (313) 699–2094
Harper–Grace Hospital 3740 John R. Detroit, Michigan 48201 3/A (Wayne State University)		Kenneth B. Frisof, M.D. Family Practice Residency 3740 John R. Detroit, Michigan 48201 (313) 577–0882
St. John's Hospital 22101 Moross Detroit, Michigan 48236 2/A (Wayne State University)		John L. Lehtinen, M.D. Family Medicine Center 17700 Mack Grosse Point, Michigan 48224 (313) 886–1672
Mount Carmel Mercy Hospital and Medical Center 6071 West Outer Drive Detroit, Michigan 48235 2/A (Wayne State University)		Fred Caumartin, M.D. Family Practice Center 6071 West Outer Drive Detroit, Michigan 48235 (313) 341–5565

FAMILY PRACTICE TEACHING PROGRAMS—CONTINUED

SPONSORING INSTITUTION	CHAIRMAN OF MEDICAL SCHOOL DEPARTMENT (IF APPLICABLE)	DIRECTOR OF RESIDENCY PROGRAM AND FAMILY PRACTICE CENTER ADDRESS AND PHONE NUMBER
St. Joseph Hospital 302 Kensington Avenue Flint, Michigan 48502 2/A (Michigan State University)		Robert M. Weber, M.D. Family Practice Residency 302 Kensington Ave. Flint, Michigan 48502 (313) 238-2601
Grand Rapids Area Medical Education Center 220 Cherry Street, Southeast Grand Rapids, Michigan 49503 1/A		Charles E. Morrill, M.D. Family Practice Residency 220 Cherry Street, Southeast Grand Rapids, Michigan 49503 (616) 459-2837
Bon Secours Hospital 468 Cadieux Road Grosse Point, Michigan 48230 2/A (Wayne State University)		Archie W. Bedell, M.D. Family Health Center 25901 Jefferson St. Claire Shores, Michigan 48081 (313) 774-7800
Southwestern Michigan A.H.E.C. 252 East Lovell Street Kalamazoo, Michigan 49006 1/A		Donald E. DeWitt, M.D. Family Practice Residency Program Stryker Building 1521 Gull Road Kalamazoo, Michigan 49001 (616) 383-7363
Edward West Sparrow Hospital 1215 East Michigan Avenue P.O. Box 30480 Lansing, Michigan 48909 2/A (Michigan State University)		Harold E. Crow, M.D. Family Practice Residency 1215 E. Michigan Avenue P.O. Box 30480 Lansing, Michigan 48909 (517) 487-9200
St. Lawrence Hospital 1210 West Saginaw Street Lansing, Michigan 48914 2/A (Michigan State University)		Dwight M. Schroeder, M.D. Director FPC St. Lawrence Hospital 1210 West Saginaw Street/ P.O. Box 19038 Lansing, Michigan 48914 (517) 372-3610 and James G. O'Brien, M.D. —Room B100 Clinical Center College of Human Medicine Michigan State University P.O. Box 19038 East Lansing, Michigan 48823 (517) 353-0770

FAMILY PRACTICE TEACHING PROGRAMS—CONTINUED

SPONSORING INSTITUTION	CHAIRMAN OF MEDICAL SCHOOL DEPARTMENT (IF APPLICABLE)	DIRECTOR OF RESIDENCY PROGRAM AND FAMILY PRACTICE CENTER ADDRESS AND PHONE NUMBER
Upper Peninsula Medical Education Program 540 West Kaye Ave. Marquette, Michigan 49855 2–A (Michigan State University)		Israel Fradkin, M.D. Family Practice Residency Program 540 West Kaye Ave. Marquette, Michigan 49855 (906) 228–7970
Midland Hospital Center 4009 Orchard Drive Midland, Michigan 48640 2/A (Michigan State University)		Robert J. LaChance, M.D. Family Practice Residency 4009 Orchard Drive Midland, Michigan 48640 (517) 631–7700
Pontiac General Hospital Seminole at West Huron Pontiac, Michigan 48053 2/A (Wayne State University)		Esly S. Caldwell, II, M.D. Family Practice Residency 132 Franklin Blvd. Pontiac, Michigan 48053 (313) 857–7488
Saginaw Cooperative Hospitals, Inc. 705 Cooper Street Saginaw, Michigan 48602 2/A (Michigan State University)		Robert J. Toteff, M.D. Family Practice Residency 705 Cooper Street Saginaw, Michigan 48602 (517) 754–8881
Providence Hospital 16001 West Nine Mile Road Southfield, Michigan 48075 2/A (Wayne State University)		Murray N. Deighton, M.D. Family Practice Residency 16001 West Nine Mile Road Southfield, Michigan 48075 (313) 424–3000

Minnesota

University of Minnesota Medical School 145 Owre Hall Minneapolis, Minnesota 55455	Edward W. Ciriacy, M.D. Chairman Dept. of Family Practice (612) 373–8539	
University of Minnesota School of Medicine Section of Family Practice 2205 East Fifth Street Duluth, Minnesota 55812	James E. Hoffman, M.D. Dept. of Clinical Sciences (218) 726–7571	
Mayo Medical School 200 First Street, Southwest Rochester, Minnesota 55901	Robert Avant, M.D. Chairman Division of Family Practice (507) 282–2511	

FAMILY PRACTICE TEACHING PROGRAMS—CONTINUED

SPONSORING INSTITUTION	*CHAIRMAN OF MEDICAL SCHOOL DEPARTMENT (IF APPLICABLE)*	*DIRECTOR OF RESIDENCY PROGRAM AND FAMILY PRACTICE CENTER ADDRESS AND PHONE NUMBER*
Duluth Graduate Medical Education Council, Inc. 330 North 8th Avenue East Duluth, Minnesota 55805 2/A (University of Minnesota)		Daniel J. Ostergaard, M.D. Duluth Family Practice Center 330 North 8th Avenue East Duluth, Minnesota 55805 (218) 723-1112
Hennepin County Medical Center 7th Street and Park Avenue Minneapolis, Minnesota 55415 2/A (University of Minnesota)		Eldon Berglund, M.D. Family Practice Residency 7th Street and Park Avenue Minneapolis, Minnesota 55415 (612) 347-3103
University of Minnesota Affiliated Community Hospital Program A-290 Mayo, Box 381 Minneapolis, Minnesota 55455 4-3/A (University of Minnesota)		Edward W. Ciriacy, M.D. Family Practice Residency A-290 Mayo, Box 381 Minneapolis, Minnesota 55455 (612) 373-8539
St. Paul–Ramsey Hospital 640 Jackson Street St. Paul, Minnesota 55101 2/A (University of Minnesota)		Vincent R. Hunt, M.D. Dept. of Family Medicine 640 Jackson Street St. Paul, Minnesota 55101 (612) 221-3540 Ext. 616
Mayo-Graduate Family Practice Residency Program Division of Family Practice 200 Southwest First Street Rochester, Minnesota 55901 4/A (Mayo Medical School)		Robert Avant, M.D. Family Practice Residency 200 Southwest First Street Rochester, Minnesota 55901 (507) 282-2511

Mississippi

University of Mississippi School of Medicine 2500 North State Street Jackson, Mississippi 39216	W.R. Gillis, M.D. Chairman Dept. of Family Medicine (601) 968-4900	

FAMILY PRACTICE TEACHING PROGRAMS—CONTINUED

SPONSORING INSTITUTION	CHAIRMAN OF MEDICAL SCHOOL DEPARTMENT (IF APPLICABLE)	DIRECTOR OF RESIDENCY PROGRAM AND FAMILY PRACTICE CENTER ADDRESS AND PHONE NUMBER
University of Mississippi Medical Center 2500 North State Street Jackson, Mississippi 39216 4/A (University of Mississippi)		B.F. Banahan, M.D. Department of Family Medicine—University Medical Center 2500 North State Street Jackson, Mississippi 39216 (601) 968-4900

Missouri

University of Missouri— Columbia School of Medicine 807 Stadium Road Columbia, Missouri 65201	Jack M. Colwill, M.D. Chairman Dept. of Family and Community Medicine (314) 882-2996	
University of Missouri— Kansas City School of Medicine 2411 Holmes Street Kansas City, Missouri 64108	W. Jack Stelmach, M.D. Chairman Dept. of Family and Community Medicine (816) 361-7333	
University of Missouri Medical Center 807 Stadium Road Columbia, Missouri 65201 4/A (University of Missouri— Columbia)		Jack M. Colwill, M.D. Family Practice Residency 807 Stadium Road Columbia, Missouri 65201 (314) 882-2996
Baptist Memorial Hospital 6601 Rockhill Road Kansas City, Missouri 64131 2/A (University of Missouri— Kansas City)		W.J. Stelmach, M.D. Baptist Memorial Hospital Family Practice Residency Goppert Family Care Center 6601 Rockhill Road Kansas City, Missouri 64131 (816) 361-7333
Lutheran Medical Center 2639 Miami Street St. Louis, Missouri 63118 1/A		Homer B. Matthews, M.D. Family Practice Center 3535 South Jefferson St. Louis, Missouri 63118 (314) 772-1456
St. John's Mercy Medical Center 615 South New Ballas Road St. Louis, Missouri 63141 1/A		Joseph J. Lauber, M.D. Family Practice Residency 615 South New Ballas Road St. Louis, Missouri 63141 (314) 569-6010

FAMILY PRACTICE TEACHING PROGRAMS—CONTINUED

SPONSORING INSTITUTION	CHAIRMAN OF MEDICAL SCHOOL DEPARTMENT (IF APPLICABLE)	DIRECTOR OF RESIDENCY PROGRAM AND FAMILY PRACTICE CENTER ADDRESS AND PHONE NUMBER
Nebraska		
Creighton University School of Medicine 2500 California Street Omaha, Nebraska 68178	Fred J. Pettid, M.D. Acting Chairman Dept. of Family Practice (402) 449–4175	
University of Nebraska College of Medicine 42nd Street and Dewey Avenue Omaha, Nebraska 68105	Paul R. Young, M.D. Chairman Dept. of Family Practice (402) 541–4979	
Lincoln Medical Education Foundation Family Medicine Residency Program Lincoln Area Health Education Center 4600 Valley Road Lincoln, Nebraska 68510 2/A (University of Nebraska—Omaha)		John C. Finegan, M.D. Lincoln Family Practice Center 4600 Valley Road Lincoln, Nebraska 68510 (402) 483–4571
Creighton University Medical School 25th and California Omaha, Nebraska 68178 4/A (Creighton University)		Fred J. Pettid, M.D. Dept. of Family Practice 601 North 30th Street Omaha, Nebraska 68131 (402) 449–4175
University of Nebraska Hospital 42nd and Dewey Avenue Omaha, Nebraska 68105 4/A (University of Nebraska—Omaha)		Paul R. Young, M.D. Family Practice Residency 42nd and Dewey Omaha, Nebraska 68105 (402) 541–4979
Nevada		
University of Nevada Affiliated Hospitals 410 Mill Street Reno, Nevada 89502 4/A (University of Nevada)		Charles E. Payton, M.D. Family Practice Residency Program 410 Mill Street Reno, Nevada 89502 (702) 329–1082

FAMILY PRACTICE TEACHING PROGRAMS—CONTINUED

SPONSORING INSTITUTION	*CHAIRMAN OF MEDICAL SCHOOL DEPARTMENT (IF APPLICABLE)*	*DIRECTOR OF RESIDENCY PROGRAM AND FAMILY PRACTICE CENTER ADDRESS AND PHONE NUMBER*
New Jersey		
Rutgers Medical School College of Medicine and Dentistry of New Jersey P.O. Box 101 Piscataway, New Jersey 08854	Frank C. Snope, M.D. Chairman Dept. of Family Medicine (201) 463–4608	
John F. Kennedy Medical Center James Street Edison, New Jersey 08817 2/A (Rutgers Medical School)		Samuel F. D'Ambola, M.D. Family Practice Residency James Street Edison, New Jersey 08817 (201) 321–7493
Hunterdon Medical Center Route 31 Flemington, New Jersey 08822 2/A (Rutgers Medical School)		John A. Zapp, M.D. Family Practice Residency Route 31 Flemington, New Jersey 08822 (201) 782–2121
St. Mary Hospital 308 Willow Avenue Hoboken, New Jersey 07030 1/A		Robert Verdon, M.D. Family Practice Residency 308 Willow Avenue Hoboken, New Jersey 07030 (201) 792–3300
Mountainside Hospital Bay Avenue and Highland Avenue Montclair, New Jersey 07042 2/A (Rutgers Medical School)		Alfred R. Dardis, M.D. Mountainside Family Planning Associates 331 Claremont Avenue Montclair, New Jersey 07042 (201) 783–7900
Somerset Hospital 120 Rehill Avenue Somerville, New Jersey 08876 2–A (Rutgers Medical School)		Carl F. Meier, M.D. Family Practice Residency 120 Rehill Avenue Somerville, New Jersey 08876 (201) 526–4800
Overlook Hospital 193 Morris Avenue Summit, New Jersey 07901 2/A (Columbia University, College of Physicians and Surgeons)		Donald F. Kent, M.D. Family Practice Residency 193 Morris Ave. Summit, New Jersey 07901 (201) 273–4700

FAMILY PRACTICE TEACHING PROGRAMS—CONTINUED

SPONSORING INSTITUTION	CHAIRMAN OF MEDICAL SCHOOL DEPARTMENT (IF APPLICABLE)	DIRECTOR OF RESIDENCY PROGRAM AND FAMILY PRACTICE CENTER ADDRESS AND PHONE NUMBER
West Jersey Hospital Mt. Ephraim and Atlantic Avenues Camden, New Jersey 08104 2/A (University of Pennsylvania)		S. Thomas Carter, Jr., M.D. Director Family Practice Residency Program West Jersey Hospital, Eastern Division Voorhees, New Jersey 08034 (609) 854-7011

New Mexico

University of New Mexico School of Medicine Albuquerque, New Mexico 87131	William Wiese, M.D. Chairman Dept. of Family and Community Medicine (505) 277-3253	
University of New Mexico 620 Camino De Salud Northeast Albuquerque, New Mexico 87131 4/A (University of New Mexico)		Warren A. Heffron, M.D. Family Practice Center 620 Camino De Salud Northeast Albuquerque, New Mexico 87131 (505) 277-2165

New York

Albany Medical College MS-122 47 New Scotland Avenue Albany, New York 12208	Alice E. Fruehan, M.D. Chairman Dept. of Family Practice (518) 445-5193	
State University of New York Downstate Medical Center College of Medicine 450 Clarkson Avenue Brooklyn, New York 11203	Charles M. Plotz, M.D. Chairman Dept. of Family Practice (212) 270-1000	
State University of New York School of Medicine Farber Hall, Bailey Avenue Buffalo, New York 14214	Robert H. Seller, M.D. Chairman Dept. of Family Medicine (716) 886-4400	
University of Rochester School of Medicine 601 Elmwood Avenue Rochester, New York 14642	Donald Treat, M.D. Acting Chairman Family Medicine Program (716) 442-7470	

FAMILY PRACTICE TEACHING PROGRAMS—CONTINUED

SPONSORING INSTITUTION	*CHAIRMAN OF MEDICAL SCHOOL DEPARTMENT (IF APPLICABLE)*	*DIRECTOR OF RESIDENCY PROGRAM AND FAMILY PRACTICE CENTER ADDRESS AND PHONE NUMBER*
State University of New York at Stony Brook Health Sciences Center School of Medicine Stony Brook, New York 11790	Melville G. Rosen, M.D. Chairman Dept. of Family Medicine (516) 859-3169	
State University of New York Upstate Medical Center College of Medicine 766 Irving Avenue Syracuse, New York 13210	L. Thomas Wolff, M.D. Chairman Dept. of Family Practice (315) 473-4385	
Albany Medical Center Affiliated Hospital Albany Medical College 43 New Scotland Avenue Albany, New York 12208 4/A (Albany Medical College)		Alice E. Fruehan, M.D., Chairman Department of Family Practice Albany Medical Center Hospital 43 New Scotland Avenue Albany, New York 12208 (518) 445-5193
Southside Hospital Montauk Highway Bay Shore, New York 11706 3/A (State University of New York—Stony Brook)		Daniel Friedman, M.D. Southside Hospital Family Practice Residency Montauk Highway Bay Shore, New York 11706 (516) 859-3169
Montefiore Hospital and Medical Center 111 East 210th Street Bronx, New York 10467 2/A (Albert Einstein Medical College)		Frances Siegel, M.D. Family Practice Residency 3329 Rochambeau Ave. Bronx, New York 10467 (212) 920-5523
Brookdale Hospital Medical Center Linden Boulevard at Brookdale Plaza Brooklyn, New York 11212 2/A (State University of New York—Downstate)		Seymour Falkow, M.D. Family Practice Residency Linden Boulevard at Brookdale Plaza Brooklyn, New York 11212 (212) 240-5984
Kings County Hospital— State University Box 51 450 Clarkson Avenue Brooklyn, New York 11220 4/A (State University of New York—Downstate)		Charles M. Plotz, M.D. Family Practice Residency Box 51, 450 Clarkson Ave. Brooklyn, New York 11203 (212) 270-1000

Department of Family Medicine (R700)
University of Miami School of Medicine
P. O. Box 016700
Miami, Florida 33101

FAMILY PRACTICE TEACHING PROGRAMS—CONTINUED

SPONSORING INSTITUTION	CHAIRMAN OF MEDICAL SCHOOL DEPARTMENT (IF APPLICABLE)	DIRECTOR OF RESIDENCY PROGRAM AND FAMILY PRACTICE CENTER ADDRESS AND PHONE NUMBER
Lutheran Medical Center 150–55th St. Brooklyn, New York 11220 2/A (State University of New York—Downstate)		Eugene Fanta, M.D. Family Physician Service of Lutheran Medical Center 4819 4th Avenue Brooklyn, New York 11220 (212) 492–4656
Deaconess Hospital 1001 Humboldt Parkway Buffalo, New York 14208 3/A (State University of New York—Buffalo)		Robert H. Seller, M.D. Family Practice Residency 1001 Humboldt Parkway Buffalo, New York 14208 (716) 886–4400
Nassau County Medical Center 2201 Hempstead Turnpike East Meadow, New York 11554 2/A (State University of New York—Stony Brook)		Clement Boccalini, M.D. Nassau City Medical Center— Family Practice Center 2201 Hempstead Turnpike East Meadow, New York 11554 (516) 542–3605
Peninsula Hospital Center 51–15 Beach Channel Drive Far Rockaway, New York 11691 2/A (State University of New York—Downstate)		Edward H. Davis, M.D., Director Family Practice Training Program Peninsula Hospital Center 51–15 Beach Channel Drive Far Rockaway, New York 11691 (212) 634–6885
Community Hospital at Glen Cove 110 St. Andrews Lane Glen Cove, New York 11542 2/A (State University of New York—Stony Brook)		William R. Smith, Jr., M.D. Community Hospital at Glen Cove 110 St. Andrews Lane Glen Cove, New York 11542 (516) 671–8700
Jamaica Hospital 89th Avenue and Van Wyck Expressway Jamaica, New York 11418 2/A (State University of New York—Downstate)		Morton M. Safran, M.D. Family Practice and Community Medicine Jamaica Hospital 89th Avenue and Van Wyck Expressway Jamaica, New York 11418 (212) 657–1800

FAMILY PRACTICE TEACHING PROGRAMS—CONTINUED

SPONSORING INSTITUTION	*CHAIRMAN OF MEDICAL SCHOOL DEPARTMENT (IF APPLICABLE)*	*DIRECTOR OF RESIDENCY PROGRAM AND FAMILY PRACTICE CENTER ADDRESS AND PHONE NUMBER*
Charles S. Wilson Memorial Hospital 33–57 Harrison Street Johnson City, New York 13790 1/A		Richard S. Heinig, M.D. Family Health Center 67 Broad Street Johnson City, New York 13790 (607) 773-6075
Kingston Hospital 396 Broadway Kingston, New York 12401 2/A (New York Medical College)		David N. Mesches, M.D. Ulster County Rural Family Practice Program 396 Broadway Kingston, New York 12401 (914) 331-3131
Niagara Falls Memorial Medical Center 621 Tenth Street Niagara Falls, New York 14302 1/A		Melvin B. Dyster, M.D. Family Practice Residency 501 Tenth Street Niagara Falls, New York 14302 (716) 278-4418
South Nassau Communities Hospital 2445 Oceanside Road Oceanside, New York 11572 2/A (State University of New York—Stony Brook)		Maurice Goldenhar, M.D. South Nassau Communities Hospital Family Practice Residency 2445 Oceanside Road Oceanside, New York 11572 (516) 764-2600
Brookhaven Memorial Hospital 101 Hospital Road Patchogue, New York 11772 2/A (State University of New York—Stony Brook)		Morton Jagust, M.D. Family Practice Residency 101 Hospital Road Patchogue, New York 11772 (516) 654-7095
Highland Hospital Dept. of Family Practice 885 South Avenue Rochester, New York 14620 3/A (University of Rochester)		Donald Treat, M.D., Acting Director Jacob W. Holler Family Medical Center 885 South Avenue Rochester, New York 14620 (716) 442-7470
St. Clare's Hospital 600 McClellan Street Schenectady, New York 12304 1/A		Allen C. Nadler, M.D. Family Health Center 600 McClellan Street Schenectady, New York 12304 (518) 382-2264

FAMILY PRACTICE TEACHING PROGRAMS—CONTINUED

SPONSORING INSTITUTION	CHAIRMAN OF MEDICAL SCHOOL DEPARTMENT (IF APPLICABLE)	DIRECTOR OF RESIDENCY PROGRAM AND FAMILY PRACTICE CENTER ADDRESS AND PHONE NUMBER
St. Joseph's Hospital and Health Center 301 Prospect Avenue Syracuse, New York 13203 2/A (State University of New York—Upstate)		John P. DeSimone, M.D. 301 Prospect Avenue Syracuse, New York 13203 (315) 424–5063
St. Elizabeth Hospital 2209 Genesee Street Utica, New York 13501 1/A		Reynold S. Golden, M.D. Family Practice Residency 2209 Genesee Street Utica, New York 13501 (315) 798–5344
St. Joseph's Hospital 127 South Broadway Yonkers, New York 10701 2/A (New York Medical College)		Anibal Marin, M.D. Family Practice Residency 127 South Broadway Yonkers, New York 10701 (914) 965–6700

North Carolina

University of North Carolina School of Medicine Clinical Sciences Building 2298 Chapel Hill, North Carolina 27514	Edward Shahady, M.D. Chairman Dept. of Family Medicine (919) 966–5151	
Duke University School of Medicine P.O. Box 3005 Durham, North Carolina 27710	William J. Kane, M.D. Chairman Division of Family Medicine (919) 471–2571	
East Carolina University School of Medicine Greenville, North Carolina 27834	James G. Jones, M.D. Chairman Dept. of Family Medicine (919) 757–4614	
Bowman Gray School of Medicine 300 South Hawthorne Road Winston–Salem, North Carolina 27103	Julian F. Keith, M.D. Chairman Dept. of Family Medicine (919) 727–4378	

FAMILY PRACTICE TEACHING PROGRAMS—CONTINUED

SPONSORING INSTITUTION	*CHAIRMAN OF MEDICAL SCHOOL DEPARTMENT (IF APPLICABLE)*	*DIRECTOR OF RESIDENCY PROGRAM AND FAMILY PRACTICE CENTER ADDRESS AND PHONE NUMBER*
Mountain Area Health Education Foundation 430 Biltmore Avenue Asheville, North Carolina 28801 2/A (University of North Carolina—Chapel Hill)		Richard F. Walton, M.D. Family Practice Residency 430 Biltmore Avenue Asheville, North Carolina 28801 (704) 258-0881
University of North Carolina Dept. of Family Medicine Clinical Sciences Building, Room 738 Chapel Hill, North Carolina 27514 4/A (University of North Carolina—Chapel Hill)		Edward J. Shahady, M.D. Family Practice Residency Clinical Sciences Building, Room 738 Chapel Hill, North Carolina 27514 (919) 966-5151
Charlotte Memorial Hospital and Medical Center 1000 Blythe Boulevard Charlotte, North Carolina 28234 2/A (University of North Carolina—Chapel Hill)		David S. Citron, M.D. Family Practice Center 1000 Blythe Boulevard Charlotte, North Carolina 28203 (704) 373-3172
Duke-Watts Family Medicine Program 1012 Broad Street Durham, North Carolina 27705 4/A (Duke University)		William J. Kane, M.D. Family Practice Residency 407 Crutchfield Street Durham, North Carolina 27704 (919) 286-4621
Area Health Education Center—Fayetteville Cape Fear Valley Hospital 1601-B Owen Drive Fayetteville, North Carolina 28304 2/A (Duke University)		Hans Koek, M.D. Family Practice Residency P.O. Box 64699 Fayetteville, North Carolina 28306 (919) 323-1152
Womack Army Hospital Fort Bragg, North Carolina 28307 5/A		Col. Milton T. Smith, M.C., U.S.A. Womack Army Hospital Family Practice Residency Fort Bragg, North Carolina 28307 (919) 396-1908

FAMILY PRACTICE TEACHING PROGRAMS—CONTINUED

SPONSORING INSTITUTION	CHAIRMAN OF MEDICAL SCHOOL DEPARTMENT (IF APPLICABLE)	DIRECTOR OF RESIDENCY PROGRAM AND FAMILY PRACTICE CENTER ADDRESS AND PHONE NUMBER
Moses H. Cone Memorial Hospital 1200 North Elm Street Greensboro, North Carolina 27401 2/A (University of North Carolina—Chapel Hill)		George Wolff, M.D. Family Practice Center 1200 North Elm Street Greensboro, North Carolina 27401 (919) 379–4132
Pitt County Memorial Franklin Highway P.O. Box 6028 Greenville, North Carolina 27834 4/A (East Carolina University)		James G. Jones, M.D. East Carolina Family Practice Center P.O. Box 136 Greenville, North Carolina 27834 (919) 757–4614
Bowman Gray Family Practice Program 300 South Hawthorne Road Winston–Salem, North Carolina 27103 4/A (Bowman Gray School of Medicine)		Charles H. Duckett, M.D. Dept. of Family Medicine 300 South Hawthorne Road Winston–Salem, North Carolina 27103 (919) 727–4274

North Dakota

University of North Dakota School of Medicine First Floor North, North Unit United Hospital Grand Forks, North Dakota 58201	E.P. Donatelle, M.D. Chairman Dept. of Family Medicine (701) 777–2011	
Bismarck Hospital 300 North 7th Bismarck, North Dakota 58501 3/A University of North Dakota—Grand Forks) and St. Alexius Hospital 311 North 9th Bismarck, North Dakota 58501		William M. Buckingham, M.D. Bismarck Family Practice Center Box 2093 Bismarck, North Dakota 58501 (701) 224–2757

FAMILY PRACTICE TEACHING PROGRAMS—CONTINUED

SPONSORING INSTITUTION	*CHAIRMAN OF MEDICAL SCHOOL DEPARTMENT (IF APPLICABLE)*	*DIRECTOR OF RESIDENCY PROGRAM AND FAMILY PRACTICE CENTER ADDRESS AND PHONE NUMBER*

St. Luke's Hospital
Fifth Street North and Mills
Fargo, North Dakota 58102
3/A (University of North
    Dakota—Grand Forks)
		Maurice L. Lindblom, M.D.
		Family Practice Center
		South Weible Hall
		Box 5089, North Dakota
		    State University Station
		Fargo, North Dakota 58102
		(701) 237-7777

United Hospital
1200 South Columbia Road
Grand Forks, North Dakota
    58201
3/A (University of North
    Dakota)
		Arvid J. Houglum, M.D.
		Family Practice Center
		United Hospital North Unit
		Grand Forks, North Dakota
		    58201
		(701) 777-4136

St. Joseph's Hospital
Southeast Third and Fourth
    Avenues
Minot, North Dakota 58701
3/A (University of North
    Dakota—Grand Forks)
 	
and
 	
Trinity Medical Center
Main and 4th Avenue,
    Southwest
Minot, North Dakota 58701
		Robert E. Hankins, M.D.
		Family Practice Center
		Box 1967
		Minot, North Dakota 58701
		(701) 852-3545

Ohio

Case Western Reserve University School of Medicine 2119 Abington Road Cleveland, Ohio 44106	Jack H. Medalie, M.D. Chairman Dept. of Family Medicine (216) 398-6000 Ext. 5731	
Wright State University School of Medicine St. Elizabeth Medical Center 601 Miami Boulevard, West Dayton, Ohio 45408	John Gillen, M.D. Chairman Dept. of Family Practice (513) 223-5859	
University of Cincinnati College of Medicine 231 Bethesda Avenue Cincinnati, Ohio 45267	Robert Smith, M.D. Chairman Dept. of Family Medicine (513) 872-4021	

FAMILY PRACTICE TEACHING PROGRAMS—CONTINUED

SPONSORING INSTITUTION	CHAIRMAN OF MEDICAL SCHOOL DEPARTMENT (IF APPLICABLE)	DIRECTOR OF RESIDENCY PROGRAM AND FAMILY PRACTICE CENTER ADDRESS AND PHONE NUMBER
Ohio State University College of Medicine 370 West Ninth Avenue Columbus, Ohio 43210	Tennyson Williams, M.D. Chairman Dept. of Family Practice (614) 422–0210	
Northeastern Ohio University College of Medicine Rootstown, Ohio 44272	John P. Schlemmer, M.D. Chairman Council of Chiefs of Medicine (216) 384–6047	
Medical College of Ohio C.S. No. 10008 Toledo, Ohio 43699	Harry E. Mayhew, M.D. Chairman Dept. of Family Medicine (419) 381–3569	
Akron City Hospital 525 East Market Street Akron, Ohio 44309 2/A (Northeastern Ohio University College of Medicine)		David Hoff, M.D. Family Practice Center of Akron 511 Market Street East Akron, Ohio 44304 (216) 375–3762
Akron General Medical Center 400 Wabash Avenue Akron, Ohio 44307 2/A (Northeastern Ohio University College of Medicine)		John P. Schlemmer, M.D. Westside Family Practice Center 275 Codding Street Akron, Ohio 44307 (216) 384–6047
Saint Thomas Hospital 444 North Main Street Akron, Ohio 44310 2/A (Northeastern Ohio University College of Medicine)		Glenn E. East, M.D. Family Practice Center of St. Thomas 444 North Main Street Akron, Ohio 44310 (216) 376–7232
Aultman Hospital 2600 Sixth Street, Southwest Canton, Ohio 44710 2/A (Northeastern Ohio University College of Medicine)		John W. McFadden, M.D. Family Practice Center 500 South Prospect Street Hartville, Ohio 44632 (216) 877–9388
University of Cincinnati Medical Center 231 Bethesda Avenue Cincinnati, Ohio 45267 4/A (University of Cincinnati)		Robert Smith, M.D. Family Practice Residency 231 Bethesda Avenue Cincinnati, Ohio 45267 (513) 872–4021

FAMILY PRACTICE TEACHING PROGRAMS—CONTINUED

SPONSORING INSTITUTION	CHAIRMAN OF MEDICAL SCHOOL DEPARTMENT (IF APPLICABLE)	DIRECTOR OF RESIDENCY PROGRAM AND FAMILY PRACTICE CENTER ADDRESS AND PHONE NUMBER
Case Western Reserve University School of Medicine 2119 Abington Road Cleveland, Ohio 44106 4A (Case Western Reserve University)		David D. Schmidt, M.D. Department of Family Practice 2119 Abington Road Cleveland, Ohio 44106 (216) 368-2756
Cleveland Metropolitan General Hospital 3395 Scranton Road Cleveland, Ohio 44109 3/A (Case Western Reserve University)		Jack H. Medalie, M.D. Family Practice Residency 3395 Scranton Road Cleveland, Ohio 44109 (216) 398-6000 Ext. 5731
Fairview General Hospital 18101 Lorain Ave. Cleveland, Ohio 44111 2/A (Case Western Reserve University)		Germaine R. Hahnel, M.D. Family Practice Center of Fairview General Hospital 18101 Lorain Ave. Cleveland, Ohio 44111 (216) 252-7071
Grant Hospital 309 East State Street Columbus, Ohio 43215 2/A (Ohio State University)		Gail W. Burrier, M.D. Family Practice Center 3341 East Livingston Ave. Columbus, Ohio 43227 (614) 239-0218
Mount Carmel Medical Center 793 West State Street Columbus, Ohio 43222 2/A (Ohio State University)		Richard Lutes, M.D., Acting Director Family Practice Residency 793 West State Street Columbus, Ohio 43222 (614) 225-5178
Ohio State University Affiliated Hospitals 1114 University Hospitals Clinic 456 Clinic Drive Columbus, Ohio 43210 4/A (Ohio State University)		Tennyson Williams, M.D. Ohio State University Hospital Affiliated Family Practice Residency 1114 University Hospital Center, 456 Clinic Drive Columbus, Ohio 43210 (614) 422-0210
Riverside Methodist Hospital 3535 Olentangy Road Columbus, Ohio 43214 2/A (Ohio State University)		David R. Rudy, M.D. Riverside Family Practice Center 797 Thomas Lane Columbus, Ohio 43214 (614) 261-5474

FAMILY PRACTICE TEACHING PROGRAMS—CONTINUED

SPONSORING INSTITUTION	CHAIRMAN OF MEDICAL SCHOOL DEPARTMENT (IF APPLICABLE)	DIRECTOR OF RESIDENCY PROGRAM AND FAMILY PRACTICE CENTER ADDRESS AND PHONE NUMBER
St. Elizabeth Medical Center 601 Miami Boulevard West Dayton, Ohio 45408 2/A (Wright State University)		Terence P. Torbeck, M.D. St. Elizabeth Family Medical Center and Residence 627 Miami Boulevard West Dayton, Ohio 45408 (513) 223-7344
Miami Valley Hospital 101 Wyoming Street Dayton, Ohio 45409 2/A (Wright State University)		Raymond K. Bartholomew, M.D. Family Practice Residency 101 Wyoming Street Dayton, Ohio 45409 (513) 223-9017
Good Samaritan Hospital 2157 Benson Drive Dayton, Ohio 45406 2/A (Wright State University)		William A. Stowe, M.D. Family Practice Residency 2157 Benson Drive Dayton, Ohio 45406 (513) 276-4141
Community Hospital of Springfield in Clark County 2615 East High Street Springfield, Ohio 45501 3/A (Wright State University)		John C. Gillen, M.D. Wright State University Integrated Family Practice Residency Program St. Elizabeth Medical Center 601 Miami Boulevard West Dayton, Ohio 45400 (513) 223-5859
Flower Hospital 5200 Harroun Road Sylvania, Ohio 43560 2/A (Medical College of Ohio—Toledo)		R.E. Scherbarth, M.D. 5200 Harroun Road Sylvania, Ohio 43560 (419) 885-1444
Mercy Hospital 2200 Jefferson Avenue Toledo, Ohio 43624 2/A (Medical College of Ohio—Toledo)		John H. Coleman, M.D. Family Planning Residency Program—Mercy Hospital 2200 Jefferson Avenue Toledo, Ohio 43624 (419) 259-1400
Toledo Hospital 2142 North Cove Boulevard Toledo, Ohio 43606 2/A (Medical College of Ohio—Toledo)		Frank F. Snyder, M.D. W.W. Knight Family Practice Center 2805 Oatis Street Toledo, Ohio 43606 (419) 473-4010

FAMILY PRACTICE TEACHING PROGRAMS—CONTINUED

SPONSORING INSTITUTION	*CHAIRMAN OF MEDICAL SCHOOL DEPARTMENT (IF APPLICABLE)*	*DIRECTOR OF RESIDENCY PROGRAM AND FAMILY PRACTICE CENTER ADDRESS AND PHONE NUMBER*
Riverside Family Practice Center 1530 Superior Street Toledo, Ohio 43604 3/A (Medical College of Ohio—Toledo)		Robert D. Gillette, M.D. MCO/Riverside Family Practice Center 1530 Superior Street Toledo, Ohio 43604 (419) 729-0711
Medical College of Ohio Department of Family Medicine C.S. No. 10008 Toledo, Ohio 43699 4/A (Medical College of Ohio—Toledo)		Harry E. Mayhew, M.D. Medical College of Ohio Family Practice Residency Program C.S. No. 10008 Toledo, Ohio 43699 (419) 381-3569
U.S. Air Force Medical Center/S.G.H.F. Wright–Patterson Air Force Base, Ohio 45433 5–2/A (Wright State University)		Maj. James B. Tucker, M.C., U.S.A.F. U.S. Air Force Medical Center/S.G.H.F. Wright–Patterson AFB, Ohio 45433 (419) 729-0711
St. Elizabeth Medical Center Belmont and Park Avenue Youngstown, Ohio 44501 2/A (Northeast Ohio University College of Medicine)		S.V. Squicquero, M.D. Family Practice Center St. Elizabeth Hospital Medical Center 1044 Belmont Avenue Youngstown, Ohio 44504 (216) 746-7211
Youngstown Hospital Association 345 Oak Hill Avenue Youngstown, Ohio 44501 2/A (Northeast Ohio University College of Medicine)		Richard W. Juvancic, M.D. Family Practice Residency Program The Youngstown Hospital Association 345 Oak Hill Ave. Youngstown, Ohio 44501 (216) 747-1036

Oklahoma

University of Oklahoma School of Medicine P.O. Box 26901 Oklahoma City, Oklahoma 73190	Wilson Steen, Ph.D. Acting Chairman Dept. of Family Practice and Community Medicine and Dentistry (405) 271-4033	

FAMILY PRACTICE TEACHING PROGRAMS—CONTINUED

SPONSORING INSTITUTION	CHAIRMAN OF MEDICAL SCHOOL DEPARTMENT (IF APPLICABLE)	DIRECTOR OF RESIDENCY PROGRAM AND FAMILY PRACTICE CENTER ADDRESS AND PHONE NUMBER
University of Oklahoma Tulsa Medical College 2727 East 21st Street Midway Building Tulsa, Oklahoma 74105	Roger Good, M.D. Chairman Dept. of Family Practice (918) 749–5531	
Jane Phillips Episcopal Memorial Medical Center 3500 Southeast Frank Phillips Boulevard Bartlesville, Oklahoma 74003 3/B (University of Oklahoma—Tulsa, first year at University of Oklahoma—Tulsa)		William L. Fesler, M.D., Director Family Practice Residency Program Jane Philips Episcopal Memorial Medical Center 3500 Southeast Frank Phillips Boulevard Bartlesville, Oklahoma 74003 (918) 333–6015
Garfield County Medical Society Family Practice Program 617 South Quincy Enid, Oklahoma 73701 3/B (University of Oklahoma—Oklahoma City, first year at University of Oklahoma)		Donald C. Karns, M.D. Enid Family Medicine Clinic 617 South Quincy Enid, Oklahoma 73701 (405) 242–1300
University Family Medical Clinic 1600 North Phillips Oklahoma City, Oklahoma 73104 4/A (University of Oklahoma—Oklahoma City)		Norman L. Haug, M.D. Family Practice Residency 1600 North Phillips Oklahoma City, Oklahoma 73104 (405) 271–4311
Pottawatomie County Medical Society Federal National Bank Building Shawnee, Oklahoma 74801 4/A (University of Oklahoma—Oklahoma City)		Robert B. Zumwalt, M.D. Shawnee Family Practice Residency Mission Hill Memorial Hospital 1900 Gordon–Cooper Drive Shawnee, Oklahoma 74801 (405) 275–6980

FAMILY PRACTICE TEACHING PROGRAMS—CONTINUED

SPONSORING INSTITUTION	*CHAIRMAN OF MEDICAL SCHOOL DEPARTMENT (IF APPLICABLE)*	*DIRECTOR OF RESIDENCY PROGRAM AND FAMILY PRACTICE CENTER ADDRESS AND PHONE NUMBER*
Tulsa Family Practice Clinic 1044 North Sheraton Tulsa, Oklahoma 74135 3/A (University of Oklahoma—Tulsa)		Roger C. Good, M.D. Director University of Oklahoma, Tulsa Medical College/ Family Planning Residency 2727 East 21st Street Tulsa, Oklahoma 74114 (918) 836-3926

Oregon

University of Oregon Health Sciences Center 3181 Southwest Sam Jackson Park Road Portland, Oregon 97201	Laurel G. Case, M.D. Chairman Dept. of Family Practice (503) 225-8311	
Emanuel Hospital 2801 North Gantenbein Avenue Portland, Oregon 97227 1–A		Ray E. Moore, M.D. Family Practice Health Center 501 North Graham Street Portland, Oregon 97227 (503) 280-4022
University of Oregon Health Sciences Center Family Practice Residency 3181 Southwest Sam Jackson Park Road Portland, Oregon 97201 4/A (University of Oregon)		William A. Fisher, M.D. Family Practice Residency 3181 Southwest Sam Jackson Park Road Portland, Oregon 97201 (503) 225-7590

Pennsylvania

Pennsylvania State University College of Medicine Milton South Hershey Medical Center 500 University Drive Hershey, Pennsylvania 17033	Thomas L. Leaman, M.D. Chairman Dept. of Family and Community Medicine (717) 534-8181	
Hahnemann Medical College 230 North Broad Street Philadelphia, Pennsylvania 19102	Lonnie Fuller, M.D. Director Division of Family Practice (215) 448-8651	

FAMILY PRACTICE TEACHING PROGRAMS—CONTINUED

SPONSORING INSTITUTION	CHAIRMAN OF MEDICAL SCHOOL DEPARTMENT (IF APPLICABLE)	DIRECTOR OF RESIDENCY PROGRAM AND FAMILY PRACTICE CENTER ADDRESS AND PHONE NUMBER
Jefferson Medical College of Thomas Jefferson University 1025 Walnut Street Philadelphia, Pennsylvania 19107	Paul C. Brucker, M.D. Chairman Dept. of Family Medicine (215) 829–8363	
Temple University School of Medicine 3440 North Broad Street Philadelphia, Pennsylvania 19140	James R. MacBride, M.D. Chairman Dept. of Family Practice and Community Health (215) 221–4600	
University of Pennsylvania School of Medicine 36th and Hamilton Walk Philadelphia, Pennsylvania 19174	Charles Hurtz, M.D. Director Office of Primary Care (215) 732–9001	
Abington Memorial Hospital 1200 Old York Road Abington, Pennsylvania 19001 1/A		Frederick Lytel, M.D. Family Practice Center 1200 Old York Road Abington, Pennsylvania 19001 (215) 884–2236
Sacred Heart Hospital Fourth and Chew Streets Allentown, Pennsylvania 18102 2/A (University of Pennsylvania— Philadelphia)		Paul L. Hermany, M.D. Sacred Heart Hospital Family Practice Residency Fourth and Chew Streets Allentown, Pennsylvania 18102 (215) 435–4401
Altoona Hospital 7th Street and Howard Avenue Altoona, Pennsylvania 16601 2/A (Pennsylvania State University)		John H. Gould, M.D. Acting Director Family Practice Residency 501 Howard Avenue— Building C Altoona, Pennsylvania 16601 (814) 946–2701
Bryn Mawr Hospital Bryn Mawr Avenue Bryn Mawr, Pennsylvania 19010 2/A (Jefferson Medical College)		D. Stratton Woodruff, M.D. Family Practice Residency Bryn Mawr Avenue Bryn Mawr, Pennsylvania 19010 (215) 525–4655

FAMILY PRACTICE TEACHING PROGRAMS—CONTINUED

SPONSORING INSTITUTION	CHAIRMAN OF MEDICAL SCHOOL DEPARTMENT (IF APPLICABLE)	DIRECTOR OF RESIDENCY PROGRAM AND FAMILY PRACTICE CENTER ADDRESS AND PHONE NUMBER
Geisinger Medical Center North Academy Avenue Danville, Pennsylvania 17821 2/A (Pennsylvania State University)		Robert W. Leipold, M.D. Family Practice Residency North Academy Avenue Danville, Pennsylvania 17821 (717) 275–6070
Hamot Medical Center 104 East Second Street Erie, Pennsylvania 16550 2/A (Pennsylvania State University)		Roland E. Miller, M.D. Family Practice Residency 231 State Street Erie, Pennsylvania 16512 (814) 452–3006
St. Vincent Hospital 232–West 25th Street Erie, Pennsylvania 16512 2/A (Hahnemann Medical College)		William G. Jackson, M.D. Family Practice Residency 232–West 25th Street Erie, Pennsylvania 16512 (814) 459–4000
Harrisburg Hospital School Front Street Harrisburg, Pennsylvania 17101 2/A (Pennsylvania State University)		Bradford K. Strock, M.D. Family Practice Residency Harrisburg Hospital Fifth-Floor–Bradyhall South Front Street Harrisburg, Pennsylvania 17101 (717) 782–5435
Polyclinic Hospital Third and Radnor Streets Harrisburg, Pennsylvania 17105 1/A		Thomas M. Bryan, M.D., Interim Director Kline Family Practice Center 2nd Floor Kline Building Polyclinic Hospital Third and Polyclinic Avenue Harrisburg, Pennsylvania 17105 (717) 782–2100 or 2102
Milton S. Hershey Family Practice Center 500 University Drive Hershey, Pennsylvania 17033 4/A (Pennsylvania State University)		Thomas L. Leaman, M.D. Family Practice Center 500 University Drive Hershey, Pennsylvania 17033 (717) 534–8181

FAMILY PRACTICE TEACHING PROGRAMS—CONTINUED

SPONSORING INSTITUTION	CHAIRMAN OF MEDICAL SCHOOL DEPARTMENT (IF APPLICABLE)	DIRECTOR OF RESIDENCY PROGRAM AND FAMILY PRACTICE CENTER ADDRESS AND PHONE NUMBER
Monsour Medical Center 70 Lincoln Way, East Jeannette, Pennsylvania 15644 1/A		William F. Ryckman, M.D. Family Practice Residency 70 Lincoln Way, East Jeannette, Pennsylvania 15644 (412) 527–1511 Ext. 432
Conemaugh Valley Memorial Hospital 1086 Franklin Street Johnstown, Pennsylvania 15905 1/A		C.F. Reeder, M.D. Family Practice Residency 1130 Franklin Street Johnstown, Pennsylvania 15905 (814) 535–5514
United Health and Hospital Services Medical Arts Building 534 Wyoming Avenue Kingston, Pennsylvania 18704 2/A (Hahnemann Medical College)		Gordon H. Earles, M.D. Family Practice Residency Medical Arts Building 534 Wyoming Avenue Kingston, Pennsylvania 18704 (717) 288–7451
Lancaster General Hospital 555 North Duke Street Lancaster, Pennsylvania 17604 2/A (Temple University)		Nikitas J. Zervanos, M.D. Family and Community Medicine 555 North Duke Street Lancaster, Pennsylvania 17604 (717) 299–5511
Latrobe Area Hospital Second Avenue Latrobe, Pennsylvania 15650 2/A (Jefferson Medical College)		R.S. Gordon, M.D. Joseph R. Govi, M.D., Co-Directors Family Practice Residency Second Avenue Latrobe, Pennsylvania 15650 (412) 539–0082
McKeesport Hospital 1500 Fifth Avenue McKeesport, Pennsylvania 15132 1/A		Rudolph L. Buck, M.D. McKeesport Hospital Family Practice Residency 1500 Fifth Avenue McKeesport, Pennsylvania 15132 (412) 644–2131 or 2132

FAMILY PRACTICE TEACHING PROGRAMS—CONTINUED

SPONSORING INSTITUTION	CHAIRMAN OF MEDICAL SCHOOL DEPARTMENT (IF APPLICABLE)	DIRECTOR OF RESIDENCY PROGRAM AND FAMILY PRACTICE CENTER ADDRESS AND PHONE NUMBER
Montgomery Hospital Powell and Fornance Streets Norristown, Pennsylvania 19401 2/A (Temple University)		Richard R. Loughlin, M.D. McShea Hall Family Practice Center Powell and Wood Streets Norristown, Pennsylvania 19401 (215) 275–6000 Ext. 360
Chestnut Hill Hospital 8835 Germantown Avenue Philadelphia, Pennsylvania 19118 2/A (Jefferson Medical College)		Warren D. Lambright, M.D. Family Practice Unit 8811 Germantown Ave. Philadelphia, Pennsylvania 19118 (215) 247–4145
Hahnemann Hospital 230 North Broad Street Philadelphia, Pennsylvania 19102 4/A (Hahnemann Medical College)		James B. Rondina, M.D. Hahnemann Family Medicine Residency 230 North Broad Street Philadelphia, Pennsylvania 19102 (215) 448–8651
Northeastern Hospital 2301 East Allegheny Avenue Philadelphia, Pennsylvania 19134 2/A (Temple University)		Flora Rauer, M.D. Family Practice Residency 2301 East Allegheny Ave. Philadelphia, Pennsylvania 19134 (215) 427–6470
Thomas Jefferson University Hospital 1025 Walnut Street Philadelphia, Pennsylvania 19107 4/A (Jefferson Medical College)		Paul C. Brucker, M.D. Family Practice Residency 1025 Walnut Street Philadelphia, Pennsylvania 19107 (215) 829–8363
Shadyside Hospital 5230 Center Avenue Pittsburgh, Pennsylvania 15232 1/A		Charles M. Awde, M.D. Director Family Practice Residency 5230 Center Avenue Pittsburgh, Pennsylvania 15232 (412) 622–2236

FAMILY PRACTICE TEACHING PROGRAMS—CONTINUED

SPONSORING INSTITUTION	CHAIRMAN OF MEDICAL SCHOOL DEPARTMENT (IF APPLICABLE)	DIRECTOR OF RESIDENCY PROGRAM AND FAMILY PRACTICE CENTER ADDRESS AND PHONE NUMBER
St. Margaret Memorial Hospital 265 46th Street Pittsburgh, Pennsylvania 15201 1/A		Paul W. Dishart, M.D. Family Practice Residency 265 46th Street Pittsburgh, Pennsylvania 15201 (412) 622-7165
Forbes Health System 500 Finley Street Pittsburgh, Pennsylvania 15206 1/A		Nicholas A. Toronto, Jr., M.D. Forbes Health System Columbia Health Center Penn Avenue at West St. Pittsburgh, Pennsylvania 15221 (412) 247-2596
Reading Hospital 301 South 7th Avenue Reading, Pennsylvania 19611 1/A		John Wagner, M.D. Family Practice Residency 301 South 7th Ave. Reading, Pennsylvania 19611 (215) 378-6198
Saint Joseph Hospital 12th and Walnut Reading, Pennsylvania 19603 2/A (Pennsylvania State University—Hershey)		Patrick A. Mazza, M.D. Family Health Unit Birch and Walnut Reading, Pennsylvania 19603 (215) 376-7413
Washington Hospital 155 Wilson Avenue Washington, Pennsylvania 15301 1/A		George C. Schmieler, M.D. Family Practice Residency 155 Wilson Avenue Washington, Pennsylvania 15301 (412) 225-7000
Williamsport Hospital 777 Rural Avenue Williamsport, Pennsylvania 17701 2/A (University of Pennsylvania— Philadelphia)		A.R. Taylor, M.D. Family Practice Residency 777 Rural Ave. Williamsport, Pennsylvania 17701 (717) 322-7861 Ext. 374
York Hospital 1001 South George York, Pennsylvania 17405 2/A (University of Maryland)		P.L. Roseberry, M.D. Family Practice Residency 1001 South George York, Pennsylvania 17405 (717) 771-2521

FAMILY PRACTICE TEACHING PROGRAMS—CONTINUED

SPONSORING INSTITUTION	*CHAIRMAN OF MEDICAL SCHOOL DEPARTMENT (IF APPLICABLE)*	*DIRECTOR OF RESIDENCY PROGRAM AND FAMILY PRACTICE CENTER ADDRESS AND PHONE NUMBER*
Puerto Rico		
University of Puerto Rico School of Medicine Medical Sciences Campus G.P.O. Box 5067 San Juan, Puerto Rico 00936	Chairman—To Be Named Dept. of Internal Medicine Division of Family Medicine (809) 744–0926	
University of Puerto Rico Centro de Medicina de Familia Caguas Regional Hospital P.O. Box 5999 Caguas, Puerto Rico 00625 3/A (University of Puerto Rico)		Herman G. Stubbe, M.D. Family Practice Residency Program P.O. Box 5999 Caguas, Puerto Rico 00625 (809) 744–0926 or 0922
Rhode Island		
Brown University School of Medicine 97 Waterman Street Providence, Rhode Island 02912	Louis I. Hochheiser, M.D. Associate Professor and Chairman Section of Family Medicine (401) 722–6000	
Pawtucket Memorial Hospital 89 Pond Street Pawtucket, Rhode Island 02860 2/A (Brown University)		Louis I. Hochheiser, M.D. Physician-in-Chief Family Care Center 89 Pond Street Pawtucket, Rhode Island 02860 (401) 725–0980
South Carolina		
Medical University of South Carolina College of Medicine 171 Ashley Avenue Charleston, South Carolina 29401	Hiram B. Curry, M.D. Chairman Dept. of Family Practice (803) 792–2411	
University of South Carolina School of Medicine Columbia, South Carolina 29208	J. Robert Hewson, M.D. Chairman Dept. of Family Medicine (803) 765–6118	

FAMILY PRACTICE TEACHING PROGRAMS—CONTINUED

SPONSORING INSTITUTION	CHAIRMAN OF MEDICAL SCHOOL DEPARTMENT (IF APPLICABLE)	DIRECTOR OF RESIDENCY PROGRAM AND FAMILY PRACTICE CENTER ADDRESS AND PHONE NUMBER
Anderson Memorial Hospital 800 North Fant Street Anderson, South Carolina 29621 2/A (Medical University of South Carolina)		James G. Halford, Jr., M.D. Family Practice Center 600 North Fant Street at Calhoun Anderson, South Carolina 29621 (803) 225-4193
Medical University of South Carolina Department of Family Practice 171 Ashley Ave. Charleston, South Carolina 29401 4/A (Medical University of South Carolina)		Hiram B. Curry, M.D. Medical University Family Practice Residency Program Medical University of South Carolina 171 Ashley Ave. Charleston, South Carolina 29403 (803) 792-2411
Naval Regional Medical Center Dept. of Family Practice (Code 215) Charleston, South Carolina 29408 5/A		Capt. Ira Horton, M.C., U.S.N. Naval Regional Medical Center Dept. of Family Practice (Code 215) Charleston, South Carolina 29408 (803) 743-6280
Richland Memorial Hospital 3301 Harden Street Columbia, South Carolina 29203 2/A (University of South Carolina—School of Medicine)		J. Robert Hewson, M.D. Family Practice Residency 3301 Harden Street Columbia, South Carolina 29203 (803) 765-6118
Greenville General Hospital 1200 Pendleton Street Greenville, South Carolina 29601 2/A (Medical University of South Carolina)		E.F. Gaynor, M.D. Family Practice Residency 701 Grove Road Greenville, South Carolina 29605 (803) 242-7800

FAMILY PRACTICE TEACHING PROGRAMS—CONTINUED

SPONSORING INSTITUTION	*CHAIRMAN OF MEDICAL SCHOOL DEPARTMENT (IF APPLICABLE)*	*DIRECTOR OF RESIDENCY PROGRAM AND FAMILY PRACTICE CENTER ADDRESS AND PHONE NUMBER*
Spartanburg General Hospital 101 East Wood Street Spartanburg, South Carolina 29303 2/A (Medical University of South Carolina)		David K. Stokes, Jr., M.D. Family Practice Residency Program Spartanburg General Hospital 101 East Wood Street Spartanburg, South Carolina 29303 (803) 573-6198

South Dakota

University of South Dakota School of Medicine 1800 South Summit Avenue Sioux Falls, South Dakota 57105	L.H. Amundson, M.D. Chairman Dept. of Community and Family Medicine	
Sioux Valley Hospital 1123 South Euclid Sioux Falls, South Dakota 57105 2/A (University of South Dakota) and McKennan Hospital 800 East Twenty-First Street Sioux Falls, South Dakota 57101		Lloyd J. Sweeney, M.D. Sioux Falls Family Practice Residency 1800 South Summit Avenue Sioux Falls, South Dakota 57105 (605) 339-1783

Tennessee

East Tennessee State University College of Medicine State University Station Johnson City, Tennessee 37601	Lewis E. Simoni, M.D. Chairman Dept. of Family Practice (615) 929-4493	
University of Tennessee College of Medicine 66 North Pauline—Suite 233 Memphis, Tennessee 38105	Thornton Bryan, M.D. Chairman Dept. of Family Medicine (901) 528-5899	

FAMILY PRACTICE TEACHING PROGRAMS—CONTINUED

SPONSORING INSTITUTION	CHAIRMAN OF MEDICAL SCHOOL DEPARTMENT (IF APPLICABLE)	DIRECTOR OF RESIDENCY PROGRAM AND FAMILY PRACTICE CENTER ADDRESS AND PHONE NUMBER
Meharry Medical College School of Medicine 1005 Eighteenth Avenue North Nashville, Tennessee 37208	John E. Arradondo, M.D. Chairman Dept. of Family and Community Health (615) 327–6572	
Bristol Memorial Hospital 225 Midway Bristol, Tennessee 37620 3/A (East Tennessee State University)		Lewis E. Simoni, M.D. Family Practice Residency Program—Bristol State University Station, Box 23, 320A Johnson City, Tennessee 37601 (615) 929–4493
University of Tennessee Clinical Education Center 921 East Third Street Chattanooga, Tennessee 37403 3/A (University of Tennessee)		Sandford L. Weiler, M.D. University of Tennessee Family Practice Center 921 East Third Street Chattanooga, Tennessee 37403 (615) 756–2481
Jackson–Madison County General 708 West Forest St. Jackson, Tennessee 38301 3/A (University of Tennessee—Memphis)		George W. Shannon, M.D. Family Practice Center 648 West Forest, Box 3172 Jackson, Tennessee 38301 (901) 423–1932
Holston Valley Community Hospital 102 East Ravine Road Kingsport, Tennessee 37660 3/A (East Tennessee State University)		Lewis E. Simoni, M.D. Family Practice Residency Program–Kingsport 102 East Ravine Road Kingsport, Tennessee 37660 (615) 929–4493
University of Tennessee Center of the Health Sciences 1924 Alcoa Highway Knoxville, Tennessee 37920 4/A (University of Tennessee)		George Shacklett, M.D. Family Practice Residency 1924 Alcoa Highway Knoxville, Tennessee 37920 (615) 971–3961
St. Joseph Hospital East 5959 Park Avenue Memphis, Tennessee 38117 2/A (University of Tennessee—Memphis)		Patrick J. Murphy, M.D. Family Practice Center 6005 Park Ave.—Suite 500 Memphis, Tennessee 38138 (901) 761–3630 or 2997

FAMILY PRACTICE TEACHING PROGRAMS—CONTINUED

SPONSORING INSTITUTION	*CHAIRMAN OF MEDICAL SCHOOL DEPARTMENT (IF APPLICABLE)*	*DIRECTOR OF RESIDENCY PROGRAM AND FAMILY PRACTICE CENTER ADDRESS AND PHONE NUMBER*
University of Tennessee Medical Center 66 North Pauline Suite 233 Memphis, Tennessee 38105 4/A (University of Tennessee)		Forest Wortham, M.D. University of Tennessee Medical Center Department of Family Medicine 66 North Pauline Suite 233 Memphis, Tennessee 38105 (901) 528-5899
Meharry Family Practice Residency 1005 18th Avenue, North Nashville, Tennessee 38708 4/A (Meharry Medical College)		John E. Arradondo, M.D. Meharry Family Practice Residency 1005 18th Avenue, North Nashville, Tennessee 38708 (615) 327-6572

Texas

University of Texas Southwestern Medical School 5323 Harry Hines Boulevard Dallas, Texas 75235	William F. Ross, M.D. Chairman, Division of Family Practice Dept. of Family Practice and Community Medicine (214) 688-2134	
University of Texas Medical Branch of Galveston 415 Texas Avenue Galveston, Texas 77550	M.L. Ross, M.D. Chairman Dept. of Family Medicine (806) 765-2166	
Baylor College of Medicine 1200 Moursund Avenue Houston, Texas 77030	Harold Brown, M.D. Chairman Division of Family Practice (713) 529-8779	
Memorial Hospital Medical Education Office 7600 Beechnut Houston, Texas 77074	C. Frank Webber, M.D. Chairman Dept. of Family Practice (713) 776-5160	
Texas Tech University Box 4569 Lubbock, Texas 79409	Berry N. Souyres, M.D. Chairman Dept. of Family Medicine (806) 743-2770	
University of Texas Health Sciences Center at San Antonio 7703 Floyd Curl Drive San Antonio, Texas 78289	Herschel L. Douglas, M.D. Chairman Dept. of Family Practice (512) 223-6361	

FAMILY PRACTICE TEACHING PROGRAMS—CONTINUED

SPONSORING INSTITUTION	CHAIRMAN OF MEDICAL SCHOOL DEPARTMENT (IF APPLICABLE)	DIRECTOR OF RESIDENCY PROGRAM AND FAMILY PRACTICE CENTER ADDRESS AND PHONE NUMBER
Amarillo Regional Academic Health Center 1400 Wallace Boulevard Amarillo, Texas 79106 3/A (Texas Tech University)		Richard Rehm, M.D. Peter Fagan, M.D. Co-Directors Family Practice Residency 1400 Wallace Boulevard Amarillo, Texas 79106 (806) 355-8961
Brackenridge Hospital 1500 East Avenue Austin, Texas 78701 1/A		Glen R. Johnson, M.D. Family Practice Residency Central Texas Medical Education Foundation 4920 North IH35 Austin, Texas 78751 (512) 458-9176
U.S. Air Force Regional Hospital Carswell Carswell Air Force Base Fort Worth, Texas 76217 5/A		Col. Mark F. Wildemann, M.C., U.S.A.F. Dept. of Family Practice Residency Program U.S. Air Force Regional Hospital Carswell Carswell Air Force Base, Texas 76127 (817) 738-3511 Ext. 7291
Memorial Medical Center 2606 Hospital Boulevard Corpus Christi, Texas 78405 1/A		Everett L. Holt, M.D. Family Practice Center P.O. Box 5280 Corpus Christi, Texas 78405 (512) 883-2575
St. Paul Hospital 5909 Harry Hines Boulevard Dallas, Texas 75235 2/A (University of Texas)		James Fogleman, M.D. Family Practice Residency Program St. Paul Hospital 5909 Harry Hines Boulevard Dallas, Texas 75235 (214) 689-2089
El Paso Regional Academic Health Center 4815 Alameda Avenue El Paso, Texas 79905 3/A (Texas Tech University)		James Jet, M.D. Family Practice Residency— Dept. of Family Practice 111 Fullan St. El Paso, Texas 79905 (915) 532-3940 or 3949

FAMILY PRACTICE TEACHING PROGRAMS—CONTINUED

SPONSORING INSTITUTION	*CHAIRMAN OF MEDICAL SCHOOL DEPARTMENT (IF APPLICABLE)*	*DIRECTOR OF RESIDENCY PROGRAM AND FAMILY PRACTICE CENTER ADDRESS AND PHONE NUMBER*
John Peter Smith Hospital 1500 South Main Street Fort Worth, Texas 76104 2/A (Southwestern Medical School)		Bruce K. Jacobson, M.D. Family Practice Residency 1500 South Main Street Fort Worth, Texas 76104 (817) 921-3431
Medical Branch of Galveston 415 Texas Avenue Galveston, Texas 77550 4/A (University of Texas— Medical Branch of Galveston)		Alice Anne O'Donell, M.D. Dept. of Family Medicine 415 Texas Avenue Galveston, Texas 77550 (713) 765-3126
Memorial Family Practice Center 7777 Southwest Freeway Houston, Texas 77002 3/A (University of Texas— Health Science Center— Houston)		William St. Clair, M.D. Memorial Family Practice Center 7777 Southwest Freeway Houston, Texas 77002 (713) 777-1311
St. Luke's Episcopal and Texas Children's Hospitals 6720 Bertner Houston, Texas 77025 4/A (Baylor College of Medicine)		Harold Brown, M.D. Baylor Family Practice Center 6720 Bertner Houston, Texas 77030 (713) 529-8779
Lubbock Regional Academic Health Center P.O. Box 4569 Lubbock, Texas 79409 4/A (Texas Tech University)		Clark A. Johnson, M.D. Family Practice Residency P.O. Box 4569 Lubbock, Texas 79409 (806) 743-2770
McAllen General Hospital 701 South Maine Street McAllen, Texas 78501 2/A (University of Texas— Health Science Center— San Antonio)		Forest Fitch, M.D. Family Medical Center— University of Texas 1306 Houston Street McAllen, Texas 78501 (512) 687-6155
University of Texas Teaching Hospitals Family Practice Program 7703 Floyd Curl Drive San Antonio, Texas 78289 4/A (University of Texas— Health Science Center— San Antonio)		Herschel L. Douglas, M.D. Family Practice Residency Training Program 7703 Floyd Curl Drive San Antonio, Texas 78289 (512) 223-6361

FAMILY PRACTICE TEACHING PROGRAMS—CONTINUED

SPONSORING INSTITUTION	CHAIRMAN OF MEDICAL SCHOOL DEPARTMENT (IF APPLICABLE)	DIRECTOR OF RESIDENCY PROGRAM AND FAMILY PRACTICE CENTER ADDRESS AND PHONE NUMBER
Providence Hospital 1700 Providence Drive P.O. Box 3276 Waco, Texas 76708 2/A (Baylor College of Medicine)		Christian N. Ramsey, M.D. McLennan County Family Practice Residency Program McLennan County Medical Education and Research Foundation P.O. Box 3276 Waco, Texas 76707 (817) 754–2471
University of Texas Health Science Center 1107 Brook Street Wichita Falls, Texas 76301 2/C (University of Texas— Southwestern; first year at John Peter Smith— Fort Worth)		J.J. Boluch, M.D. Family Practice Residency Program 1700 7th Street Wichita Falls, Texas 76301 (817) 626–5433

Utah

University of Utah College of Medicine 50 North Medical Drive Salt Lake City, Utah 84132	C.H. Castle, M.D. Chairman Dept. of Family and Community Medicine (801) 581–7234	
McKay–Dee Hospital 3939 Harrison Boulevard Ogden, Utah 84403 3/A (University of Utah) and Holy Cross Hospital 50 North Medical Drive Salt Lake City, Utah 84132		John M. Tudor, M.D. Dept. of Family and Community 50 North Medical Drive Salt Lake City, Utah 84132 (801) 581–7234

Vermont

University of Vermont College of Medicine 104 Rowell Building Burlington, Vermont 05401	Edward E. Friedman, M.D. Chairman Dept. of Family Practice (802) 656–4330	

FAMILY PRACTICE TEACHING PROGRAMS—CONTINUED

SPONSORING INSTITUTION	*CHAIRMAN OF MEDICAL SCHOOL DEPARTMENT (IF APPLICABLE)*	*DIRECTOR OF RESIDENCY PROGRAM AND FAMILY PRACTICE CENTER ADDRESS AND PHONE NUMBER*
University of Vermont— Dept. of Family Practice 104 Rowell Building Burlington, Vermont 05401 4/A (University of Vermont)		Edward E. Friedman, M.D. University of Vermont— Family Practice Center Villemaire Health Center Meadow Lane Milton, Vermont 05468 (802) 656–4330

Virginia

University of Virginia School of Medicine Box 157 Charlottesville, Virginia 22903	Lewis Barnett, M.D. Chairman Dept. of Family Practice (804) 296–0143	
Eastern Virginia Medical School P.O. Box 1980 Norfolk, Virginia 23501	Robert L. Cassidy, M.D. Chairman Dept. of Family Practice (804) 446–5637	
Medical College of Virginia Virginia Commonwealth University School of Medicine Box 251 Richmond, Virginia 23298	Fitzhugh Mayo, M.D. Chairman Dept. of Family Practice (804) 786–9626	
University of Virginia Medical School 1224 West Main Street Towers Office Building Charlottesville, Virginia 22901 4/A (University of Virginia— Charlottesville)		Lewis Barnett, M.D. Family Practice Residency Box 414 Charlottesville, Virginia 22901 (804) 296–0143
Fairfax Hospital 3300 Gallows Road Falls Church, Virginia 22046 2/A (Medical College of Virginia)		Robert K. Quinnell, M.D. Fairfax Family Practice Center 380 Maple Avenue West Vienna, Virginia 22180 (703) 938–5870
DeWitt Army Hospital Fort Belvoir, Virginia 22060 5/A		Col. Thomas F. Camp, Jr., M.C., U.S.A. DeWitt Army Hospital Fort Belvoir, Virginia 22060 (703) 664–4737

FAMILY PRACTICE TEACHING PROGRAMS—CONTINUED

SPONSORING INSTITUTION	CHAIRMAN OF MEDICAL SCHOOL DEPARTMENT (IF APPLICABLE)	DIRECTOR OF RESIDENCY PROGRAM AND FAMILY PRACTICE CENTER ADDRESS AND PHONE NUMBER
Lynchburg Family Practice Residency Program P.O. Box 3176 Lynchburg, Virginia 24503 2/C (University of Virginia— Charlottesville, first year spent at Roanoke Memorial Hospital)		John H. Danby, M.D. Lynchburg Family Practice Program P.O. Box 3176 Lynchburg, Virginia 24503 (804) 384-1731
Riverside Hospital J. Clyde Morris Boulevard Newport News, Virginia 23601 2-A (Medical College of Virginia)		G.S. Mitchell, Jr., M.D. Riverside Hospital—Family Practice Residency J. Clyde Morris Boulevard Newport News, Virginia 23601 (804) 599-7310
Eastern Virginia Graduate School of Medicine Family Practice Program P.O. Box 1980 Norfolk, Virginia 23501 4/A (East Virginia Medical School)		Robert L. Cassidy, M.D. Family Practice Residency Ghent Family Practice Center P.O. Box 1980 Norfolk, Virginia 23501 (804) 446-5263
Roanoke Memorial Hospital Bellview and Jefferson Streets Roanoke, Virginia 24014 2/A (University of Virginia— Charlottesville)		Gene Clapsaddle, M.D. Family Practice Residency Bellview and Jefferson Streets Roanoke, Virginia 24014 (703) 981-7228
Chippenham Hospital Inc. 7101 Jahnke Road Richmond, Virginia 23225 2/A (Medical College of Virginia)		Darrell K. Gilliam, M.D. Chesterfield Family Practice Center 2500 Pocoshock Place Richmond, Virginia 23235 (804) 276-9305
Medical College of Virginia Family Practice Program 1200 East Broad Street Richmond, Virginia 23225 4/A (Medical College of Virginia)		A. Epes Harris, Jr., M.D. Blackstone Family Practice Center 820 South Main Street Blackstone, Virginia 23824 (804) 292-7261

FAMILY PRACTICE TEACHING PROGRAMS—CONTINUED

SPONSORING INSTITUTION	CHAIRMAN OF MEDICAL SCHOOL DEPARTMENT (IF APPLICABLE)	DIRECTOR OF RESIDENCY PROGRAM AND FAMILY PRACTICE CENTER ADDRESS AND PHONE NUMBER
General Hospital of Virginia Beach 1060 First Colonial Road Virginia Beach, Virginia 23454 2/C (Medical College of Virginia, first year spent at Riverside Hospital— Newport News, Virginia)		James P. Charlton, M.D. First Colonial Family Planning Center 1120 First Colonial Road— Suite 100 Virginia Beach, Virginia 23454 (804) 481-2333

Washington

University of Washington School of Medicine Seattle, Washington 98195	John Geyman, M.D. Chairman Dept. of Family Medicine (206) 543-3101	
Doctor's Hospital 909 University Seattle, Washington 98101 2/A (University of Washington)		Joseph N. Scardapane, M.D. Doctor's Hospital Family Practice Residency 1106 Summit Avenue Seattle, Washington 98101 (206) 447-4111
Group Health Cooperative of Puget Sound 200–15th Avenue East Seattle, Washington 98112 2/A (University of Washington)		Robert B. Monroe, M.D. Family Practice Residency 200–15th Avenue East Seattle, Washington 98112 (206) 326-6724
Providence Family Medical Center 1715 East Cherry Street Seattle, Washington 98112 2-A (University of Washington)		Richard H. Layton, M.D. Providence Family Practice Residency 1715 East Cherry Street Seattle, Washington 98112 (206) 326-5581
University Hospital 1959 Northeast Pacific Street Seattle, Washington 98195 4/A (University of Washington)		Ronald Schneeweiss, M.D. Family Medicine Residency Program Dept. of Family Medicine RF-30 University of Washington Seattle, Washington 98195 (206) 543-9425

FAMILY PRACTICE TEACHING PROGRAMS—CONTINUED

SPONSORING INSTITUTION	CHAIRMAN OF MEDICAL SCHOOL DEPARTMENT (IF APPLICABLE)	DIRECTOR OF RESIDENCY PROGRAM AND FAMILY PRACTICE CENTER ADDRESS AND PHONE NUMBER
Inland Empire Hospital Services Association South 511 Pine Street Spokane, Washington 99202 2/A (University of Washington)		Kenneth E. Gudgel, M.D. Family Medicine Spokane South 511 Pine Street Spokane, Washington 99202 (509) 624-2313
Madigan Army Medical Center Box 828 Tacoma, Washington 98431 5/A		Col. Kenneth E. Holtzapple, M.D. Madigan Army Medical Center Box 373 Tacoma, Washington 98431 (206) 967-6673
Tacoma General Hospital 315 South Kay Street Tacoma, Washington 98405 2/A (University of Washington)		Roy W. Virak, M.D. Family Practice Residency Foundation Tacoma Family Medicine Allemore Medical Center 19th and Union Tacoma, Washington 98405 (206) 383-5855
Family Medicine Yakima Valley 421 South 47th Avenue Yakima, Washington 98902 2/C (University of Washington; first year spent at Family Medicine Spokane)		Douglas O. Corpron, M.D. Family Medicine Yakima Valley 421 South 47th Avenue Yakima, Washington 98908 (509) 966-9480

West Virginia

Marshall University School of Medicine Huntington, West Virginia 25701	Roy Kessel, M.D. Chairman Dept. of Family Practice (304) 696-2331	
West Virginia University School of Medicine Morgantown, West Virginia 26506	John W. Traubert, M.D. Chairman Dept. of Family Medicine (304) 293-5204	

FAMILY PRACTICE TEACHING PROGRAMS—CONTINUED

SPONSORING INSTITUTION	*CHAIRMAN OF MEDICAL SCHOOL DEPARTMENT (IF APPLICABLE)*	*DIRECTOR OF RESIDENCY PROGRAM AND FAMILY PRACTICE CENTER ADDRESS AND PHONE NUMBER*
West Virginia University Medical Center (Charleston Division) Charleston, West Virginia 25325	C. Carl Tully, M.D. Chairman Dept. of Family Practice (304) 768–3941	
Charleston Area Medical Center Charleston, West Virginia 3/A (West Virginia University—Charleston Division) and Herbert J. Thomas Memorial Hospital South Charleston, West Virginia 25309		C. Carl Tully, M.D. Kanawha Valley Family Practice Center 4605 MacCorkle Ave., Southwest South Charleston, West Virginia 25309 (304) 768–3941
United Hospital Center, Inc. Hospital Plaza—P.O. Box 2290 Clarksburg, West Virginia 26301 1/A		L. Dale Simmons, M.D. Family Practice Residency P.O. Box 2290 Clarksburg, West Virginia 26301 (304) 624–7598
Marshall Family Practice Center 1801 Sixth Avenue Huntington, West Virginia 25701 3/A (Marshall University)		Ray Kessel, M.D. Marshall Family Practice Center 1801 Sixth Avenue Huntington, West Virginia 25701 (304) 696–2331
West Virginia University Hospital Morgantown, West Virginia 26506 4/A (West Virginia University—Morgantown)		John W. Traubert, M.D. West Virginia University Hospital Morgantown, West Virginia 26506 (304) 293–5204
Wheeling Hospital Medical Park Wheeling, West Virginia 26003 1/A		George M. Kellas, M.D. Family Health Center Suite 105 Professional Center, Medical Park Wheeling, West Virginia 26003 (304) 242–7870

FAMILY PRACTICE TEACHING PROGRAMS—CONTINUED

SPONSORING INSTITUTION	CHAIRMAN OF MEDICAL SCHOOL DEPARTMENT (IF APPLICABLE)	DIRECTOR OF RESIDENCY PROGRAM AND FAMILY PRACTICE CENTER ADDRESS AND PHONE NUMBER
Wisconsin		
Medical College of Wisconsin 561 North 15th Street Milwaukee, Wisconsin 53233	Donald J. Welter, M.D. Chairman Dept. of Family Practice (414) 933–0700	
University of Wisconsin— Madison Center for Health Sciences 777 South Mills Street Madison, Wisconsin 53715	William Scheckler, M.D. Acting Chairman Dept. of Family Medicine and Practice (608) 263–4550	
Eau Claire Regional Education Consortium Box 861 611 South Farwell Street Eau Claire, Wisconsin 54701 3/A (University of Wisconsin—Madison)		Larry L. Hanley, M.D. Eau Claire Family Practice Residency Program Box 861 611 South Farwell Street Eau Claire, Wisconsin 54701 (715) 839–5175
St. Francis Hospital 709 South Tenth La Crosse, Wisconsin 54601 2/A (Mayo Medical School)		Ted L. Thompson, M.D. Family Practice Residency 709 South Tenth La Crosse, Wisconsin 54601 (608) 785–0940 Ext. 2696
St. Mary's Hospital Medical Center 777 South Mills Street Madison, Wisconsin 53715 3/A (University of Wisconsin—Madison)		Lynn Phelps, M.D. Family Practice Residency 777 South Mills Street Madison, Wisconsin 53715 (608) 263–4550
Deaconess Hospital 610 North 19th Street Milwaukee, Wisconsin 53233 2/A (Medical College of Wisconsin)		Thomas F. Garland, M.D. Deaconess Family Practice Residency Program 610 North 19th Street Milwaukee, Wisconsin 53233 (414) 933–3600
Lutheran Hospital 2200 West Kilbourn Avenue Milwaukee, Wisconsin 53233 2/A (Medical College of Wisconsin)		Glenn A. Dall, M.D. Family Practice Residency Program Lutheran Hospital of Milwaukee 2200 West Kilbourn Avenue Milwaukee, Wisconsin 53233 (414) 933–0700

FAMILY PRACTICE TEACHING PROGRAMS—CONTINUED

SPONSORING INSTITUTION	CHAIRMAN OF MEDICAL SCHOOL DEPARTMENT (IF APPLICABLE)	DIRECTOR OF RESIDENCY PROGRAM AND FAMILY PRACTICE CENTER ADDRESS AND PHONE NUMBER
Milwaukee County General Hospital 8700 West Wisconsin Avenue Milwaukee, Wisconsin 53226 2/A (Medical College of Wisconsin) (414) 257-7996		To be named (program not operational)
St. Luke's Hospital 2900 West Oklahoma Avenue Milwaukee, Wisconsin 53215 2/A (Medical College of Wisconsin)		John A. Palese, M.D. Family Practice Residency 2900 W. Oklahoma Avenue Milwaukee, Wisconsin 53215 (414) 647-6558
St. Mary's Hospital 2323 North Lake Drive Box 503 Milwaukee, Wisconsin 53201 3/A (Medical College of Wisconsin)		Werner F. Cryns, M.D. Family Practice Program 2320 North Lake Drive St. Mary's Hospital, Box 503 Milwaukee, Wisconsin 53201 (414) 271-2346
St. Michael Hospital 2400 West Villard Avenue Milwaukee, Wisconsin 53209 2/A (Medical College of Wisconsin)		Norbert G. Bauch, M.D. Family Practice Residency 2400 W. Villard Avenue Milwaukee, Wisconsin 53209 (414) 263-8000
Waukesha Memorial Hospital 1111 Delafield Street Waukesha, Wisconsin 53186 3/A (University of Wisconsin—Madison)		John L. Raschbacher, M.D. Family Practice Residency 434 Madison Waukesha, Wisconsin 53186 (414) 549-4284
Wausau Hospital, Inc. Maple Hill Wausau, Wisconsin 54401 3/A (University of Wisconsin—Madison)		Thomas H. Peterson, M.D. Wausau Family Practice Residency Program Ridgewood Building Maple Hill Wausau, Wisconsin 54401 (715) 845-4610

Wyoming

SPONSORING INSTITUTION	CHAIRMAN OF MEDICAL SCHOOL DEPARTMENT (IF APPLICABLE)	DIRECTOR OF RESIDENCY PROGRAM AND FAMILY PRACTICE CENTER ADDRESS AND PHONE NUMBER
Memorial Hospital of Natrona County 1233 East 2nd Street Casper, Wyoming 82601 3/A (University of Wyoming)		Charles W. Huff, M.D. Family Practice Residency 1522 E. A Street Casper, Wyoming 82601 (307) 265-3926

* Newly approved residency programs as a result of action taken by Liaison Committee on Graduate Medical Education since the last printing.

ACOG–AAFP Agreement for Curriculum and Hospital Privileges in Obstetrics–Gynecology[*]

I. Core curriculum

The ultimate concern of all physicians must be the welfare of the patient. There may be different approaches to care by reason of the patient's age, background, or illness, but the appropriate history, examination, and the social, psychological, and human sexuality aspects of care must be an integral part of training.

The knowledge and skills acquired in residency training are a necessary base, although they will not necessarily translate into the practice of every family physician.

    A. Cognitive knowledge

        1. Normal growth and development, and variants

        2. Gynecology

            Physiology of menstruation
            Abnormal uterine bleeding

---

[*] Developed by a joint ad hoc committee of the American Academy of Family Physicians, the American College of Obstetricians and Gynecologists, and the Council on Resident Education in Obstetrics and Gynecology.

Diagnosis of pediatric gynecologic problems
Infections of the female reproductive tract and urinary systems
Sexual assault
Trauma
Benign and malignant neoplasms of the female reproductive
tract
Pelvic tissue injury
Menopause and geriatric gynecology
Assessment of surgical needs

3. Obstetrics

Antepartum care
Labor and delivery
Postpartum care
Care of the normal newborn
Obstetric complications; diagnosis and management, including
emergency breech delivery and postpartum hemorrhage
Pregnancy risk assessment systems and their implementation

4. Family life education

Family planning and fertility problems
Interconceptional care
Family and sexual counseling

5. Process of examination

Pediatric female reproductive examination
Adult female reproductive examination

6. Consultation and Referral

Individual patient consultation and referral
Women's health care delivery systems
Maternal and perinatal health regional planning

B. Skills

Emotional preparation and performance of the gynecologic examination at all ages.

1. Gynecology

Obtaining vaginal and cervical cytology
Endometrial biopsy
Cervical biopsy and polypectomy

Culdocentesis
Cryosurgery/cautery for benign disease
Microscopic diagnosis of urine and vaginal smears
Bartholin cyst drainage or marsupialization
D and C
Conization (II)

2. Conception Control

Oral contraceptive counseling
IUD insertion and removal and counseling
Diaphragm fitting and counseling
Voluntary interruption of pregnancy to 10 weeks gestation

3. Pregnancy

First examination—evaluation of pelvic adequacy
Use of risk assessment protocols
Evaluation of fetal maturity and fetoplacental adequacy
Amniocentesis for diagnosis (II)
Normal cephalic delivery including outlet forceps
Exploration of vagina, cervix, uterus
Manual removal of placenta
Episiotomy and repair
Pudendal and paracervical block anesthesia
Fetal monitoring
Induction of labor (II)
Third-degree perineal repair
Cesarean section (II)

4. Surgery

Assist at common major surgical procedures
Tubal ligation with cesarean section (II)

II. Implementation

Core cognitive ability and skill should require a minimum of three months
experience in a structured obstetric–gynecologic educational program, with
supervised management of at least 30 vaginal deliveries. Residents will
obtain substantial additional obstetric–gynecologic experience throughout the
three years of their experience in family practice centers and will return
to the family practice centers for their scheduled times even during the
obstetric–gynecologic rotation.

For those family practice residents electing additional training in obstetrics–
gynecology, particularly those residents who are planning to practice in

communities without readily available specialist consultation, an additional minimum of three months experience in a structured obstetric–gynecologic educational program is strongly recommended. This program should include experience in induction of labor, cesarean section (a minimum of ten procedures) and tubal ligation if appropriate to physician beliefs, and gynecologic procedures such as conization. These advanced skills are identified by (II).

A structured educational program is defined as one which provides the specified cognitive knowledge and skills, appropriate supervision, and continuing interrelationship of the resident with the family practice center.

Every educational institution sponsoring graduate medical education should assume corporate responsibility for the overall program.

Programs for family practice residents should have a joint training committee composed of equal numbers of obstetrician–gynecologists and family physicians, with members of the committee approved by chairmen of the respective departments in the sponsoring educational institution. It shall be the responsibility of the joint training committee to develop objectives commensurate with the above goals, to monitor the residents' experience, and to evaluate the residents' attainment of these objectives. It shall also be the responsibility of this committee to assess the capabilities of the faculty for family practice resident education in obstetrics–gynecology.

III. Hospital privileges

If a resident satisfactorily fulfills the above criteria, that resident may be recommended by the joint training committee to a hospital or hospitals. The assignment of hospital privileges remains the responsibility of the individual hospital.

The following statement is from the recommendations of the AMA Interspecialty Advisory Council Committee on Jurisdiction. It has been approved by the Board of Directors of the American Academy of Family Physicians:

Interdepartmental Relationships

Interdepartmental relationships in the provision of medical care should be defined. If a staff member, who is a member of one clinical department, applies for privileges for which he is qualified in another department, his privileges should be recommended by the first department with the concurrence and approval of the second department. The exercise of the clinical privileges granted in each department shall be the responsibility of the respective department in consultation with the original department.

The Virginia Study

David W. Marsland, M.D., Maurice Wood, M.B.,
Fitzhugh Mayo, M.D.

PART I: RANK ORDER OF DIAGNOSIS BY
FREQUENCY   446

PART II: DIAGNOSIS BY DISEASE CATEGORY
AND AGE/SEX DISTRIBUTION   462

PART I. RANK ORDER OF DIAGNOSES BY FREQUENCY

Rank	RCGP Number	Description	Male		Female		Total	Total	Percent
							FREQUENCY	CUMULATIVE	
1	511	Other medical exam for preventive and presymptomatic purposes	20,206	+	23,745	=	43,951	43,951	8.353
2	218	Benign or unspecified hypertension w/wo heart and/or renal disease	9,965	+	20,270	=	30,235	74,186	14.099
3	483	Lacerations, amputations, contusions, and abrasions	12,675	+	8,462	=	21,137	95,323	18.115
4	242	Pharyngitis (including febrile sore throat and tonsillitis)	8,387	+	11,789	=	20,176	115,499	21.950
5	247	Bronchitis, acute	5,724	+	7,787	=	13,511	129,010	24.517
6	480	Sprains and strains	6,664	+	6,166	=	12,830	141,840	26.956
7	91	Diabetes mellitus	3,812	+	8,623	=	12,435	154,275	29.319
8	240	Coryza (nonfebrile common cold)	4,389	+	6,562	=	10,951	165,226	31.400
9	101	Obesity	1,928	+	8,751	=	10,679	175,905	33.430
10	241	Febrile cold and influenzalike illness	4,466	+	4,900	=	9,366	185,271	35.209
11	183	Otitis media, acute	4,513	+	4,632	=	9,145	194,416	36.947
12	134	Depressive neurosis	1,486	+	6,347	=	7,833	202,249	38.436
13	500	Cervical smear	0		7,706	=	7,706	209,955	39.900
14	352	Normal pregnancy prenatal care	0		7,189	=	7,189	217,144	41.267
15	130	Anxiety neurosis	1,691	+	4,954	=	6,645	223,789	42.529
16	221	Arteriosclerosis (including cardiovascular disease)	2,800	+	3,813	=	6,613	230,402	43.786
17	335	Vulvitis, vaginitis, and cervicitis (non-venereal)	0		6,324	=	6,324	236,726	44.988
18	306	Abdominal pain other than colic	1,735	+	3,903	=	5,638	242,364	46.060
19	215	Congestive heart failure	1,966	+	3,086	=	5,052	247,416	47.020
20	313	Urinary infection (cystitis)	494	+	4,358	=	4,852	252,268	47.942
21	243	Sinusitis (acute)	1,717	+	2,997	=	4,714	256,982	48.838
22	272	Other sign, symptom, or incomplete diagnosis (Category 8)	1,766	+	2,587	=	4,353	261,335	49.665
23	409	Other forms of arthritis and rheumatism	1,334	+	2,899	=	4,233	265,568	50.469
24	464	Other sign, symptom, or incomplete diagnosis (Category 16)	1,383	+	2,729	=	4,112	269,680	51.251
25	246	Pneumonia pneumonitis	1,982	+	2,068	=	4,050	273,730	52.020
26	135	Physical disorders of presumably psychogenic origin	996	+	2,927	=	3,923	277,653	52.766
27	454	Headache	1,010	+	2,475	=	3,485	281,138	53.428
28	380	Dermatitis, contact	1,563	+	1,916	=	3,479	284,617	54.089
29	111	Iron-deficiency (hypochromic) anemia (male and female)	1,156	+	2,293	=	3,449	288,066	54.745
30	86	Asthma (Category 3)	1,367	+	2,021	=	3,388	291,454	55.389
31	316	Other infections of urinary system including prostatitis	1,972	+	1,410	=	3,382	294,836	56.031
32	256	Other disease process not included above (Category 8)	1,539	+	1,655	=	3,194	298,030	56.638
33	257	Rhinitis, vasomotor or allergic	1,308	+	1,794	=	3,102	301,132	57.228
34	505	Other prophylactic procedures	1,260	+	1,837	=	3,097	304,229	57.816

35	406	Osteoarthritis	791 +	2,192 =	2,983	307,212	58.383
36	372	Other cellulitis without mention of lymphangitis	1,391 +	1,525 =	2,916	310,128	58.937
37	273	Acute gastritis or duodenitis	1,279 +	1,585 =	2,864	312,992	59.482
38	425	Back pain alone	1,168 +	1,669 =	2,837	315,829	60.021
39	155	Vascular lesions	1,134 +	1,620 =	2,754	318,583	60.544
40	585	Oral contraceptive advice	0 +	2,721 =	2,721	321,304	61.061
41	317	Other diseases of the urinary tract	763 +	1,935 =	2,698	324,002	61.574
42	377	Other local infections of skin and subcutaneous tissue	1,297 +	1,252 =	2,549	326,551	62.059
43	95	Specific allergies	992 +	1,540 =	2,532	329,083	62.540
44	381	Other dermatitis	1,016 +	1,488 =	2,504	331,587	63.016
45	398	Rash	1,033 +	1,290 =	2,323	333,910	63.457
46	182	Otitis externa	1,026 +	1,278 =	2,304	336,214	63.895
47	568	Other disease inoculations	992 +	1,268 =	2,260	338,474	64.324
48	245	Influenza epidemic	925 +	1,312 =	2,237	340,711	64.749
49	28	Other recognized disease not included above (Category 1)	693 +	1,542 =	2,235	342,946	65.174
50	217	Other heart disease	1,184 +	997 =	2,181	345,127	65.589
51	285	Other diseases of intestines and peritoneum	801 +	1,361 =	2,162	347,289	66.000
52	415	Other disease process not mentioned above (Category 13)	913 +	1,172 =	2,085	349,374	66.396
53	170	Conjunctivitis and ophthalmia	938 +	1,089 =	2,027	351,401	66.781
54	405	Rheumatoid arthritis	645 +	1,382 =	2,027	353,428	67.166
55	25	Viral warts (infectious)	942 +	1,071 =	2,013	355,441	67.549
56	427	Other sign, symptom, or incomplete diagnosis (Category 13)	830 +	1,149 =	1,979	357,420	67.925
57	420	Bursitis	819 +	1,057 =	1,876	359,296	68.281
58	200	Vertigo	629 +	1,216 =	1,845	361,141	68.632
59	212	Other ischemic heart disease	885 +	949 =	1,834	362,975	68.981
60	190	Other diseases of ear and mastoid process	763 +	1,041 =	1,804	364,779	69.323
61	211	Acute myocardial infarction	1,179 +	613 =	1,792	366,571	69.664
62	5	Diarrhea and/or vomiting intestinal infectious disease	778 +	982 =	1,760	368,331	69.998
63	304	Diarrhea and/or vomiting (afebrile)	674 +	1,039 =	1,713	370,044	70.324
64	214	Heart block and other disorders of rhythm	715 +	996 =	1,711	371,755	70.649
65	543	Group diphtheria, whooping cough, and tetanus prophylaxis	886 +	783 =	1,669	373,424	70.966
66	280	Functional gastric disorders	637 +	1,010 =	1,647	375,071	71.279
67	331	Other diseases of female genitalia	0 +	1,576 =	1,576	376,647	71.579
68	226	Phlebitis and thrombophlebitis	490 +	1,015 =	1,505	378,152	71.865
69	147	Tension headache	294 +	1,173 =	1,467	379,619	72.144
70	231	Precordial pain	772 +	683 =	1,455	381,074	72.420
71	394	Insect bites	718 +	733 =	1,451	382,525	72.696
72	303	Diarrhea and/or vomiting (febrile)	638 +	810 =	1,448	383,973	72.971
73	244	Laryngitis and tracheitis	584 +	835 =	1,419	385,392	73.241
74	225	Hemorrhoids	692 +	725 =	1,417	386,809	73.510

PART I. Continued

			FREQUENCY			CUMULATIVE	
Rank	RCGP Number	Description	Male	Female	Total	Total	Percent
75	428	Pain in joint (arthralgia)	550 +	857 =	1,407	388,216	73.777
76	408	Fibrositis and muscular rheumatism	548 +	820 =	1,368	389,584	74.037
77	465	Foreign body entering not through orifice	754 +	614 =	1,368	390,952	74.297
78	230	Angina of effort	724 +	616 =	1,340	392,292	74.552
79	112	Other specific anemias (male and female)	394 +	942 =	1,336	393,628	74.806
80	141	Abuse of alcohol	944 +	389 =	1,333	394,961	75.059
81	387	Disease of nail and nail bed	632 +	700 =	1,332	396,293	75.312
82	74	All other benign neoplasms (Category 2)	514 +	816 =	1,330	397,623	75.565
83	267	Cough	533 +	764 =	1,297	398,920	75.811
84	495	Other fractures not included above	658 +	639 =	1,297	400,217	76.058
85	486	Burns, second degree	735 +	557 =	1,292	401,509	76.303
86	375	Impetigo	667 +	608 =	1,275	402,784	76.546
87	4	Gonorrhea	740 +	509 =	1,249	404,033	76.783
88	389	Disease of sweat and sebaceous glands	672 +	575 =	1,247	405,280	77.020
89	158	Epilepsy (Category 6)	583 +	639 =	1,222	406,502	77.252
90	399	Other sign, symptom, or incomplete diagnosis (Category 12)	517 +	704 =	1,221	407,723	77.484
91	704	Family relationship problems	290 +	913 =	1,203	408,926	77.713
92	237	Other sign, symptom, or incomplete diagnosis (Category 7)	542 +	636 =	1,178	410,104	77.937
93	187	Wax in ear	634 +	527 =	1,161	411,265	78.157
94	326	Amenorrhea	0 +	1,137 =	1,137	412,402	78.373
95	255	Emphysema without bronchitis	956 +	177 =	1,133	413,535	78.589
96	476	Fracture, carpal, metacarpal, tarsal, or metatarsal bones	668 +	451 =	1,119	414,654	78.801
97	379	Dermatitis, atopic (eczema)	338 +	729 =	1,117	415,771	79.014
98	284	Other hernias of abdominal cavity	426 +	689 =	1,115	416,886	79.226
99	290	Constipation	394 +	721 =	1,115	418,001	79.437
100	344	Other sign, symptom, or incomplete diagnosis (Category 10)	296 +	818 =	1,114	419,115	79.649
101	493	Other known injury not included above	554 +	551 =	1,105	420,220	79.859
102	275	Diseases of teeth and supporting structures	423 +	655 =	1,078	421,298	80.064
103	369	Acne	459 +	607 =	1,066	422,364	80.267
104	93	Gout (Category 3)	728 +	334 =	1,062	423,426	80.468
105	329	Menopausal symptoms	0 +	1,026 =	1,026	424,452	80.663
106	223	Peripheral arterial disease	538 +	484 =	1,022	425,474	80.858
107	494	Other sign, symptom, or incomplete diagnosis (Category 17)	569 +	450 =	1,019	426,493	81.051
108	271	Pleuritic pain	356 +	647 =	1,003	427,496	81.242

448

109	400	Cervical injury, e.g., whiplash (excluding fracture or disk)	380 +	623 =	1,003	428,499	81.432
110	31	Pyrexia of unknown origin	510 +	480 =	990	429,489	81.621
111	23	Epidemic winter vomiting (viral gastroenteritis)	441 +	545 =	986	430,475	81.808
112	234	Edema	241 +	727 =	968	431,443	81.992
113	233	Syncope	324 +	641 =	965	432,408	82.175
114	248	Bronchitis, chronic	467 +	491 =	958	433,366	82.357
115	293	Nausea	296 +	659 =	955	434,321	82.539
116	184	Otitis media, chronic	432 +	521 =	953	435,274	82.720
117	276	Other diseases of buccal cavity	425 +	506 =	931	436,205	82.897
118	421	Tenosynovitis	401 +	526 =	927	437,132	83.073
119	477	Fracture of phalanges	574 +	349 =	923	438,055	83.248
120	27	Other virus infection	380 +	537 =	917	438,972	83.423
121	181	Other diseases of the eye	444 +	467 =	911	439,883	83.596
122	125	Schizophrenia	341 +	563 =	904	440,787	83.768
123	227	Other disease of circulatory system	429 +	473 =	902	441,689	83.939
124	2	Tuberculosis (other forms)	517 +	384 =	901	442,590	84.110
125	544	Poliomyelitis prophylaxis	457 +	433 =	890	443,480	84.279
126	169	Other diseases of peripheral nerves or ganglia	358 +	510 =	868	444,348	84.444
127	322	Breast diseases, other than neoplasm	78 +	766 =	844	445,192	84.605
128	88	Hyperthyroidism	98 +	741 =	839	446,031	84.764
129	87	Allergic dermatosis, urticaria	326 +	511 =	837	446,868	84.923
130	308	Other sign, symptom, or incomplete diagnosis (Category 9)	357 +	472 =	829	447,697	85.081
131	21	Dermatophytosis	491 +	325 =	816	448,513	85.236
132	328	Menorrhagia and metrorrhagia	0 +	814 =	814	449,327	85.391
133	311	Pyelitis and pyelonephritis	189 +	618 =	807	450,134	85.544
134	224	Varicose veins of lower extremities	240 +	562 =	802	450,936	85.606
135	278	Duodenal ulcer	476 +	315 =	791	451,727	85.847
136	374	Cellulitis and abscess with lymphangitis	414 +	360 =	774	452,501	85.994
137	210	Rheumatic heart disease	291 +	471 =	762	453,263	86.138
138	70	Breast (Category 2—benign)	69 +	690 =	759	454,022	86.283
139	813	Hypertension (Category 21)	284 +	470 =	754	454,776	86.426
140	370	Boil and carbuncle	405 +	338 =	743	455,519	86.567
141	89	Hypothyroidism	109 +	621 =	730	456,249	86.706
142	457	Weight loss	303 +	422 =	725	456,974	86.844
143	302	Melena	368 +	353 =	721	457,695	86.981
144	327	Irregular menstruation	0 +	717 =	717	458,412	87.117
145	159	Migraine	130 +	576 =	706	459,118	87.251
146	73	Skin (Category 2—benign)	272 +	420 =	692	459,810	87.383
147	904	Other psychotropic drugs (Category 22)	148 +	538 =	686	460,496	87.513
148	283	Hernia, inguinal or femoral	524 +	161 =	685	461,181	87.643

	DIAGNOSIS		FREQUENCY			CUMULATIVE	
Rank	RCGP Number	Description	Male	Female	Total	Total	Percent
149	289	Cirrhosis of liver	431 +	248 =	679	461,860	87.772
150	288	Other diseases of liver, gallbladder, and pancreas	278 +	379 =	657	462,517	87.897
151	315	Urethritis, nonvenereal	571 +	86 =	657	463,174	88.022
152	94	Other recognized disease not included above (Category 3)	235 +	418 =	653	463,827	88.146
153	110	Pernicious (megaloblastic) anemia	238 +	411 =	649	464,476	88.269
154	321	Other diseases of male genitalia	647 +	0 =	647	465,123	88.392
155	157	Parkinsonism	376 +	261 =	637	465,760	88.513
156	385	Other hypertrophic and atrophic skin conditions	245 +	390 =	635	466,395	88.634
157	250	Sinusitis (chronic)	181 +	445 =	626	467,021	88.753
158	485	Burns, first degree	328 +	288 =	616	467,637	88.870
159	469	Fracture of tibia and/or fibula (Potts)	339 +	274 =	613	468,250	88.986
160	343	Hematuria (Category 10)	362 +	242 =	604	468,854	89.101
161	281	Other diseases of esophagus, stomach, and duodenum	276 +	323 =	599	469,453	89.215
162	251	Pleurisy	231 +	356 =	587	470,040	89.327
163	128	Organic psychoses	223 +	348 =	571	470,611	89.435
164	446	Debility or fatigue	193 +	370 =	563	471,174	89.542
165	323	Salpingitis and oophoritis	0 +	561 =	561	471,735	89.649
166	279	Pyloric, juxtapyloric, prepyloric ulcer	332 +	228 =	560	472,295	89.755
167	14	Herpes zoster	207 +	345 =	552	472,847	89.860
168	17	Infectious mononucleosis	245 +	306 =	551	473,398	89.965
169	504	Health education counseling	235 +	316 =	551	473,949	90.069
170	541	Tuberculosis prophylaxis	224 +	326 =	550	474,499	90.174
171	150	Other special sign or symptom not coded elsewhere (Category 5)	253 +	296 =	549	475,048	90.278
172	160	Other diseases of CNS	243 +	304 =	547	475,595	90.382
173	390	Chronic ulcer of skin	278 +	268 =	546	476,141	90.486
174	484	Foreign body entering through orifice	355 +	185 =	540	476,681	90.589
175	424	Backache with other neuritis	192 +	340 =	532	477,213	90.690
176	277	Gastric ulcer	267 +	258 =	525	477,738	90.789
177	263	Epistaxis	246 +	267 =	513	478,251	90.887
178	383	Pruritus	167 +	341 =	508	478,759	90.983
179	471	Fracture of ribs	285 +	220 =	505	479,264	91.079
180	586	Other contraceptive advice	6 +	494 =	500	479,764	91.174
181	805	Carcinoma (Category 21)	251 +	249 =	500	480,264	91.269
182	378	Dermatitis, seborrheic	199 +	293 =	492	480,756	91.363

183	496	Adverse effect of other drugs	151	+	341	=	492	481,248	91.456
184	466	Sweating	227	+	253	=	480	481,728	91.548
185	407	Lumbago (backache) not attributed to disk lesion	198	+	273	=	471	482,199	91.637
186	475	Colles' fracture	232	+	233	=	465	482,664	91.726
187	371	Cellulitis of finger and toe	203	+	245	=	448	483,112	91.811
188	213	Myocardial degeneration from other causes	214	+	233	=	447	483,559	91.896
189	67	Leukemia, all types	181	+	258	=	439	483,998	91.979
190	625	Other abnormal biochemistry	213	+	224	=	437	484,435	92.062
191	401	Torticollis	174	+	259	=	433	484,868	92.144
192	68	All other malignant neoplasms	197	+	235	=	432	485,300	92.226
193	85	Hay fever (Category 3)	193	+	231	=	424	485,724	92.307
194	325	Dysmenorrhea	0	+	424	=	424	486,148	92.388
195	312	Calculi of kidneys and ureters	302	+	119	=	421	486,569	92.468
196	391	Dermatitis herpetiformis, pemphigus, lichen, etc	178	+	235	=	413	486,982	92.546
197	161	Labyrinthitis	131	+	278	=	409	487,391	92.624
198	13	Chicken pox	215	+	190	=	405	487,796	92.701
199	20	Oxyuriasis	164	+	235	=	399	488,195	92.777
200	309	Anal fissure and fistula	179	+	216	=	395	488,590	92.852
201	16	Infectious hepatitis	239	+	154	=	393	488,983	92.926
202	337	Dysuria and/or strangury	109	+	281	=	390	489,373	93.000
203	219	Malignant hypertension	118	+	269	=	387	489,760	93.074
204	57	Bronchus, lung and trachea (Category 2—malignant)	192	+	186	=	378	490,138	93.146
205	114	Other recognized disease not included above (Category 4)	170	+	208	=	378	490,516	93.218
206	334	Other disorders of menstruation	0	+	375	=	375	490,891	93.289
207	207	Other sign, symptom, or incomplete diagnosis (Category 6)	168	+	202	=	370	491,261	93.359
208	310	Nephritis and nephrosis	140	+	226	=	366	491,627	93.429
209	301	Colic	137	+	217	=	354	491,981	93.496
210	411	Other internal derangements of the knee	191	+	163	=	354	492,335	93.563
211	249	Tonsillar and adenoidal hypertrophy	151	+	202	=	353	492,688	93.630
212	318	Prostatic hypertrophy (benign)	353	+	0	=	353	493,041	93.697
213	473	Fracture of clavicle	244	+	106	=	350	493,391	93.764
214	287	Cholecystitis and/or cholangitis without calculus	56	+	289	=	345	493,736	93.829
215	274	Esophagitis	129	+	213	=	342	494,078	93.894
216	177	Keratitis, with or without corneal ulcer	221	+	119	=	340	494,418	93.959
217	905	Thiazide diuretics (Category 22)	142	+	198	=	340	494,758	94.024
218	388	Disease of hair and hair follicle	137	+	199	=	336	495,094	94.087
219	294	Heartburn	144	+	183	=	327	495,421	94.150
220	58	Breast (Category 2—malignant)	3	+	316	=	319	495,740	94.210
221	229	Pulmonary embolism	137	+	180	=	317	496,057	94.270
222	644	Other abnormal procedure (Category 19)	80	+	237	=	317	496,374	94.331

PART 1. Continued

		DIAGNOSIS	FREQUENCY				CUMULATIVE	
Rank	RCGP Number	Description	Male	Female		Total	Total	Percent
223	105	Other sign, symptom, or incomplete diagnosis (Category 21)	116 +	198	=	314	496,688	94.390
224	133	Obsessive–compulsive neurosis	80 +	225	=	305	496,993	94.448
225	179	Cataract	103 +	202	=	305	497,298	94.506
226	801	Anemia (including hemoglobinopathies) (Category 21)	54 +	249	=	303	497,601	94.564
227	320	Epididymitis and/or orchitis	299 +	0	=	299	497,900	94.621
228	3	Syphilis (infectious and sequelae)	161 +	136	=	297	498,197	94.677
229	468	Fracture of femur	39 +	257	=	296	498,493	94.733
230	146	Insomnia	148 +	146	=	294	498,787	94.789
231	807	Diabetes (Category 21)	124 +	170	=	294	499,081	94.845
232	148	Enuresis	158 +	135	=	293	499,374	94.901
233	15	Mumps	161 +	131	=	292	499,666	94.956
234	456	Dehydration	60 +	231	=	291	499,957	95.012
235	136	Neurasthenia	77 +	206	=	283	500,240	95.065
236	127	Senile and presenile dementia	71 +	205	=	276	500,516	95.118
237	140	Mental retardation	138 +	138	=	276	500,792	95.170
238	336	Colic (renal)	211 +	55	=	266	501,058	95.221
239	152	Impotence	265 +	0	=	265	501,323	95.271
240	286	Cholelithiasis	54 +	204	=	258	501,581	95.320
241	412	Displacement of intervertebral disk	136 +	121	=	257	501,838	95.369
242	382	Psoriasis	89 +	162	=	251	502,089	95.417
243	90	Other thyroid disease (Category 3)	37 +	212	=	249	502,338	95.464
244	129	Other and unspecified psychoses	101 +	148	=	249	502,587	95.511
245	546	Measles prophylaxis	120 +	127	=	247	502,834	95.558
246	444	Lymphadenopathy, enlargement of lymph nodes	94 +	151	=	245	503,079	95.605
247	139	Drug abuse	143 +	101	=	244	503,323	95.651
248	82	Other sign, symptom, or incomplete diagnosis (Category 2)	64 +	177	=	241	503,564	95.697
249	123	Excessive smoking	129 +	112	=	241	503,805	95.743
250	901	Steroids (Category 22)	103 +	137	=	240	504,045	95.788
251	314	Cystitis, chronic	23 +	216	=	239	504,284	95.834
252	295	Dysphagia	101 +	137	=	238	504,522	95.879
253	423	Backache with sciatica	110 +	128	=	238	504,760	95.924
254	474	Fracture of humerus	104 +	133	=	237	504,997	95.969
255	345	Genitourinary infection during pregnancy	0 +	235	=	235	505,232	96.014
256	368	Pityriasis rosea	95 +	139	=	234	505,466	96.058

257	467	Fracture of spine	118 +	104 =	222	505,688	96.100
258	612	Abnormal blood test	132 +	89 =	221	505,909	96.142
259	168	Sciatica	90 +	129 =	219	506,128	96.184
260	180	Glaucoma	74 +	145 =	219	506,347	96.226
261	1	Tuberculosis (respiratory system including late effects)	90 +	128 =	218	506,565	96.267
262	386	Other dermatoses	114 +	104 =	218	506,783	96.309
263	206	Paraesthesiae	89 +	126 =	215	506,998	96.349
264	458	Pyrexia of unknown origin	105 +	110 =	215	507,213	96.390
265	350	Abortion, spontaneous	0 +	214 =	214	507,427	96.431
266	340	Frequency (Category 10)	71 +	140 =	211	507,638	96.471
267	282	Appendicitis	126 +	83 =	209	507,847	96.511
268	481	Intracranial injury	127 +	78 =	205	508,052	96.550
269	437	Congenital malformation of bone and joint	112 +	91 =	203	508,255	96.588
270	235	Dyspnea (Category 7)	76 +	126 =	202	508,457	96.627
271	902	Antidepressives (Category 22)	48 +	153 =	201	508,658	96.665
272	545	Rubella prophylaxis	101 +	94 =	195	508,853	96.702
273	292	Anorexia	64 +	129 =	193	509,046	96.739
274	172	Hordeolum or stye	86 +	103 =	189	509,235	96.774
275	197	Convulsions	122 +	67 =	189	509,424	96.810
276	189	Other forms of deafness	90 +	97 =	187	509,611	96.846
277	460	Albuminuria	93 +	93 =	186	509,797	96.881
278	72	Other female genitourinary organs (Category 2—benign)	0 +	183 =	183	509,980	96.916
279	265	Dyspnea (Category 8)	84 +	98 =	182	510,162	96.951
280	351	Normal delivery	0 +	180 =	180	510,342	96.985
281	730	Other legal problems	129 +	51 =	180	510,522	97.019
282	487	Burns, third degree	119 +	58 =	177	510,699	97.053
283	384	Corns and callosities	60 +	116 =	176	510,875	97.086
284	149	Cardiac arrhythmia	99 +	75 =	174	511,049	97.119
285	908	Other cardiac drugs (Category 22)	77 +	97 =	174	511,223	97.152
286	338	Retention of urine	108 +	63 =	171	511,394	97.185
287	339	Incontinence of urine	44 +	127 =	171	511,565	97.217
288	71	Uterus (Category 2—benign)	0 +	169 =	169	511,734	97.249
289	631	Abnormal chest x-ray	76 +	93 =	169	511,903	97.281
290	53	Colon (Category 2—malignant)	35 +	133 =	168	512,071	97.313
291	96	Addison's disease, serum lipid abnormalities	111 +	57 =	168	512,239	97.345
292	113	Hemorrhagic conditions (male and female)	88 +	78 =	166	512,405	97.377
293	44	Pediculosis	81 +	84 =	165	512,570	97.408
294	174	Other inflammatory diseases of the eye	84 +	81 =	165	512,735	97.439
295	61	Prostate (Category 2—malignant)	164 +	0 =	164	512,899	97.471
296	635	Abnormal findings at other instrumental test	63 +	97 =	160	513,059	97.501

			FREQUENCY			CUMULATIVE	
Rank	RCGP Number	Description	Male	Female	Total	Total	Percent
297	488	Effects of alcohol poisoning	108 +	49 =	157	513,216	97.531
298	559	Tetanus alone prophylaxis	77 +	80 =	157	513,373	97.561
299	299	Jaundice (Category 9)	88 +	68 =	156	513,529	97.590
300	151	Other sign, symptom, or incomplete diagnosis (Category 5)	70 +	84 =	154	513,683	97.620
301	22	Scabies	75 +	76 =	151	513,834	97.648
302	620	Abnormal sugar	67 +	84 =	151	513,985	97.677
303	332	Cervical erosion	0 +	150 =	150	514,135	97.705
304	367	Abortion, induced	0 +	149 =	149	514,284	97.734
305	362	Other complications of pregnancy, delivery, and puerperium	0 +	147 =	147	514,431	97.762
306	32	Other sign, symptom, or incomplete diagnosis (Category 1)	78 +	65 =	143	514,574	97.789
307	131	Hysterical neurosis	27 +	116 =	143	514,717	97.816
308	137	Other and unspecified neurosis	50 +	93 =	143	514,860	97.843
309	417	Scoliosis, kyphoscoliosis	39 +	99 =	138	514,998	97.869
310	30	Pyrexia with rash (any site)	62 +	75 =	137	515,135	97.895
311	64	Skin (Category 2—malignant)	71 +	64 =	135	515,270	97.921
312	422	Synovitis	68 +	67 =	135	515,405	97.947
313	482	Internal injury of chest, abdomen, and pelvis	69 +	64 =	133	515,538	97.972
314	438	Other congenital malformation not included above (Category 14)	72 +	59 =	131	515,669	97.997
315	602	Abnormal urinalysis	73 +	58 =	131	515,800	98.022
316	138	Personality disorders and sexual deviation	42 +	86 =	128	515,928	98.046
317	171	Blepharitis	65 +	63 =	128	516,056	98.070
318	205	Tinnitus	72 +	56 =	128	516,184	98.095
319	258	Bronchiolitis	60 +	67 =	127	516,311	98.119
320	319	Hydrocele	127 +	0 =	127	516,438	98.143
321	907	Cardiac glycosides (Category 22)	60 +	64 =	124	516,562	98.167
322	463	Senility	32 +	88 =	120	516,682	98.189
323	156	Multiple sclerosis	42 +	74 =	116	516,798	98.211
324	252	Pneumothorax, spontaneous	79 +	36 =	115	516,913	98.233
325	99	Electrolyte disturbance	28 +	86 =	114	517,027	98.255
326	270	Hoarseness	42 +	72 =	114	517,141	98.277
327	298	Hepatomegaly	53 +	60 =	113	517,254	98.298
328	122	Other sign, symptom, or incomplete diagnosis (Category 4)	44 +	68 =	112	517,366	98.319
329	640	Abnormal sigmoidoscopy	44 +	68 =	112	517,478	98.341
330	126	Affective psychoses	57 +	54 =	111	517,589	98.362

331	342	Dyspareunia	0 +	109 =	109	517,698	98.382
332	165	Facial nerve paralysis	34 +	74 =	108	517,806	98.403
333	261	Catarrh	33 +	72 =	105	517,911	98.423
334	66	Hodgkin's disease	75 +	29 =	104	518,015	98.443
335	542	Smallpox prophylaxis	50 +	53 =	103	518,118	98.462
336	373	Infantile eczema	37 +	62 =	99	518,217	98.481
337	453	Failure to thrive	57 +	40 =	97	518,314	98.499
338	587	Intrauterine device	0 +	97 =	97	518,411	98.518
339	906	Specific hypotensives (Category 22)	53 +	44 =	97	518,508	98.536
340	707	Pregnancy and birth out of wedlock (parent and child)	0 +	95 =	95	518,603	98.554
341	624	Abnormal liver function	56 +	38 =	94	518,697	98.572
342	903	Hypnotics (Category 22)	43 +	51 =	94	518,791	98.590
343	731	Adopted child	42 +	50 =	92	518,883	98.607
344	59	Cervix uteri (Category 2—malignant)	0 +	91 =	91	518,974	98.625
345	436	Congenital malformation of genitourinary system	76 +	14 =	90	519,064	98.642
346	630	Abnormal EKG	53 +	37 =	90	519,154	98.659
347	397	Pigmentation (Category 12)	29 +	60 =	89	519,243	98.676
348	416	Genu valgum or varum	52 +	37 =	89	519,332	98.693
349	479	Dislocation, shoulder	67 +	22 =	89	519,421	98.710
350	209	Cor pulmonale	51 +	37 =	88	519,509	98.726
351	426	Frozen shoulder	33 +	55 =	88	519,597	98.743
352	472	Fracture of pelvis	46 +	42 =	88	519,685	98.760
353	102	Glycosuria	49 +	38 =	87	519,772	98.776
354	558	Cholera prophylaxis	41 +	45 =	86	519,858	98.793
355	176	Refractive errors	43 +	42 =	85	519,943	98.809
356	413	Flat foot	49 +	36 =	85	520,028	98.825
357	429	Anencephaly, microcephaly, or monstrosity	30 +	55 =	85	520,113	98.841
358	703	Educational problems	49 +	36 =	85	520,198	98.857
359	10	Poliomyelitis (acute and sequelae)	20 +	63 =	83	520,281	98.873
360	450	Sleep disturbance	46 +	37 =	83	520,364	98.889
361	712	Other high-risk individual (Category 20)	41 +	42 =	83	520,447	98.905
362	296	Hematemesis	23 +	56 =	79	520,526	98.920
363	404	Cervical spondylosis	55 +	24 =	79	520,605	98.935
364	198	Tremor	37 +	41 =	78	520,683	98.949
365	6	Scarlet fever	31 +	45 =	76	520,759	98.964
366	307	Wind	37 +	39 =	76	520,835	98.978
367	578	Sterilization, male and female	24 +	52 =	76	520,911	98.993
368	324	Uterovaginal prolapse	0 +	73 =	73	520,984	99.007
369	727	Alcoholism in parent or child	51 +	21 =	72	521,056	99.020
370	220	Raynaud's disease	23 +	48 =	71	521,127	99.034

PART I. Continued

		DIAGNOSIS		FREQUENCY			CUMULATIVE	
Rank	RCGP Number	Description	Male	Female	Total	Total	Percent
371	264	Hemoptysis	42 +	29 =	71	521,198	99.047
372	346	Toxemias of pregnancy	0 +	71 =	71	521,269	99.061
373	395	Erythema	20 +	51 =	71	521,340	99.074
374	452	Feeding problems	47 +	23 =	70	521,410	99.087
375	132	Phobic neurosis	14 +	55 =	69	521,479	99.101
376	433	Congenital malformation of circulatory system	26 +	43 =	69	521,548	99.114
377	563	Other chronic adult situational reaction	39 +	30 =	69	521,617	99.127
378	12	Rubella	28 +	39 =	67	521,684	99.140
379	366	Other signs, symptoms, or complications of pregnancy	0 +	66 =	66	521,750	99.152
380	260	Pleural effusion	28 +	37 =	65	521,815	99.164
381	11	Measles	30 +	34 =	64	521,879	99.177
382	166	Trigeminal neuralgia	20 +	44 =	64	521,943	99.189
383	706	Other high-risk family situations (Category 20)	18 +	46 =	64	522,007	99.201
384	462	Uremia (raised BUN)	28 +	35 =	63	522,070	99.213
385	451	Other causes of perinatal morbidity	20 +	42 =	62	522,132	99.225
386	55	Pancreas (Category 2—malignant)	49 +	10 =	59	522,191	99.236
387	62	Bladder and other urinary organs (Category 2—malignant)	31 +	28 =	59	522,250	99.247
388	291	Splenomegaly	37 +	22 =	59	522,309	99.258
389	330	Disorders of menarche	0 +	59 =	59	522,368	99.269
390	470	Fracture of skull	35 +	24 =	59	522,427	99.281
391	124	Paranoid states	22 +	36 =	58	522,485	99.292
392	705	Legal problems	13 +	45 =	58	522,543	99.303
393	142	Delusions and hallucinations	32 +	25 =	57	522,600	99.313
394	403	Congenital talipes	16 +	41 =	57	522,657	99.324
395	97	Cushing's syndrome	20 +	36 =	56	522,713	99.335
396	178	Strabismus	39 +	16 =	55	522,768	99.345
397	561	Chronic adult marital situational reaction	12 +	43 =	55	522,823	99.356
398	601	Abnormal urinoscopy	21 +	34 =	55	522,878	99.366
399	54	Rectum (Category 2—malignant)	26 +	27 =	53	522,931	99.376
400	29	Aseptic meningitis due to enterovirus	24 +	27 =	51	522,982	99.386
401	92	Hypovitaminosis	9 +	42 =	51	523,033	99.396
402	254	Bronchiectasis	7 +	43 =	50	523,083	99.405
403	143	Hyperkinesis	36 +	13 =	49	523,132	99.415
404	556	Typhoid, paratyphoid prophylaxis	26 +	23 =	49	523,181	99.424

405	566	Acute adolescent situational reaction	8 +	41 =	49	523,230	99.433
406	610	Abnormal hematocrit	21 +	27 =	48	523,278	99.442
407	300	Ascites (Category 9)	22 +	25 =	47	523,325	99.451
408	216	Left ventricular failure (acute)	10 +	36 =	46	523,371	99.460
409	414	Hallux valgus or varus	30 +	16 =	46	523,417	99.469
410	611	Abnormal blood count	22 +	24 =	46	523,463	99.477
411	199	Ataxia	30 +	15 =	45	523,508	99.486
412	410	Torn meniscus of knee	28 +	17 =	45	523,553	99.494
413	236	Ascites (Category 7)	29 +	15 =	44	523,597	99.503
414	173	Iritis	24 +	19 =	43	523,640	99.511
415	808	Drug reaction	14 +	29 =	43	523,683	99.519
416	51	Esophagus (Category 2—malignant)	22 +	20 =	42	523,725	99.527
417	560	Acute adult marital situational reaction	4 +	38 =	42	523,767	99.535
418	702	Medical care problems	18 +	24 =	42	523,809	99.543
419	185	Mastoiditis	11 +	30 =	41	523,850	99.551
420	186	Meniere's disease	6 +	35 =	41	523,891	99.559
421	803	Bleeding disorder (Category 21)	16 +	25 =	41	523,932	99.566
422	50	Buccal cavity and pharynx, including lip (Category 2—malignant)	17 +	23 =	40	523,972	99.574
423	461	Hematuria (Category 16)	18 +	22 =	40	524,012	99.582
424	144	Mental disorders, not psychotic, associated with physical condition	20 +	19 =	39	524,051	99.589
425	333	Ovulation pain	0 +	39 =	39	524,090	99.596
426	26	Other helminth infection	19 +	19 =	38	524,128	99.604
427	65	Brain (Category 2—malignant)	17 +	21 =	38	524,166	99.611
428	439	Other sign, symptom, or incomplete diagnosis (Category 14)	21 +	16 =	37	524,203	99.618
429	604	Abnormal urine test	7 +	30 =	37	524,240	99.625
430	700	Economic problems	13 +	23 =	36	524,276	99.632
431	7	Erysipelas	11 +	24 =	35	524,311	99.638
432	228	Other venous embolism and thrombosis	13 +	22 =	35	524,346	99.645
433	491	Effects of aspirin poisoning	13 +	22 =	35	524,381	99.652
434	717	Other employment problems (Category 20)	18 +	16 =	34	524,415	99.658
435	816	Kidney disease (Category 21)	18 +	15 =	33	524,448	99.664
436	455	Malingering	12 +	20 =	32	524,480	99.670
437	297	Hiccough	25 +	6 =	31	524,511	99.676
438	440	Birth injury due to difficult labor	16 +	15 =	31	524,542	99.682
439	81	Pleural effusion	12 +	18 =	30	524,572	99.688
440	222	Chilblains	14 +	16 =	30	524,602	99.694
441	418	Osteoporosis	9 +	21 =	30	524,632	99.699
442	562	Other acute adult situational reaction (Category 5)	5 +	25 =	30	524,662	99.705
443	253	Pneumoconiosis	25 +	4 =	29	524,691	99.711
444	708	Social isolation	11 +	17 =	28	524,719	99.716

Rank	RCGP Number	Description	Male	Female	Total	Total	Percent
				FREQUENCY		CUMULATIVE	
445	713	Out of work, acute	13 +	15 =	28	524,747	99.721
446	728	Drug abuse in parent or child	18 +	10 =	28	524,775	99.726
447	195	Coma and stupor	10 +	17 =	27	524,802	99.732
448	201	Meningismus	12 +	15 =	27	524,829	99.737
449	621	Abnormal urea (BUN)	15 +	12 =	27	524,856	99.742
450	634	Other abnormal x-ray (Category 19)	10 +	17 =	27	524,883	99.747
451	19	Bornholm disease	9 +	17 =	26	524,909	99.752
452	824	Tuberculosis	12 +	14 =	26	524,935	99.757
453	341	Polyuria	16 +	9 =	25	524,960	99.762
454	196	Delirium	19 +	5 =	24	524,984	99.766
455	204	Photophobia	8 +	16 =	24	525,008	99.771
456	52	Stomach (Category 2—malignant)	12 +	11 =	23	525,031	99.775
457	203	Nystagmus	7 +	16 =	23	525,054	99.779
458	567	Chronic adolescent situational reaction	6 +	17 =	23	525,077	99.784
459	804	Blindness (Category 21)	12 +	11 =	23	525,100	99.788
460	167	Brachial neuritis (Category 6)	11 +	11 =	22	525,122	99.792
461	348	Ectopic pregnancy	0 +	22 =	22	525,144	99.796
462	353	Placenta previa	0 +	22 =	22	525,166	99.801
463	812	Heart disease (Category 21)	12 +	10 =	22	525,188	99.805
464	419	Brachial neuritis (Category 13)	5 +	16 =	21	525,209	99.809
465	489	Effects of carbon monoxide poisoning	13 +	8 =	21	525,230	99.813
466	202	Diplopia	11 +	9 =	20	525,250	99.817
467	432	Congenital hydrocephalus	12 +	8 =	20	525,270	99.820
468	478	Dislocation, jaw	12 +	8 =	20	525,290	99.824
469	722	Other social problems, family and individual	3 +	17 =	20	525,310	99.828
470	145	Frigidity	0 +	19 =	19	525,329	99.832
471	106	Erythema multiforme	7 +	11 =	18	525,347	99.835
472	434	Cleft palate and harelip	6 +	12 =	18	525,365	99.838
473	435	Congenital malformation of digestive system	7 +	11 =	18	525,383	99.842
474	550	Dependent (including pseudo dependent symbiotic and maternal maturing)	6 +	12 =	18	525,401	99.845
475	823	Thyroid disease (Category 21)	7 +	11 =	18	525,419	99.849
476	56	Larynx (Category 2—malignant)	10 +	7 =	17	525,436	99.852
477	441	Atelectasis, other asphyxia of newborn	9 +	8 =	17	525,453	99.855

			+	=			
478	622	Abnormal electrolytes	5	12	17	525,470	99.858
479	120	Purpura, secondary or unspecified	6	10	16	525,486	99.861
480	347	Ante partum hemorrhage	0	16	16	525,502	99.864
481	364	Caesarean section (all indications)	0	16	16	525,518	99.867
482	709	Occupational maladjustment	10	6	16	525,534	99.870
483	802	Asthma	7	9	16	525,550	99.874
484	820	Neurological disorders (Category 21)	8	8	16	525,566	99.877
485	825	Other familial, genetic, or otherwise significant disease (Category 21)	4	12	16	525,582	99.880
486	9	Meningococcal infections	9	6	15	525,597	99.882
487	37	Malaria	5	10	15	525,612	99.885
488	175	Lacrimal apparatus	7	8	15	525,627	99.888
489	188	Otosclerosis	2	13	15	525,642	99.891
490	305	Appendicular pain	7	8	15	525,657	99.894
491	459	Rigors	6	9	15	525,672	99.897
492	553	Passive aggressive	8	7	15	525,687	99.899
493	557	Yellow fever prophylaxis	9	6	15	525,702	99.902
494	701	Housing problems	3	12	15	525,717	99.905
495	721	Divorce proceedings	3	12	15	525,732	99.908
496	100	Exophthalmos	3	11	14	525,746	99.911
497	104	Polyuria	10	4	14	525,760	99.913
498	402	Congenital dislocated hip	6	8	14	525,774	99.916
499	445	Umbilical sepsis	13	1	14	525,788	99.921
500	449	Immaturity, dysmaturity	6	8	14	525,802	99.921
501	490	Effects of barbiturate poisoning	9	5	14	525,816	99.924
502	98	Coeliac disease	4	9	13	525,829	99.926
503	60	Corpus uteri (Category 2—malignant)	0	12	12	525,841	99.929
504	724	High-risk pregnancy	0	12	12	525,853	99.931
505	726	High-risk physical violence	3	9	12	525,865	99.933
506	268	Sputum, noninfected	7	4	11	525,876	99.935
507	361	Puerperal mastitis	0	11	11	525,887	99.937
508	357	Prolonged labor	0	10	10	525,897	99.939
509	623	Abnormal PBI	3	7	10	525,907	99.941
510	711	Chronic physical disability	6	4	10	525,917	99.943
511	729	Other social/personal problem	9	1	10	525,927	99.945
512	809	Epilepsy (Category 21)	3	7	10	525,937	99.947
513	811	Hay fever (Category 21)	2	8	10	525,947	99.949
514	8	Whooping cough	8	1	9	525,956	99.950
515	492	Motion sickness	4	5	9	525,965	99.952
516	821	Rheumatic fever (Category 21)	3	6	9	525,974	99.954
517	266	Stridor	5	3	8	525,982	99.955

PART I. Continued

Rank	RCGP Number	Description	FREQUENCY			CUMULATIVE	
			Male	Female	Total	Total	Percent
518	363	Postpartum hemorrhage	0 +	8 =	8	525,990	99.957
519	430	Spina bifida and meningocele with hydrocephalus	5 +	3 =	8	525,998	99.958
520	552	Angry aggressive	1 +	7 =	8	526,006	99.960
521	564	Acute childhood situational reaction	3 +	5 =	8	526,014	99.961
522	632	Abnormal GI series	5 +	3 =	8	526,022	99.963
523	710	Dependency	4 +	4 =	8	526,030	99.964
524	63	Other genital organs (Category 2—malignant)	4 +	3 =	7	526,037	99.966
525	262	Cyanosis (Category 7)	3 +	4 =	7	526,044	99.967
526	356	Malposition and/or disproportion affecting second stage labor	0 +	7 =	7	526,051	99.968
527	826	Atopy (Category 21)	3 +	4 =	7	526,058	99.970
528	80	Ascites (Category 2)	1 +	5 =	6	526,064	99.971
529	103	Pigmentation (Category 3)	2 +	4 =	6	526,070	99.972
530	154	Stammer and/or stutter	4 +	2 =	6	526,076	99.973
531	232	Cyanosis (Category 8)	3 +	3 =	6	526,082	99.974
532	497	Dislocation of radial head	5 +	1 =	6	526,088	99.975
533	551	Masochistic	1 +	5 =	6	526,094	99.977
534	732	Foster child	5 +	1 =	6	526,100	99.978
535	41	Hydatidosis	1 +	4 =	5	526,105	99.979
536	355	Forceps delivery (all indications)	0 +	5 =	5	526,110	99.980
537	358	Laceration or episiotomy	0 +	5 =	5	526,115	99.980
538	714	Out of work, chronic	1 +	4 =	5	526,120	99.981
539	810	Gout (Category 21)	5 +	0 =	5	526,125	99.982
540	815	Jaundice (Category 21)	4 +	1 =	5	526,130	99.983
541	365	Pyrexia of childbirth and puerperium	0 +	4 =	4	526,134	99.984
542	431	Spina bifida and meningocele without hydrocephalus	1 +	3 =	4	526,138	99.985
543	643	Abnormal lumbar puncture	3 +	1 =	4	526,142	99.986
544	716	Unemployable because of illness	3 +	1 =	4	526,146	99.986
545	42	Filarial infection	2 +	1 =	3	526,149	99.987
546	269	Sputum, infected	2 +	1 =	3	526,152	99.987
547	354	Retained placenta	0 +	3 =	3	526,155	99.988
548	360	Puerperal thrombophlebitis	0 +	3 =	3	526,158	99.989
549	718	Imprisonment	3 +	0 =	3	526,161	99.989
550	725	High-risk accident	0 +	3 =	3	526,164	99.990
551	806	Deafness (Category 21)	1 +	2 =	3	526,167	99.990

552	818	Mental illness (Category 21)	0 +	3 =	3	526,170	99.991
553	35	Amoebiasis	0 +	2 =	2	526,172	99.991
554	36	Yaws	1 +	1 =	2	526,174	99.992
555	43	Ancylostomiasis	0 +	2 =	2	526,176	99.992
556	443	Birth injury to brain, spinal cord, bone, or nerve	0 +	2 =	2	526,178	99.992
557	565	Chronic childhood situational reaction	0 +	2 =	2	526,180	99.993
558	603	Abnormal urine culture	1 +	1 =	2	526,182	99.993
559	642	Abnormal cystoscopy	1 +	1 =	2	526,184	99.993
560	719	Prosecution or impending litigation	1 +	1 =	2	526,186	99.994
561	814	Infection, recurrent (Category 21)	2 +	0 =	2	526,188	99.994
562	819	Mental retardation (Category 21)	1 +	1 =	2	526,190	99.994
563	822	Stroke (Category 21)	1 +	1 =	2	526,192	99.995
564	39	Trypanosomiasis	0 +	1 =	1	526,193	99.995
565	40	Schistosomiasis	1 +	0 =	1	526,194	99.995
566	448	Hemorrhagic disease	0 +	1 =	1	526,195	99.995
567	715	Medical absenteeism	1 +	0 =	1	526,196	99.996

PART II. DIAGNOSES BY DISEASE CATEGORY AND AGE/SEX DISTRIBUTION

Diagnosis Category 1—Communicable Diseases

DIAGNOSES (DESCRIPTION AND RCGP NUMBER)	0 – 4 M	0 – 4 F	5 – 9 M	5 – 9 F	10 – 14 M	10 – 14 F	15 – 24 M	15 – 24 F	25 – 34 M	25 – 34 F	35 – 44 M	35 – 44 F	45 – 54 M	45 – 54 F	55 – 64 M	55 – 64 F	65+ M	65+ F	Total M	Total F
28—Other recognized disease not included above (Category 1)	227	215	75	65	39	46	133	393	60	291	62	211	29	138	27	91	41	92	693	1,542
25—Viral warts (infectious)	16	34	77	79	191	144	296	401	152	164	91	72	75	94	26	59	18	24	942	1,071
5—Diarrhea and/or vomiting intestinal infectious disease	231	180	56	43	51	42	98	183	109	186	51	92	47	69	61	56	74	131	778	982
4—Gonorrhea	2	3	3	0	6	8	419	347	246	102	35	28	10	1	9	7	10	13	740	509
31—Pyrexia of unknown origin	168	154	77	69	43	28	47	61	41	37	21	11	17	10	20	12	76	98	510	480
23—Epidemic winter vomiting (viral gastroenteritis)	136	120	58	47	40	31	64	85	53	64	23	45	29	46	17	37	21	70	441	545
27—Other virus infection	89	111	61	43	38	38	71	118	51	107	25	32	22	31	13	31	10	26	380	537
2—Tuberculosis (other forms)	18	17	49	15	18	22	42	45	50	61	77	64	122	49	70	70	71	41	517	384
21—Dermatophytosis	33	22	26	21	37	28	150	86	79	42	46	33	57	38	39	19	24	36	491	325
14—Herpes zoster	8	0	4	7	8	5	47	29	21	16	14	35	11	41	38	66	56	146	207	345
17—Infectious mononucleosis	4	4	25	19	32	54	165	208	17	14	1	1	0	3	1	1	0	2	245	306
13—Chicken pox	76	61	100	63	29	35	3	18	2	4	1	3	2	1	0	0	2	3	215	190
20—Oxyuriasis	68	91	55	80	21	32	6	12	7	15	4	4	1	1	0	0	2	0	164	235
16—Infective hepatitis	1	4	1	0	2	1	104	74	52	25	49	10	14	23	9	11	7	8	239	154
3—Syphilis (infectious and sequelae)	0	4	0	0	0	2	57	27	28	17	14	8	11	16	13	21	38	41	161	136
15—Mumps	17	21	86	46	35	30	9	16	6	6	5	4	2	2	0	2	0	1	161	131
1—Tuberculosis (respiratory system including late effects)	6	6	2	2	5	1	3	11	5	6	4	19	21	20	26	8	18	55	90	128
44—Pediculosis	2	5	4	4	5	11	40	34	18	23	7	1	1	0	1	2	3	4	81	84
22—Scabies	5	14	3	4	8	10	34	27	13	4	5	7	6	6	1	1	0	3	75	76
32—Other sign, symptom, or incomplete diagnosis (Category 1)	1	7	1	3	5	3	41	33	19	11	4	2	3	3	2	3	2	0	78	65
30—Pyrexia with rash (any site)	30	26	13	13	7	4	5	6	2	14	4	4	1	6	0	0	0	2	62	75
10—Poliomyelitis (acute and sequelae)	0	12	0	0	0	5	0	16	4	6	4	6	0	10	7	1	1	7	20	63
6—Scarlet fever	6	12	11	13	3	5	6	6	2	9	1	0	0	0	2	0	0	0	31	45
12—Rubella	13	11	3	3	6	3	1	12	2	5	1	0	0	5	1	0	0	0	28	39
11—Measles	19	17	5	4	1	1	1	3	2	0	0	0	2	5	0	0	0	3	30	34
29—Aseptic meningitis due to enterovirus	2	3	3	3	1	1	5	9	9	8	1	1	2	0	0	2	1	0	24	27
26—Other helminth infection	5	10	1	2	4	4	5	1	2	0	0	0	0	0	1	1	1	1	19	19
7—Erysipelas	1	0	3	3	1	0	1	6	4	2	0	2	0	0	0	2	1	5	11	24
19—Bornholm disease	0	1	0	0	0	0	3	6	0	1	4	0	1	1	0	0	0	4	9	17
9—Meningococcal infections	0	0	1	1	0	0	1	2	0	1	0	0	1	1	0	0	0	0	5	6
37—Malaria	0	0	0	0	2	0	1	0	1	2	0	0	1	1	0	3	0	0	5	10
8—Whooping cough	8	1	0	0	0	0	0	0	0	0	0	0	0	0	0	0	0	0	8	1
41—Hydatidosis	1	0	0	0	1	0	0	1	0	0	0	0	0	1	0	0	0	0	1	4
42—Filarial infection	0	0	0	0	1	0	0	0	0	1	0	0	1	0	0	0	0	0	2	1
35—Amoebiasis	0	1	0	0	0	0	0	1	0	0	0	0	0	0	0	0	0	0	0	2

Diagnosis Category 1 (continued)

	22	34	17	13	17	22	73	112	71	139	63	106	98	143	67	125	86	122	514	816
36—Yaws	0	0	0	0	0	0	0	0	0	0	0	0	0	0	0	0	0	0	1	1
43—Ancylostomiasis	0	0	0	1	0	0	0	0	0	0	0	1	0	0	0	0	0	0	0	2
39—Trypanosomiasis	0	0	0	0	0	0	0	0	0	0	0	0	0	0	0	0	0	0	0	1
40—Schistosomiasis	0	0	0	0	0	0	1	0	0	0	0	0	0	0	0	0	0	0	1	0
38—Leishmaniasis	0	0	0	0	0	0	0	0	0	0	0	0	0	0	0	0	0	0	0	0

Diagnosis Category 2—Neoplasms, Including Reticuloses

	22	34	17	13	17	22	73	112	71	139	63	106	98	143	67	125	86	122	514	816
74—All other benign neoplasms (Category 2)	0	3	0	5	9	15	14	159	11	120	16	162	4	101	11	64	4	61	69	690
70—Breast (Category 2—benign)	5	3	9	5	10	27	42	57	66	90	33	67	43	72	36	39	28	60	272	420
73—Skin (Category 2—benign)	2	1	2	0	0	9	26	0	17	0	0	0	0	3	53	167	97	74	181	258
67—Leukemia, all types	1	2	6	0	18	5	40	18	0	1	11	6	13	41	30	40	61	109	197	235
68—All other malignant neoplasms	0	0	0	0	0	0	3	0	0	0	2	1	30	74	74	39	83	72	192	186
57—Bronchus, Lung, and trachea (Category 2—malignant)	0	0	0	0	0	0	0	0	0	0	0	14	0	0	0	0	0	0	3	316
58—Breast (Category 2—malignant)	4	0	0	0	0	0	0	3	0	7	0	14	0	76	1	59	2	157	64	177
82—Other sign, symptom, or incomplete diagnosis (Category 2)	0	2	2	4	6	7	10	27	3	35	13	32	9	23	7	24	10	23	0	183
72—Other female genitourinary organs (Category 2—benign)	0	4	0	0	0	2	0	53	0	35	0	36	0	29	0	10	0	14	0	169
71—Uterus (Category 2—benign)	0	0	0	0	0	0	0	5	0	34	0	52	0	59	6	11	0	8	35	133
53—Colon (Category 2—malignant)	0	0	0	0	0	1	0	5	2	3	1	9	3	10	0	30	23	75	164	0
61—Prostate (Category 2—malignant)	1	0	0	0	0	0	0	1	0	0	0	0	0	0	18	7	145	0	71	64
64—Skin (Category 2—malignant)	0	0	0	0	0	0	30	1	1	0	12	4	14	7	14	7	29	45	75	29
66—Hodgkin's disease	0	0	0	0	5	0	0	15	21	0	0	6	1	6	15	1	3	1	0	91
59—Cervix uteri (Category 2—malignant)	0	0	0	0	0	0	1	1	0	6	0	15	0	35	0	12	22	22	49	10
55—Pancreas (Category 2—malignant)	0	0	0	0	0	0	0	0	0	2	0	1	0	1	10	3	38	3	10	28
62—Bladder and other urinary organs (Category 2—malignant)	0	0	0	0	0	0	1	1	2	0	3	4	5	8	11	8	9	7	31	27
54—Rectum (Category 2—malignant)	0	0	0	0	0	0	0	0	0	1	1	1	2	6	4	4	19	15	26	20
51—Esophagus (Category 2—malignant)	0	0	0	0	0	0	0	0	0	3	0	19	1	19	13	1	8	8	22	23
50—Buccal cavity and pharynx including lip (Category 2—malignant)	0	0	0	0	0	0	0	0	0	0	0	3	1	3	14	7	2	13	17	21
65—Brain (Category 2—malignant)	1	0	1	0	0	0	0	0	0	1	0	2	0	1	7	1	7	16	17	18
81—Pleural effusion	0	0	0	1	0	0	0	1	1	1	1	0	0	3	7	13	3	1	12	11
52—Stomach (Category 2—malignant)	0	0	0	0	0	0	0	0	1	0	0	0	0	0	2	2	8	8	12	7
56—Larynx (Category 2—malignant)	0	0	0	0	0	0	0	0	0	1	1	1	4	1	1	0	4	4	10	12
60—Corpus uteri (Category 2—malignant)	0	0	0	0	0	0	0	1	0	0	1	1	0	2	0	3	4	0	0	3
63—Other genital organs (Category 2—malignant)	0	0	0	0	0	0	1	0	1	1	0	0	0	2	0	0	3	2	4	5
80—Ascites	0	0	0	0	0	0	0	0	0	0	0	0	0	3	1	2	0	0	1	5

PART II. Continued

Diagnosis Category 3—Allergic, Endocrine, Metabolic, and Nutritional Disorders

AGE GROUPS

DIAGNOSES (DESCRIPTION AND RCGP NUMBER)	0 – 4		5 – 9		10 – 14		15 – 24		25 – 34		35 – 44		45 – 54		55 – 64		65 +		Total	
	M	F	M	F	M	F	M	F	M	F	M	F	M	F	M	F	M	F	M	F
91—Diabetes mellitus	11	14	6	24	18	46	107	239	252	414	349	619	903	1,734	950	2,440	1,216	3,093	3,812	8,623
101—Obesity	45	41	31	72	77	183	213	1,167	406	1,651	370	1,626	412	1,927	229	1,423	145	661	1,928	8,751
86—Asthma	179	88	253	89	148	154	296	275	215	231	55	307	185	375	152	313	119	168	1,367	2,021
95—Specific allergies	109	111	121	101	196	105	143	275	200	330	55	176	86	234	52	98	30	110	992	1,540
93—Gout	0	0	0	0	0	0	11	3	31	11	111	25	197	69	203	106	172	120	728	334
88—Hyperthyroidism	1	0	0	5	1	12	10	100	11	125	7	133	12	109	15	99	41	158	98	741
87—Allergic dermatosis, urticaria	55	25	35	44	53	38	61	94	36	82	19	53	34	61	21	53	12	61	326	511
89—Hypothyroidism	1	4	1	2	1	7	5	37	13	79	18	77	27	171	17	138	26	106	109	621
94—Other recognized disease not included above (Category 3)	29	21	8	8	9	11	12	59	40	57	21	42	50	80	32	53	34	87	235	418
85—Hay fever	10	7	21	10	29	26	52	46	34	38	16	39	19	36	6	14	6	14	193	231
105—Other sign, symptom, or incomplete diagnosis (Category 3)	4	6	10	8	12	12	18	34	14	28	11	29	15	24	18	21	14	36	116	198
90—Other thyroid disease	1	0	0	0	1	0	4	22	5	33	7	36	9	55	3	44	7	19	37	212
96—Addison's disease, serum lipid abnormalities	0	0	0	0	1	0	1	0	18	4	27	10	41	9	9	9	14	25	111	57
99—Electrolyte disturbance	1	0	1	0	0	0	7	0	1	4	5	10	5	16	1	19	8	37	28	86
102—Glycosuria	1	0	2	1	2	0	4	9	3	3	7	0	8	7	10	8	12	10	49	38
97—Cushing's syndrome	0	0	0	0	0	0	2	0	3	5	1	3	6	8	1	16	7	4	20	36
92—Hypovitaminosis	1	0	0	0	0	3	4	6	0	5	0	3	2	11	0	3	2	8	9	42
106—Erythema multiforme	0	2	0	0	0	3	2	2	1	2	1	1	2	1	0	0	1	0	7	11
100—Exophthalmos	0	0	0	0	0	0	2	2	1	1	0	5	0	1	0	1	0	1	3	11
104—Polyuria	0	0	0	0	0	0	0	2	6	0	2	1	0	0	0	0	0	1	10	4
98—Coeliac disease	0	0	0	0	0	0	0	1	2	8	1	0	0	0	0	0	0	0	4	9
103—Pigmentation	1	0	0	0	0	0	0	1	0	0	1	3	0	0	0	0	0	0	2	4

Diagnosis Category 4—Diseases of Blood and Blood-Forming Organs

DIAGNOSES	0 – 4		5 – 9		10 – 14		15 – 24		25 – 34		35 – 44		45 – 54		55 – 64		65 +		Total	
	M	F	M	F	M	F	M	F	M	F	M	F	M	F	M	F	M	F	M	F
111—Iron-deficiency (hypochromic) anemia (male and female)	446	328	95	111	138	138	14	352	21	216	77	264	41	258	70	226	268	451	1,156	2,293
112—Other specific anemias (male and female)	95	111	45	50	24	26	48	91	6	116	41	126	23	79	46	77	66	266	394	942
110—Pernicious (megaloblastic) anemia (male and female)	8	3	1	8	0	1	4	6	12	1	3	22	14	5	64	168	132	204	238	411
114—Other recognized disease not included above	14	11	13	8	9	1	27	33	18	18	10	13	30	16	27	60	22	48	170	208
113—Hemorrhagic conditions (male and female)	6	1	35	1	2	3	4	2	3	8	6	10	20	2	2	37	10	14	88	78

Diagnosis																		
122—Other sign, symptom, or incomplete diagnosis (Category 4)	2	2	5	5	5	10	5	5	7	24	10	6	9	4	6	23	44	68
120—Purpura, secondary or unspecified	1	0	0	1	0	0	1	0	2	0	0	1	2	0	2	2	6	10

Diagnosis Category 5—Mental Illness, Personality Disorders, and Psychoneurosis

Diagnosis																		
134—Depressive neurosis	3	11	5	2	7	24	153	687	212	1,191	260	1,196	308	1,268	274	998	1,486	6,347
130—Anxiety neurosis	12	16	7	21	50	46	238	652	286	967	302	947	322	927	274	692	1,691	4,954
135—Physical disorders of presumably psychogenic origin	5	9	21	19	25	35	136	391	237	680	195	641	218	553	101	310	996	2,927
147—Tension headache	4	4	8	3	18	17	52	266	66	300	63	264	49	181	26	61	294	1,173
141—Abuse of alcohol	3	1	4	0	3	1	34	10	120	42	231	108	283	141	186	25	944	389
125—Schizophrenia			0	0	0	1	23	13	59	77	42	65	56	231	87	94	341	563
128—Organic psychoses	3	0	0	1	1	3	14	13	3	12	9	4	27	31	21	272	223	348
150—Other special sign or symptom not coded elsewhere (Category 5)	51	38	68	33	55	15	25	56	7	27	11	24	11	19	8	42	253	296
133—Obsessive-compulsive neurosis	0	0	2	2	1	1	19	33	11	41	14	70	18	28	5	30	80	225
146—Insomnia	7	3	5	2	5	41	15	15	21	21	13	19	20	28	18	37	148	146
148—Enuresis	19	29	67	44	32	3	16	8	2	3	1	7	1	0	13	7	158	135
136—Neurasthenia	1	0	1	4	1	0	13	48	3	35	28	45	15	34	8	13	77	206
127—Senile and presenile dementia	0	0	0	0	0	0	1	2	0	2	0	3	1	10	3	179	71	205
140—Mental retardation	20	6	14	10	18	12	33	29	19	25	11	21	8	14	10	9	138	138
152—Impotence	0	0	0	0	1	1	17	19	30	0	54	0	85	0	49	0	265	0
129—Other and unspecified psychoses	1	5	4	0	1	1	7	8	13	26	12	22	19	34	23	26	101	148
139—Drug abuse	0	0	0	0	0	2	10	7	13	14	25	17	34	30	39	6	143	101
123—Excessive smoking	0	0	0	0	0	0	34	33	38	28	25	21	16	26	11	1	129	112
149—Cardiac arrhythmia	0	0	1	1	1	0	2	0	12	1	12	10	17	20	23	33	99	75
151—Other sign, symptom, or incomplete diagnosis	6	3	6	1	5	1	19	10	6	14	6	17	7	17	10	11	70	84
131—Hysterical neurosis	0	0	0	0	0	0	7	22	6	36	7	39	2	11	3	2	27	116
137—Other and unspecified neurosis	2	1	0	0	2	0	10	25	6	16	5	13	9	16	9	10	50	93
138—Personality disorders and sexual deviation	3	5	0	10	0	3	20	27	4	12	8	14	5	9	1	3	42	86
126—Affective psychoses	2	1	16	0	3	0	11	5	1	3	4	6	3	11	2	19	57	54
132—Phobic neurosis	1	0	2	1	1	23	1	8	2	8	2	3	4	4	1	5	14	55
563—Other chronic adult situational reaction	2	2	15	4	10	3	4	3	2	7	0	1	0	0	0	9	39	30
124—Paranoid states	0	0	0	0	0	0	1	4	3	5	5	7	3	6	6	9	22	36
142—Delusions and hallucinations	0	0	1	0	1	13	13	3	3	3	5	3	1	0	3	14	32	25
561—Chronic adult marital situational reaction	0	0	0	0	0	1	1	4	4	8	1	21	5	7	1	1	12	43
143—Hyperkinesis	1	2	19	0	8	3	3	0	2	1	1	7	0	1	0	1	36	13
566—Acute adolescent situational reaction	0	0	0	1	5	12	0	26	0	0	0	0	0	1	0	0	8	41
560—Acute adult marital situational reaction	0	0	0	0	0	0	0	9	1	14	0	10	2	3	0	0	4	38
144—Mental disorders not psychotic associated with physical condition	1	0	0	2	1	0	6	0	1	4	2	4	2	3	4	7	20	19

PART II. Continued

Diagnosis Category 5—Continued

DIAGNOSES (DESCRIPTION AND RCGP NUMBER)	0 - 4		5 - 9		10 - 14		15 - 24		25 - 34		35 - 44		45 - 54		55 - 64		65 +		Total	
	M	F	M	F	M	F	M	F	M	F	M	F	M	F	M	F	M	F	M	F
562—Other acute adult situational reaction	0	0	0	0	0	0	0	4	1	9	1	7	2	2	1	0	0	3	5	25
567—Chronic adolescent situational reaction	0	0	0	2	0	1	4	12	0	2	2	0	0	0	0	0	0	0	6	17
145—Frigidity	0	0	0	0	0	0	0	3	0	7	0	3	0	5	0	0	0	1	0	19
550—Dependent (including pseudo-dependent symbiotic and maternal maturing)	0	0	0	0	0	0	0	3	0	1	0	0	5	0	1	1	0	7	6	12
553—Passive aggressive	0	0	0	0	0	0	0	0	0	0	5	2	0	0	0	1	3	4	8	7
552—Angry aggressive	0	0	0	0	0	0	0	3	0	3	0	0	0	0	0	1	1	0	1	7
564—Acute childhood situational reaction	0	1	0	0	1	0	0	0	0	1	1	1	1	1	0	1	0	0	3	5
551—Masochistic	0	0	0	0	0	1	1	1	0	0	0	2	0	1	0	0	0	0	1	5
154—Stammer and/or stutter	0	0	0	0	2	1	0	0	0	0	0	0	1	1	0	0	1	0	4	2
565—Chronic childhood situational reaction	0	1	0	0	0	0	0	0	0	1	0	0	0	0	0	0	0	0	0	2
555—Narcissistic	0	0	0	0	0	0	0	0	0	0	0	0	0	0	0	0	0	0	0	0

Diagnosis Category 6—Diseases of Nervous System and Sense Organs

DIAGNOSES (DESCRIPTION AND RCGP NUMBER)	0 - 4		5 - 9		10 - 14		15 - 24		25 - 34		35 - 44		45 - 54		55 - 64		65 +		Total	
	M	F	M	F	M	F	M	F	M	F	M	F	M	F	M	F	M	F	M	F
183—Otitis media, acute	2,384	2,058	853	783	375	381	325	480	213	395	136	217	100	150	66	98	61	70	4,513	4,632
155—Vascular lesions	5	5	1	1	3	2	4	7	7	14	19	11	65	43	240	148	791	1,392	1,134	1,620
182—Otitis externa	99	86	111	113	187	194	221	292	125	197	81	104	79	148	81	84	42	60	1,026	1,278
170—Conjunctivitis and ophthalmia	220	183	125	82	83	90	130	162	95	143	81	91	68	117	57	96	79	125	938	1,089
200—Vertigo	5	5	5	2	8	23	72	134	85	148	68	137	106	206	113	202	167	360	629	1,216
190—Other diseases of ear and mastoid process	119	95	140	120	78	116	106	232	96	156	50	95	65	103	51	58	58	66	763	1,041
158—Epilepsy	39	36	27	32	18	57	86	101	86	80	112	88	110	91	58	96	47	58	583	639
187—Wax in ear	21	17	53	40	22	35	109	87	88	84	82	60	70	59	73	41	116	104	634	527
184—Otitis media, chronic	133	120	117	82	35	35	41	86	35	64	28	33	20	42	15	28	8	31	432	521
181—Other diseases of the eye	49	33	22	28	29	20	63	53	50	56	55	42	70	67	49	85	57	83	444	467
169—Other diseases of peripheral nerves or ganglia	3	2	4	3	4	10	33	43	36	72	61	54	80	149	77	95	60	82	358	510
159—Migraine	0	0	3	0	8	5	26	89	22	165	49	148	18	125	4	34	0	10	130	576
157—Parkinsonism	0	0	0	0	0	0	0	0	0	4	6	1	10	13	45	30	315	213	376	261
160—Other diseases of CNS	12	8	9	3	11	7	31	34	23	37	53	36	36	32	45	55	23	92	243	304
161—Labyrinthitis	1	1	1	3	0	3	10	24	12	41	26	46	21	61	36	38	24	61	131	278
207—Other sign, symptom, or incomplete diagnosis (Category 6)	1	4	2	4	1	3	14	23	21	26	7	27	44	24	32	32	46	59	168	202
177—Keratitis, with or without corneal ulcer	10	11	13	4	25	14	37	20	57	20	19	13	20	13	19	14	21	19	221	119

179—Cataract	1	2	2	1	1	0	0	1	3	1	3	7	4	6	27	12	33	72	129	103	202
168—Sciatica	0	0	0	0	0	0	2	8	6	11	19	7	25	27	50	22	17	12	20	90	129
180—Glaucoma	0	0	0	1	3	1	1	9	9	2	18	7	8	17	17	18	36	26	72	74	145
206—Paraesthesiae	1	1	0	3	1	0	3	5	5	18	12	12	29	16	38	24	13	17	20	89	126
172—Hordeolum or stye	11	6	6	4	8	18	20	19	9	2	15	8	16	8	14	7	7	5	5	86	103
197—Convulsions	14	14	4	4	4	5	4	2	8	5	14	22	4	22	3	21	7	2	22	122	67
189—Other forms of deafness	2	2	9	10	5	1	1	12	11	4	8	8	9	9	19	14	7	31	35	90	97
174—Other inflammatory diseases of the eye	8	6	6	1	9	3	19	16	15	11	10	15	9	11	6	9	9	5	9	84	81
171—Blepharitis	7	8	7	4	5	5	12	7	5	7	4	5	7	4	2	6	18	18	7	65	63
205—Tinnitus	0	1	0	0	0	6	4	8	6	25	2	9	10	10	8	18	17	72	56
156—Multiple sclerosis	0	0	0	1	0	3	6	19	37	19	7	7	8	6	3	42	74
165—Facial nerve paralysis	4	1	1	0	17	1	8	6	11	6	2	7	11	13	13	2	13	34	74
176—Refractive errors	0	7	2	6	7	9	5	0	4	10	7	5	5	4	7	4	4	5	43	42
198—Tremor	0	1	0	0	2	5	4	11	3	2	6	5	6	6	8	8	12	37	41
166—Trigeminal neuralgia	0	0	0	0	11	3	2	9	10	2	5	7	0	8	1	2	15	20	44
178—Strabismus	22	3	3	5	3	2	3	3	0	2	1	3	1	0	1	1	39	16
199—Ataxia	4	0	3	1	2	1	0	0	2	7	2	2	2	10	1	3	30	15
173—Iritis	2	0	0	1	1	0	4	4	4	4	3	4	8	2	0	4	24	19
185—Mastoiditis	0	1	1	2	3	4	14	3	4	0	4	8	6	1	0	11	30
186—Meniere's disease	0	4	0	2	0	0	0	0	10	0	2	2	2	3	4	10	6	35
195—Coma and stupor	0	0	1	2	1	1	1	1	1	0	0	4	1	3	1	5	7	10	17
201—Meningismus	4	4	0	2	0	0	2	2	4	1	1	0	0	3	1	2	2	12	15
196—Delirium	0	1	0	2	0	0	4	1	1	1	0	0	0	17	19	5
204—Photophobia	0	0	0	0	1	3	8	3	2	0	2	0	0	0	2	2	8	16
203—Nystagmus	2	2	0	0	0	1	5	1	1	0	5	0	3	1	2	1	7	16
167—Brachial neuritis	0	0	0	0	3	0	1	0	4	0	2	2	4	4	2	1	3	11	11
202—Diplopia	0	0	3	0	0	0	0	2	3	0	1	2	4	1	0	1	0	11	9
175—Lacrimal apparatus	4	2	1	0	1	0	1	0	3	1	1	0	2	2	1	1	0	7	8
188—Otosclerosis	0	2	0	0	0	1	2	0	2	0	0	3	0	0	0	1	3	2	13

Diagnosis Category 7—Diseases of the Circulatory System

218—Benign or unspecified hypertension w/wo heart and/or renal disease	25	31	14	22	14	23	259	271	756	1,048	1,474	2,392	2,532	5,044	2,631	5,156	2,260	6,283	9,965	20,270
221—Arteriosclerosis (including cardiovascular disease)	0	0	0	0	5	0	6	2	3	6	66	26	341	112	569	408	1,810	3,259	2,800	3,813
215—Congestive heart failure	4	12	3	4	4	0	4	13	17	23	46	62	140	219	480	639	1,268	2,114	1,966	3,086
217—Other heart disease	77	79	96	65	44	40	61	99	42	41	87	73	163	94	227	149	387	357	1,184	997
212—Other ischemic heart disease	0	4	4	1	1	0	0	8	6	11	45	16	180	227	248	249	402	608	885	949
211—Acute myocardial infarction	0	0	3	0	0	0	0	3	4	8	67	26	313	62	363	185	432	329	1,179	613
214—Heart block and other disorders of rhythm	5	6	3	1	4	4	22	39	30	69	50	88	80	111	180	209	341	469	715	996
226—Phlebitis and thrombophlebitis	0	0	0	0	0	0	12	80	33	139	25	126	73	244	169	146	178	280	490	1,015
231—Precordial pain	1	3	3	0	13	6	51	55	85	77	139	93	187	155	156	114	137	180	772	683
225—Hemorrhoids	0	0	0	0	5	1	129	91	180	184	130	130	124	131	71	96	53	92	692	725
230—Angina of effort	0	0	0	0	0	0	0	6	3	5	58	44	242	107	207	186	214	268	724	616

PART II. Continued

Diagnosis Category 7—Continued

DIAGNOSES (DESCRIPTION AND RCGP NUMBER)	0 – 4		5 – 9		10 – 14		15 – 24		25 – 34		35 – 44		45 – 54		55 – 64		65 +		Total	
	M	F	M	F	M	F	M	F	M	F	M	F	M	F	M	F	M	F	M	F
Total	1,318	1,233	1,641	1,722	1,264	1,605	1,972	3,404	1,067	1,925	609	830	253	524	165	302	98	244	8,387	11,789
237—Other sign, symptom, or incomplete diagnosis (Category 7)	5	6	7	5	5	18	29	50	57	62	78	94	98	122	138	127	125	152	542	636
223—Peripheral arterial disease	0	0	0	1	0	1	4	6	13	13	31	29	68	73	148	85	274	276	538	484
234—Edema	11	8	5	2	9	8	6	47	8	95	15	96	19	141	51	124	117	206	241	727
233—Syncope	1	3	0	6	15	21	51	114	53	80	21	69	50	83	41	49	92	216	324	641
227—Other disease of circulatory system	3	4	3	0	4	2	21	30	19	30	31	45	46	77	96	85	206	199	429	473
224—Varicose veins of lower extremities	0	0	0	2	1	0	7	9	17	51	13	90	48	126	73	111	81	173	240	562
210—Rheumatic heart disease	4	2	15	21	11	45	51	54	19	48	36	101	46	87	53	34	56	79	291	471
213—Myocardial degeneration from other causes	0	1	1	1	2	0	4	0	21	5	42	12	27	41	33	42	84	131	214	233
219—Malignant hypertension	0	0	0	0	0	0	2	3	8	9	27	49	24	73	31	66	26	69	118	269
229—Pulmonary embolism	0	0	0	0	0	0	1	7	4	4	14	11	11	16	39	53	68	89	137	180
235—Dyspnea (Category 7)	0	0	1	0	4	3	8	21	6	32	4	11	14	19	14	13	25	27	76	126
209—Cor pulmonale	0	0	0	0	0	1	1	0	1	0	1	0	5	11	18	2	25	23	51	37
220—Raynaud's disease	0	0	0	0	0	1	0	4	1	12	2	9	6	8	5	4	9	10	23	48
216—Left ventricular failure (acute)	0	0	0	0	0	0	0	2	3	0	0	13	1	2	2	9	4	10	10	36
236—Ascites	0	0	0	1	0	0	0	0	1	2	7	2	2	4	8	5	11	1	29	15
228—Other venous embolism and thrombosis	0	0	0	0	0	0	1	0	1	1	1	4	0	4	5	1	5	12	13	22
222—Chilblains	0	0	0	0	0	0	2	1	0	1	2	1	3	1	3	2	4	10	14	16
232—Cyanosis	3	1	0	0	0	1	0	0	0	0	0	1	0	0	0	0	0	0	3	3

Diagnosis Category 8—Diseases of the Respiratory System

DIAGNOSES (DESCRIPTION AND RCGP NUMBER)	0 – 4		5 – 9		10 – 14		15 – 24		25 – 34		35 – 44		45 – 54		55 – 64		65 +		Total	
	M	F	M	F	M	F	M	F	M	F	M	F	M	F	M	F	M	F	M	F
242—Pharyngitis (including febrile sore throat and tonsillitis)	885	631	563	503	378	399	777	1,137	667	1,218	594	1,016	566	1,095	572	763	722	1,025	5,724	7,787
247—Bronchitis, acute	1,493	1,392	642	575	318	466	625	1,316	492	1,043	281	581	216	506	157	346	165	337	4,389	6,562
240—Coryza (nonfebrile common cold)	832	722	601	477	402	356	705	925	686	833	461	527	307	425	242	300	230	335	4,466	4,900
241—Febrile cold and influenzalike illness	27	30	55	49	76	87	350	488	430	806	310	596	197	462	166	262	106	217	1,717	2,997
243—Sinusitis (acute)	535	542	207	226	152	179	191	459	210	418	142	276	108	166	111	157	110	164	1,766	2,587
272—Other sign, symptom, or incomplete diagnosis (Category 8)																				
246—Pneumonia pneumonitis	328	218	171	186	130	206	108	138	235	243	144	151	209	249	169	119	488	558	1,982	2,068
256—Other disease process not included above (Category 8)	381	271	186	206	105	103	198	266	114	212	87	124	105	156	144	154	219	163	1,539	1,655
257—Rhinitis, vasomotor or allergic	191	141	188	136	174	97	245	351	146	324	101	224	111	187	73	109	79	183	1,308	1,794
245—Influenza epidemic	82	98	97	71	97	86	139	242	189	258	105	161	83	130	70	144	63	122	925	1,312

Diagnosis																				
244—Laryngitis and tracheitis	206	142	81	60	46	29	54	116	49	119	32	104	45	106	37	83	34	76	584	835
267—Cough	140	132	61	50	48	44	76	122	56	106	47	77	23	63	36	73	46	97	533	764
255—Emphysema without bronchitis	7	1	1	2	0	0	2	3	4	4	30	1	170	42	289	70	453	89	956	177
271—Pleuritic pain	1	0	8	4	16	16	62	129	67	114	64	97	71	113	44	119	23	104	356	647
248—Bronchitis, chronic	22	8	4	5	8	7	14	29	15	42	20	33	94	115	106	58	184	124	467	491
250—Sinusitis (chronic)	1	1	2	5	2	1	9	23	20	42	22	48	43	65	39	46	43	149	181	445
251—Pleurisy	2	4	5	5	4	3	28	52	40	69	43	45	47	26	51	39	15	75	231	356
263—Epistaxis	17	15	24	44	30	30	44	30	26	16	16	15	38	5	31	3	20	52	246	267
249—Tonsillar and adenoidal hypertrophy	60	34	31	35	17	20	16	54	15	36	7	7	20	14	12	14	1	8	151	202
265—Dyspnea (Category 8)	20	12	3	0	1	2	3	23	6	10	5	7	0	15	20	0	14	16	84	98
258—Bronchiolitis	41	16	1	5	2	2	7	7	1	14	4	8	3	15	3	0	0	0	60	67
252—Pneumothorax, spontaneous	2	1	1	2	0	0	8	9	3	13	9	11	15	0	15	12	5	2	79	36
270—Hoarseness	4	2	2	0	1	2	1	9	7	9	4	13	2	14	9	13	12	12	42	72
261—Catarrh	2	4	4	2	3	4	0	8	5	12	1	5	4	3	4	3	10	21	33	72
264—Hemoptysis	0	0	0	0	2	1	6	0	10	3	4	3	5	6	8	6	7	12	42	29
260—Pleural effusion	0	0	0	0	1	0	2	1	1	1	3	3	1	3	3	3	5	24	28	37
254—Bronchiectasis	0	2	4	4	0	0	3	3	1	3	16	8	0	4	0	8	1	14	7	43
253—Pneumoconiosis	0	0	0	1	0	0	1	1	1	2	1	0	3	0	0	0	15	1	25	4
268—Sputum, noninfected	0	0	1	0	0	0	2	0	1	1	2	1	0	1	0	1	0	1	7	4
266—Stridor	0	0	0	0	0	0	0	1	0	0	0	0	0	0	3	1	0	0	5	3
262—Cyanosis	0	0	1	0	2	0	1	1	0	0	0	0	0	0	0	2	0	0	3	4
269—Sputum, infected	0	0	0	0	0	0	1	0	0	0	0	1	1	0	0	0	0	0	2	1

Diagnosis Category 9—Diseases of the Digestive System

Diagnosis																				
306—Abdominal pain other than colic	51	91	146	159	163	203	300	964	235	695	192	516	231	470	198	338	219	467	1,735	3,903
273—Acute gastritis or duodenitis	116	109	92	79	84	92	246	316	194	301	147	164	144	215	154	159	102	150	1,279	1,585
285—Other diseases of intestines and peritoneum	27	24	18	22	52	15	74	141	73	186	97	131	84	233	171	207	205	402	801	1,361
304—Diarrhea and/or vomiting (afebrile)	132	112	55	42	34	29	122	179	110	193	66	106	54	102	52	141	49	135	674	1,039
280—Functional gastric disorders	30	16	25	31	36	39	117	240	106	222	109	145	78	135	55	81	81	101	637	1,010
303—Diarrhea and/or vomiting (febrile)	201	172	53	52	31	39	92	136	73	97	47	65	40	77	56	83	45	89	638	810
284—Other hernias of abdominal cavity	88	87	11	13	6	2	16	16	44	36	47	58	59	186	77	141	78	150	426	689
290—Constipation	82	77	29	22	14	20	23	125	20	76	19	47	27	77	36	66	144	211	394	721
275—Diseases of teeth and supporting structures	55	51	54	34	19	44	99	145	61	109	41	76	32	85	26	50	36	61	423	655
293—Nausea	36	41	38	28	28	23	35	149	34	107	19	62	26	54	27	55	53	140	296	659
276—Other diseases of buccal cavity	146	98	22	34	27	17	58	96	48	66	39	40	19	51	26	34	40	70	425	506
308—Other sign, symptom, or incomplete diagnosis (Category 9)	14	20	13	10	13	9	45	62	47	54	47	62	57	79	60	68	61	108	357	472
278—Duodenal ulcer	1	0	3	0	7	1	34	25	79	44	63	67	77	61	103	51	109	66	476	315
302—Melena	14	5	7	5	3	7	28	41	45	64	58	52	62	50	39	42	112	87	368	353
283—Hernia, inguinal or femoral	58	12	25	8	21	3	56	7	36	2	30	12	87	15	84	25	127	77	524	161
289—Cirrhosis of liver	3	1	1	0	0	0	1	1	22	18	187	26	97	108	71	34	50	60	431	248
288—Other diseases of liver, gallbladder, and pancreas	1	0	0	3	0	2	29	63	48	50	56	73	60	71	45	61	39	56	278	379
281—Other diseases of esophagus, stomach, and duodenum	10	5	11	10	7	6	37	53	51	62	46	45	35	44	35	26	44	72	276	323

Diagnosis Category 9—Continued

AGE GROUPS

DIAGNOSES (DESCRIPTION AND RCGP NUMBER)	0 – 4		5 – 9		10 – 14		15 – 24		25 – 34		35 – 44		45 – 54		55 – 64		65	+	Total	
	M	F	M	F	M	F	M	F	M	F	M	F	M	F	M	F	M	F	M	F
279—Pyloric, juxtapyloric, prepyloric ulcer	3	0	0	1	3	0	27	25	51	47	71	32	70	41	45	40	62	42	332	228
277—Gastric ulcer	0	5	3	0	2	4	9	15	51	16	37	35	38	41	66	53	61	89	267	258
309—Anal fissure and fistula	29	10	7	6	7	3	28	52	32	41	29	31	13	33	21	18	13	22	179	216
301—Colic	33	27	3	1	3	1	17	41	12	35	18	24	11	29	12	20	28	39	137	217
287—Cholecystitis and/or cholangitis without calculus	0	0	2	0	0	1	1	21	5	52	7	53	10	72	10	45	21	45	56	289
274—Esophagitis	3	7	2	4	4	0	17	23	37	33	16	26	22	40	10	36	18	44	129	213
294—Heartburn	0	0	1	1	5	0	22	30	34	34	16	30	23	39	22	17	21	32	144	183
286—Cholelithiasis	0	1	3	4	0	1	0	16	7	19	2	17	17	35	14	26	11	86	54	204
295—Dysphagia	3	1	3	3	2	2	14	16	17	24	9	19	19	26	20	24	14	22	101	137
282—Appendicitis	1	2	9	7	30	13	39	26	21	10	6	5	9	17	6	0	5	3	126	83
292—Anorexia	3	5	3	33	1	3	7	24	2	15	4	3	5	8	15	16	24	22	64	129
299—Jaundice	10	12	2	1	1	0	4	9	9	1	6	11	13	4	16	13	29	26	88	68
298—Hepatomegaly	1	2	1	2	0	1	0	4	7	12	13	11	15	5	11	11	5	12	53	60
296—Hematemesis	0	0	0	2	0	1	6	14	5	5	5	2	3	5	3	4	1	23	23	56
307—Wind	2	5	3	1	0	0	1	2	1	8	4	6	17	7	3	6	8	7	37	39
291—Splenomegaly	0	0	8	6	6	2	19	3	1	0	1	3	2	3	0	0	0	0	37	22
300—Ascites	0	1	1	0	0	0	1	4	1	3	10	4	3	2	2	7	4	5	22	25
297—Hiccough	0	1	0	0	0	0	4	0	5	0	2	1	6	0	3	3	5	1	25	6
305—Appendicular pain	1	0	0	0	3	0	1	6	1	0	0	1	0	0	0	1	1	0	7	8

Diagnosis Category 10—Diseases of the Genitourinary System

DIAGNOSES (DESCRIPTION AND RCGP NUMBER)	0 – 4		5 – 9		10 – 14		15 – 24		25 – 34		35 – 44		45 – 54		55 – 64		65	+	Total	
	M	F	M	F	M	F	M	F	M	F	M	F	M	F	M	F	M	F	M	F
335—Vulvitis, vaginitis, and cervicitis (nonvenereal)	0	59	0	56	0	79	0	2,674	0	1,813	0	804	0	389	0	228	0	222	0	6,324
313—Urinary infection (cystitis)	12	71	7	144	21	114	79	1,098	86	865	67	561	52	395	53	412	117	698	494	4,358
316—Other infections of urinary system including prostatitis	17	54	16	54	11	35	157	276	246	210	289	171	344	166	270	133	622	311	1,972	1,410
317—Other diseases of the urinary tract	20	77	33	64	9	40	109	463	72	301	63	193	77	202	108	221	272	374	763	1,935
331—Other diseases of female genitalia	0	24	0	14	0	18	0	486	0	422	0	202	0	199	0	92	0	119	0	1,576
326—Amenorrhea	0	0	0	0	0	23	0	685	0	289	0	85	0	51	0	2	0	2	0	1,137
344—Other sign, symptom, or incomplete diagnosis (Category 10)	16	23	14	31	13	31	60	199	28	158	19	103	22	100	53	54	71	119	296	818
329—Menopausal symptoms	0	0	0	0	0	0	0	0	0	37	3	147	9	574	5	225	0	43	0	1,026
322—Breast diseases other than neoplasm	2	5	0	0	20	19	21	165	7	187	3	176	9	100	5	46	11	42	78	766
328—Menorrhagia and metrorrhagia	0	0	0	0	0	17	0	268	0	210	0	170	0	123	0	15	11	0	0	814
311—Pyelitis and pyelonephritis	4	9	5	17	20	19	24	157	36	113	17	79	36	52	17	91	30	81	189	618

Diagnosis																				Total
327—Irregular menstruation	0	0	0	1	14	0	339	0	177	0	112	0	59	0	0	10	0	0	5	0	717
315—Urethritis, nonvenereal	6	4	4	5	2	237	14	176	19	74	9	34	7	13	14	22	13	571	86
321—Other diseases of male genitalia	103	0	55	42	5	136	0	99	0	64	0	44	0	37	67	67	0	647	0
343—Hematuria	4	6	23	16	2	73	30	51	49	31	34	68	30	43	36	53	43	362	242
323—Salpingitis and oophoritis	0	9	0	0	28	0	261	0	207	0	69	0	19	0	1	0	1	0	561
325—Dysmenorrhea	0	0	0	1	0	0	271	0	70	0	41	0	8	0	0	4	0	0	424
312—Calculi of kidneys and ureters	1	0	0	1	0	22	21	72	12	81	16	59	21	35	13	32	35	302	119
337—Dysuria and/or strangury	4	15	0	1	5	29	21	20	60	6	33	12	29	9	45	15	35	109	281
334—Other disorders of menstruation	0	0	0	2	0	0	169	0	101	0	62	0	24	0	7	0	1	0	375
310—Nephritis and nephrosis	1	1	9	14	9	17	23	9	38	14	13	24	26	31	39	20	70	140	226
318—Prostatic hypertrophy (benign)	0	1	0	0	0	3	0	6	0	14	0	32	0	61	0	237	0	353	0
320—Epididymitis and/or orchitis	0	0	3	8	0	58	0	63	0	46	0	54	0	27	0	40	0	299	0
336—Colic (renal)	0	0	0	0	0	5	4	64	4	47	5	49	23	32	10	14	9	211	55
314—Cystitis, chronic	4	9	0	2	3	3	36	2	30	4	25	9	20	7	25	3	65	23	216
340—Frequency	5	11	0	9	7	7	37	10	30	9	8	8	15	17	13	14	15	71	140
338—Retention of urine	1	1	0	8	2	1	15	1	9	2	8	8	5	2	7	72	20	108	63
339—Incontinence of urine	3	7	4	5	7	2	13	0	9	2	19	9	23	20	2	23	27	44	127
332—Cervical erosion	0	0	0	1	0	1	50	0	59	0	22	0	11	0	5	0	2	0	150
319—Hydrocele	45	7	0	0	1	0	0	4	0	5	0	19	0	9	0	28	2	127	0
342—Dyspareunia	0	0	0	0	0	9	42	0	32	0	13	0	6	0	3	0	7	0	109
324—Uterovaginal prolapse	0	0	0	0	6	0	6	0	2	0	10	0	11	0	11	0	33	0	73
330—Disorders of menarche	0	0	0	0	11	0	16	0	18	0	10	0	2	1	0	0	0	0	59
333—Ovulation pain	0	0	0	1	0	4	17	0	12	0	4	0	0	0	0	0	1	0	39
341—Polyuria	5	1	1	0	0	2	3	1	2	1	0	3	1	3	0	0	1	16	9

Diagnosis Category 11—Pregnancy, Parturition, and Puerperium

Diagnosis																				Total
352—Normal pregnancy prenatal care	0	0	0	0	81	0	4,791	0	1,904	0	392	0	21	0	0	0	0	0	0	0	7,189
345—Genitourinary infection during pregnancy	0	0	0	0	0	0	167	0	57	0	11	0	0	0	0	0	0	0	0	0	235
350—Abortion, spontaneous	0	0	0	0	3	0	131	0	66	0	12	0	2	0	0	0	0	0	0	0	214
351—Normal delivery	0	0	0	0	3	0	125	0	44	0	7	0	0	0	0	0	0	0	0	0	180
367—Abortion, induced	0	0	0	0	5	0	92	0	36	0	16	0	0	0	0	0	0	0	0	0	149
362—Other complications of pregnancy, delivery, and puerperium	0	0	0	0	0	0	89	0	45	0	12	0	1	0	0	0	0	0	0	0	147
346—Toxemias of pregnancy	0	0	0	0	0	0	47	0	22	0	2	0	0	0	0	0	0	0	0	0	71
366—Other signs, symptoms, or complications of pregnancy	0	0	0	0	0	0	36	0	20	0	9	0	1	0	0	0	0	0	0	0	66
348—Ectopic pregnancy	0	0	0	0	0	0	13	0	8	0	1	0	0	0	0	0	0	0	0	0	22
353—Placenta previa	0	0	0	0	0	0	13	0	9	0	0	0	0	0	0	0	0	0	0	0	22
347—Ante partum hemorrhage	0	0	0	0	0	0	11	0	4	0	0	1	0	0	0	0	0	0	0	0	16
364—Caesarean section (all indications)	0	0	0	0	0	0	13	0	2	0	0	1	0	0	0	0	0	0	0	0	16
361—Puerperal mastitis	0	0	0	0	0	0	6	0	5	0	0	0	0	0	0	0	0	0	0	0	11
357—Prolonged labor	0	0	0	0	0	0	7	0	2	0	1	0	0	0	0	0	0	0	0	0	10
363—Postpartum hemorrhage	0	0	0	0	1	0	7	0	0	0	0	0	0	0	0	0	0	0	0	0	8
356—Malposition and/or disproportion affecting second stage	0	0	0	0	0	0	4	0	3	0	0	0	0	0	0	0	0	0	0	0	7
355—Forceps delivery (all indications)	0	0	0	0	0	0	4	0	1	0	0	0	0	0	0	0	0	0	0	0	5

Diagnosis Category 11—Continued

DIAGNOSES (DESCRIPTION AND RCGP NUMBER)	0-4 M	0-4 F	5-9 M	5-9 F	10-14 M	10-14 F	15-24 M	15-24 F	25-34 M	25-34 F	35-44 M	35-44 F	45-54 M	45-54 F	55-64 M	55-64 F	65+ M	65+ F	Total M	Total F
358—Laceration or episiotomy	0	0	0	0	0	0	0	2	0	3	0	0	0	0	0	0	0	0	0	5
365—Pyrexia of childbirth and puerperium	0	0	0	0	0	1	0	0	0	3	0	0	0	0	0	0	0	0	0	4
354—Retained placenta	0	0	0	0	0	0	0	2	0	0	0	0	0	0	0	1	0	0	0	3
360—Puerperal thrombophlebitis	0	0	0	0	0	0	0	2	0	0	0	1	0	0	0	0	0	0	0	3
349—Malposition of fetus in uterus	0	0	0	0	0	0	0	0	0	0	0	0	0	0	0	0	0	0	0	0
359—Puerperal sepsis	0	0	0	0	0	0	0	0	0	0	0	0	0	0	0	0	0	0	0	0

Diagnosis Category 12—Diseases of Skin and Cellular Tissue

DIAGNOSES (DESCRIPTION AND RCGP NUMBER)	0-4 M	0-4 F	5-9 M	5-9 F	10-14 M	10-14 F	15-24 M	15-24 F	25-34 M	25-34 F	35-44 M	35-44 F	45-54 M	45-54 F	55-64 M	55-64 F	65+ M	65+ F	Total M	Total F
380—Dermatitis, contact	92	95	213	143	264	212	339	441	220	323	145	223	127	171	83	150	80	158	1,563	1,916
372—Other cellulitis without mention of lymphangitis	57	41	91	63	120	70	271	265	241	263	188	202	146	172	131	259	146	190	1,391	1,525
377—Other local infections of skin and subcutaneous tissue	121	104	70	75	105	80	273	272	237	183	162	115	122	115	53	131	154	177	1,297	1,252
381—Other dermatitis	222	232	88	103	87	118	193	273	104	218	97	152	78	118	56	95	91	179	1,016	1,488
398—Rash	338	301	125	102	74	96	150	250	102	164	67	122	50	97	55	64	72	94	1,033	1,290
394—Insect bites	123	91	134	121	92	54	123	149	72	92	69	68	37	57	42	41	26	60	718	733
387—Disease of nail and nail bed	15	13	22	30	114	71	205	172	105	77	40	64	48	92	33	64	50	117	632	700
375—Impetigo	228	212	209	200	104	61	68	67	27	30	11	14	9	9	7	10	4	5	667	608
389—Disease of sweat and sebaceous glands	26	25	7	7	28	9	129	115	137	106	72	83	113	86	89	73	71	71	672	575
399—Other sign, symptom, or incomplete diagnosis (Category 12)	43	34	39	37	35	37	96	148	85	100	52	98	50	72	51	89	66	89	517	704
379—Dermatitis, atopic (eczema)	99	85	51	81	26	59	56	179	32	93	22	62	31	62	21	44	50	64	388	729
369—Acne	0	0	14	3	49	82	347	375	27	118	5	19	10	6	3	2	4	2	459	607
374—Cellulitis and abscess with lymphangitis	15	29	40	37	57	21	104	112	73	51	54	35	40	42	12	18	19	15	414	360
370—Boil and carbuncle	12	16	11	1	19	21	116	110	91	75	62	47	43	29	24	25	27	14	405	338
385—Other hypertrophic and atrophic skin conditions	10	16	10	10	13	29	40	75	26	51	39	55	33	54	26	30	48	70	245	390
390—Chronic ulcer of skin	5	5	0	0	2	2	14	8	9	15	32	15	44	34	45	63	127	126	278	268
383—Pruritus	10	13	11	19	5	14	18	52	30	48	17	42	20	48	28	47	28	58	167	341
378—Dermatitis, seborrheic	58	46	5	18	11	22	23	43	30	48	17	28	18	32	13	20	24	36	199	293
371—Cellulitis of finger and toe	10	14	19	13	15	16	47	37	26	58	25	29	24	30	19	25	18	23	203	245
391—Dermatitis herpetiformis, pemphigus, lichen, etc.	16	8	7	6	12	16	51	53	25	40	17	44	21	35	11	16	18	17	178	235
388—Disease of hair and hair follicle	26	16	11	5	10	8	32	40	11	51	21	23	15	19	4	25	7	12	137	199
382—Psoriasis	0	0	0	5	4	5	10	26	10	24	24	33	24	12	12	10	5	44	89	162
368—Pityriasis rosa	5	2	8	14	12	11	27	59	27	21	7	18	1	8	5	4	3	2	95	139

Diagnosis																				
386—Other dermatoses	9	1	5	4	7	6	32	21	11	16	11	13	8	8	11	14	20	21	114	104
384—Corns and callosities	1	0	1	1	4	2	4	9	5	18	9	14	4	22	10	17	22	33	60	116
373—Infantile eczema	16	4	4	3	3	4	2	21	3	4	1	12	7	7	3	2	2	9	37	62
397—Pigmentation	2	8	1	4	4	2	3	15	4	7	2	7	4	5	1	11	5	1	29	60
395—Erythema	3	1	3	4	4	11	2	6	2	5	3	6	1	9	1	8	1	1	20	51

Diagnosis Category 13—Diseases of Bones and Organs of Movement

Diagnosis																				
409—Other forms of arthritis and rheumatism	3	16	5	9	15	13	64	87	83	139	103	191	261	630	360	742	440	1,072	1,334	2,899
406—Osteoarthritis	3	1	1	1	2	5	10	11	12	24	23	84	120	254	227	559	393	1,253	791	2,192
425—Back pain alone	2	7	4	3	13	15	179	250	248	311	231	303	217	390	177	219	97	171	1,168	1,669
415—Other disease process not mentioned above (Category 13)	64	73	23	20	100	53	167	142	104	179	101	156	133	210	120	177	101	162	913	1,172
405—Rheumatoid arthritis	2	30	3	1	5	2	54	51	14	48	59	208	156	375	172	315	180	352	645	1,382
427—Other sign, symptom, or incomplete diagnosis (Category 13)	23	27	20	21	65	37	141	134	120	191	105	183	130	215	112	146	114	195	830	1,149
420—Bursitis	1	3	3	1	19	7	56	71	83	100	152	217	213	279	172	192	120	187	819	1,057
428—Pain in joint (arthralgia)	9	8	20	22	35	29	77	101	95	154	77	131	89	160	83	120	65	132	550	857
408—Fibrositis and muscular rheumatism	5	0	6	10	23	17	74	104	100	148	97	122	101	199	80	99	62	121	548	820
400—Cervical injury, e.g., whiplash (excluding fracture or disk)	1	1	1	1	2	8	78	140	119	177	75	112	35	88	55	45	14	51	380	623
421—Tenosynovitis	0	0	5	4	18	23	61	48	71	82	75	110	100	135	48	79	23	45	401	526
424—Backache with other neuritis	0	0	0	1	2	8	21	61	26	56	25	46	56	83	34	57	28	28	192	340
407—Lumbago (backache) not attributed to disk lesion	0	0	0	0	1	0	18	36	47	48	36	70	59	70	24	23	13	26	198	273
401—Torticollis	6	1	8	2	5	12	25	35	27	68	33	69	32	19	19	31	19	22	174	259
411—Other internal derangements of the knee	2	1	1	4	32	17	67	47	31	15	22	20	19	21	11	22	6	16	191	163
412—Displacement of intervertebral disk	0	0	0	0	0	0	4	3	21	13	38	47	44	25	23	11	6	22	136	121
423—Backache with sciatica	0	0	0	0	0	0	1	8	30	21	35	52	16	26	17	11	11	10	110	128
417—Scoliosis, kyphoscoliosis	1	2	2	5	13	13	13	37	0	12	8	8	1	8	3	4	6	14	39	99
422—Synovitis	0	0	1	1	2	6	0	12	9	9	9	5	12	4	14	15	6	15	68	67
416—Genu valgum or varum	42	28	2	2	2	1	2	0	0	9	15	7	4	1	0	0	5	2	52	37
426—Frozen shoulder	0	2	0	2	0	0	7	1	4	7	7	5	7	20	10	14	3	8	33	55
413—Flat foot	24	13	0	6	7	7	0	6	4	0	0	2	1	4	1	3	0	1	49	36
404—Cervical spondylosis	3	0	0	0	0	0	2	0	0	1	2	1	21	2	15	4	15	11	55	24
414—Hallux valgus or varus	0	8	0	0	0	2	0	0	1	1	1	0	1	3	1	3	20	0	30	16
410—Torn meniscus of knee	3	0	0	0	1	0	0	5	10	3	2	3	1	2	3	2	1	2	28	17
418—Osteoporosis	0	0	0	0	0	0	0	0	1	0	3	1	2	3	1	4	2	13	9	21
419—Brachial neuritis	0	1	0	0	0	0	0	4	0	3	2	0	2	5	1	2	0	1	5	16

Diagnosis Category 14—Congenital Malformation

Diagnosis																				
437—Congenital malformation of bone and joint	56	47	16	6	3	3	12	10	5	3	4	0	6	3	3	2	3	17	112	91
438—Other congenital malformation not included above	28	8	16	6	3	3	15	12	2	1	3	21	1	6	3	0	1	2	72	59

PART II. Continued

Diagnosis Category 14—Continued

DIAGNOSES (DESCRIPTION AND RCGP NUMBER)	0 – 4		5 – 9		10 – 14		15 – 24		25 – 34		35 – 44		45 – 54		55 – 64		65 +		Total	
	M	F	M	F	M	F	M	F	M	F	M	F	M	F	M	F	M	F	M	F
436—Congenital malformation of genitourinary system	35	3	22	1	5	0	5	3	0	1	2	1	0	2	1	1	6	2	76	14
429—Anencephaly, microcephaly, or monstrosity	7	12	7	1	1	4	3	11	4	10	3	2	2	5	1	5	2	5	30	55
433—Congenital malformation of circulatory system	8	15	6	10	4	2	1	8	1	6	2	1	2	0	0	0	2	1	26	43
403—Congenital talipes	2	2	0	1	2	4	1	0	5	10	3	6	1	10	1	1	1	7	16	41
439—Other sign, symptom, or incomplete diagnosis (Category 14)	12	4	1	2	2	1	1	2	1	2	1	1	1	2	0	1	2	1	21	16
432—Congenital hydrocephalus	6	6	1	0	2	0	1	1	2	0	0	0	0	0	0	0	0	1	12	8
434—Cleft palate and harelip	4	0	0	1	0	0	1	0	0	6	1	1	0	3	0	0	0	1	6	12
435—Congenital malformation of digestive system	7	2	0	1	0	0	0	5	0	0	0	2	0	0	0	0	0	1	7	11
402—Congenital dislocated hip	5	4	1	1	0	1	0	1	0	0	0	1	0	0	0	0	0	0	6	8
430—Spina bifida and meningocele with hydrocephalus	1	2	0	0	1	0	1	1	0	0	0	0	0	0	2	0	0	0	5	3
431—Spina bifida and meningocele without hydrocephalus	0	0	0	0	0	0	1	3	0	0	0	0	0	0	0	0	0	0	1	3

Diagnosis Category 15—Certain Diseases of Early Infancy

DIAGNOSES (DESCRIPTION AND RCGP NUMBER)	0 – 4		5 – 9		10 – 14		15 – 24		25 – 34		35 – 44		45 – 54		55 – 64		65 +		Total	
	M	F	M	F	M	F	M	F	M	F	M	F	M	F	M	F	M	F	M	F
453—Failure to thrive	53	38	4	2	0	0	0	0	0	0	0	0	0	0	0	0	0	0	57	40
452—Feeding problems	43	23	3	0	1	0	0	0	0	0	0	0	0	0	0	0	0	0	47	23
451—Other causes of perinatal morbidity	18	42	1	0	1	0	0	0	0	0	0	0	0	0	0	0	0	0	20	42
440—Birth injury due to difficult labor	5	6	0	3	0	0	2	0	2	0	0	0	2	1	2	1	3	4	16	15
441—Atelectasis other asphyxia of newborn	8	3	0	4	1	1	0	0	0	0	0	0	0	0	0	0	0	0	9	8
445—Umbilical sepsis	13	1	0	0	0	0	0	0	0	0	0	0	0	0	0	0	0	0	13	1
449—Immaturity dysmaturity	6	8	0	0	0	0	0	0	0	0	0	0	0	0	0	0	0	0	6	8
443—Birth injury to brain, spinal cord, bone, or nerve	0	0	0	0	0	1	0	1	0	0	0	0	0	0	0	0	0	0	0	2
448—Hemorrhagic disease	0	0	0	0	0	0	0	1	0	0	0	0	0	0	0	0	0	0	0	1
447—Hemolytic disease	0	0	0	0	0	0	0	0	0	0	0	0	0	0	0	0	0	0	0	0

Diagnosis Category 16—Signs, Symptoms, and Ill-Defined Conditions

Diagnosis																			
464—Other sign, symptom, or incomplete diagnosis (Category 16)	162	162	97	93	73	112	193	172	357	109	333	190	428	181	350	206	457	1,383	2,729
454—Headache	13	13	61	59	98	94	196	220	576	155	405	118	374	87	211	68	142	1,010	2,475
457—Weight loss	18	1	1	2	8	9	31	40	64	16	45	68	48	40	62	85	93	303	422
446—Debility or fatigue	1	0	5	2	3	8	51	32	63	26	49	23	43	28	29	24	84	193	370
466—Sweating	33	52	13	17	24	50	39	31	25	28	26	32	15	16	7	11	18	227	253
456—Dehydration	9	10	2	0	2	0	1	2	17	12	3	7	9	8	5	24	172	60	231
444—Lymphadenopathy, enlargement of lymph nodes	17	14	11	17	13	20	25	10	21	8	16	7	12	2	5	1	12	94	151
458—Pyrexia of unknown origin	37	28	21	8	8	7	4	9	13	4	7	4	4	8	0	7	10	105	110
460—Albuminuria	23	22	19	13	6	5	19	8	0	4	4	2	7	6	8	6	4	93	93
463—Senility	7	0	0	6	0	0	0	1	13	1	0	2	1	1	5	27	82	32	88
450—Sleep disturbance	7	10	0	1	1	0	2	0	1	4	2	7	4	9	1	14	13	46	37
462—Uremia (raised BUN)	1	2	0	0	0	0	1	2	1	2	1	1	4	4	2	19	23	28	35
461—Hematuria	0	0	1	0	2	2	1	3	2	0	1	6	0	0	2	1	3	18	22
455—Malingering	0	0	0	0	1	2	2	1	0	0	1	3	10	3	0	3	1	12	20
459—Rigors	0	1	0	0	0	0	2	0	2	0	2	1	0	3	0	0	1	6	9

Diagnosis Category 17—Accidents, Poisoning, and Violence

Diagnosis																				
483—Lacerations, amputations, contusions, and abrasions	1,038	706	1,356	817	1,716	874	3,333	1,791	1,897	1,064	1,162	811	1,022	887	626	597	525	915	12,675	8,462
480—Sprains and strains	91	57	149	146	629	493	2,049	1,389	1,339	1,091	974	1,023	679	890	473	543	281	534	6,664	6,166
465—Foreign body entering not through orifice	31	25	49	19	79	48	175	177	151	95	80	73	69	73	66	51	54	53	754	614
495—Other fractures not included above	12	14	59	48	116	83	157	87	91	47	42	49	59	66	47	46	75	199	658	639
486—Burns, second degree	111	67	44	27	53	46	120	131	97	79	92	59	109	49	83	33	26	66	735	557
476—Fracture, carpal, metacarpal, tarsal, or metatarsal bones	12	3	44	23	116	48	219	65	102	55	54	59	43	61	51	55	27	82	668	451
493—Other known injury not included above	71	80	53	40	87	36	136	112	55	66	43	59	45	69	38	47	26	42	554	551
494—Other sign, symptom, or incomplete diagnosis (Category 17)	75	55	60	71	64	40	120	74	62	67	55	33	59	30	26	20	48	60	569	450
477—Fracture of phalanges	8	8	26	12	109	59	127	61	90	83	64	29	92	30	43	40	15	27	574	349
485—Burns, first degree	46	29	18	14	10	15	72	92	51	34	36	26	53	36	33	22	9	20	328	288
469—Fracture of tibia and/or fibula (Potts)	25	7	15	16	41	30	87	39	39	28	29	32	53	35	17	20	33	67	339	274
484—Foreign body entering through orifice	44	37	45	17	31	19	83	37	72	26	30	20	28	19	14	5	8	5	355	185
471—Fracture of ribs	1	0	4	0	1	2	18	15	40	23	23	19	14	14	48	42	57	80	285	220
496—Adverse effect of other drugs	19	24	6	8	57	11	29	47	13	40	48	34	67	19	46	25	37	106	151	341
475—Colles' fracture	8	6	28	19	41	29	52	17	39	8	13	19	10	46	28	32	2	81	232	233
473—Fracture of clavicle	48	31	38	20	57	23	81	8	12	8	8	10	13	26	6	5	2	7	244	106
468—Fracture of femur	3	0	2	32	0	5	4	0	0	3	3	13	4	0	4	5	2	128	39	257
474—Fracture of humerus	8	4	20	12	26	10	17	4	3	1	1	8	4	7	2	88	17	39	104	133
467—Fracture of spine	0	0	2	0	1	1	16	3	2	16	3	4	7	21	6	2	17	61	118	104
481—Intracranial injury	8	8	11	5	26	4	41	24	17	2	14	16	3	14	4	18	39	75	127	78
487—Burns, third degree	15	8	12	3	4	2	9	9	15	11	6	22	2	13	1	24	13	5	8	119	58

James M. Gall, M.D., C.C.F.P.
Department of Family Medicine
University of Miami School of Medicine
P. O. Box 016700
Miami, Florida 33101

PART II   Continued   *(continued)*

Diagnosis Category 17—Continued

DIAGNOSES (DESCRIPTION AND RCGP NUMBER)	0-4 M	0-4 F	5-9 M	5-9 F	10-14 M	10-14 F	15-24 M	15-24 F	25-34 M	25-34 F	35-44 M	35-44 F	45-54 M	45-54 F	55-64 M	55-64 F	65 + M	65 + F	Total M	Total F
488—Effects of alcohol poisoning	1	1	0	0	0	0	5	3	16	2	23	4	10	32	20	2	33	5	108	49
482—Internal injury of chest, abdomen, and pelvis	1	0	2	5	1	2	26	15	9	10	12	11	6	8	7	3	5	10	69	64
479—Dislocation, shoulder	1	0	0	1	2	0	33	4	7	3	18	5	3	3	3	3	0	3	67	22
472—Fracture of pelvis	0	0	0	1	7	0	2	0	3	0	0	1	0	1	5	0	29	39	46	42
470—Fracture of skull	4	7	1	1	3	4	8	2	0	0	4	2	10	4	1	0	4	4	35	24
491—Effects of aspirin poisoning	4	7	0	0	0	1	2	4	0	8	4	1	0	1	3	0	0	0	13	22
489—Effects of carbon monoxide poisoning	2	1	2	0	0	0	4	0	0	6	4	0	1	1	0	0	0	0	13	8
478—Dislocation, jaw	0	0	2	0	2	2	6	2	1	0	0	3	0	0	0	0	1	1	12	8
490—Effects of barbiturate poisoning	2	0	0	0	0	0	0	1	1	0	0	0	4	1	1	0	1	3	9	5
492—Motion sickness	0	0	0	0	0	1	0	1	1	0	1	1	0	1	1	0	1	1	4	5
497—Dislocation of radial head	1	1	0	0	1	0	2	0	0	0	0	0	1	0	0	0	0	0	5	1

Diagnosis Category 18—Prophylactic Procedures

DIAGNOSES (DESCRIPTION AND RCGP NUMBER)	0-4 M	0-4 F	5-9 M	5-9 F	10-14 M	10-14 F	15-24 M	15-24 F	25-34 M	25-34 F	35-44 M	35-44 F	45-54 M	45-54 F	55-64 M	55-64 F	65 + M	65 + F	Total M	Total F
511—Other medical exam for preventive and presymptomatic purposes	5,869	5,386	1,930	1,721	1,683	1,217	4,126	4,851	1,773	2,639	1,324	2,003	1,098	1,949	824	1,488	1,579	2,491	20,206	23,745
500—Cervical smear	0	27	0	11	0	22	0	1,979	0	1,972	0	1,400	0	1,066	0	675	0	554	0	7,706
505—Other prophylactic procedures	168	195	129	94	95	101	134	252	105	167	98	147	125	230	154	239	252	412	1,260	1,837
585—Oral contraceptive advice	0	0	0	3	0	29	0	1,681	0	790	0	165	0	53	0	0	0	0	0	2,721
568—Other disease inoculations	138	134	128	87	90	97	208	201	124	111	37	251	68	107	82	99	117	181	992	1,268
543—Group diphtheria, whooping cough, and tetanus prophylaxis	441	423	100	103	33	29	106	81	58	38	31	28	31	14	21	10	65	57	886	783
544—Poliomyelitis prophylaxis	297	293	63	73	16	12	25	14	1	5	1	1	1	1	1	2	52	32	457	433
504—Health education counseling	18	16	6	6	9	9	43	88	38	70	26	32	32	45	41	32	22	18	235	316
541—Tuberculosis prophylaxis	70	77	31	26	10	8	37	70	26	68	13	28	16	30	6	13	15	6	224	326
586—Other contraceptive advice	0	0	0	1	0	6	1	207	4	208	0	62	1	10	0	0	0	0	6	494
546—Measles prophylaxis	100	106	16	16	1	0	0	5	0	0	0	0	0	0	2	0	1	0	120	127
545—Rubella prophylaxis	74	57	21	19	2	4	1	7	0	6	1	0	0	1	1	0	1	0	101	94
559—Tetanus alone prophylaxis	5	8	1	1	11	9	24	36	12	6	6	4	10	4	2	4	6	8	77	80
542—Smallpox prophylaxis	10	8	16	9	6	2	6	13	4	8	0	4	3	3	1	2	4	4	50	53
587—Intrauterine device	0	0	0	0	0	2	0	46	0	44	0	6	0	0	0	0	0	0	0	97
558—Cholera prophylaxis	0	0	0	3	0	2	22	24	6	3	8	7	3	4	1	1	1	1	41	45
578—Sterilization, male and female	0	0	0	0	0	0	2	8	11	24	7	15	3	4	0	0	1	1	24	52
556—Typhoid, paratyphoid prophylaxis	0	2	0	0	0	0	16	9	4	5	2	3	3	2	1	0	0	2	26	23
557—Yellow fever prophylaxis	0	2	4	2	2	2	1	0	0	0	0	0	0	0	2	0	0	0	9	6

Department of Family Medicine (R700)
University of Miami School of Medicine
P. O. Box 016700
Miami, Florida 33101

Diagnosis Category 19—Procedures Performed

Procedure																						
625—Other abnormal biochemistry	3	3	0	0	0	0	3	3	13	29	18	34	16	16	64	47	46	63	34	61	213	224
644—Other abnormal procedure	1	4	5	11	6	6	48	9	54	13	44	10	30	15	16	18	5	15	15	13	80	237
612—Abnormal blood test	6	9	8	3	2	17	3	17	3	27	11	16	15	33	17	12	12	11	16		132	89
631—Abnormal chest x-ray	1	0	1	3	2	2	2	4	12	17	16	13	10	21	23	8	8	11	15	16	76	93
635—Abnormal findings at other instrumental test	0	0	0	0	1	1	1	4	15	17	23	9	21	20	11	10	9	2	7		63	97
620—Abnormal sugar	2	0	1	5	1	2	1	10	8	13	5	8	18	14	21	17	11	19			67	85
602—Abnormal urinalysis	2	1	5	7	6	8	27	18	7	3	5	8	11	7	7	2	2	2			73	58
640—Abnormal sigmoidoscopy	0	0	0	0	0	5	6	2	17	12	6	14	19	5	9	6	6	11			44	68
624—Abnormal liver function	2	0	0	2	0	6	6	9	1	10	1	7	9	6	10	11	16	11			56	38
630—Abnormal EKG	0	0	0	2	7	5	7	1	6	18	9	0	11	3	3	3	8	11			53	37
601—Abnormal urinoscopy	2	2	2	10	3	7	3	6	5	2	4	4	0	3	2	1	0	2			21	34
610—Abnormal hematocrit	1	3	2	6	2	2	0	3	0	1	3	2	4	3	2	1	0	2			21	34
611—Abnormal blood count	2	3	3	2	4	0	1	1	5	5	5	1	0	2	3	2	2	1			22	24
604—Abnormal urine test	0	0	1	0	3	4	4	12	1	10	4	1	1	0	3	3	0	3			7	30
621—Abnormal urea (BUN)	0	1	0	2	2	0	2	0	1	0	0	1	1	4	1	1	4	3			15	12
634—Other abnormal x-ray	0	0	0	1	0	3	1	3	0	0	1	2	2	3	6	4	2	4			10	17
622—Abnormal electrolytes	0	0	0	0	0	0	0	0	2	1	2	2	3	2	4	2	3	3			5	12
623—Abnormal PBI	0	0	0	0	0	0	0	0	1	0	1	1	0	0	0	0	0	0			3	7
632—Abnormal GI series	0	0	0	0	0	0	1	0	0	1	1	0	1	0	0	1	0	1			5	3
643—Abnormal lumbar puncture	0	0	1	0	0	0	0	0	0	2	0	0	0	0	0	0	0	0			10	3
603—Abnormal urine culture	0	0	0	0	1	0	1	0	0	0	1	0	0	0	0	0	0	0			3	1
642—Abnormal cystoscopy	0	0	0	0	0	0	0	0	0	0	1	0	0	0	0	1	1	0			1	1
641—Abnormal esophagoscopy	0	0	0	0	0	0	0	0	0	0	0	0	0	0	0	0	0	0			0	0

Diagnosis Category 20—Problems Other Than Specific Diagnostic/Symptomatic

Problem																				
704—Family relationship problems	25	21	12	9	11	26	43	181	53	259	55	232	56	93	21	59	14	33	290	913
730—Other legal problems	0	0	1	3	0	0	1	5	10	6	35	13	32	12	41	8	9	4	129	51
707—Pregnancy and birth out of wedlock (parent and child)	0	0	0	0	0	4	0	78	0	8	0	5	0	0	0	0	0	0	0	95
731—Adopted child	6	3	3	6	3	2	20	20	3	12	2	3	3	2	1	0	1	2	42	50
703—Educational problems	1	0	28	13	9	10	6	7	0	0	0	3	3	1	0	3	2	2	49	36
712—Other high-risk individual	3	1	4	2	1	1	9	21	13	8	5	5	5	2	0	3	4	4	41	42
727—Alcoholism in parent or child	0	0	0	0	0	1	1	7	1	8	10	4	4	4	14	1	1	1	51	21
706—Other high-risk family situations	7	9	1	1	1	0	2	3	2	9	4	11	3	8	1	3	2	2	18	46
705—Legal problems	0	0	1	1	0	2	2	11	5	7	1	4	3	7	2	13	0	1	13	45
702—Medical care problems	1	0	0	1	2	0	0	0	1	0	5	4	3	7	2	0	6	9	18	24
700—Economic problems	0	1	2	2	0	0	2	3	4	3	4	3	2	8	1	4	1	1	13	23
717—Other employment problems	0	0	0	0	0	0	3	2	1	6	6	1	5	1	0	1	2	0	18	16
708—Social isolation	0	0	2	1	1	1	1	4	2	3	1	0	1	2	0	8	0	2	11	17
713—Out of work, acute	1	1	0	0	4	1	9	4	5	3	0	0	2	3	5	0	5	1	13	15
728—Drug abuse in parent or child	0	0	0	0	2	2	0	5	2	2	0	0	2	2	1	0	1	0	18	10
722—Other social problems, family and individual	0	0	0	0	0	0	0	5	0	0	2	2	3	0	0	0	0	1	3	17

PART II. Continued

Diagnosis Category 20—Continued

DIAGNOSES (DESCRIPTION AND RCGP NUMBER)	AGE GROUPS																			
	0 – 4		5 – 9		10 – 14		15 – 24		25 – 34		35 – 44		45 – 54		55 – 64		65 +		Total	
	M	F	M	F	M	F	M	F	M	F	M	F	M	F	M	F	M	F	M	F
709—Occupational maladjustment	1	0	1	0	0	0	2	2	2	2	2	1	1	2	1	0	0	0	10	6
701—Housing problems	0	0	1	0	1	0	0	2	2	2	0	2	0	4	0	0	1	2	3	12
724—High-risk pregnancy	0	0	0	0	0	0	0	4	0	5	0	5	0	0	0	0	0	0	0	12
726—High-risk physical violence	1	1	0	0	0	0	1	3	0	3	0	1	0	0	0	1	0	0	3	9
711—Chronic physical disability	0	0	0	0	1	0	0	1	0	0	1	0	0	1	0	0	0	0	6	4
729—Other social/personal problem	0	0	0	0	0	5	0	1	1	0	0	2	3	1	0	0	0	0	6	10
710—Dependency	0	0	2	1	0	0	1	0	0	0	1	2	0	0	0	0	0	0	4	4
732—Foster child	0	0	3	1	1	0	0	0	0	0	0	0	0	0	0	0	0	0	5	1
714—Out of work, chronic	0	0	0	0	0	0	1	0	0	0	0	0	0	0	1	3	1	0	1	4
716—Unemployable because of illness	0	0	0	0	0	0	3	0	0	0	1	0	0	1	0	1	0	0	3	1
718—Imprisonment	0	0	0	0	1	0	2	0	0	0	0	0	0	0	0	0	0	0	3	0
725—High-risk accident	0	0	0	0	0	2	0	0	0	0	0	1	0	0	0	0	0	0	0	3
719—Prosecution or impending litigation	0	0	0	0	0	0	0	0	1	0	0	0	0	0	1	0	0	0	1	1
715—Medical absenteeism	0	0	0	0	0	0	0	0	1	0	0	0	0	0	0	0	0	0	1	0
720—Other problem with alcohol	0	0	0	0	0	0	0	0	0	0	0	0	0	0	0	0	0	0	0	0
723—High-risk infant	0	0	0	0	0	0	0	0	0	0	0	0	0	0	0	0	0	0	0	0

Diagnosis Category 21—Family History of Selected Diseases

DIAGNOSES (DESCRIPTION AND RCGP NUMBER)	0 – 4		5 – 9		10 – 14		15 – 24		25 – 34		35 – 44		45 – 54		55 – 64		65 +		Total	
	M	F	M	F	M	F	M	F	M	F	M	F	M	F	M	F	M	F	M	F
813—Hypertension	1	2	0	0	0	1	18	2	21	21	44	63	60	87	73	122	67	172	284	470
805—Carcinoma	0	10	0	0	0	0	2	4	1	10	11	10	38	22	38	87	161	116	251	249
801—Anemia (including hemoglobinopathies)	5	5	5	5	2	2	3	22	0	20	12	30	3	33	2	20	24	107	54	249
807—Diabetes	0	3	0	1	3	3	13	11	12	22	11	26	18	22	15	40	54	43	124	170
808—Drug reaction	2	1	0	1	2	2	3	8	3	4	3	3	0	5	1	4	1	2	14	29
803—Bleeding disorder	0	2	1	0	1	1	2	3	2	8	3	3	2	2	2	2	4	5	16	25
816—Kidney disease	0	5	0	0	0	0	0	4	4	0	3	2	2	1	2	2	7	2	18	15
824—Tuberculosis	1	0	0	0	2	2	1	0	0	4	2	4	2	0	0	1	4	3	12	14
804—Blindness	0	0	0	0	0	0	1	1	1	1	1	3	2	2	1	0	6	8	12	11
812—Heart disease	0	1	1	0	0	0	3	2	5	1	1	3	2	2	0	0	2	2	12	10
823—Thyroid disease	0	0	0	0	0	0	1	1	0	3	2	3	1	2	2	2	0	0	7	11
802—Asthma	0	0	2	0	1	1	1	2	0	2	1	1	0	1	1	2	2	0	7	9
820—Neurological disorders	1	0	0	0	0	1	1	2	0	0	3	0	0	1	1	0	2	5	8	8
825—Other familial, genetic, or otherwise significant disease	2	1	1	2	2	0	0	2	0	1	1	2	1	1	1	2	0	1	4	12
809—Epilepsy	0	0	0	0	0	0	1	0	0	1	1	0	0	3	0	1	2	0	3	7
811—Hay fever	1	3	0	1	1	2	0	0	0	0	0	0	0	0	0	0	0	0	2	8
821—Rheumatic fever	0	1	1	0	2	1	1	0	0	2	0	1	0	0	0	0	0	0	3	6

826—Atopy	3	3	0	0	0	0	0	0	0	0	0	16	0	0	0	0	0	3	4
810—Gout	0	0	0	0	0	0	1	0	0	0	0	1	1	0	0	0	0	5	0
815—Jaundice	0	1	0	0	0	0	0	0	0	2	0	0	1	0	0	0	0	4	1
806—Deafness	0	0	0	0	0	0	0	0	0	0	0	0	0	1	0	0	1	1	2
818—Mental illness	0	1	0	0	0	0	0	0	0	0	0	1	0	0	0	1	0	0	3
814—Infection, recurrent	0	0	0	0	0	0	0	0	0	0	1	0	0	0	0	0	0	2	0
819—Mental retardation	0	0	0	0	0	0	0	0	0	1	0	0	0	0	0	0	0	1	1
822—Stroke	0	0	0	0	0	0	0	0	0	0	0	1	1	0	0	0	1	1	1
817—Malformation	0	0	0	0	0	0	0	0	0	0	0	0	0	0	0	0	0	0	0

Diagnosis Category 22—Selective Therapeutic Index

904—Other psychotropic drugs	7	4	4	4	4	3	16	86	33	129	33	76	24	155	16	27	11	54	148	538
905—Thiazide diuretics	0	0	0	0	0	1	1	4	7	4	19	18	18	51	42	49	55	71	142	198
901—Steroids	1	2	3	4	7	6	14	22	11	17	5	20	16	39	20	14	26	13	103	137
902—Antidepressives	0	0	1	0	1	0	3	27	10	50	15	6	6	18	6	5	7	4	48	153
908—Other cardiac drugs	0	0	0	0	0	0	0	0	0	0	3	1	11	1	9	16	54	79	77	97
907—Cardiac glycosides	0	0	0	0	0	0	0	3	4	1	0	5	2	10	9	20	45	25	60	64
906—Specific hypotensives	0	0	0	0	0	0	0	2	1	3	7	0	19	11	18	7	8	21	53	44
903—Hypnotics	1	1	0	1	2	1	9	18	15	10	4	7	6	3	5	3	1	7	43	51

Conversion Code from RCGP to ICHPPC Classification System[*]

Ronald Schneeweiss, M.B., H. Winston Stuart, Jr, Jack Froom, M.D., Maurice Wood, M.B., Herbert L. Tindall, M.D., and Jenny D. Williamson

RCGP Code	RCGP Rubric	ICHPPC Equiv- alent(s)	RCGP Code	RCGP Rubric	ICHPPC Equiv- alent(s)
	RCGP CATEGORY 1— COMMUNICABLE DISEASES		14—Herpes Zoster		053—
			15—Mumps		072—
1—Tuberculosis (Respiratory System, Including Late Effects)		011—	16—Infective Hepatitis		070—
			17—Infectious Mononucleosis		075—
2—Tuberculosis (Other Forms)		011—	19—Bornholm's Disease		136—
3—Syphilis (Infectious and Sequelae)		090—	20—Oxyuriasis		127—
			21—Dermatophytosis		110—
4—Gonorrhea		098—	22—Scabies		133—
5—Intestinal Infectious Disease		009—	23—Epidemic Winter Vomiting (Viral, Acute, or Gastroenteric)		136—
6—Scarlet Fever		034—			
7—Erysipelas		034—	25—Viral Warts		0791
8—Whooping Cough		033—	26—Other Helminth Infection		127—
9—Meningococcal Infections		136—	28—Other Recognized Disease Not Included Here (Category 01)		136—
10—Poliomyelitis (Acute and Sequelae)		040—	29—Aseptic Meningitis due to Enterovirus		040—
11—Measles		055—	30—Pyrexia with Rash (Any Site)		057—
12—Rubella		056—	31—Pyrexia without Rash		7888
13—Chicken Pox		052—			

[*] For further background on the use and value of this conversion code see Schneeweiss, R., Stuart, H. W. Jr., Froom, J., et al.: A conversion code from the RCGP to the ICHPPC classification system. *Journal of Family Practice* 5:415, 1977.

RCGP Code	RCGP Rubric	ICHPPC Equiv- alent(s)
32—Other Sign, Symptom, or Incomplete Diagnosis (Category 01)		7889
35—Amoebiasis		008–
36—Yaws		136–
38—Leishmaniasis		136–
39—Trypanosomiasis		136–
40—Schistosomiasis		136–
41—Hydatidosis		127–
42—Filarial Infection		136–
43—Ancylostomiasis		127–
44—Pediculosis		132–
27—Other Virus Infection		0799
37—Malaria		084–

RCGP CATEGORY 2—
NEOPLASMS, INCLUDING RETICULOSES

RCGP Code	RCGP Rubric	ICHPPC Equiv- alent(s)
80—Ascites		199–
50—Buccal Cavity, Pharynx, or Lip		199–
51—Esophagus		151–
52—Stomach		151–
53—Colon		151–
54—Rectum		151–
55—Pancreas		199–
56—Larynx		162–
57—Bronchus, Lung, or Trachea		162–
58—Breast		174–
59—Cervix Uteri		180–
60—Corpus Uteri		180–
61—Prostate		188–
62—Bladder or Other Urinary Organs		188–
63—Other Genital Organs		188–
64—Skin		173–
65—Brain		199–
66—Hodgkin's Disease		201–
68—All Other Malignant Neoplasms, Including Blood and Lymph		199–
70—Breast		217–
71—Uterus		218–
72—Other Female Genitourinary Organs		228–
73—Skin		216–
74—All Other Benign Neoplasms		228–
67—Leukemia		201–
81—Pleural Effusion		0122
82—Other Sign, Symptom, or Incomplete Diagnosis (Category 02)		239–

RCGP CATEGORY 3—
ALLERGIC, ENDOCRINE, METABOLIC, AND NUTRITIONAL PROBLEMS

RCGP Code	RCGP Rubric	ICHPPC Equiv- alent(s)
85—Hay Fever		507–
86—Asthma		493–

RCGP Code	RCGP Rubric	ICHPPC Equiv- alent(s)
87—Allergic Dermatosis and Urticaria		708–
88—Hyperthyroidism		242–
89—Hypothyroidism Including Myxedema and Cretinism		244–
90—Other Thyroid Disease		240–
91—Diabetes Mellitus		250–
92—Hypovitaminosis		260–
93—Gout		274–
94—Other Recognized Disease Not Included Here (Category 03)		279–
95—Specific Allergies		691–
95A—Penicillin		977–
95B—Foods		692–
95C—Contact Allergies		692–
95D—Drugs		977–
95E—Other		977–
96—Serum Lipid Abnormalities		272–
97—Cushing's Syndrome		279–
98—Coeliac Disease		260–
99—Electrolyte Disturbance		7889
100—Exophthalmos		7889
101—Obesity		277–
102—Glycosuria		789–
103—Pigmentation		709–
104—Polyuria		7864
105—Other Sign, Symptom, or Incomplete Diagnosis (Category 03)		7889
106—Erythema Multiforme		709–

RCGP CATEGORY 4—
DISEASES OF BLOOD AND
BLOOD FORMING ORGANS

RCGP Code	RCGP Rubric	ICHPPC Equiv- alent(s)
110—Pernicious (Megaloblastic) Anemia		281–
111—Iron Deficiency (Hypochromic) Anemia		280–
112—Other Specific Anemias		285–
114—Other Recognized Disease Not Included Here (Category 04)		2899
120—Purpura, Secondary or Unspecified		287–
112—Other Sign, Symptom, or Incomplete Diagnosis (Category 04)		7889
113—Hemorrhagic Conditions Including Purpura		287–

RCGP CATEGORY 5—
MENTAL, PERSONALITY, AND
PSYCHONEUROTIC DISORDERS

RCGP Code	RCGP Rubric	ICHPPC Equiv- alent(s)
123—Excessive Smoking		3049
124—Paranoid States		295–

RCGP Code	RCGP Rubric	ICHPPC Equiv- alent(s)
124—Paranoid Personality Disorder		301–
125—Schizophrenia		295–
125—Schizoid Personality Disorder		301–
126—Affective Psychoses		296–
127—Senile and Presenile Dementia		294–
128—All Other Organic Psychoses		294–
129—Other and Unspecified Psychoses		298–
130—Anxiety Neurosis		3000
131—Hysterical Neurosis		3001
132—Phobic Neurosis		3009
133—Obsessive-Compulsive Neurosis		3009
134—Depressive Neurosis		3004
135—Neurosis Related to Physical Disorders		3001
136—Neurasthenia		3009
137—Other and Unspecified Neurosis		3009
138—Personality Disorders and Sexual Deviations (Psychological and Social)		301–
139—Drug Abuse		3048
140—Mental Retardation		315–
141—Abuse of Alcohol		3031
142—Delusions and Hallucinations		298–
143—Hyperkinesis		308–
144—Mental Disorders Associated with Physical Condition		309–
145—Frigidity		3056
146—Insomnia		3064
147—Tension Headache		3068
148—Enuresis		7862
148A—Encopresis		7889
149—Cardiac Arrhythmia		3001
150—Other Special Symptoms Not Elsewhere Classified		309–
151—Other Sign, Symptom, or Incomplete Diagnosis (Category 05)		7889
152—Impotence		3056
154—Stammer		309–
550—Dependent Personality Including Symbiotic and Maternal Maturing		301–
551—Masochistic		309–
552—Angry Aggressive		301–
553—Passive Aggressive		301–
554—Paranoid		301–
555—Narcissistic		309–
560—Acute Adult Marital Situation Reaction		307–
561—Chronic Adult Marital Situation Reaction		Y84–
562—Other Acute Adult Marital Situation Reaction		307–
563—Other Chronic Adult Marital Situation Reaction		Y94–
564—Acute Childhood Situation Reaction		307–

RCGP Code	RCGP Rubric	ICHPPC Equiv- alent(s)
565—Chronic Childhood Situation Reaction		Y94–
566—Acute Adolescent Situation Reaction		307–
567—Chronic Adolescent Situation Reaction		Y94–

RCGP CATEGORY 6— DISEASES OF NERVOUS SYSTEM AND SENSE ORGANS

RCGP Code	RCGP Rubric	ICHPPC Equiv- alent(s)
155—Vascular Lesions (Central Nervous System)		438–
156—Multiple Sclerosis (Diffuse Systemic)		340–
157—Parkinsonism		342–
158—Epilepsy		345–
159—Migraine		346–
160—Other Diseases of Central Nervous System		355–
161—Labyrinthitis		385–
165—Facial Nerve Paralysis		355–
166—Trigeminal Neuralgia		355–
167—Brachial Neuritis		355–
168—Sciatica		725–
169—Other Diseases of Peripheral Nerves or Ganglia		355–
170—Conjunctivitis and Ophthalmia		360–
171—Blepharitis		361–
172—Hordeolum or Stye		361–
173—Iritis		378–
174—Other Inflammatory Diseases of the Eye		378–
175—Lacrimal Apparatus (Including Tear Duct) Disease		378–
176—Refractive Errors		370–
177—Keratitis with or without Corneal Ulcer		378–
177A—Corneal Abrasion		918–
177B—Corneal Ulcer		378–
178—Strabismus		378–
179—Cataract		374–
180—Glaucoma		375–
181—Other Diseases of the Eye		378–
182—Otitis Externa		380–
183—Otitis Media (Acute)		3810
184—Otitis Media (Chronic)		3811
185—Mastoiditis		3879
186—Meniere's Disease		385–
187—Wax in Ear		3871
188—Otosclerosis		386–
189—Other Forms of Deafness		386–
190—Other Diseases of the Ear or Mastoid Process		3879
190A—Secretory Otitis		384–
195—Coma and Stupor		7889
196—Delirium		7889

RCGP Code	RCGP Rubric	ICHPPC Equiv- alent(s)
197—Convulsions		7802
198—Tremor		7803
199—Ataxia		7889
200—Vertigo		7805
201—Meningismus		7889
202—Diplopia		7889
203—Nystagmus		7889
204—Photophobia		7889
205—Tinnitus		7813
206—Paraesthesiae		7816
207—Other Sign, Symptom, or Incomplete Diagnosis (Category 06)		7889

RCGP CATEGORY 7— DISEASES OF CIRCULATORY SYSTEM

RCGP Code	RCGP Rubric	ICHPPC Equiv- alent(s)
209—Cor Pulmonale		426–
210—Rheumatic Heart Disease		390–
211—Acute Myocardial Infarction		410–
212—Other Ischemic Heart Disease		412–
213—Myocardial Degeneration from Other Causes		429–
214—Heart Block and Other Disorders of Rhythm		429–
215—Congestive Heart Failure		4270
216—Left Ventricular Failure (Acute)		4270
217—Other and Ill-Defined Heart Disease		429–
218—Benign Hypertension with or without Renal Disease		401–
219—Malignant Hypertension with or without Heart Disease		400–
220—Reynaud's Disease		443–
221—Arteriosclerosis		440–
222—Chilblains		443–
223—Peripheral Arterial Disease		443–
224—Varicose Veins of Lower Extremities		454–
225—Hemorrhoids		455–
226—Phlebitis and Thrombophlebitis		451–
227—Other Diseases of Circulatory System		4589
228—Other Venous Embolism and Thrombosis		451–
229—Pulmonary Embolism		450–
230—Angina of Effort		412–
231—Precordial Pain		7820
232—Cyanosis		7889
233—Syncope		7825
234—Edema		7826
235—Dyspnea		7832
236—Ascites		7889
237—Other Sign, Symptom, or Incomplete Diagnosis (Category 07)		7889

RCGP CATEGORY 8— DISEASES OF RESPIRATORY SYSTEM

RCGP Code	RCGP Rubric	ICHPPC Equiv- alent(s)
240—Coryza (Nonfebrile Common Cold)		460–
241—Febrile Cold and Influenza-like Illness		460–
242—Pharyngitis Including Febrile Sore Throat, and Tonsillitis		463–
242A—Acute Pharyngitis and Other Throat Infections		460–
242B—Streptococcal Throat Infection		034–
242C—Vincent's Infection		136–
243—Sinusitis Acute		461–
244—Laryngitis and Tracheitis		464–
245—Influenza Epidemic		470–
246—Pneumonia, Pneumonitis		486–
247—Bronchitis (Acute)		466–
248—Bronchitis (Chronic)		491–
249—Tonsillar and Adenoidal Hypertrophy		500–
250—Sinusitis (Chronic)		461–
251—Pleurisy		511–
252—Spontaneous Pneumothorax		519–
253—Pneumoconiosis		519–
254—Bronchiectasis		492–
255—Emphysema without Mention of Bronchitis		492–
256—Other Recognized Disease Not Included Here (Category 08)		519–
257—Rhinitis, Vasomotor or Allergic		507–
258—Bronchiolitis		466–
260—Pleural Effusion		0122
261—Catarrh		519–
262—Cyanosis		7889
263—Epistaxis		7830
264—Hemoptysis		7831
265—Dyspnea		7832
266—Stridor		7889
267—Cough		7833
268—Sputum (Noninfected)		7889
269—Sputum (Infected)		7889
270—Hoarseness		7835
271—Pleuritic Pain		7837
272—Other Sign, Symptom, or Incomplete Diagnosis (Category 08)		7889

RCGP CATEGORY 9— DISEASES OF DIGESTIVE SYSTEM

RCGP Code	RCGP Rubric	ICHPPC Equiv- alent(s)
273—Acute Gastritis		536–
274—Esophagitis		530–
275—Diseases of Teeth or Supporting Structures		520–

RCGP Code	RCGP Rubric	ICHPPC Equiv-alent(s)
276—Other Diseases of Buccal Cavity		528–
276A—Herpes Stomatitis		054–
276B—Herpangina		136–
276C—Oral Thrush		112–
277—Gastric Ulcer		533–
278—Duodenal Ulcer		532–
279—Pyloric, Juxtapyloric, or Prepyloric Ulcer		533–
280—Functional Gastric Disorders		536–
281—Other Diseases of Esophagus, Stomach, or Duodenum		536–
282—Appendicitis		540–
283—Hernia (Inguinal or Femoral)		550–
284—Other Hernias of Abdominal Cavity		553–
285A—Regional Enteritis (Crohn's Disease)		563–
285B—Ulcerative Colitis		563–
285C—Diverticulosis, Diverticulitis		562–
285D—Other Diseases of Intestines or Peritoneum		578–
286—Cholelithiasis		574–
287—Cholecystitis and Cholangitis without Calculus		574–
288—Other Diseases of Liver, Gall Bladder, or Pancreas		578–
289—Cirrhosis of the Liver		571–
290—Constipation		5640
291—Splenomegaly		7851
292—Anorexia		7840
293—Nausea		7841
294—Heartburn		7843
295—Dysphagia		7889
296—Hematemesis		7845
297—Hiccough		7889
298—Hepatomegaly		7851
299—Jaundice		7889
300—Ascites		7889
301—Colic		7855
302—Melena		7845
303—Diarrhea and/or Vomiting		7841
304—Emotionally Determined Digestive Disorder		564–
304A—Emotionally Determined Dyspepsia		536–
304B—Emotionally Determined Alteration of Large Bowel Function		564–
305—Appendicular Pain		7855
306—Abdominal Pain other than Colic		7855
307—Wind		7847
308—Other Sign, Symptom, or Incomplete Diagnosis (Category 09)		7889
309—Anal Fissure and Fistula		565–

RCGP CATEGORY 10—
DISEASES OF GENITOURINARY SYSTEM

RCGP Code	RCGP Rubric	ICHPPC Equiv-alent(s)
310—Nephritis and Nephrosis Including Glomerulo, Chronic		580–
311—Pyelitis and Pyelonephritis		5901
312—Calculi of Kidneys or Ureters		592–
313—Cystitis, Acute		595–
314—Cystitis, Chronic		595–
315—Urethritis Nonvenereal		597–
316—Other Infections of Urinary System Including Prostate		601–
317—Other Diseases of Urinary Tract		599–
318—Prostatic Hypertrophy (Benign)		600–
319—Hydrocele		603–
320—Epididymitis and Orchitis		604–
321—Other Diseases of Male Genitalia		607–
322—Breast Diseases other than Neoplasm		611–
323—Salpingitis and Oophoritis		612–
324—Uterovaginal Prolapse		623–
325—Dysmenorrhea		6263
326—Amenorrhea		6260
327—Irregular Menstruation		6264
328—Menorrhagia and Metrorrhagia		6262
329—Menopausal Symptoms		627–
330—Disorders of Menarche		629–
331—Other Diseases of Female Genitalia		629–
332—Cervical Erosion		620–
333—Ovulation Pain		6263
334—Other Disorders of Menstruation		6269
335—Vulvitis, Vaginitis, and Cervicitis, (Non venereal)		6221
336—Colic (Renal)		7860
337—Dysuria and Strangury		7860
338—Retention of Urine		7889
339—Incontinence of Urine		7863
340—Frequency		7864
341—Polyuria		7864
342—Dyspareunia		7867
343—Hematuria		789–
344—Other Sign, Symptom, or Incomplete Diagnosis (Category 10)		7889

RCGP CATEGORY 11—
PREGNANCY, PARTURITION, AND PUERPERIUM

RCGP Code	RCGP Rubric	ICHPPC Equiv-alent(s)
345—Genitourinary Infection during Pregnancy		635–
346—Toxemias of Pregnancy		637–

RCGP Code	RCGP Rubric	ICHPPC Equiv-alent(s)
347—Antepartum Hemorrhage		632–
348—Ectopic Pregnancy		631–
349—Malposition of Fetus in Uterus		649–
350—Abortion Spontaneous		643–
351—Normal Delivery		650–
352—Normal Pregnancy (Prenatal Care)		Y61–
352A—Normal Pregnancy		Y60–
352B—Multiple Pregnancy		649–
353—Placenta Previa		632–
354—Retained Placenta		677–
355—Forceps Delivery (All Indications)		661–
356—Malposition and/or Disproportion Affecting 2nd Stage		661–
357—Prolonged Labor		661–
358—Laceration and Episiotomy		661–
359—Puerperal Sepsis		677–
360—Puerperal Thrombophlebitis		677–
361—Puerperal Mastitis		678–
362—Other Complications of Pregnancy, Delivery, or Puerperium		649–
363—Postpartum Hemorrhage		661–
364—Cesarean Section (All Indications)		661–
365—Pyrexia of Childbirth and Puerperium		677–
367—Abortion Induced		640–
366—Other Sign, Symptom, or Incomplete Diagnosis (Category 11)		649–

RCGP CATEGORY 12—
DISEASES OF SKIN AND
CELLULAR TISSUE

RCGP Code	RCGP Rubric	ICHPPC Equiv-alent(s)
368—Pityriasis Rosea		6963
369—Acne		7061
370—Boil and Carbuncle		680–
371—Cellulitis of Finger and Toe		681–
372—Other Cellulitis without Mention of Lymphangitis		680–
373—Infantile Eczema		691–
374—Cellulitis and Abcess with Lymphangitis		683–
375—Impetigo		684–
377—Other Infections of Skin and Subcutaneous Tissue		685–
378—Seborrheic Dermatitis		690–
379—Atopic Dermatitis (Eczema)		691–
380—Contact Dermatitis		692–
381—Other Dermatitis		692–
382—Psoriasis		6961
383—Pruritis		698–

RCGP Code	RCGP Rubric	ICHPPC Equiv-alent(s)
384—Corns and Callosities		700–
385—Other Hypertrophic and Atrophic Conditions of Skin		709–
386—Other Dermatoses		709–
387—Disease of Nail and Nail Bed		703–
388—Disease of Hair and Hair Follicle		704–
389—Disease of Sweat and Sebaceous Glands		705–
390—Chronic Ulcer of Skin		707–
391—Dermatitis Herpetiformis, Pemphigus, and Erythema		709–
394—Insect Bites		910–
395—Erythema		709–
397—Pigmentation		709–
398—Rash		7882
399—Other Sign, Symptom, or Incomplete Diagnosis (Category 12)		7889

RCGP CATEGORY 13—
DISEASES OF BONE AND ORGANS
OF MOVEMENT

RCGP Code	RCGP Rubric	ICHPPC Equiv-alent(s)
400—Cervical Injury (eg, Whiplash, Excluding Fractured Disc)		8470
401—Spasm of Neck Muscle with or without Torticollis		720–
404—Cervical Spondylosis		7131
405—Rheumatoid Arthritis		712–
406—Osteoarthritis		713–
407—Backache Not Attributed to Disc Lesion		7289
408—Fibrositis and Muscular Rheumatism		7179
409—Other Forms of Arthritis and Rheumatism		715–
410—Torn Meniscus of Knee		724–
411—Other Internal Derangements of Knee		724–
412—Displacement of Intervertebral Disc		725–
413—Flat Foot		738–
414—Hallux Valgus or Varus		738–
415—Other Recognized Disease Not Included Here (Category 13)		739–
415A—Femoral Anteversion		754–
416—Genu Valgum or Varum		738–
416A—Tibial Torsion		738–
417—Scoliosis and Kyphoscoliosis		735–
418—Osteoporosis		7230
420—Bursitis		731–
421—Tenosynovitis		731–
422—Synovitis		731–
423—Backache with Sciatica		725–
424—Backache with Other Neuritis		7289

RCGP Code	RCGP Rubric	ICHPPC Equiv- alent(s)
425—Back Pain Alone		7289
426—Frozen Shoulder		717–
427—Other Sign, Symptom, or Incomplete Diagnosis (Category 13)		7889
428—Pain in Joint (Arthralgia)		7873

RCGP CATEGORY 14— CONGENITAL MALFORMATIONS

RCGP Code	RCGP Rubric	ICHPPC Equiv- alent(s)
402—Congenital Dislocated Hip		754–
403—Congenital Talipes		754–
429—Anencephaly, Microcephaly, and Monstrosity		758–
430—Spina Bifida and Meningocele with Hydrocephalus		758–
431—Spina Bifida and Meningocele without Hydrocephalus		758–
432—Congenital Hydrocephalus		758–
433—Congenital Malformations of Circulatory System		746–
434—Cleft Palate and Hair Lip		758–
435—Congenital Malformation of Digestive System		758–
436—Congenital Malformation of Genitourinary System		758–
437—Congenital Malformation of Bone and Joint		758–
438—Other Recognized Disease Not Included Here (Category 14)		758–
438A—Chromosomal Abnormality		758–
439—Other Imprecisely Defined Congenital Abnormality		758–

RCGP CATEGORY 15— CERTAIN DISEASES OF EARLY INFANCY

RCGP Code	RCGP Rubric	ICHPPC Equiv- alent(s)
5—Diarrhea of Newborn		778–
170—Ophthalmia Neonatorum		778–
246—Pneumonia of Newborn		778–
440—Birth Injury due to Difficult Labor		778–
441—Respiratory Distress Syndrome		778–
443—Birth Injury to Brain, Spinal Cord, Bone, or Nerve		778–
445—Umbilical Sepsis		778–
447—Hemolytic Disease		778–
448—Hemorrhagic Disease		778–
449—Immaturity, Dysmaturity		778–
451—Other Recognized Disease Not Included Here (Category 15)		778–
452—Feeding Problems		2699
453—Failure to Thrive		778–

RCGP CATEGORY 16— SYMPTOMS, SIGNS, AND ILL-DEFINED CONDITIONS

RCGP Code	RCGP Rubric	ICHPPC Equiv- alent(s)
444—Lymphadenopathy, Enlargement of Lymph Nodes		7827
446—Debility and Fatigue		7901
450—Sleep Disturbance		3064
454—Headache		791–
455—Malingering		7889
456—Dehydration		7889
457—Weight Loss		7884
458—Pyrexia of Unknown Origin		7888
459—Rigors		7889
460—Albuminuria		789–
462—Uremia (Raised BUN)		251–
463—Senility		794–
464—Other Sign, Symptom, or Incomplete Diagnosis (Category 16)		7889
466—Sweating		7881

RCGP CATEGORY 17— ACCIDENTS, POISONING, AND VIOLENCE

RCGP Code	RCGP Rubric	ICHPPC Equiv- alent(s)
465—Foreign Body Not Entering Through Orifice		888–
467—Fracture of Spine		805–
468—Fracture of Femur		820–
469—Fracture of Tibia and/or Fibula		823–
470—Fracture of Skull		802–
471—Fracture of Ribs		807–
472—Fracture of Pelvis		829–
473—Fracture of Clavicle		810–
474—Fracture of Humerus		812–
475—Colles' Fracture		813–
476—Fracture of Carpal, Metacarpal, Tarsal, or Metatarsal		814–
477—Fracture of Phalanges		816–
478—Dislocation of Jaw		839–
479—Dislocation of Shoulder		839–
480—Sprains and Strains		848–
481—Intracranial Injury Excluding Fracture of Skull		850–
482—Internal Injury of Chest, Abdomen, or Pelvis		959–
483—Lacerations, Amputations, Contusions, and Abrasions		889–
484—Foreign Body Entering Through Orifice		939–
485—Burns, First-Degree		949–
486—Burns, Second-Degree		949–
487—Burns, Third-Degree		949–
488—Effects of Alcohol Poisoning		989–
489—Effects of Carbon Monoxide Poisoning		989–

RCGP Code	RCGP Rubric	ICHPPC Equivalent(s)
490—Effects of Barbiturate Poisoning		977–
491—Effects of Aspirin Poisoning		977–
492—Motion Sickness		994–
493—Other Recognized Disease Not Included Here (Category 17)		959–
494—Other Sign, Symptom, or Incomplete Diagnosis (Category 17)		7889
495—Other Fractures Not Included Here		829–
496—Adverse Effects of Other Drugs		977–
497—Dislocation of Radial Head		839–
497—Adverse Effects of Hallucinogens		977–

RCGP CATEGORY 18— PROPHYLACTIC PROCEDURES

RCGP Code	RCGP Rubric	ICHPPC Equivalent(s)
500—Cervical Smear		Y00–
504—Health Education and Counseling		Y71–
505—Other Prophylactic Procedures		Y00–
510—Routine Medical Examination Including Geriatric		Y00–
511—Other Preventive or Presymptomatic Examination		Y00–
511A—Medical Examination for Administrative Purposes		Y00–
511B—Well-Baby Check		Y00–
541—TB (BCG)		Y02–
542—Smallpox		Y02–
543—Diptheria		Y02–
543—Whooping Cough		Y02–
543—Tetanus		Y02–
544—Poliomyelitis		Y02–
545—Rubella		Y02–
546—Measles		Y02–
556—Typhoid or Paratyphoid		Y02–
557—Yellow Fever		Y02–
558—Cholera		Y02–
559—Tetanus Alone		Y02–
568—Other Disease Immunization		Y02–
578—Sterilization Male or Female		Y40–
578A—Vasectomy		Y40–
578B—Female Sterilization		Y40–
585—Oral Contraceptive Advice		Y41–
586—Other Contraceptive Advice		Y43–
587—Intrauterine Device (IUD)		Y42–

RCGP CATEGORY 19— ABNORMAL FINDINGS OF INVESTIGATIONAL PROCEDURES

RCGP Code	RCGP Rubric	ICHPPC Equivalent(s)
601—Abnormal Urine Examination		789–
602—Abnormal Urinalysis		789–
603—Abnormal Urine Culture		789–
604—Abnormal Urine Test		789–
610—Abnormal Hematology		2896
611—Abnormal Blood Count		2896

RCGP Code	RCGP Rubric	ICHPPC Equivalent(s)
612—Abnormal Blood Test		2896
620—Abnormal Blood Sugar		251–
621—Abnormal Blood Urea		251–
622—Abnormal Electrolytes		251–
623—Abnormal Thyroid Function		251–
624—Abnormal Liver Function		251–
625—Other Abnormal Biochemistry		251–
630—Abnormal ECG		429–
631—Abnormal Chest X-Ray		7887
632—Abnormal GI Series X-Ray		7887
637—Abnormal Other X-Ray		7887
635—Abnormal Findings at Other Instrumental Tests		7887
640—Abnormal Findings at Sigmoidoscopy		7887
641—Abnormal Findings at Esophagoscopy		7887
642—Abnormal Findings at Cystoscopy		7887
643—Abnormal Findings at Lumbar Puncture		7887
644—Abnormal Findings at Other Procedure		7887
645—Abnormal PAP Smear		7887

RCGP CATEGORY 20— PSYCHOSOCIAL AND FAMILY PROBLEMS

RCGP Code	RCGP Rubric	ICHPPC Equivalent(s)
700—Economic Problems		Y80–
701—Housing Problems		Y81–
702—Medical Care Problems		Y83–
703—Educational Problems		Y90–
704—Family Relationship Problems		Y89–
704A—Marital Conflict		Y84–
704B—Parent/Child Conflict		Y85–
704C—In-law Problems		Y86–
704D—Other Family Relationship Problems		Y89–
705—Legal Problems		Y96–
706—Other High-Risk Family Situations		Y89–
707—Pregnancy and Birth Out-Of-Wedlock in Parent or Child		Y91–
708—Social Isolation		Y92–
709—Occupational Maladjustment		Y93–
710—Dependency		Y95–
711—Physical Disability Chronic		Y94–
712—Other High-Risk Individual		Y17–
713—Out of Work, Acute		Y93–
714—Out of Work, Chronic		Y93–
715—Medical Absenteeism		Y93–
716—Unemployment due to Illness		Y93–
717—Other Employment Problems		Y93–
718—Imprisonment		Y96–
719—Prosecution or Impending Litigation		Y96–

RCGP Code	RCGP Rubric	ICHPPC Equiv- alent(s)
721—Divorce Proceedings		Y96–
722—Other Social Problems in Family or Individual		Y95–
723—High-Risk Infant		Y17–
724—High-Risk Pregnancy		Y17–
725—High-Risk Accident		Y17–
726—High-Risk Physical Violence		Y17–
727—Alcoholism in Parent or Child		Y85–
728—Drug Abuse in Parent or Child		Y85–
729—Other Social and Personal Problems		Y95–
730—Other Legal Problems		Y96–
731—Adopted Child		Y85–
732—Foster Child		Y85–

RCGP CATEGORY 21—
FAMILY HISTORY OF SELECTED DISEASES

These RCGP codes have no equivalents in the ICHPPC. A parallel classification can be maintained with a modifying letter, e.g.,

819—Mental Retardation		F315–

RCGP CATEGORY 22—
SELECTED DRUG INDEX

RCGP Code	RCGP Rubric	ICHPPC Equiv- alent(s)
585—Birth Control Pills		Y41–
901—Corticosteroids or ACTH		Y16–
902—Antidepressives		Y16–
903—Hypnotics		Y16–
904—Other Psychotropic Drugs		Y16–
905—Thiazide Diuretics		Y16–
906—Specific Hypotensives		Y16–
907—Cardiac Glycosides		Y16–
908—Other Cardiac Drugs		Y16–
909—Birth Control Pills		Y41–
910—Antibiotics and Other Anti-Infective Agents		Y16–
911—Oral Hypoglycemics		Y16–
912—Insulin		Y16–
913—Hormones other than Listed Above		Y16–
914—Anticoagulants		Y16–
915—L-Dopa		Y16–
916—Other Drugs Presenting a Risk		Y16–

Preventive Medicine Approaches
A LIFETIME HEALTH-MONITORING PROGRAM—GOALS AND PROFESSIONAL SERVICES *

For each of the ten age groups, a set of distinct health goals and professional services is desirable.

PREGNANCY AND PERINATAL PERIOD

Health Goals

1. To provide the mother a healthy, full-term pregnancy and rapid recovery after a normal delivery.
2. To facilitate the live birth of a normal baby, free of congenital or developmental damage.
3. To help both mother and father achieve the knowledge and capacity to provide for the physical, emotional, and social needs of the baby.

Professional Services

1. Prior education and appropriate counseling for parents expecting their first baby in physical, emotional, and social aspects of childbearing and infant care, including family planning.

---

* From: Breslow, L., and Somers, A. R.: The lifetime health-monitoring program: A practical approach to preventive medicine. *New England Journal of Medicine* 296:601, 1977.

2. Antenatal and postnatal care for mother and baby, education/counseling for both parents, and risk assessment throughout the perinatal period, as needed.
3. Delivery services, including specialized perinatal care, as needed.

INFANCY (FIRST YEAR)

Health Goals

1. To establish immunity against specified infectious diseases.
2. To detect and prevent certain other diseases and problems before irreparable damage occurs.
3. To facilitate growth and development to the infant's optimal potential.
4. To provide a basis for lifetime emotional stability, especially through a loving relation with mother, father, and other family members.

Professional Services

1. Before discharge from the hospital, tests for inherited metabolic and certain other congenital disorders; parent counseling.
2. Four postdischarge professional visits with the healthy infant during the year for observation, specified immunizations, and parent counseling.

PRESCHOOL CHILD (1 TO 5 YEARS)

Health Goals

1. To facilitate the child's optimal physical, emotional and social growth and development.
2. To begin the process of socialization through happy and effective family relations and gradual introduction to school and other facets of the outside world.

Professional Services

1. Two professional visits with the healthy child and mother (ideally, the father also) at 2 to 3 years and at school entry for compliance with immunization schedule and for observation and counseling about nutrition, activity, vision, hearing, speech, dental health, accident prevention, and general physical, emotional, and social development.
2. For special high-risk groups, blood tests for anemia, lead poisoning, and tuberculosis.

SCHOOL CHILD (6 TO 11 YEARS)

Health Goals

1. To facilitate the child's optimal physical/mental/emotional/social growth and development, including a positive self image.
2. To establish healthy behavioral patterns for nutrition, exercise, study, recreation, and family life as a foundation for a healthy lifetime lifestyle.

Professional Services

1. Two professional visits with the healthy child (at 6 to 7 and 9 to 10 years of age), including one complete physical/mental/behavioral/social examination, with appropriate tests for, and follow-up observation of, any physical or mental impairment, including obesity, vision and hearing defects, muscular incoordination and learning disabilities, and completion of any necessary immunizations.
2. Mandatory school health education and individual counseling, as needed, for physical fitness, nutrition, exercise, study, accident prevention, sexual development, and use of cigarettes, drugs, and alcohol.
3. Annual dental examination and prophylaxis.

ADOLESCENCE (12 TO 17 YEARS)

Health Goals

1. To continue optimal physical/mental/emotional/social growth and development.
2. To reinforce healthy behavior patterns, and discourage negative ones, in physical fitness, nutrition, exercise, study, work, recreation, sex, individual relations, driving, smoking, alcohol, and drugs as foundation for healthy lifetime lifestyle, including marriage, parenthood, and career or job.

Professional Services

1. Mandatory school health education and individual counseling, as needed, for the above subjects, including a course in sex, marriage, and family relations as a prerequisite to graduation from high school.
2. One professional visit with the healthy adolescent (at about 13 years of age) with attention to emotional status, vision and hearing, skin, blood pressure, blood cholesterol, and contraception.
3. Annual dental examination and prophylaxis.

YOUNG ADULTHOOD (18 TO 24 YEARS)

Health Goals

1. To facilitate transition from dependent adolescence to mature, independent adulthood with maximum physical, mental, and emotional resources.
2. To achieve useful employment and maximum capacity for a healthy marriage, parenthood, and social relations.

Professional Services

1. One professional visit with the healthy adult, including complete physical examination; tetanus booster if not received within 10 years; tests for syphilis, gonorrhea, malnutrition, cholesterol, and hypertension; and medical and behavioral history. This visit may be provided upon entrance into college, the armed forces, or first full-time job, but should be before marriage.
2. Health education and individual counseling, as needed, for nutrition, exercise, study, career, job, occupational hazards and problems, sex, contraception, marriage and family relations, alcohol, drugs, smoking, and driving.
3. Dental examination and prophylaxis every two years.

YOUNG MIDDLE AGE (25 TO 39 YEARS)

Health Goals

1. To prolong the period of maximum physical energy and to develop full mental, emotional, and social potential.
2. To anticipate and guard against the onset of chronic diseases through good health habits and early detection and treatment where effective.

Professional Services

1. Two professional visits with the healthy person—at about 30 and 35—including tests for hypertension, anemia, cholesterol, and cervical and breast cancer and instruction in self examination of breasts, skin, testes, neck, and mouth.
2. Professional counseling regarding nutrition, exercise, smoking, alcohol, marriage, parental relations, and other aspects of health-related behavior and lifestyle.
3. Dental examination and prophylaxis every two years.

OLDER MIDDLE AGE (40 TO 59 YEARS)

Health Goals

1. To prolong the period of maximum physical energy and optimum mental and social activity, including menopausal adjustment.
2. To detect as early as possible any of the major chronic diseases, including hypertension, heart disease, diabetes, and cancer, as well as vision, hearing, and dental impairments.

Professional Services

1. Four professional visits with the healthy person, once every five years—at about 40, 45, 50, and 55—with complete physical examination and medical history, tests for specific chronic conditions, appropriate immunizations and counseling regarding changing nutritional needs; physical activities; occupational, sex, marital, and parental problems; and use of cigarettes, alcohol, and drugs.
2. For those over 50, annual tests for hypertension, obesity, and certain cancers.
3. Annual dental prophylaxis.

THE ELDERLY (60 TO 74 YEARS)

Health Goals

1. To prolong the period of optimum physical/mental/social activity.
2. To minimize handicapping and discomfort from onset of chronic conditions.
3. To prepare in advance for retirement.

Professional Services

1. Professional visits with the healthy adult at 60 years of age and every two years thereafter, including the same tests for chronic conditions as in older middle age, and professional counseling regarding changing lifestyle related to retirement, nutritional requirements, absence of children, possible loss of spouse, and probable reduction in income, as well as reduced physical resources.
2. Annual immunization against influenza (unless the person is allergic to vaccine).
3. Annual dental prophylaxis.
4. Periodic podiatry treatments as needed.

OLD AGE (75 YEARS AND OVER)

Health Goals

1. To prolong period of effective activity and ability to live independently, and to avoid institutionalization so far as possible.
2. To minimize inactivity and discomfort from chronic conditions.
3. When illness is terminal, to assure as little physical and mental distress as possible and to provide emotional support to patient and family.

Professional Services

1. Professional visit at least once a year, including complete physical examination and medical and behavioral history, and professional counseling regarding changing nutritional requirements, limitations on activity and mobility, and living arrangements.
2. Annual immunization against influenza (unless the person is allergic to vaccine).
3. Periodic dental and podiatry treatments as needed.
4. For low-income and other persons not sick enough to be institutionalized but not well enough to cope entirely alone, counseling regarding sheltered housing, health visitors, home helps, day care and recreational centers, meals-on-wheels, and other measures designed to help them remain in their own homes and as nearly independent as possible.
5. Professional assistance with family relations and preparations for death, if needed.

FLOW SHEET FOR HEALTH SCREENING OF ADULTS

See chart on facing page.

TEST	AGE	21	22	23	24	25	26	27	28	29	30	31	32	33	34	35	36	37	38	39	40	41	42	43	44	45	46	47	48	49	50	51	52	53	54	55	56	57	58	59	60	61	62	63	64	65	66	67	68	69	70
Complete History and Physical Examination		●	●	●																																															
History of Rheumatic Fever																																																			
Smoking History		●	●	●																	●										●										●										●
History of Alcohol Use		●	●	●	●		●		●		●		●		●		●		●		●			●		●			●		●			●		●			●		●		●		●		●		●		●
Blood Pressure		●	●		●		●		●		●		●		●		●		●		●	●		●	●		●		●		●		●		●		●		●		●		●		●		●		●		●
Weight and Height		●	●		●		●		●		●		●		●		●		●		●		●		●		●		●		●		●		●		●		●		●		●		●		●		●		●
Pap Smear		●					●	●	●			●			●		●		●		●			●	●			●			●		●		●		●		●		●				●						
Cholesterol		●					●										●				●																														
VDRL		●																																																	
PPD		●																																																	
Stool for Occult Blood																					●		●		●		●		●		●		●		●		●		●		●		●	●	●	●	●	●	●	●	●
Teach Self Palpation Breast, Neck, Testes		●									●										●										●										●										
Teach to Report Mouth Sores or Lesions																					●										●										●										
Teach to Report Post Menopausal Bleeding																															●										●										
Tonometry and Funduscopy																																	●				●								●				●		
Proctosigmoidoscopy																																			●	●															
Physician Breast Check		●	●		●		●		●		●						●				●						●				●		●		●		●		●		●			●	●		●		●	●	●

Source: Frame PS, Carlson SJ: A critical review of periodic health screening using specific screening criteria. J. Fam Pract 2:289, 1975.

497

Department of Family Medicine (R700)
University of Miami School of Medicine
P. O. Box 016700
Miami, Florida 33101

APPENDIX EIGHT

James M. Gall M. D., C. C. F. P.
Department   mily Medicine
University   i School of Medicine
P. O. Bo
Miami   33 01

Community Resources:
AVAILABLE COMMUNITY RESOURCES*

HEALTH DEPARTMENTS

- Child health clinics
- Immunization clinics
- Family planning clinics
- Tuberculosis clinics
- WIC (women–infants–children) food supplement programs
- Public health nurses
- Children's dental services
- Children and youth clinics
- Venereal disease clinics

HOME CARE AGENCIES

Nationwide Agencies

- Visiting nurse service (and other Medicare and state-certified home health agencies)

* Source: Werblun M. N., Twersky, R. K.: Use of Community Resources. In Rosen, G. M., Geyman, J. P., Layton, R. H. (eds.): Behavioral Science in Family Practice. New York, Appleton, 1980.

- Medical personnel pool
- Manpower medical services
- Homemakers, Inc.
- We Sit Better
- Others—usually listed in the yellow pages under "Nurses"

SOCIAL SERVICES—PUBLIC AGENCIES

Health and Welfare Agencies

DIVISION OF PUBLIC ASSISTANCE
- Information and referral service
- Financial aid
  - ACD (aid to families with dependent children)
  - GAU (general assistance to the unemployed)
  - Food stamp program
  - Medicaid
- Case work services
  - Child care
  - Homemaker services
- Child welfare services (foster care)
- Child protective services

STATE SERVICES FOR THE BLIND
BUREAU OF DEVELOPMENTAL DISABILITIES—
EMPLOYMENT SERVICES
- Job services
- Unemployment compensation

COUNSELING SERVICES

Community Mental Health Centers

- Individual
- Group
- Day treatment
- Crisis outreach teams
- Growth groups, e.g., family life education

Family Agencies (should be members of the Family Service Association of America)

- Individual

- Group
- Family life education classes

Other

- Sexual assault centers
- Private practice counselors, e.g., psychiatrists, psychologists, and social workers

DISEASE-RELATED AGENCIES

- American Cancer Society
- Cancer Life-Line
- American Diabetes Association
- Cerebral Palsy Center
- Childbirth Education Association
- Association for Retarded Citizens
- Multiple Sclerosis Association
- Muscular Dystrophy Association
- Spastic Children's Clinic
- State Lung Association
- Speech and Hearing Clinics

SHORT-TERM EMERGENCY ASSISTANCE

- American Red Cross (disaster relief; servicemen's families)
- Salvation Army Welfare Service
- Milk Fund (funds for food in households with children)

INFORMATIONAL AND REFERRAL SERVICES

- United Way
- Department of Social and Health Services
- Easter Seals (handicapped services)
- Senior Services (over 60 age group)
- Alcoholism Agency
- Center for Addiction Services
- Medicare Information—Social Security Office
- Crisis clinics

SELECTED LIST OF VOLUNTARY HEALTH AGENCIES*

Alcoholics Anonymous World Service, Inc.
305 East 45 Street
New York, New York 10017

National Council on Alcoholism, Inc.
New York Academy of Medicine
2 East 103 Street
New York, New York 10029

The Allergy Foundation of America
801 Second Avenue
New York, New York 10017

The Arthritis Foundation
1212 Avenue of the Americas
New York, New York 10036

The American Foundation for the Blind
15 West 16 Street
New York, New York 10011

The National Society for the Prevention of
Blindness, Inc.
16 East 40 Street
New York, New York 10016

Braille Institute of America, Inc.
741 North Vermont Avenue
Los Angeles, California 90029

The Brain Research Foundation
39 South LaSalle Street
Chicago, Illinois

The American Cancer Society
219 East 42 Street
New York, New York 10017

The United Cerebral Palsy Association
321 West 44 Street
New York, New York 10036

The Association for the Aid of Crippled
Children
345 46 Street
New York, New York 10017

The National Society for Crippled
Children and Adults
2023 West Ogden Avenue
Chicago, Illinois 60612

The National Foundation
800 Second Avenue
New York, New York 10017

The National Cystic Fibrosis Research
Foundation
521 Fifth Avenue
New York, New York 10017

The American Diabetes Association
1 East 45 Street
New York, New York 10017

National Council on Family Relations
1219 University Avenue, S.E.
Minneapolis, Minnesota 55414

Family Service Association of America
44 East 23 Street
New York, New York 10010

The Margaret Sanger Research Bureau
17 West 16 Street
New York, New York 10011

American Association of Marriage Counselors, Inc.
285 Madison Avenue
New York, New York 10017

Planned Parenthood—World Population
515 Madison Avenue
New York, New York 10022

National Association on Service to
Unmarried Parents
44 East 23 Street
New York, New York 10010

The American Hearing Society
919 18 Street N.W.
Washington, D.C. 20006

* Source: Farley, E. S., Treat D. F.: Utilization of Community Resources. In Conn, H. F., Rakel, R. E., Johnson, T. W. (eds): Family Practice. Philadelphia, Saunders, 1973, p. 125.

American Speech and Hearing Association
1001 Connecticut Avenue N.W.
Washington, D.C.

The American Heart Association
44 East 23 Street
New York, New York 10010

The National Hemophilia Foundation
175 Fifth Avenue, Room 1012
New York, New York 10010

The National Kidney Foundation
342 Madison Avenue
New York, New York 10017

The Leukemia Society, Inc.
211 East 43 Street
New York, New York

The American Association for Maternal
  Child Health
116 South Michigan Avenue
Chicago, Illinois

The Maternity Center Association
48 East 92 Street
New York, New York 10028

Medic Alert Foundation International
Turlock, California 95380

The National Association for Mental
  Health
10 Columbus Circle
New York, New York 10019

The National Multiple Sclerosis Society
257 Park Avenue South
New York, New York

Muscular Dystrophy Association of
  America, Inc.
1790 Broadway
New York, New York 10019

The Myasthenia Gravis Foundation, Inc.
2 East 103 Street
New York, New York 10029

Narcotics Education
6830 Laurel Avenue
Washington, D.C. 20012

Synanon Foundation
1910 Ocean Front
Santa Monica, California 90406

The National Foundation for Neuro-
  muscular Disease, Inc.
250 West 57 Street
New York, New York 10029

American Association of Poison Control
  Centers
New York City Department of Health
125 North Street
New York, New York 10013

American Psychological Association
1200 17th Street N.W.
Washington, D.C. 20036

The American National Red Cross
17 and D Streets N.W.
Washington, D.C. 20026

The National Rehabilitation Association
1029 Vermont Avenue
Washington, D.C.

The Sister Elizabeth Kenny Foundation,
  Inc.
1800 Chicago Avenue
Minneapolis, Minnesota 55404

The National Association for Retarded
  Children, Inc.
420 Lexington Avenue
New York, New York 10017

American Association of Retired Persons
1225 Connecticut Avenue N.W.
Washington, D.C. 20036

National Safety Council
425 North Michigan Avenue
Chicago, Illinois 60611

The American Social Health Association
1790 Broadway, Room 1402
New York, New York 10019

The National Tuberculosis Association
1790 Broadway
New York, New York 10019

Veterans' Administration
Washington, D.C.

COMMUNITY RESOURCE QUESTIONNAIRE*

We are seeking to identify resources for our patients and therefore are asking your help in telling us about the services your organization offers.

Please answer the following questions as completely as possible and then return this questionnaire in the enclosed self-addressed envelope.

1. Name of your organization:_____

2. Address:_____
   (street)

   Phone:_____   _____
                            (city)   (state)   (zip code)

3. Director of the organization:_____
                                (name)   (title)

   Phone:_____
                                              (business address)

4. What is the purpose of your organization?

   _____

5. List the services provided for patients with chronic conditions: (use the back if needed)

   _____

6. What geographical area do these services cover?

   _____

7. Source of financial support:_____

8. Fees charged for services: Yes_____   No_____

   If yes, amount for use of services: _____
9. Hours and/or days services available:

   _____

10. Management (Board of Directors, Executive Committee, etc. & Number)

   _____

11. To whom should one direct applications or requests for information?

_____

Thank you for your cooperation.

         _____

              (Doctor's name)

         _____

                (Address)

         _____

            (City, state, zip code)

         _____

                 (Date)

CONSENT FOR MUTUAL EXCHANGE OF INFORMATION*

I hereby give permission for a mutual exchange of information between

_____

Street address   City   State   Zip code

and _____ M.D., including any and all
information regarding the history, diagnostic, and treatment records and similar
information from the record of

_____

Patient name   Patient Birthdate

Approximate dates of service _____

_____

Signature of Person Giving Consent

_____   _____

Relationship   Date

_____   _____

Signature of Witness   Title

         (Name of Physician)

* Source: Werblun, M. N., Twersky, R. K.: Use of Community Resources. In Rosen, G. M., Geyman, J. P., Layton, R. H. (eds.): Behavioral Science in Family Practice. New York, Appleton, 1980.

Glossary for Primary Care
REPORT OF THE NORTH AMERICAN PRIMARY CARE RESEARCH GROUP (NAPCRG) COMMITTEE ON STANDARD TERMINOLOGY*

The recent upsurge of interest in primary health care within the academic medical community and government agencies has underscored the need for accurate ambulatory health care data. Essential to collection of such data are precise definitions of terms describing the process of primary care. Whenever possible, uniform, unambiguous definitions are required by research workers as well as by agencies concerned with reimbursement and health care planning.

In response to these needs in North America, an ad hoc committee of the North American Primary Care Research Group (NAPCRG) was formed in 1976. The product of the collaborative efforts of this committee, with suggestions from the general NAPCRG membership, is presented here in the form of a glossary of terms defining the process of primary health care delivery.

The definitions provided are intended as guidelines rather than absolute dicta for primary care providers and researchers who desire comparability. New knowledge, drifts in use of language with time, and new processes will inevitably require revision of definitions and the addition of new terms. Countries other than the United States and Canada may wish to make use of the glossary with certain modifications or they may feel that differences in definition of included terms are sufficient to preclude its use. A comprehensive dictionary is, however,

* Originally published in *The Journal of Family Practice*: 5, 633, 1977.

beyond the scope of this work. Included are terms most commonly used in the United States and Canada.

I. GENERAL

A. *Primary Care*—Primary care is a type of health care which emphasizes first-contact care and assumes ongoing responsibility for the patient in both health maintenance and therapy of illness; it is personal care involving a unique interaction and communication and includes the overall coordination of care of the patient's health problems with the appropriate use of consultants and community resources (modified American Medical Association definition).

B. *Health*—The state of optimal physical, mental, and social well-being and not merely the absence of disease or infirmity (modified World Health Organization definition).

C. *Health Care*—The provision of advice, therapy, education, etc., by qualified professionals to improve or maintain the health of one or more patients.

D. *Health Care System*—*Health Services System*—The organizational structure through which health care is provided.

E. *Recorder*—The individual transcribing the information under study.

F. *Practice Register*—The listing of all registered patients in a practice.

G. *Age–Sex Register*—The listing by age and sex of all registered patients in a practice.

H. *Problem Index* (Morbidity Index, Diagnostic Index, Disease Index, E Book are synonymous terms)—a compilation of lists of patients by problem or diagnosis.

II. PROVIDER DESCRIPTORS

Health Care Provider—Any individual who renders health services within the field of his/her qualifications.

Classification of Health Care Providers

A. *Physician*

1. Family Physician—The family physician provides health care in the discipline of family practice. His or her training and experience qualify him/her to practice in several fields of medicine and surgery.

The family physician is educated and trained to develop and bring to bear in practice unique attitudes and skills that qualify him or her to provide continuing, comprehensive health maintenance and medical care to the entire family regardless of sex, age, or type of problem, be it biological, behavioral, or social. This physician serves as the patients' or families' advocate in all health-related matters, including the appropriate use of consultants and community resources (American Academy of Family Physicians).

2. Other Primary Care Specialists—Practice limited by patient age, patient sex, or patient problem, or terms of physician's employment. (The Committee invites other primary care physician groups to submit definitions which describe their discipline.)

3. Physician in Graduate Training—Intern, Resident, Fellow.

4. Consultant—A physician having in-depth knowledge of a particular area of medicine who provides services related to this area on the request of another health care provider.

5. Specialist—A physician with in-depth knowledge and education in a particular area of medicine.

B. *Other Health Care Providers*—Include, for example, dentist, pharmacist, physicians associate, medex, nurse practitioner, graduate nurse, public health nurse, psychologist, social worker, pastor, etc. (The Committee invites these provider groups to submit definitions which describe their discipline.)

C. *Health Care Team*—Group of health care providers working cooperatively to provide health care is a health care team.

III. PRACTICE DESCRIPTORS

Practice—The organizational framework in which one or more physicians provide or supervise the health care for a discrete population of patients.

Manpower Classification of Practices

A. *Solo*—A practice where the population is cared for by a single physician.

B. *Group*—A practice where the population is cared for by more than one physician. The principal responsibility for subgroups (of the population) may be assigned to one or more physicians, but the ultimate responsibility rests with the group (physicians sharing only office space or some personnel, but not patients, shall be called an association of practices).

1. Single-Specialty Group—A practice where the population is cared for by a group of physicians each of whom has the same specialty.

2. Multispecialty Group—A practice where the population is cared for by a group of physicians representing more than one specialty.

Geographic Classification of Practices

A. *Central City*—A practice serving a discrete population, a majority of which are located in the central business district or downtown area of a city of 50,000 or more population.

B. *Urban*—A practice serving a discrete population, a majority of which are located in a city of 50,000 or more population.

C. *Suburban*—A practice serving a discrete population, a majority of which are located in a residential area adjacent to a city of 50,000 or more population, usually part of Standard Metropolitan Statistical Area or similar conurbation.

D. *Small City*—A practice serving a discrete population, a majority of which are located in a city with a population greater than 2500 but less than 50,000 and not part of Standard Metropolitan Statistical Area or similar conurbation.

E. *Rural*—A practice serving a discrete population, a majority of which are located in a farming area or town of less than 2500 population.

Income Classification of Practices

A. *Fee For Service*—Practice receives a fee for each service provided (either from patient or from third party).

B. *Prepaid*—The practice receives an advance payment to provide specified health services to a particular patient during a specified time period.

C. *Capitation*—Payment is based on the number of registered patients.

Special Function Practices

A. *Teaching*

B. *Institutional health services*

IV. PATIENT DESCRIPTORS

Family

A group of persons sharing a common household. A relationship (not necessarily by blood or marriage ties) is implied. For purposes of definition this includes persons who temporarily reside away from the household and single patients living alone.

A. *Registered Family*—A family containing at least one individual who has contracted for health care from a practice.

B. *Active Family*—A registered family containing at least one member who has received health care at least one time in the preceding two years.

C. *Attending Family*—A registered family containing at least one member who has received health care in the preceding year.

D. *Inactive Family*—A registered family containing at least one member who has received medical care in the past, but none who has received health care within the preceding two years.

E. *Former Family*—A previously registered family which is no longer considered (by the practice or by personal determination) to be part of the practice population and is removed from the register.

James M. Gall, M.D., C.C.F.P.
Department of Family Medicine
University of Miami School of Medicine
P. O. Box 016700
Miami, Florida 33101

Patient

A person who receives or contracts for professional advice or services from a health care provider.

    A. *Temporary or Transient Patient*—Patient who receives one or more services from the practice but who usually receives his/her health care elsewhere.

    B. *Registered Patient*—Patient who has contracted for ongoing health care from a practice (excludes former, temporary, or transient patient.)

    C. *Former Patient*—Patient (excluding temporary or transient) who has previously been registered but who is no longer considered (by the practice or by personal determination) to be part of the practice population and is removed from the register.

FOR PRACTICES REGISTERING BY FAMILIES

A. *Active Patient*—A registered patient who has received services from the practice at least one time *and* who belongs to a family, one member of which has received services within the last two years.

    B. *Inactive Patient*—A registered patient who has received services from the practice at least one time, but neither he/she nor any members of his/her family have received services within the last two years.

FOR PRACTICES NOT REGISTERING BY FAMILIES

A. *Visiting Patient*—A registered patient who has received services from the practice at least one time in the last two years. This includes attending patients.

    B. *Attending Patient*—A registered patient who has personally received services from the practice in the past year.

    C. *Nonvisiting Patient*—A registered patient who has received no services from the practice within the last two years.

Department of Family Medicine (R700)
University of Miami School of Medicine
P. O. Box 016700
Miami, Florida 33101

Statistics and Analysis

The following demographic data are desirable for statistical and analytical purposes:

    A. *Patient Identification*—Should be unique.

    B. *Residence*—There are several options for the classification of residence, which include address and census tract, postal or zip code, grid, or municipal jurisdiction.

    C. *Date of Birth*—Should be collected in such a way that age may be calculated to the nearest year.

    D. *Sex*—Male or female.

    E. *Marital Status*—Married (includes common-law), single, separated, divorced, or widowed.

    F. *Race*—Black, white, other (patient determined).

V. POPULATION DESCRIPTORS

A. *Study Population*—All patients included in a study during the period of a project.

B. *Registered Population*—The total of patients registered in a practice taken at the midpoint of the study. *Note:* 1. This population is usually difficult to determine in North American practices. 2. Current evidence indicates that it may be possible to calculate the practice population by reference to portions of encounter data. It should be clearly stated in any reports or papers if this method has been employed.

C. *Standard Age Groups*—< 1; 1–4; 5–14; 15–44; 45–64; $\geqslant 65$. These groups may be further subdivided into smaller cohorts provided the standard division points are retained.

VI. MORBIDITY DESCRIPTORS

A. *Problem*—A provider-determined assessment of anything that concerns the patient, the provider, or both. Problems should be recorded at the level of specificity determined at the time of that particular visit. The *International Classification of Health Problems for Primary Care* (ICHPPC) should be used to classify and code problems.

B. *New Problem*—The first presentation of a problem by a patient to a health care provider. This includes the first visit for a recurrence of a previously resolved problem, but excludes the presentation of a previously assessed problem to a different provider.

C. *Continuing Problem*—A previously assessed problem which requires ongoing care. It includes follow-up for a problem, or initial presentation to the provider of a problem previously assessed by another provider, and may be subdivided into old problem and follow-up for a problem.

D. *Episode*—The occurrence of a specific problem or illness in a patient extending over a period of time from its onset to its resolution.

E. *Diagnosis*—A formal statement of the provider's understanding of the patient's problem.

F. *Diagnostic Criteria*—Those facts and observations that lead to a diagnosis.

VII. ENCOUNTER DESCRIPTORS

A. *Encounter*—Any professional interchange between a patient and one or more members of the health care team.

B. *Indirect Encounter*—An encounter in which there is no physical or face-to-face meeting between the patient and the professional. These encounters may be subdivided by the mode of communication; that is, telephone encounter or written encounter.

C. *Direct Encounter*—An encounter in which there is a face-to-face meeting of the patient and professional. A direct encounter is the same as a visit.

D. *Classification of Direct Encounters*

1. Office visit—A direct encounter occurring in the provider's office.
2. Home visit—A direct encounter occurring at the patient's residential location (this includes home of a friend where a patient is visiting, hotel room, etc.).
3. Hospital visit—A direct encounter in the hospital setting. Count one encounter for each patient visited.
   a. Hospital inpatient visit—A direct encounter with an inpatient;
   b. Outpatient visit—A direct encounter with an outpatient in either the emergency room or the outpatient clinic.
4. Other direct encounters—These include accident scene, extended-care facility, and professional visits in a social setting, etc. *Note:* When more than one person is seen for problems of a single patient, the encounter is counted as one visit. When more than one person is seen for a shared problem, the encounter is counted as one visit.

E. *Classification of Reasons for Encounter*—A suitable classification of patient's reason for encounter has not yet been developed.

F. *Problem Contact*—A patient/provider transaction in regard to one problem. There may be several problem contacts during each encounter.

VIII. SERVICE DESCRIPTORS

A. *Service*—An action taken by the provider in order to improve or maintain the patient's and/or the family's health and well being. Health services may be classified into three large areas. They are as follows:

1. Diagnostic (investigative) services—These include a general assessment of any problem, annual health assessments, laboratory examinations performed both within and outside of the office setting, and others.
2. Therapeutic services—These include pharmacological therapy, surgical therapy, physical therapy, psychotherapy, and others.
3. Preventive services—These include immunizations, screening tests, education, pre- and postnatal checkups, well-baby care, family planning, and others.

Several items in the above classification may be classified in more than one section. A diagnostic service could be therapeutic or even preventive. Data items within this section must be defined carefully.

IX. STANDARD REPORTING

Acceptance of the preceding definitions should permit comparisons in the same terms. Allowance must also be made for the size of the study population and the duration of the report period, often a year. In all cases, *duration of the period should be stated*.

The effective size of the study population presents particular problems in North America because of nonattendance, absence of registration systems, and/or multiple attendances to different practices or teams. Thus, the effective size of the study population may be unknown.

Rates

Rates are defined as the number of events occurring to a study population as recorded by a given health care team, divided by the size of the study population. According to the previous definitions, the study population may be made up of any one of the following groups: registered patients, active patients, visiting patients, attending patients, etc.

Rates per 100 or per 1000 are typical, but this may change to 10,000 or 100,000 as the frequency of the event decreases.

For some rates the study population of patients may not constitute the denominator, which instead may refer to the provider, e.g., the number of patients seen per week per provider. Thus, we may construct rates with one of the following numerators: problems, encounters or services, patients, families, etc., and one of the following denominators: provider, team, practice, study population, registered practice population, attending practice population, etc.

Adjusted Rates

Two practices may still generate different rates for reasons unconnected with the underlying morbidity or operation of the practice. Thus, the direct encounter rate per hundred patients, in an attending population, will vary according to the age and sex composition of the attending population. To compare crude rates between practices it is necessary to standardize them by age and sex. The "adjusted rates" become comparable in spite of age and sex differences of the study population. Rates may also be standardized for other parameters measured in the study population.

Incidence

Incidence expresses the number of new episodes (cases) of a specific disease occurring in a population per year.

$$\begin{array}{c} \text{Incidence} \\ \text{(episodes per} \\ \text{1000 population)} \end{array} = \dfrac{\begin{array}{c}\text{new episodes}\\\text{reported during}\\\text{the year}\end{array}}{\begin{array}{c}\text{survey population}\\\text{at midpoint}\\\text{of the year}\end{array}} \times 1000$$

Prevalence

This is defined as the number of all episodes (cases) of a specific disease existing in a population at the designated time.

$$\begin{array}{c} \text{Point} \\ \text{prevalence} \\ \text{rate} \end{array} = \dfrac{\begin{array}{c}\text{all episodes}\\\text{of a particular}\\\text{disease at one}\\\text{point in time}\end{array}}{\begin{array}{c}\text{study population}\\\text{at that point}\\\text{in time}\end{array}} \times 1000$$

Examples of Crude Rates

1. *Incidence rate in attending population*—This rate will show the frequency of new events occurring in the attending population during a given period of time—traditionally a year.

2. *Prevalence rate in active patient population*—This rate will show the total number of episodes known to be existent in the active patients during a given period of time—traditionally a year.

$$\begin{array}{c} \text{3. } \textit{Annual direct} \\ \textit{encounter rate} \\ \text{per 100} \\ \text{active patients} \end{array} = \dfrac{\begin{array}{c}\text{number of direct}\\\text{encounters arising from}\\\text{the active patients}\\\text{in a given year}\end{array}}{\begin{array}{c}\text{number in 100s}\\\text{of the active patients}\\\text{in that year}\end{array}}$$

4. Specific subpopulation rates of incidence, prevalence, frequency of encounter, etc, may be determined for subsets of the population by substituting the number of events which have occurred within this subgroup in the numerator and the number of patients in the population subset in the denominator. Reports

should clearly indicate that this has been done, e.g., incidence among Caucasians, point prevalence for females, etc.

5. Specific rates may be computed for different combinations of sex, age, disease, and other factors.

Note: By changing the denominator from the "attending population" to the "registered population" similar rates "per 100 patients" are still generated. There is, however, a considerable difference between these rates, and the phrase "per patient" or "per active patient" should be chosen carefully to correspond with the appropriate denominator.

ACKNOWLEDGMENTS

The committee is grateful to the several members who carefully reviewed the revisions and who made suggestions, many of which were incorporated in the final manuscript. The general membership of NAPCRG approved the glossary at its 1977 Annual Meeting in Williamsburg, Virginia.

- John E. Anderson, M.D.—Queens University
- Martin Bass, M.D.—University of Western Toronto
- Russell M. Boyle—Medical College of Virginia
- Donald M. Freeman, M.D.—Baylor College of Medicine
- James Kilpatrick, Ph.D—Medical College of Virginia
- Maurice Wood, M.D.—Medical College of Virginia
- Jack Froom, M.D.—University of Rochester, Committee Chairman

Research Workbook:

A GUIDE FOR INITIAL PLANNING OF CLINICAL, SOCIAL, AND BEHAVIORAL RESEARCH PROJECTS

Michael J. Gordon, Ph.D.*

INTRODUCTION

Research has often been described as organized curiosity. But the skills and techniques of organizing one's curiosity seldom come naturally. The purpose of this workbook is to provide the clinician–researcher with an explicit approach to thinking about and recording each element in the initial development of a unique research plan.

The workbook is not a do-it-yourself manual for inexperienced researchers. It will provide useful questions, suggestions, and approaches to guide and stimulate the inventive thinking of the researcher, but it provides no answers, no assistance in making decisions, and no technical expertise. For these essentials, the clinician–researcher must rely on colleagues and competent research consultants.

An earlier version of the workbook has been used productively by numerous

Source: Originally published in The Journal of Family Practice: 7, 145, 1977.

* Dr. Michael J. Gordon is Research Associate Professor Department of Family Medicine, University of Washington, Seattle, Washington.

family practice residents, faculty, and other health science students. The current version has been included in this monograph at the suggestion of family physicians who were delighted to find that a simple, nontechnical aid, in conjunction with their own professional training, experience, and resourcefulness, could take them so far in organizing their curiosity.

I.　SELECT A RESEARCHABLE QUESTION

Begin by stating a question of great interest to you in a simple, nontechnical interrogative sentence.

_____

_____

_____

_____

As you complete the workbook exercises from this point through the development of your hypothesis (section IV), you will find it useful to rewrite your research question several times. Each revision should reflect greater precision and probably narrower scope in your search for an answer.

The research will require access to these resources.

1. _____   4. _____

2. _____   5. _____

3. _____   6. _____

Is the research feasible?　　Yes____　No____

Define the important terms in your statement of the research question.

	Terms		*Definitions*
1.	_____	1.	_____
			_____
2	_____	2.	_____
			_____
3.	_____	3.	_____
			_____

4.   ————————————   4.   ————————————

                                    ————————————

5.   ————————————   5.   ————————————

                                    ————————————

II.   SEARCH FOR RELATED WORK

List questions you hope are already
answered by previous research.

————————————————

————————————————

————————————————

————————————————

————————————————

Likely sources of information
(not necessarily in journals).

————————————————

————————————————

————————————————

————————————————

————————————————

List relevant theories or models.

————————————————

————————————————

————————————————

————————————————

————————————————

Likely sources of information

————————————————

————————————————

————————————————

————————————————

————————————————

Other background information
you could use.

————————————————

————————————————

————————————————

————————————————

————————————————

————————————————

Likely sources of information

————————————————

————————————————

————————————————

————————————————

————————————————

————————————————

III.   JUSTIFYING THE STUDY

Who cares about the answer?

How is present opinion divided?

How important is it to have the right answer?

What are the implications of various possible answers?

Write a paragraph justifying your study. Consider the questions above but feel free to modify or add to them.

_____

_____

_____

_____

_____

_____

_____

_____

_____

_____

_____

_____

_____

_____

IV.   HYPOTHESES

Hypotheses require the investigator to predict an answer to the research question based on knowledge of the field, logical analysis, and/or anecdotal observations. Purely descriptive studies do not require formal hypotheses. Even so, it is wise to commit yourself to a set of expectations regarding results.

Initial statement of hypotheses.

_____

_____

_____

General relationships implied by your hypotheses.

_____ is related to _____

_____ is related to _____

_____ is related to _____

Can you identify specific alternative relationships or explanations which would serve as competing or rival hypotheses?

_____

_____

_____

Revised statement of hypotheses, considering (if possible) specific competing alternatives to the hypothesized relationships.

_____

_____

_____

V.   INSTRUMENTS AND DATA SOURCES

Complete this inventory of measurements or counts to be made. Then list your proposed instruments or data sources for measuring or counting.

Things to be measured or counted	*Proposed instruments or data sources*	*Available?*
1. _____	_____	_____
2. _____	_____	_____
3. _____	_____	_____
4. _____	_____	_____

5. _____   _____   _____

6. _____   _____   _____

7. _____   _____   _____

8. _____   _____   _____

For items above for which an adequate instrument is *not* readily available, indicate critical characteristics of instruments to be found or developed.

Proposed Instruments   *Critical Characteristics*

_____   _____

_____   _____

_____   _____

_____   _____

_____   _____

Instrument reliability and validity

For each instrument, both of these questions should be addressed:

Reliability: How closely do repeated observations (by different people, at different times, etc) of the same thing agree with each other?

Validity: With what assurance do we know that the instrument is measuring what we believe it is measuring?

Mark each instrument with an ⓇⓇ? if you believe reliability is a problem and a Ⓥ? if you believe validity is a problem.

PREPARING THE RESEARCH DESIGN

The design of the study refers to the way in which relationships are to be studied. It is wise to seek competent help in preparing a research design, since design options are numerous. Choices among designs will always require compromises between the practical and the ideal. Well-designed research, like anything else designed well, should be more efficient and better suited to your needs than a haphazard approach. Poorly designed research may be inefficient or, even worse, may make it impossible for you to analyze the data legitimately!

You can identify the issues which your design should address by considering carefully each of the items in sections VI through VIII.

VI.   SAMPLING

Describe the characteristics of the people (or other subjects) who will be eligible for participation in the study.

_____

_____

_____

_____

Describe the population (beyond your sample) to which you wish to generalize conclusions.

_____

_____

_____

_____

Now review the two descriptions critically and revise either or both descriptions so that they fit together.

Sample Size

The most important considerations in determining sample size are often how much money you have to spend and how much time you can commit.

Increases in sample size increase the precision of the research. Small samples do *not* of themselves introduce bias. A large sample should enable you to detect more subtle (but perhaps less important) relationships. When other design features have been worked out, a research consultant should be able to help you arrive at a reasonable sample size. The most helpful information in this decision comes from the results of similar studies and your estimate of the strength of the relationships you expect to find.

VII.   DEVELOPING THE RESEARCH PROTOCOL

How will you select your sample? _____

_____

_____

_____

_____

Will you divide your sample into groups? If so, how? _____

_____

_____

_____

Describe what will happen to each subject. (Feel free to use a list, flow chart, or diagram.)

Who will gather the data and how? _____

_____

_____

_____

_____

_____

_____

_____

_____

VIII. ELIMINATING PROCEDURAL BIAS

Bias refers to sources of systematic error which may affect study results. Unless adequately controlled, bias may render your results uninterpretable. With a general protocol in mind, specific attention should be given to each of the following potential sources of bias. The design should evolve as you add controls for the most serious of these. Those mentioned below are adapted from "Experimental and Quasi-Experimental Design for Research," Campbell DT and Stanley JC, Chicago, Rand McNally College Publishing, 1966.

1. Effects of Historical Events—Can you anticipate events such as personnel changes, remodeling plans, interference by nonparticipants, etc, which will take place during your data collection phase and which might affect the results?

No____   Yes____   (If yes, describe problem.)

_____

_____

_____

2. Effects of Maturation—If subjects are to be observed over time, are there changes which might result merely by normal development, growth, natural course of illness, etc?

     No_____   Yes_____ (If yes, describe problem.)

_____

_____

_____

3. Effects of Repeated Measurement—If the same measurements are repeated on subjects, are subjects likely to remember past responses, prepare differently for the next session, relax procedures?

     No_____   Yes_____ (If yes, describe problem.)

_____

_____

_____

4. Instrument Decay—Is it likely that test equipment will wear out, observers get bored, protocols get short-cut by investigators, etc?

     No_____   Yes_____ (If yes, describe problem.)

_____

_____

_____

5. Effects of Statistical Regression—If subjects are chosen because they lie at the extremes of a distribution (eg, high blood pressure, low compliance with therapy), subsequent measurements will tend to be more nearly average, for purely statistical reasons. Are your subjects chosen or assigned to groups on the basis of their "extremeness"?

     No_____   Yes_____ (If yes, describe problem.)

_____

_____

_____

6. Subject Selection—Is there anything in the selection of your sample or assignment of subjects to groups which makes one group of subjects unintentionally different from other groups?

     No_____   Yes_____ (If yes, describe problem.)

_____

_____

_____

7. Loss of Subjects—Subjects lost to attrition may be different from those who remain. Is your study jeopardized by this possibility?

No_____   Yes_____ (If yes, describe problem.)

_____

_____

_____

8. Investigator Bias—Are you in a position to unintentionally "shade" results to confirm your hypotheses or to influence subjects by your attention, attitude, etc?

No_____   Yes_____ (If yes, describe problem.)

_____

_____

_____

IX.   IDENTIFY THE LIMITATIONS OF THE STUDY

After struggling to achieve a design which is feasible and provides control of the most troublesome sources of bias, you may be left with inadequate controls over other sources of bias. Use the space below to identify these.

Potential Sources of Bias Remaining

_____

_____

_____

_____

_____

_____

_____

_____

Even unbiased studies have limitations in their generalizability. To what kinds of people beyond your study sample can you justify generalizing your conclusions. (It may be easier to identify individuals for whom your conclusions do not necessarily apply.)

Limitations to Generalizability

_____

_____

_____

_____

_____

_____

_____

_____

_____

X.   DATA COLLECTION FORMS

Use the space below to sketch forms you will use to record the data of the study. Alternatively, you may list and describe the forms below and then attach specimens.

XI.   REPORTING OF RESULTS

Use the space below to sketch summary data tables and/or graphs which you would expect to use in presenting your results. You may include simulated results of the kind you hope to find.

XII.   STATISTICAL ANALYSIS

Design and analysis are two sides of the same inferential coin. *Always* seek competent consultation in the design phase or there may never be any analysis worth doing.

You may begin to organize the analysis by listing below all of the variables considered in your design. Separate the variables into the three categories described.

A. Demographic variables which describe characteristics of subjects such as age, sex, race, previous hospitalizations, etc.

_____

_____

_____

_____

_____

_____

B. Variables of the study under the control of the investigator, such as type of instruction given, therapy options, duration of treatment, or other exposures or treatments to which the investigator can *assign* subjects.

_____

_____

_____

_____

_____

_____

C. Outcome variables or effects potentially related to or caused by A or B above, such as adherence to instructions, speed of recovery, or client satisfaction.

_____

_____

_____

_____

_____

_____

XIII. DISCUSSIONS, INTERPRETATIONS, OR CONCLUSIONS

No workbook exercises are included for this phase of research. Instead it is suggested that the researcher should maintain a notebook or diary in which to capture anecdotes, remarks of subjects, comments by others involved in the project, or any other facts or ideas which might help to make sense out of the phenomena under study. It is often the serendipity of the alert and curious researcher which leads to insightful interpretations and fruitful new hypotheses.

XIV. ADMINISTRATIVE ARRANGEMENTS

The most elegantly designed studies have sometimes collapsed for lack of attention to administrative details. Use the space below to outline your administrative duties.

Touch Base With	*Regarding*
Human Subjects Review Committee	*Protection of subjects*
_____	_____
_____	_____
_____	_____
_____	_____
_____	_____
_____	_____
_____	_____

Describe other administrative arrangements, eg, money, equipment, supplies, space, printing, consultation, postage, telephone, computer programing.

_____

_____

_____

_____

_____

_____

_____

_____

_____

_____

_____

INDEX

Page numbers in *italics* indicate illustrations.
Page numbers followed by *t* indicate tables.

A

Abridged Index Medicus as research tool
    for family practice, 304
Academic discipline, family practice as, evo-
    lution of, 329–30
Accessibility of primary care, 72–73*t*, 74
Accountability of primary care, 74*t*, 77
Adolescence, health-monitoring program
    for, 493
Adult, health-monitoring program for,
    494–95
Advisors in undergraduate teaching pro-
    gram for family practice, 148
Age-sex register as research tool for family
    practice, 302, *303*
Age spectrum of practice in family practice

compared with other specialties,
    264, 267, 268*t*
Alpert, J., 70, 80, 82
American Academy of Family Physicians
    (AAFP), 331
    and American College of Obstetricians
    and Gynecologists, agreement of,
    for curriculum and hospital priv-
    ileges in obstetrics-gynecology,
    441–44
American Academy of General Practice,
    10–11
American Board of Family Practice
    (ABFP), 17–18
    certification and recertification by, 196–
    97
    development of, 330–31

American College of Obstetricians and Gynecologists (ACOG) and American Academy of Family Physicians, agreement of, for curriculum and hospital privileges in obstetrics-gynecology, 444–44

Anlyan, W., 116, 117

APGAR scoring system for family functioning, 242–43, 244*t*, 245*t*

Assessment, self, in CME in medical practice, 194

Association of Chairmen of Departments of Family Medicine, functions of, 331, 333

Audit, medical, increasing use of, in CME in family practice, 194

B

Bauman, M., 225

Beck, J., 134

Behavior, illness, family dynamics in, 238–39

Behavioral sciences, requirements for training in, in family practice residency, 364

Brown, C., 188

Bryan, J., 7, 9, 20

Burstin, B., 238, 239

Byrne, P., 299

C

Cardiac catherization of, national health planning guidelines for, 356–57

Care. *See also* Health care; Medical care; Primary care

continuity of, in family practice residencies, 170–71

Career, family practice as, 277–95

misconceptions about, 278–83

personal satisfactions in, 283–87

requisites for 287–91

selection of residency training for, 291–93

Carmichael, L., 226

Catheterization, cardiac, national health planning guidelines for, 356–57

Certifications and recertification by American Board of Family Practice, 196–97

Chase, R., 118, 119

Chest pain, patterns of, research on, 309, 312*t*

Child

preschool, health-monitoring program for, 492

school, health-monitoring program for, 493

Citizens Commission on Graduate Medical Education in evolution of family practice as specialty, 15–16

City, no need for family physician in, as misconception about family practice, 280–81

Classification system

RCGP to ICHPPC, conversion code for, 481–89

as tool for research in family practice, 300–1

Clinical content of family practice, 203–22

comparative, by specialty, 215, 217, 218*t*, 219–20*t*

studies of, 206–14

variables affecting, 204–6

Cohen, W., 120, 121

Collaboration in research in family medicine, 307

Community

family physician as part of, satisfaction due to, 285–86

hospital in, benefits of family practice residency program for, 181

involvement of medical education with, 131–33

resources of

available, 499–505

questionnaire on, 504–5

utilization of, family physician and, 259, 261

as setting for undergraduate education for family practice, 143

Community medicine, requirements for training in, in family practice residency, 365–66

Comprehensiveness of primary care, 73*t*, 74–76, 79–82

Computed tomographic scanners, national health planning guidelines for, 358–59

Consultation
in family practice, 214–15, 216*t*, 261–62
request form for, *263*
in research in family medicine, 307

Consumer-related barriers to health care, 51–59

Continuing medical education (CME) in family practice, 185–200
approaches to, 191–97
coordination of, with undergraduate and graduate medical education, 133–34
departments for family practice in, 197–99
generic problems of, 186–90
expansion of medical information as, 187
ineffective teaching methods as, 189
irrelevance of content as, 188
lack of clear goals and methods as, 189–90
lack of correlation between knowledge and performance as, 188
logistic barriers as, 188
implications of, for family physician, 199–200
learning through reading in, 195–96
learning through teaching in, 196
medical audit in, 194
problem-oriented medical record in, 193
profiling and indexing of practice experience in, 192, 193*t*
requisites for, 191
research and evaluation of, 198
self-assessment in, 194
self-instruction in, 194–95
small-group teaching in, 194–95

Continuity of primary care, 73–74*t*, 77

Coordinating Council on Medical Education (CCME)
purpose of, 133–34
recommendations of, 41–42

Coordination of primary care, 73*t*, 76–77

Costs of family practice residencies, 172–73

Counseling
community services for, 500–1
for family problems, 244–46

Cousins, N., 277

Crises, transitional, in family, 229, 233, 235, 236*t*

Cultural barriers to health care, 58–59

Curriculum for family practice residencies, 167–70

Curry, H., 1, 228

D

Decisiveness as requisite for family physician, 288

Dennis, J., 24, 141, 203

Diagnostic index as research tool in family practice, 302, *303*

Distribution of physicians
geographic, 35, 36*t*, 37–38, 39*t*
by specialty, 38, 40–41

E

Economic function of American family, changes in, 226–27

Education
maternal, infant mortality rates by, *55*
medical. *See* Medical education

Educational barrier to health care, 58

Educational function of American family, changes in, 227

Educational goals of family practice residencies, 165–67

Edwards, C., 27

Elderly
health care barriers for, special, 63, *64*
health-monitoring program for, 495–96

Emergency assistance, community agencies for, 501

Encounter form as research tool in family practice, 304, *305–6*

English, J., 63

Environment, effect of, on clinical content of family practice, 205

Evaluation
  in family practice residencies, 171–72,
      174–76*t*
  of family practice residencies, 293

F

Faculty
  for family practice program
    need for, 333
    recruitment of, 323–26
  for family practice residencies, 163, 165,
      166*t*
Family
  changing roles of, in America, 226–28
  in family practice, 225–47
  impact of individual illness on, 239–42
  life cycle of, 228–29, 230–32*t, 233*
  nature of illness in, 235–42. *See also*
      Illness in family
  as object of care, 242–47
    diagnostic approaches to, 242–44,
        245–46*t*
    management approaches to, 244–47
  stress and transitional crises in, 229, 233,
      235, 236*t*
Family medicine. *See also* Family practice
  definition of, 19–20
  requirements for training in, in family
      practice residency, 363–64
Family physician(s)
  assistant to, 258, 259*t*
  consultation with, 214–15, 216*t*
  definition of, 19
  extenders of, 256, 258, 259*t, 260*, 274
  implications of CME for, 199–200
  practice patterns of, 249–75. *See also*
      Family practice, patterns of
  practicing
    collaborative research with, in CME,
        199
    as teachers in CME, 198
  as primary care physicians, 78, 79*t*
  referrals by, 214–15, 216*t*
  requisites for, 287–91
  workloads of, by setting, 251, 252*t*
Family practice
  age spectrum of, compared with other
      specialties, 264, 267, 268*t*

Family Practice (*cont.*)
  American Board of, 17–18
  base for, in medical schools, need to
      strengthen, 334
  as career, 277–95. *See also* Career, fam-
      ily practice as center for, in fam-
      ily practice residencies, 160–61
  clinical content of, 203–22. *See also*
      Clinical content of family prac-
      tice
  consultation in, 214–15, 216*t*, 261–62,
      263
  continuing education in, 185–200. *See
      also* Continuing medical educa-
      tion (CME) in family practice
  definition of, 19
  department of
    roles for, 197–99
    for undergraduate teaching program,
        145–46
  duration of office visits in, compared
      with other specialties, 267–68,
      269*t*
  family in, 225–47
  functional elements of, 20–24
  graduate education for, 159–82. *See also*
      Graduate medical education for
      family practice; Residency(ies),
      family practice
  group
    growth in, 250–51
    pros and cons of, 252
  hospital, clinical content of, 20, 78, 212–
      13
  location of, selection of, factors affecting,
      253–54, 255–56*t*
  misconceptions about, 278–83
  obstetric care in, 222
  office, clinical content of, 207, 208*t,*
      209–12*t, 213t*
  organizational structures of, 250–53
  patterns of, 250–64
    comparison of, with other specialties,
        264–74
    group as, 250–52
    partnership as, 252–53
    solo practice as, 253
    team as, 254, 256–59
  personal satisfactions in, 283–87

Family Practice (*cont.*)

preventive medicine in, 220, 222

problem-solving approaches in, compared with other specialties, 268–70

programs for, funding of, need for, 334

progress in, in 1970s, 321–38

measures of, 322–33

distribution of graduates as, 327, 328*t*

evolution as academic discipline as, 329–30

faculty recruitment as, 323–26

organization of teaching programs as, 322–23, *324–25t*

organizational development as, 330–33

patient care as, 327, 329

research progress as, 330, 331

student interest as, 326–27

referral in, 214–15, 216*t,* 261–62

research in, 297–318. *See also* Research in family practice

research as career option in, 294

residencies in, 160–73. *See also* Residency(ies), family practice

role models for, in undergraduate teaching program, 147–48

satisfaction with, compared with other specialties, 271–73*t*

settings for, 253–54, 255–56*t*

as specialty, 13–25

evolution of, 14–17

teaching as career option in, 294

teaching of, continuum of, incorporating continuing education into, 199–98

teaching programs for, 369–439*t*

team, 254, 256–59, *260,* 274

undergraduate education for, 141–57. *See also* Undergraduate medical education for family practice

utilization of community resources by, 259, 261

Virginia study of, 213–14, 445–79*t*

Federal government in funding of medical education, 127

Fein, R., 105, 106

Flexibility as requisite for family physician, 290

Flexner Report in reform of medical education, 2

Folsom Commission on Community Health Services in evolution of family practice as specialty, 15

Foreign medical graduates

influence of

on geographic distribution of physicians, 35, 37

on specialty distribution of physicians, 40

influx of, implications of, 31, 34

restricted entry to, to stabilize physician supply, 129

Freidson, E., 342

Fuchs, V., 99, 100

Funding

for family practice programs, need for, 334

for family practice residencies, 172–73

for medical education, constraints of, 126–27

G

Geiger, J., 61

General practice

American Academy of, 10–11, 15

decline of, 5–8

impact of, on primary care, 9–10

growth of specialization and, 3–5

historical perspective on, 2–3

history of, 1–11

General practitioner

as primary care physician, 78, 79*t*

and specialist, relationship between, history of, 1–2

Generic problems of continuing medical education, 186–90

Geographic barrier to health care, 59

Geographic distribution of physicians, 35, 36*t,* 37–38, 39*t*

Goals, lack of, as problem of continuing medical education, 189–91

Government, federal, in funding medical education, 127

Grace, N., 225

Graduate medical education
    for family practice, 158–82. *See also*
        Residency(ies), family practice
    coordination of, with undergraduate
        and continuing medical educa-
        tion, 133–34
    at Medical College of Virginia, 173,
        176–78
    and undergraduate education, linkage
        of, 144–45
    at University of Washington, 178–80
    and geographic maldistribution of phy-
        sicians, 35
    redistribution of, 44, 45*t*
    and specialty maldistribution of physi-
        cians, 40
Graduates of family practice program, dis-
        tribution of, 327, 328*t*
Gross National Product (GNP), health ex-
        penditures related to, 90, *91*
Group, family practice
    alternatives for, 83
    growth of, 250–51
    pros and cons of, 252
Gynecology, requirements for training in,
        in family practice residency, 365

H

Haggerty, R., 6
Health, lifetime monitoring program for,
        491–97
Health agencies, voluntary, 502–3
Health care
    barriers to, 51–66, 95–96
        background of, 52–53
        consumer-related, 52–59
        cultural, 58–59
        educational, 58
        for elderly, 63, *64*
        geographic, 59
        informational, 58
        for poor, 61–63
        provider-related, 59–61
        psychologic, 58
        racial, 59, 60
        for rural inhabitants, 63–65
        socioeconomic, 53–57, 95–96

Health Care (*cont.*)
    cost of, increasing, 57, 96–97, 98*t*
    expenditures on, related to GNP, 90, *91*
    industry for, expanding, 90–95
    and medical care, distinction between,
        79–80
    need and demand for, relationship be-
        tween, 29
    primary, 69–87. *See also* Primary care
    third-party-payers for, increasing, 92, 94
    utilization of, by income level, *55*
Health care services, fragmented, as barrier
        to health care, 59–60
Health care system
    changing, 89–112
    problems of, 95–101
        approaches to
            current, 105–111
            recent, 101–105
        duplication and waste as, 97–99
        increasing cost as, 96–97, 98*t*
        limited access as, 95–96
        marginal outcomes as, 99–101
Health departments, community, 499
Health insurance
    national, controversy over, 109–11
    private
        coverage by, 92, 95
        percent of persons with, *54*
Health Maintenance Organization
        (HMOs), 84
    services of, 108–9
Health manpower plan, coordinated, lack
        of, 126
Health planning, national guidelines for,
        345–60
Health Professions Educational Assistance
        Act of 1976, provisions of, 42
Health status, index of, as research tool in
        family practice, 304, *307*
Health Systems Agencies, functions of,
        106–7
Heart, catheterization of, national health
        planning guidelines for, 356–57
Holman, H., 89
Home care agencies, community, 499–500
Hospital(s)
    community, benefits of family practice
        residency program for, 181

Hospital(s) (*cont.*)
general
bed supply in, national health planning guidelines for, 348–50
occupancy rate of, national health planning guidelines for, 350–51
utilization of, 93, 96
Hospital practice, clinical content of, 207–8, 212–13
Hospital privileges, problems with, as misconception about family practice, 279–80, 281
Hospital-sponsored primary-care group practice, 84
Hospital training in family practice residencies, 161–63, 164*t*
Huntly, R., 13

I

Illness
in family
incidence of, 236–37
nature of, 235–42
presentation of, 238–39
of individual, impact of, on family, 239–42
presentation of, research on, 313–14, 315*t*
Income level
chronic conditions related to, 62
health care utilization by, 55, 97
infant mortality rates by, 55
physician visits by, 56
Index
diagnostic, as research tool in family practice, 302, 303
of health status as research tool in family practice, 304, 307
Index Medicus, Abridged, as research tool in family practice, 304
Indexing and profiling of practice experience in CME in family practice, 192, 193*t*
Industry, health care, expanding, 90–95
Infancy, health-monitoring program for, 492

Infant mortality rates, 99, *100*
by income and maternal education, 55
Information
medical
expansion of, as problem of continuing medical education, 187
and performance, lack of correlation between, as problem of continuing medical education, 188
mutual exchange of, consent for, 505
Informational barrier to health care, 58
Instruction, self, increased use of, in CME in medical practice, 194–95
Insurance, health
national, controversy over, 109–11
private
coverage by, 92, 95
percent of persons with, 54
Intellectual challenge, lack of, as misconception about family practice, 278–79
Interests, broad, as requisite for family physician, 287–88
Internal medicine, requirements for training in, in family practice residency, 364
Interpersonal relationships, ease with, as requisite for family physician, 290

J

James, G., 22, 25
James stages of health care, 22–23
Jason, H., 121, 125
Judgment as requisite for family physician, 287

K

Knouss, R., 40, 47
Knowledge, medical
expansion of, as problem of continuing medical education, 187
and performance, lack of correlation between, as problem of continuing medical education, 188
Knowles, J., 28

L

Lead poisoning, screening for, research on, 312–13, 214*t*

Leaman, T., 142

Learning
through reading in CME in medical practice, 195–96
through teaching in CME in medical practice, 196

Lee, P., 80

Levinson, D., 86

Lewis, C., 89, 104, 109

Liaison Committee on Graduate Medical Education (LCGME), 41

Library services as research tool in family practice, 304, 307

Licensure of physicians, changes in, trends in medical education and, 134–35

Lifetime health-monitoring program, 491–97

M

Macy Commission, report of, on physician manpower planning, 43

Magraw, R., 24, 79, 254, 255

Malerich, J., 206

McWhinney, I., 14, 23, 187, 282, 295, 299

Mechanic, D., 27, 29, 51, 52, 65, 100, 101, 110

Medex as physician extender 258, 259*t*

Medical audit, increasing use of, in CME in family practice, 194

Medical care and health care, distinction between, 79–80

Medical College of Virginia, graduate education program for family medicine of, 173, 176–78

Medical education
basic problems in, 119–27
changing trends in, 115–38
continuing. *See* Continuing medical education for family practice
evolution of medical schools in, 116–17
funding for, constraints of, 126–27
future projections for, 136–38

Medical Education (*cont.*)
graduate. *See* Graduate medical education
growth of teaching programs in, 117, 118*t, 119–20*
historical perspective on, 116–19
limited relevance of, to medical practice, 121, 125–26
major trends in, 129–36
changes in licensure as, 134–35
changing medical student as, 135–36
community involvement as, 131–33
coordination of undergraduate, graduation and continuing medical education as, 133–34
decentralization as, 131–33
emphasis on primary care as, 130–31
shift from teaching to learning as, 136
stabilization of growth as, 127–30
specialization in, 117–19
undergraduate. *See* Undergraduate medical education for family practice

Medical information
expansion of, as problem of continuing medical education, 187
and performance, lack of correlation between, as problem of continuing medical education, 188

Medical practice, limited relevance of medical education to, 121, 125–26

Medical record, problem-oriented
increasing use of, in CME in family practice, 193
as research tool in family practice, 301

Medical schools
base for family practice in, need to strengthen, 334
evolution of, 116–17
product of, and public need, imbalance between, as problem of medical education, 119–21, 122–25*t*

Medical student, changing characteristics of, 135–36

Medicine
building primary care base of, 105–06
family. *See also* Family practice
definition of, 19–20
requirements for training in, in family practice residency, 363–64

MEDLINE as tool for research in family practice, 304, 307

Metropolitan area, no need for family physician in, as misconception about family practice, 280–81

Miller, G., 189, 191

Millis Commission in evolution of family practice as specialty, 15–16

Millis, J., 20, 342

Multispecialty group practice, 83

N

National Commission on Community Health Services in evolution of family practice as specialty, 15

National health insurance, controversy over, 109–11

National health planning guidelines, 345–60

National Health Planning and Resources Development Act, provisions of, 106–7

Neonatal special care units, national health planning guidelines for, 353–54

North American Primary Care Research Group
   Committee on Standard Terminology, report of, 507–16
   functions of, 333

Nurse practitioner as physician extender, 258, 259*t*, 274

O

Obstetric care in family practice, 222

Obstetrical services, national health planning guidelines for, 351–53

Obstetrics, requirements for training in, in family practice residency, 365

Office practice, clinical content of, 207, 208*t*, 209–12*t*, 213*t*

Office visit, duration of, in family practice compared with other specialties, 267–68, 269*t*

Ogburn, W., 226, 227

Olsen, E., 239, 241, 242

Open heart surgery, national health planning guidelines for, 355–56

P

Pain, chest, patterns of, research on, 309, 312*t*

Partnership family practice, 252–53

Patient care, changes in family practice related to, 327, 329

Patient population, effect of, on clinical content of family practice, 205

Pediatric inpatient services, national health planning guidelines for, 354–55

Pediatrics, requirements for training in, in family practice residency, 364

Pellegrino, E., 13, 142, 143, 341, 343

People, interest in, as requisite for family physician, 287

Performance, clinical, and knowledge, lack of correlation between, as problem of continuing medical education, 188

Perinatal period, health-monitoring program for, 491–92

Personal satisfactions in family practice, 283–87

Petersdorf, R., 46

Phillips, T., 3

Physicians
   aggregate number of, 30–31, 32–33*t*, 34–35
   assistants to, in primary care, 84–86
   distribution of
      geographic, 35, 36*t*, 37–38
      specialty, 38, 40–41
   family. *See* Family physician(s)
   licensure of, changes in, trends in medical education and, 134–35
   manpower problems involving, approaches to, 41–44
   primary care, 69–87. *See also* Primary care
   range of services offered by, 81*t*
   shortage of, reports on, 32–33*t*
   supply of
      and distribution of, 27–47
      increased, projected, *31*
      variables affecting, 28–30

Physicians (*cont.*)
    variables related to, effect of, on clinical content of family practice, 205
Poisoning, lead, screening for, research on, 312–13, 314*t*
Poor, health care barriers for, special, 61–63
Practice experience, profiling and indexing of, in CME in family practice, 192, 193*t*
Practice patterns of family physician, 249–75. *See also* Family practice, patterns of
Practitioners, middle-level, in primary care, 84–86
Pregnancy, health-monitoring program for, 491–92
Preventive medicine in family practice, 220–222
Primary care
    accessibility of, 72–73*t*, 74
    accountability of, 74*t*, 77
    base for, of medicine, building, 105–6
    checklist for, 72–74*t*
    comprehensiveness of, 73*t*, 74–76, 79–82
    continuity of, 73–74*t*, 77
    coordination of, 73*t*, 76–77
    definition of, 70–72
    elements of, 72–77
    emphasis on, in medical education, 130–31
    functions of, 72
    issues in, 77–86
    limited relevance of medical education to, 125–26
    organization of, alternatives for, 82–84
    perspectives in, 69–87
    providers of, 77–79
    role of middle-level practitioners in, 84–86
Problem-oriented medical record
    increasing use of, in CME in family practice, 193
    as research tool in family practice, 301
Problem-solving approaches in family practice compared with other specialties, 268–70

Professional Standards Review Organizations, functions, 107–8
Profiling and indexing of practice experience in CME in family practice, 192, *193t*
Protective function of American family, changes in, 227
Provider-related barriers to health care, 59–61
Psychiatry, requirements for training in, in family practice residency, 364
Psychologic barrier to health care, 58
Psychosocial factors in illness in family, 237
Public Law 93-222 and HMOs, 108–9
Public Law 93-641, provisions of, 106–7
Public Law 94-484, provisions of, 42

R

Racial barriers to health care, 59, 60
Radiation therapy, national planning guidelines for, 357–58
RCGP to ICHPPC classification system, conversion code for, 481–89*t*
Reading, learning through, in CME in medical practice, 195–96
Record, medical, problem-oriented
    increasing use of, in CME in family practice, 193
    as research tool in family practice, 301
Recreational function of American family, changes in, 227
Referral services, community, 501
Referrals by family physicians, 214–15, 216*t*, 261–62
Regional differences, effect of, on clinical content of family practice, 205
Relationships, interpersonal, ease with, as requisite for family physician, 290
Religious function of American family, changes in, 227
Renal disease, end-stage, national health planning guidelines for, 359–60

Research
  as career option in family practice, 294
  clinical, social, and behavioral, projects
      in, initial planning of, guide for,
      517–30
  definition of, 298–99
  in family practice, 297–318
    background of, 298–99
    base for, development of, need for,
        334
    basic approaches and methods for,
        300–7
    climate for, favorable, 300
    collaboration in, 307
    consultation in, 307
    content areas in, 308, 310–11*t*
    opportunities for involvement in,
        315–17
    progress of, 330, *331*
    tools for, 300–7
  requirements for training in, in family
      practice residency, 366
Residency(ies), family practice
  common features of, 160–73
  content of, 363–66
  continuity of care in, 170–71
  costs and funding of, 172–73
  curriculum for, 167–70
  educational goals of, 165–67
  essentials for, 361–67
  evaluation in, 171–72, 174–76*t*
  evaluation of, 293
  faculty for, 163, 165, 166*t*
  family practice center in, 160–61
  hospital training in, 161–63, 164*t*
  at Medical College of Virginia, 173,
      176–78
  organization of, 361–63
  program size for, 163
  selection of, 291–94
  types of, *162*
  at University of Washington, 178–80
Residency positions, increase in, 117, *119–
    20*
Responsibility, ability to assume, as requi-
    site for family physician, 288–
    89

Roy, W., 112
Ruhe, W., 137, 138
Rural inhabitants, health care barriers for,
    special, 63–65

S

Sanazaro, P., 190
Scanners, computed tomographic, national
    health planning guidelines for,
    358–59
Scherger, J., 148
Schools, medical
  base for family practice in, need to
      strengthen, 334
  evolution of, 116–17
  product of, and public need, imbalance
      between, as problem of medical
      education, 119–21, 122–25*t*
Screening for lead poisoning, research on,
    312–13, 314*t*
Self-assessment in CME in medical practice,
    194
Self-instruction, increased use of, in CME
    in medical practice, 194–95
Sensitivity–objectivity mix as requisite for
    family physician, 289
Sheps, C., 115, 126
Single-specialty group practice, 83
Social service agencies, community, 500
Society of Teachers of Family Medicine
    (STFM), evolution of, 331
Socioeconomic barrier to health care, 53–
    57, 95–96
Solo family practice, 82–83, 253
Somers, A., 46, 69, 93, 94, 99, 105, 110
Southern Illinois University, undergraduate
    teaching program for family
    practice of, 151–52
Specialists
  and general practitioners, relationship be-
      tween, history of, 1–2
  geographic distribution of, 36*t*
  as primary care physicians, 78, 79*t*
Specialization
  growth of, 3–5
  in medical education, 117–19

Specialty(ies)
  comparative content of family practice
      by, 215, 217, 218*t*, 219–20*t*
  comparative practice patterns among,
      264–74
  family practice as, 13–25
    evolution of, 14–17
  maldistribution of physicians by, 38, 40–
      41
Spitzer, W., 308
Stability as requisite for family physician,
      289
Stambler, H., 29, 35
Staphylococcus aureus, susceptibility pat-
      terns of, research on, 309, 312,
      313*t*
Starr, P., 94, 95, 109
Status-conferring function of American
      family, changes in, 227
Stephens, G., 285
Stevens, R., 126
Stress in family, 229, 233, 235, 236*t*
Students
  interest of, in family practice, 326–27
  medical, changing characteristics of, 135–
      36
Surgery, requirements for training in, in
      family practice residency, 365

                    T

Teaching
  as career option in family practice, 294
  learning through, in CME in medical
      practice, 196
  methods of, ineffective, as problem of
      continuing medical education,
      189
  small-group, increased use of, in CME
      in medical practice, 194–95
Teaching programs
  in family practice
    need for, 333–34, 335*t*
    organization of, 322–23, 324–25*t*
    refinement of quality-control mecha-
        nisms in, need for, 334
  in medical education, growth of, 117,
      118*t, 119–20*

Team practice, family, 254, 256–59, *260*,
      274
Tomographic scanners, computed, national
      health planning guidelines for,
      358–59
Training, hospital, in family practice resi-
      dencies, 161–63, 164*t*
Transitional crises in family, 229, 233, 235,
      236*t*

                    U

Undergraduate medical education for fam-
      ily practice, 141–57
  content of, 142–43
  coordination of, with graduate and con-
      tinuing medical education, 133–
      34
  curriculum organization in, 144
  and graduate education, linkage of, 144–
      45
  logistic problems in, 145
  programs for
    at Southern Illinois University, 151–
        52
    at University of Washington, 152–54
  requisites for, 145–48
    advising program as, 148
    coordinating four-year curriculum as,
        146–47
    department of family practice as, 145–
        46
    evaluation system as, 148, 149–50*t*
    exemplary clinical settings as, 146
    family practice role models as, 147–
        48
  site of, 142–43
University
  benefits of family practice residency pro-
      gram for, 181
  as setting for undergraduate education
      for family practice, 143
  of Washington
    graduate education program for fam-
        ily medicine of, 178–80
    undergraduate teaching program for
        family practice of, 152–54

Urban area, no need for family physician in, as misconception about family practice, 280–81

V

Virginia, Medical College of, graduate education program for family medicine of, 173, 176–78
Virginia study of family practice, 213–14, 445–79*t*

W

Washington, University of
  graduate education program for family medicine of, 178–80

undergraduate teaching program for family practice of, 152–54
Watts, M., 185
Weiss, P., 187
Wesson, A., 38
White, K., 111, 297, 308
Whitehead, A., 146
Willard Report in evolution of family practice as specialty, 16–17
Women, unsuitability of, for family practice as misconception, 282–83
Wood, M., 299, 318
Worby, C., 229
Workload
  excessive, as misconception about family practice, 281
  of family practice compared with other specialties, 264, 265–67*t*, 268*t*
Wright, 145

James M. Gall, M.D., C.C.F.P.
Department of Family Medicine
University of Miami School of Medicine
P. O. Box 016700
Miami, Florida 33101

Department of Family Medicine (R700)
University of Miami School of Medicine
P. O. Box 016700
Miami, Florida 33101